Bell's Orofacial Pains:

The Clinical Management of Orofacial Pain

Sixth Edition

Bell's

OROFACIAL PAINS

The Clinical Management
of Orofacial Pain

Sixth Edition

Jeffrey P. Okeson, DMD

Director
Orofacial Pain Center
Chairman
Department of Oral Health Science
University of Kentucky
College of Dentistry
Lexington, Kentucky

Quintessence Publishing Co, Inc

Chicago, Berlin, Tokyo, Copenhagen, London, Paris, Milan, Barcelona, Istanbul, São Paulo, New Delhi, Moscow, Prague, and Warsaw

Library of Congress Cataloging-in-Publication Data

Okeson, Jeffrey P.
  Bell's orofacial pains : the clinical management of orofacial pain /
Jeffrey P. Okeson.-- 6th ed.
      p. ; cm.
  Includes bibliographical references and index.
  ISBN 0-86715-439-X (hardcover)
  1. Orofacial pain.
  [DNLM: 1. Facial Pain. 2. Temporomandibular Joint Disorders. 3.
Pain--physiopathology. WU 140 O41b 2004] I. Title: Orofacial pains. II.
Bell, Welden E. Orofacial pains. III. Title.

  RK322.B44 2005
  617.5'2--dc22
                                        2004015986

**quintessence
books**

©2005 Quintessence Publishing Co, Inc

Quintessence Publishing Co, Inc
551 Kimberly Drive
Carol Stream, IL 60188
www.quintpub.com

Editor: Lindsay Harmon
Cover and internal design: Dawn Hartman
Production: Susan Robinson

Printed in Canada

This book is dedicated to the memory of
Dr Welden E. Bell (1910–1990)

My teacher,
my mentor,
and
my friend

and to his devoted wife of 58 years
Lucy Bell (1910–2003)

With special recognition to my wife
Barbara
"the light of my life"

Table of Contents

Foreword *xiii*
Preface *xv*

Section One: The Nature of Pain

1 Defining the Problem 3
Pain as a Clinical Complaint
The Dental Practitioner's Responsibility
Historical Note
Changing Concepts of Pain
The Emergency Nature of Pain
Levels of Pain Processing
Phylogenic Considerations
Anatomic Considerations of the Human
Neural Pathways of Pain

2 The Neural Anatomy of Orofacial Pain 13
Neural Structures
Functional Neuroanatomy
The Trigeminal System
The Autonomic Nervous System
Peripheral Nociceptive Pathways
General Considerations of Peripheral Nociceptive Pathways

3 The Neurophysiology of Orofacial Pain 45
Nerve Action Potential
The Synapse
The Ion Channels
Neurotransmitters
Elimination of the Transmitter from the Synapse
The Neurochemistry of Nociception
Neuronal Sensitization
The Axon Transport System
Transmission of Afferent Impulses to the Cortex
Summary

4 The Processing of Pain at the Brainstem Level   63
The Initiation of Nociception in the Peripheral Tissues
The Central Processing of Nociception
The Experience of Pain
The Modulation Concept
State-Dependent Sensory Processing
Summary

5 The Processing of Pain at the Supraspinal Level   95
Factors That Influence the Pain Experience
Psychologic Factors Influence All Pains
Acute Pain Versus Chronic Pain
Emotional Significance of Orofacial Pains
Psychologic Considerations of Orofacial Pains

Section Two: Clinical Considerations of Orofacial Pain

6 The Various Presentations of Pain   107
Not All Pains Are Alike
Normal Neural Activities: Central and Peripheral Mechanisms
Inflammatory Pain
Noninflammatory Pain
Other Causes of Orofacial Pains
The Contribution of Neuroplasticity to Chronic Pain Conditions
Other Considerations

7 Category Classification of Orofacial Pains   129
Pain Diagnosis
Categories of Orofacial Pains

8 Principles of Pain Diagnosis   141
Evaluation of the Pain Condition
Preliminary Interview
History for Orofacial Pain
Clinical Examination for Orofacial Pain
Establishing the Pain Category
Choosing the Correct Pain Disorder
Confirmation of the Clinical Diagnosis
Multiple Categories of Pain

9 General Considerations in Managing Orofacial Pains   *197*

Cause-Related Therapy
Therapeutic Modalities
Considerations Related to Chronic Orofacial Pain

Section Three: Clinical Pain Syndromes

10 Cutaneous and Mucogingival Pains   *243*

Behavior of Cutaneous and Mucogingival Pains
Types of Cutaneous and Mucogingival Pains
Differential Diagnosis
Therapeutic Options

11 Pains of Dental Origin   *259*

Behavior of Dental Pains
Types of Dental Pains
Differential Diagnosis
Therapeutic Options

12 Pains of Muscle Origin   *287*

Behavior of Muscular Pain
Types of Masticatory Muscle Pains
Masticatory Muscle Pain Model
Chronic Myalgic Pain Disorders
Muscular Toothache
Referred Pain Mistaken for Masticatory Pain
Differentiating Various Masticatory Muscle Pains
Differential Diagnosis
Therapeutic Options

13 Temporomandibular Joint Pains   *329*

Behavior of TMJ Pains
Normal Anatomy and Function of the TMJ
Types of TMJ Pains
Diagnostic Considerations
Differential Diagnosis
Therapeutic Options for Disc-Interference Disorders
Other Therapeutic Options

14 Other Musculoskeletal Pains   *381*

Osseous Pains
Periosteal Pains
Soft Connective Tissue Pains
Differential Diagnosis
Therapeutic Options

15 Visceral Pains   *387*

Behavior of Visceral Pains
Pains Emanating from Visceral Mucosa
Glandular Pains
Ocular Pains
Auricular Pains
Differential Diagnosis
Therapeutic Options

16 Vascular and Neurovascular Pains   *401*

Behavior of Vascular and Neurovascular Pain
Neurovascular Pains of the Mouth and Face
Vascular Pains of the Mouth and Face
Differential Diagnosis

17 Neuropathic Pains   *449*

Behavior of Neuropathic Pains
Episodic Neuropathic Pains: Paroxysmal Neuralgias
Continuous Neuropathic Pains
Summary

18 Psychologic Factors and Orofacial Pain: Axis II   *519*

Acute Pain Versus Chronic Pain and the Biopsychosocial Model
The Psychologic Significance of Orofacial Pains
Axis II: Classification of Mental Disorders
General Therapeutic Considerations
The Concept of Physical Self-Regulation
A Closing Note

Terminology   *545*
Index   *549*

List of Cases

The number following each case refers
to the page on which it is located.

Case 1   278

Heterotopic pain, felt as toothache,
referred from the masseter muscle

Case 2   280

Heterotopic pain, felt as toothache,
referred from the cardiac muscle

Case 3   302

Cycling masticatory muscle pain secondary
to chronic ear pain

Case 4   303

Masticatory muscle pain expressed as
spasm in the lateral pterygoid muscle

Case 5   309

Myofascial pain of the masticatory muscles secondary to a cervical pain condition

Case 6   310

Masticatory muscle pain expressed as
significant co-contraction and cyclic
muscle pain

Case 7   312

Masticatory muscle pain expressed as
chronic centrally mediated myalgia

Case 8   346

Temporomandibular arthralgia originating
in the retrodiscal tissues

Case 9   349

Acute retrodiscitis secondary to trauma

Case 10   351

Temporomandibular arthralgia expressed
as capsular pain

Case 11   352

Capsular pain arising from inflamed
capsular fibrosis

Case 12   358

Temporomandibular arthralgia expressed as
degenerative joint disease or osteoarthritis

Case 13   359

Temporomandibular arthralgia expressed as
arthritic pain secondary to hyperuricemia

Case 14   361

Temporomandibular arthralgia expressed
as arthritic pain secondary to inflamed
fibrous ankylosis

Case 15   362

Temporomandibular arthralgia expressed
as arthritic pain secondary an invasive
malignant tumor

Case 16 *394*
Heterotopic pain felt as toothache and referred from an inflamed nasal mucosa (so-called sinus headache)

Case 17 *396*
Heterotopic pain felt as preauricular pain and referred from an inflamed sub-mandibular gland

Case 18 *398*
Heterotopic pain felt as preauricular pain due to a trigger point affecting the sterno-cleidomastoid muscle

Case 19 *432*
Heterotopic pain felt as a toothache secondary to a neurovascular pain source

Case 20 *434*
Cyclic masticatory muscle pain in the masseter secondary to neurovascular pain

Case 21 *435*
Neurovascular pain disorder mistaken for masticatory pain

Case 22 *454*
Paroxysmal neuralgia of the auriculo-temporal nerve

Case 23 *455*
Paroxysmal neuralgia of the maxillary branch of the trigeminal nerve

Case 24 *456*
Paroxysmal neuralgia of the mandibular branch of the trigeminal nerve

Case 25 *458*
Paroxysmal neuralgia of the glossopharyngeal nerve

Case 26 *474*
Peripheral neuritis secondary to maxillary sinusitis, expressed as toothache

Case 27 *476*
Neuritic pain of the inferior alveolar nerve, expressed as a mandibular toothache

Case 28 *477*
Neuritis of the glossopharyngeal nerve due to a fractured styloid process, mistaken for masticatory pain

Case 29 *480*
Herpes zoster involving the mandibular nerve, expressed intraorally

Case 30 *483*
Deafferentation pain expressed as toothache

Case 31 *486*
Traumatic neuroma pain located in eden-tulous mucogingival tissue (postsurgical)

Case 32 *487*
Traumatic neuroma pain in the TMJ as a result of trauma

Case 33 *504*
Sympathetically maintained pain felt in a tooth

Case 34 *505*
Deafferentation pain, maintained by sympathetic activity

Case 35 *534*
Clinical presentation of a somatoform pain disorder with some possibility of a posttraumatic stress disorder

Foreword

This sixth edition of *Bell's Orofacial Pains* is essential reading for those interested in clinical approaches to orofacial pain conditions and in their underlying neural mechanisms. Like the preceding editions, this book covers a very important topic in clinical dentistry. Pain in the face and mouth is very common and in fact is one of the main reasons for patients to seek dental care. In addition, it can take many forms, and there is a wide variety of treatment options, many of which do not have a strong scientific or evidence basis. Furthermore, this region of the body has special emotional, psychological, and social meaning to the individual. It is little wonder, then, that a patient with orofacial pain, in particular pain that has become chronic, can represent a significant challenge to the clinician trying to diagnose and manage the pain effectively. Indeed, Dr Okeson points out on the very first page of this book that the dental profession has become very effective in managing most acute orofacial pains, but chronic orofacial pain is more problematic.

To deal effectively with pain disorders, the clinician must have a good understanding of the mechanisms underlying the disorders. The knowledge base is still limited, but there have been several insights into these processes since the last edition of this book as a consequence of an enhanced research focus into pain mechanisms through the use of molecular and cellular techniques as well as animal models of pain. These mechanisms encompass peripheral sensitization, central sensitization, pain-modulatory influences, and genetic and molecular processes. There has also been an increased research effort in the behavioral and psychosocial factors influencing pain.

A particular feature of this book is the emphasis that Dr Okeson places on these recent advances within the context of the diagnosis and management of orofacial pains, so that a more comprehensive understanding of pain and the rationale for management approaches can be appreciated by the reader. The research advances and clinical approaches that are presented are supported by an extensive list of references. Furthermore, there are several features that differentiate this edition from earlier editions of the book. These include an updated overview of pain mechanisms and expanded outlines of the utility of local anesthetic techniques and general therapeutic considerations, as well as a new classification scheme for orofacial pain conditions.

Dr Okeson has divided the text into three major sections. The first section outlines the nature of pain and the mechanisms that underlie its expression and modulation, and thereby provides the reader with a firm basis upon which to understand and manage pain conditions. The second section outlines the principles of pain diagnosis and general aspects of pain management, and thus provides the crucial underpinning for the third section, which deals with the differential diagnosis and management options for each orofacial pain disorder.

Like its predecessors, this book should prove to be an invaluable resource not only to dental clinicians and other clinical practitioners wanting to have a basic understanding of pain mechanisms and clinical approaches currently available to diagnose and manage orofacial pain problems, but also to basic and clinical pain scientists who are interested in an up-to-date and comprehensive review of the diagnostic and management issues in the orofacial pain field.

Barry J. Sessle, BDS, MDS, BSc, PhD, DSc (hc), FRSC
Professor and Canada Research Chair
Faculty of Dentistry
University of Toronto

Preface

In the early spring of 1982, I first had the opportunity to listen to Dr Welden E. Bell lecture on the subject of orofacial pain. Through his written work I had already known him as an international authority on this subject. I will never forget the first words from his mouth: "Pain is not a sensation," he proclaimed. I remember squinting slightly, thinking that I had misheard his statement, but then he repeated the seemingly ridiculous remark. I thought, why, of course pain is a sensation. How could such an authority make such a misleading statement? He then went on to say that "pain is far more than a simple sensation; pain is an experience." I must admit that at that time in my professional development I really did not appreciate what he was saying. Following that course and after much further reading of his and other texts, I began to better appreciate his words. There is an old saying that "when the student is ready, the teacher will appear." At that moment, Dr Bell became my teacher and later my mentor.

As my career progressed, I learned more and more from Dr Bell. He continued to write even after his retirement from practice, completing seven editions of his two classic texts on orofacial pains and temporomandibular disorders. As I grew to know him personally, my admiration grew even stronger.

In 1985, I published my first textbook on occlusion and temporomandibular disorders. The first letter that I received commenting on this new text came from Dr Bell. His praise and compliments meant more to me then he would ever know. Later he honored me by writing the foreword to the second edition of that text.

In October 1989, I received a letter from Dr Bell informing me that he had just finished the fourth edition of *Orofacial Pains*. He was then 79 years old and asked if I would consider coauthoring the fifth edition of this text when the time came. His letter provoked two very different emotions in me. I immediately felt that I had just received the greatest professional compliment of my career; yet at the same time, I was confronted with the most difficult task I had ever been asked to accomplish. I dared to say yes, but I certainly could not say no. I immediately called Dr Bell to discuss his proposal. I told him of my feelings and he comforted me by explaining that although he would like for me to take the major responsibilities, he would be there for direction and continuity. With a certain amount of pride and a great deal of insecurity, I accepted his invitation.

In the spring of 1990, I had the privilege to meet with Dr Bell on three occasions; two were during meetings that were dedicated to him for his outstanding contributions to the professions. I had the privilege to speak at both of these meetings and I felt so proud to have him in the audience. During those three meetings, we were able to take some quiet time to discuss new research findings that altered the current views of muscle pain. He contributed greatly to the muscle pain model you see in this text.

In May of 1990, shortly after the publication of the third edition of his textbook on temporomandibular disorders, Dr Bell became suddenly ill and died. His death was a tragic loss to his family and especially his wonderful wife of 58 years, Lucy. His passing was also a tremendous loss to the profession. I personally felt as though I had lost my professional father, and, in fact, I had. During the next year I considered and reconsidered how I would accomplish the monumental task of rewriting this text. At times I even considered not attempting it at all, but my admiration for Dr Bell would not let me linger long on such thoughts. As such, the fifth edition was published in 1995.

After Dr Bell's death I kept in close personal contact with Lucy Bell. During the writing of the fifth edition I sent her chapters as I completed them, for her review. I wanted her to be a part of the project, as she had been with Dr Bell. She was always so kind and would only compliment me on my writings. Whenever I was in Dallas I tried to meet with her for lunch and conversation. She was a very special person, one of the finest I have ever known. I know how Dr Bell found the strength to dedicate so much work to the profession; it was because of Lucy's love and support. Even 13 years after Dr Bell's death, she was still mourning his loss. In December 2003 she left this life to once again join him. It is truly a match made in heaven. I miss her greatly.

My goal in writing the sixth edition is an attempt to update the clinician with the latest findings related to pain. This text is divided into three major sections. The first section presents the normal neuroanatomy and function of the trigeminal system. With a clear understanding of normal function, the clinician can begin to understand and manage dysfunction. The second major section presents a classification of the various orofacial pain disorders and describes the history and examination procedures that can be used to differentiate each disorder. This process, called *diagnosis*, is the most important aspect of orofacial pain management. The third major section presents management considerations for each orofacial pain disorder. It is hoped that this sequence of information will allow the reader to improve his or her skills in the complicated field of orofacial pain.

The work involved in this edition is a labor of love dedicated to Dr Welden Bell. It would not have been possible, however, without the love and support of my wonderful wife of 34 years, Barbara. None of my accomplishments would have been possible without her love, understanding, and constant support. Dr Bell dedicated his books to Lucy, "the light of my life." Barbara is the light of my life and I am indebted to her greatly. She is "the rock on which I stand" and "the wind beneath my wings." Thanks, honey, for all you are and do.

Jeffrey P. Okeson, DMD

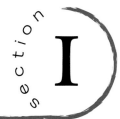

The Nature
of Pain

Defining the Problem

Pain is an unpleasant experience that perhaps motivates an individual far greater than any other life experience. Pain seriously impairs the lives of millions of people around the world. In 1984, Bonica[1] reported that nearly one third of the population in industrialized nations suffers to some extent from chronic pain. At that time he estimated that chronic pain cost the American people more than $65 billion annually for health care services, loss of work, decreased productivity, and disability compensation. It is likely that this represents only a fraction of the cost today. Andersson et al[2] found that 55% of a general population in Sweden had perceived persistent pain for more than 3 months, and 49% had experienced this for 6 months or longer. Among individuals with chronic pain, 90% localized their pain to the musculoskeletal system to a variable extent and 13% reported their pain problem to be associated with reduced functional capacity.

The clinical management of orofacial pain is a primary concern of health professionals all over the world. It is interesting to note that the profession has become extremely effective in the management of acute pain secondary to surgical procedures. The same, however, cannot be said regarding clinical or pathologic pain.

There are reasons for this. The cause of surgical pain is obvious, and its management consists of either suppressing the passage of nociceptive impulses or making the patient insensible to them. Therefore, an effective solution lies within the grasp of the clinician. Clinical pain, however, presents with different circumstances. For example, the cause of clinical pain may not be easily identified. In fact, in some cases the initiating cause may no longer even be present. The mechanisms that are involved with clinical pain appear to be different from those that cause surgical pain and are certainly not as well understood. As a rule, orofacial pain from an obvious cause such as a toothache is managed with no difficulty at all. But when a pain occurs spontaneously or without evidence of structural cause, the clinician may become confused and frustrated. For the clinician to effectively manage clinical pain, he or she must have a basic understanding of the mechanisms that create this unpleasant experience. These mechanisms are certainly not easy to understand, since our knowledge base falls short of being complete. The purpose of this text is to present the latest information regarding our understanding of clinical pain. The explosion of information in the area of pain is so great that keeping a text updated is an extremely difficult task. I hope the information provided in this text will assist the clinician in managing orofacial pain disorders. However, the reader must constantly access current research findings that may shed new light on this most complex problem.

The specific goals of this textbook are: (1) to supply sufficient documented information concerning pain behavior so that one may better understand what pain is, how it behaves, and what means are available to manage it; (2) to develop a more useful classification of orofacial pain disorders; (3) to offer practical diagnostic criteria by which the different pain disorders can be identified on a clinical level; and (4) to suggest guidelines for the effective management of patients who suffer pain about the mouth and face.

Pain as a Clinical Complaint

Pain, especially chronic pain, is a major health problem. According to The Nuprin Pain Report,[3] of the 1,254 persons questioned, 27% reported having experienced dental pain and 73% reported headaches during the previous 12 months. Twelve percent of the patients who reported headache sought care for the pain from a dental practitioner. The sample was constructed statistically in such a manner as to allow these figures to reflect the entire adult population of the United States. This report indicates that the task of managing head and neck pain is a very real one indeed. The problem crosses the lines that demarcate the professions; therefore, it should be the concern of all health care professionals.

As a clinical symptom, pain is an experience that cannot be shared. It is wholly personal, belonging to the sufferer alone. Different individuals sensing identical noxious stimulation feel pain in different ways and react at different levels of suffering. It is impossible for one person to sense exactly what another feels. Therefore, the examiner is faced with the task of securing from the patient enough information to understand how the pain feels and what meaning it has for the patient. The ability to diagnose and treat a person afflicted with pain rests largely on knowledge of the mechanisms and behavioral characteristics of pain in its various manifestations.

The Dental Practitioner's Responsibility

A great burden of responsibility rests upon the dental practitioner for the proper management of pains in and about the mouth, face, and neck. He or she must therefore learn to differentiate between pains that stem from dental, oral, and masticatory sources and those that emanate elsewhere. The dental practitioner must become an expert in pain diagnosis so as to choose the complaints that are manageable on a dental level with dental methods and techniques. He or she must be able to positively identify complaints that, although they may relate to oral and masticatory functioning, in fact stem from causes that cannot reasonably be resolved by ordinary dental procedures.

The dental practitioner's responsibility in managing pain problems of the mouth and face is twofold. The initial responsibility is diagnostic, ie, identification of those complaints that are correctable by dental therapy. To do this, the dentist must have accurate knowledge of pain problems arising from sources that are not oral or masticatory. If a proper diagnosis cannot be made, it becomes the dentist's responsibility to refer the patient to someone perceived to be competent in that field of practice.

The second responsibility of the dental clinician relates to therapy. Once the pain complaint is correctly identified as a condition amenable to dental therapy, treatment by the dentist is in order. Whether or not a consultation with another practitioner is needed should be considered during the treatment planning. If therapy at any point does not prove effective as planned, it becomes the dentist's responsibility to seek the cause of failure by using, if needed, the aid of colleagues. If the condition presented is clearly one that would not be amenable to dental therapy, the patient should be referred to the appropriate health care practitioner.

Many pain problems are such that interdisciplinary management is needed. Such problems require a good working relationship among the therapists. It is important that the dental clinician understand what his or her responsibilities in treatment are so that he or she can conduct his or her portion of the therapy effectively. The dental practitioner should exercise care not to attempt more than his or her fraction of responsibility—nor should any responsibilities of the dentist be relinquished. A positive, confident competence tempered by a reasonable and cooperative attitude should properly equip the dentist to work effectively in any multidisciplinary environment, whether it is wholly dental or dental and medical combined.

In recent years there has been an increase in the dental profession's interest in orofacial pain disorders. This interest has motivated some universities to initiate specialized programs in the field of orofacial pain. A new type of clinician is developing with unique experience in managing orofacial pain disorders. This clinician must have a sound understanding of the principles of medicine as well as dentistry. The role of this professional in the management of pain is being established at this time. Today

is certainly an exciting time to be in this field of study.

Historical Note

Merskey[4] reviewed some of the historical background of modern pain concepts. In ancient times, Homer thought that pain was the result of arrows shot by the gods. The feeling that pain is inflicted from an outside source seems to be a primitive instinct that has persisted to some degree through the ages. Aristotle, who probably was the first to distinguish the five physical senses, considered pain to be a "passion of the soul" that somehow resulted from the intensification of other sensory experience. Plato contended that pain and pleasure arose from within the body, an idea that perhaps gave birth to the concept that pain is an emotional experience more than a localized body disturbance.

The Bible makes reference to pain not only in relationship to injury and illness but also as anguish of the soul. Hebrew words used to express grief, sorrow, and pain are used rather interchangeably in the scriptures[5]; this implies that the early Hebrews considered pain to be a manifestation of concerns that led also to grief and sorrow. However, as knowledge of anatomy and physiology increased, it became possible to distinguish between pains that were the result of physical or emotional causes.

During the 19th century, the developing knowledge of neurology fostered the concept that pain was mediated by specific pain pathways and was not simply a result of excessive stimulation of the special senses. Later it was recognized that strict specificity of neural structures for the exclusive mediation of pain did not exist. In recent years, however, some specialization of nociceptive pathways has been identified.[6] Freud developed the idea that physical symptoms could result from thought processes. He considered that such symptoms as pain could develop as a solution to emotional conflicts.

Therefore, it can be seen that, until very recently, concepts concerning pain changed little since ancient times.

Changing Concepts of Pain

The definition of pain found in the medical dictionary summarizes very well the traditional understanding of what pain is like:

> A more or less localized sensation of discomfort, distress, or agony, resulting from the stimulation of specialized nerve endings. It serves as a protective mechanism insofar as it induces the sufferer to remove or withdraw from the source.[7]

This definition identifies pain as a localized sensation that occurs as the result of noxious stimulation. It suggests that pain is mediated by way of specialized neural structures that are made for that purpose and indicates that pain is a protective mechanism against injury. Being external to the body, the presumed noxious agent could be avoided by proper evasive action. Such a definition actually describes only one type of pain: superficial somatic pain, which is pain that occurs as the result of noxious stimulation of cutaneous structures by an environmentally located agent that affects the exteroceptive nociceptors.

In recent years, quite a different concept of pain has evolved. Although the usefulness of pain as a protective mechanism is recognized with regard to purely exterocep-

tive noxious stimulation, most pain occurs too late to have much protective value. Instead, it has to do with events that have already taken place.

Although pain is now recognized as being more an experience than a sensation, it does have a sensory dimension that registers the nature of the initiating stimulus, including its quality, intensity, location, and duration. But pain also has other dimensions: *(1)* cognitive, which represents the subject's ability to comprehend and evaluate the significance of the experience; *(2)* emotional, which represents the feelings that are generated; and *(3)* motivational, which has to do with the drive to terminate it. In humans, pain actively involves neocortical processes that have to do with the recognition and interpretation of the consequences of the experience, thus exerting a good measure of influence on the pain and the suffering that is generated by it.[8] Pain is thought to be more like other "need states" such as hunger and thirst; it initiates a drive for action. Pain cannot be sensed in a detached manner; it comes in combination with dislike, anxiety, fear, and urgency.[9] Although pain does result from noxious stimulation, it can also result from nonnoxious stimuli or even occur spontaneously with no stimulus at all. The source of stimulation need not be external to the body.

This revised concept of what constitutes pain is expressed in the definition proposed by the Subcommittee on Taxonomy of the International Association for the Study of Pain: "An unpleasant sensory and emotional experience associated with actual or potential tissue damage, or described in terms of such damage."[10] By this definition, pain is understood to represent a subjective psychologic state rather than an activity that is induced solely by noxious stimulation. It should be noted that if the subject reports his or her experience as pain, it should be accepted as pain.

Perhaps an even more complete definition of pain is

an unpleasant sensation associated with actual or potential tissue damage and mediated by specific nerve fibers to the brain, where its conscious appreciation may be modified by various factors.[11]

This definition recognizes that pain may have a noxious transmission component, a psychologic component, and a very important modulatory component. As will be discussed in this text, the ability to modulate ascending transmission as it passes through the higher centers is a very important part of understanding the pain experiences.

More precisely, pain as presently conceived has a sensory-discriminative dimension to identify the form of energy (thermal, mechanical, and chemical) and the spatial, temporal, and intensive aspects of the stimulus. It also has a motivational-affective property by which the consequences of the experience become manifested as escape and avoidance behavior, which includes reflex somatic and autonomic motor responses.[12]

When an identifiable cause can be established for pain, management usually entails measures to eliminate this cause, if possible. Some pains, however, have a significant central component that makes them more complex. Such pains may confuse a clinician who is oriented to the stimulus-response concept and thinks only in terms of cause. Many times, however, the consequences of the experience become the paramount issue in managing the pain problem. In such cases, the proper manipulation of various environmental factors may help the patient unlearn his or her pain behavior.[13]

It is also interesting to note that the more severe the pain and the more distressed the patient, the more emotional are the responses and the greater the impact on the ability to function.[14] The pressure to seek aid for a pain problem increases when the patient is under greater-than-usual stress. It seems that those who find their life situation satisfactory tend to ignore symptoms.[15]

It is interesting to note that the degree of pain and suffering that a patient experiences is not related to the amount of tissue injury experienced. It has been observed that the intensity of pain from physical injury relates to the attention given at the time. Pain and injury may be coincident only when attention is directed to the injury. If one's attention is fully absorbed at the time of injury, no pain may be felt. The subject may remain relatively free of pain if he or she is distracted by events having to do with self-preservation, fighting back, escaping, or obtaining aid. Pain may not become an issue until the consequences of the injury induce feelings of concern and anxiety that relate more to therapy and recovery processes than to the injury itself.[16,17]

With the changing concepts of pain represented in body, mind, and person, the diagnosis and management of such problems require a broad understanding of people on the part of the attending clinician. Good therapy begins with an attitude of caring and concern for the person more than for his or her body. Human beings are more than patients who have to be treated.[18]

The Emergency Nature of Pain

Pain creates an emergency for the patient and therefore becomes a prime motivating cause for seeking aid. When the suffering occurs in and about the mouth, the dental practitioner is usually the first to be called. When it occurs about the ears, face, head, or neck, a physician may be consulted. The actual location of the symptom may well determine who the patient sees first. Yet the location of the pain can mislead both patient and practitioner as to its true source and significance. In the case of obscure pain, the patient may visit several doctors and receive conflicting opinions and treatments. The alarm with which a patient naturally regards his or her own discomfort is increased when a clinician fails to give prompt and lasting relief, so ineffective therapy may intensify the pain and magnify the task of the next therapist to be consulted. It therefore behooves every clinician to become familiar with the mechanisms of pain and the technique of examining patients with pain complaints.

The emergency nature of pain relates to the significance the patient attaches to it. If the cause is obvious, such as a cut finger, little or no alarm ensues because the subject is able to recognize the cause of his suffering and evaluate it realistically. If, however, the pain is located in an area of greater significance, as, for example, the eye, the alarm mounts because it represents a greater threat. Similarly, if the discomfort arises from deeper structures where its cause is less obvious and its seriousness less certain, the patient becomes more concerned. The emergency nature of pain relates more to the fear that it generates than to the actual intensity of the discomfort.

The importance of prompt and effective therapy should not be underestimated, for in this area the therapist proves himself or utterly fails. Whereas competent therapy has as its prime attribute the means of furnishing consolation to a suffering patient, it can be said conversely that incompetence can intensify the patient's alarm. Perhaps there is no area of practice in which this is more likely to occur than in the diagnosis and treatment of obscure pain—nor is any complaint more adversely affected by professional failure. Minor discomfort assumes major significance if the patient feels he or she has a problem so dreadful that it escapes even the "magical abilities" of the doctor.

Levels of Pain Processing

Early in a discussion of pain it is important to distinguish the differences between four terms: *nociception*, *pain*, *suffering*, and *pain behavior*. *Nociception* refers to the noxious stimulus originating from the sensory receptor. This information is carried into the central nervous system (CNS) by the primary afferent neuron.

Pain is an unpleasant sensation perceived in the cortex, usually as a result of incoming nociceptive input. However, the presence or absence of nociceptive input does not always relate closely to pain. As will be discussed in detail in chapter 4, the CNS has the ability to alter or modulate nociceptive input before it reaches the cortex for recognition. Therefore, nociceptive input entering the CNS can be modified in such a manner that the cortex never perceives it as pain. One can quickly appreciate that this ability of the CNS to modulate noxious stimulation is an extremely important function. As will be discussed later, modulation of nociceptive input can either increase or decrease the perception of pain.

The term *suffering* refers to still another phenomenon: how the human reacts to the perception of pain. When pain is perceived by the cortex, a very complex interaction of many factors begins. Factors such as past experiences, expectations, perceived threat of the injury, and attention drawn to the injury determine to what degree the subject will suffer. Suffering, therefore, may not be proportionally related to nociception or pain. Patients experiencing little pain may suffer greatly, while others with significant pain may suffer less.

Pain behavior is still another term with a different meaning. Pain behavior refers to the individual's audible and visible actions that communicate his suffering to others.

Pain behavior is the only communication the clinician receives regarding the pain experience. This behavior is as individual as people themselves.

It is important for the clinician to recognize that the information related to the therapist by the patient is not nociception or pain or even suffering. The patient only relates his or her pain behavior. Yet it is through this communication that the clinician must gain insight into the patient's pain problem; thus, one can easily see the difficulty of the clinician's task when attempting to manage pain disorders.

Phylogenic Considerations

It is interesting to note that the human being has a brain system that can be functionally divided into three components. The first component is made up of the spinal cord and medulla. This might be thought of as the basic reptilian brain, since it functions on a very primitive level and likely represents the only functional brain of the reptile. This portion of the brain provides protective reflex activity against challenges from the environment. For example, if you were to accidentally touch a hot stove, your hand would quickly pull away. This reflex activity occurs without thought or cerebral function. The same activity occurs if you strike a snake with a stick. The snake will coil up or quickly slither away. There is no evidence in reptiles that pain is felt. This primitive brain serves a valuable protective function for the individual.

The second functional brain in humans is the mammalian brain. The mammalian brain is made up of the limbic structures wrapped around the upper portion of the medulla and spinal cord. The limbic structures provide the individual with instinctive drives and emotions. This portion of the brain is made up of various centers that instinctively drive the individual toward certain behaviors. These drives do not function on a totally conscious level but rather represent basic needs of the individual, eg, hunger, thirst, sleep, sexual activity. There appears to be a pain/pleasure center in the limbic structures that strongly motivates the individual. When pain is felt, the individual will instinctively direct behavior toward activities that will reduce the pain and when possible stimulate the pleasure side of this center. Stimulating the pleasure side of the pain/pleasure center is a basic drive and can powerfully direct behavior. In fact, addictions to drugs, alcohol, food, and sexual activities are common behaviors that represent instinctive drives to stimulate the pleasure center of the limbic system.

The third functional component of the human brain is the most complex structure: the cortex. A human not only has the medulla and spinal cord (the primate brain) with the limbic structures (the mammalian brain), but attached to these structures is the cortex. The cortex provides the human with the ability to reason and think. It is at this level that the human who experiences pain begins to apply meaning and consequence to the sensation. For example, the human experiencing pain will evaluate the meaning of this condition as to how it will affect relationships, such as those with a spouse or other family members, or how it might influence the ability to work or to socialize. It is this phenomenon that makes suffering as we know it so different from that experienced by lower animal life. It is through this mechanism that factors such as attention, anxiety, and fear influence the level of suffering. The effect of one's mental awareness or state of arousal, one's concern for the outcome, and the emotional and/or physical stability of the individual become the dominant modulating influences in every painful experience. We may consider therefore that clinical pain as we know it is an experience unique to humans.

Anatomic Considerations of the Human

The human being is a phenomenal organism, with complexity far beyond the imagination of the best scientific minds. Perhaps it is best to begin a discussion of anatomy from a very broad prospective. The human being is a musculoskeletal system that is encompassed by an envelope that separates it from the environment. The basic structures or cells of the musculoskeletal system as well as the envelope need to receive food or nutrients, and so a supply system is present to carry out this task. The functions of all these systems are very complex; therefore a communication system is needed to coordinate activities of the entire organism.

We have just described the basic systems of the human being. The musculoskeletal system is made up of muscle, bones, and associated structures such as ligaments and tendons. These structures provide the individual with mobility so that food can be procured. The envelope consists of the cutaneous (skin) and mucogingival structures that surround the musculoskeletal system. These structures provide input to the individual from the environment, so that appropriate actions can be carried out to preserve the organism.

The supply system is able to take in food and air and convert it into energy that can be utilized by the cells. The supply system then transports these essential elements to each individual cell throughout the organism. The supply system is comprised of the digestive, pulmonary, and circulatory systems.

Because of the complexity of these systems, a master control system is in place to coordinate all these activities. This system is known as the *nervous system* and is divided into several functional parts. The *peripheral nervous system* carries information from the musculoskeletal and cutaneous (envelope) structures. There is also a separate nervous system that coordinates activities of the supply system. This is called the *autonomic nervous system*, and it is predominantly responsible for the regulation of blood flow, breathing, and digestion. Coordination of the peripheral and autonomic nervous systems is carried out by the *central nervous system*, which is made up of the brainstem and the cortex. The cortex can be thought of as the master computer that stores the data necessary to carry out function of the individual.

One of the basic concepts in understanding pain is to appreciate that the manner in which the master computer communicates with each of these structures is perceived by individuals differently. As soon as the clinician appreciates this concept, the patient's description of the pain complaint becomes meaningful. As will be discussed in latter chapters, pains originating in each structure have certain clinical characteristics to help differentiate them from each other.

In general, the medical and dental professions do not refer to the various systems with such terms as supply system or envelope. The terms that will be used in this text will be as follows: *Somatic structures* include all the structures that make up the body (soma) other than the neurologic structures. Somatic structures are divided into two types, the *superficial somatic structures*, which represent the envelope (skin and mucogingival tissues), and the *deep somatic structures*, which make up the remainder of the body tissues. The deep somatic structures are then divided into the *musculoskeletal structures* and the *visceral structures* (ie, supply structures). The nervous system is divided into the three components that have already been presented (peripheral, central, and autonomic).

Neural Pathways of Pain

Fields[19] has noted that the subjective experience of pain arises by four distinct processes: *transduction, transmission, modulation,* and *perception.*

Transduction is the process by which noxious stimuli lead to electrical activity in the appropriate sensory nerve endings. The body has several types of sensory organs that initiate the process of nociception. These receptors will be discussed in detail in chapter 2.

The second process is called *transmission* and refers to the neural events that carry the nociceptive input into the CNS for proper processing. There are three basic components to the transmission system. The first is the peripheral sensory nerve: the *primary afferent neuron.* This neuron carries the nociceptive input from the sensory organ in to the spinal cord. The second component of the transmission process is the *second-order neuron,* which carries the input to the higher centers. Actually, this portion of the transmission process can involve a number of neurons that interact as the input is sent up to the thalamus. The third component of the transmission system represents interactions of neurons between the thalamus, the cortex, and the limbic system as the nociceptive input reaches these higher centers. This process of transmission will be discussed in detail in chapters 2 and 3.

The third process involved in the subjective experience of pain is called *modulation.* Modulation refers to the ability of the CNS to control the pain-transmitting neurons. Several areas of the cortex and brainstem have been identified that can either enhance or reduce nociceptive input arriving by way of the transmitting neurons. The phenomena of modulation will be discussed in chapter 4.

The final process involved in the subjective experience of pain is *perception.* If nociceptive input reaches the cortex, perception occurs; this immediately initiates a complex interaction of neurons between the higher centers of the brain. It is at this point that suffering and pain behavior begin. This is the least understood aspect of pain and the most variable between individuals. This will be discussed in chapters 5 and 6.

The remaining chapters of this text will review the etiologic, diagnostic, and treatment considerations of orofacial pain disorders.

References

1. Bonica J. Pain research and therapy: Recent advances and future needs. In: Kruger L, Liebeskind CJ (eds). Neural Mechanisms of Pain, vol 6, Advances in Pain Research and Therapy. New York: Raven Press, 1984:1–22.
2. Andersson HI, Ejlertsson G, Leden I, Rosenberg C. Chronic pain in a geographically defined general population: Studies of differences in age, gender, social class, and pain localization. Clin J Pain 1993;9:174–182.
3. Sternbach RA. Survey of pain in the United States: The Nuprin Pain Report. Clin J Pain 1986;2:49–53.
4. Merskey H. Some features of the history of the idea of pain. Pain 1980;9:3–8.
5. Strong J. Strong's Exhaustive Concordance of the Bible. Nashville, TN: Abingdon, 1986.

6. Dubner R. Specialization of nociceptive pathways: Sensory discrimination, sensory modulation, and neural connectivity. In: Fields HL, Dubner R, Cervero F (eds). Proceedings of the Fourth World Congress on Pain: Seattle, vol 9, Advances in Pain Research and Therapy. New York: Raven Press, 1985:111–137.

7. Dorland WAN. Dorland's Illustrated Medical Dictionary, ed 27. Philadelphia: Saunders, 1988:1724.

8. Melzack R. Psychological concepts and methods for the control of pain. In: Bonica JJ (ed). International Symposium on Pain, vol 4, Advances in Neurology. New York: Raven Press, 1974:275–280.

9. Wall P. Why do we not understand pain? In: Duncan R, Weston-Smith M (eds). The Encyclopaedia of Ignorance. Oxford: Pergamon Press, 1977:361–368.

10. Merskey H. Pain terms: A list with definitions and notes on usage. Pain 1979;6:249–252.

11. Stedman TL. Stedman's Medical Dictionary, ed 27. Baltimore: Lippincott Williams & Wilkins, 2000:1297.

12. Price DD, Dubner R. Neurons that subserve the sensory-discriminative aspects of pain. Pain 1977;3:307–338.

13. Fordyce W. Pain viewed as learned behavior. In: Bonica JJ (ed). International Symposium on Pain, vol 4, Advances in Neurology. New York: Raven Press, 1974:415–422.

14. Lipton JA, Marbach JJ. Components of the response to pain and variables influencing the response in three groups of facial pain patients. Pain 1983;16:343–359.

15. Marbach JJ, Lipton JA. Aspects of illness behavior in patients with facial pain. J Am Dent Assoc 1976;96:630-638.

16. Wall PD. On the relation of injury to pain. Pain 1979;6:253–261.

17. Bonica J. Letters to the editor. Pain 1975;7:203–207.

18. Degenaar J. Some philosophical considerations on pain. Pain 1979;7:281–304.

19. Fields H. Pain. New York: McGraw-Hill, 1987.

The Neural Anatomy of Orofacial Pain

The most essential element in the management of a patient's pain problem is an understanding of normal function of the system. This is true in managing any condition. A clinician cannot effectively treat a disorder until he has a sound understanding of order. This basic fact needs to be appreciated by all clinicians. When a patient reports to an office with some type of dysfunction, the clinician's therapy should be directed toward re-establishing normal function, and the clinician cannot expect to be successful if he or she lacks a sound understanding of normal function. The management of pain disorders is far too complex to develop a simple "cookbook" of therapies. The clinician must understand the unique characteristics of the system so that therapy can be designed appropriately for each patient.

As mentioned in chapter 1, the functional processing of pain can be grossly separated into four categories: transduction, transmission, modulation, and perception. *Transduction* is the process by which noxious stimuli lead to electrical activity in the appropriate sensory nerve endings. The body has several types of sensory organs that initiate the process of nociception.

The second process, *transmission,* refers to the neural events that carry the nociceptive input into the central nervous system for proper processing. The neuroanatomy of transduction and transmission will be discussed in this chapter. Modulation and perception will be discussed in chapters 3 and 4.

Neural Structures

Neuron (Nerve Cell)

A nerve is a cordlike structure that has the ability to convey electrical and chemical impulses. It consists of a connective tissue sheath, called the *epineurium,* that encloses bundles (fasciculi) of nerve fibers, each bundle being surrounded by its own connective tissue sheath, the *perineurium.* Within each

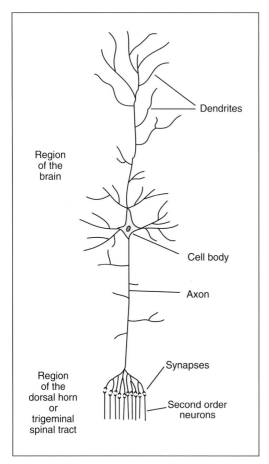

Dendrites

Region of the brain

Cell body

Axon

Synapses

Region of the dorsal horn or trigeminal spinal tract

Second order neurons

Fig 2-1 The structure of a large neuron of the brain. (Adapted from Guyton AC. Textbook of Medical Physiology, ed 8. Philadelphia: Saunders, 1991:479. Used with permission.)

rolemma (primary sheath or sheath of Schwann). Some of these fibers also have a layer of fatty nerve tissue called the *myelin sheath* (medullary sheath or white substance of Schwann). Fibers with myelin sheaths form the "white nerves," and those without myelin sheaths are the "gray nerves." Constrictions called *nodes of Ranvier* occur in myelinated nerves at intervals of about 1 mm. These nodes are caused by the absence of myelin material, so that only neurolemma covers the nerve fiber. Nerve fibers in the central nervous system (CNS) have no neurolemma. Those situated in the white substance are myelinated, whereas those in the gray substance are unmyelinated.

Myelination of a nerve fiber affects the resting and action potential of the neuron. The myelin acts as insulation, so that the action potential of a transferring impulse is expressed only at the node of Ranvier. Therefore the impulse travels from node to node, requiring less time to move down the nerve fiber,[1] so that myelination increases the conduction velocity of the fiber. The ultrastructure of the primary trigeminal neuron has been well described[2] by use of electron microscopic techniques.

The structural unit of the nervous system is the nerve cell, or *neuron*. It is composed of a mass of protoplasm termed the *nerve cell body* (perikaryon), which contains a spherical nucleus (karyon) and gives off one or more processes. The nerve cell bodies located in the spinal cord are found in the gray substance of the CNS. Cell bodies found outside the CNS are grouped together in *ganglia*. The term *nucleus*, as applied to the gross structure of the CNS, is used to designate a group of nerve cells that bear a direct relationship to the fibers of a particular nerve. Protoplasmic processes from the nerve cell body are called *dendrites* and *axons* (Fig 2-1). A dendrite (from the Greek word *dendron*, meaning tree) is a branched arborizing process that conducts impulses toward the cell body. An axon (from the Greek word *axon*, meaning axle or

bundle the nerve fibers are separated by interstitial connective tissue called the *endoneurium*.

An individual nerve fiber consists of a central bundle of neurofibrils in a matrix of nerve protoplasm, called the *axoplasm*, which is enclosed in a thin nerve tissue plasma membrane called the *axolemma*. Each peripheral nerve fiber is covered by a cellular nerve tissue sheath called the *neu-*

axis) or axis-cylinder is the central core that forms the essential conducting part of a nerve fiber and is an extension of cytoplasm from a nerve cell.

Depending on the number of axons present, a nerve cell is *unipolar, bipolar,* or *multipolar.* Peripheral sensory neurons are unipolar. The single axon leaves the nerve cell body, located in the dorsal root ganglion, and branches into two parts: a peripheral branch that extends to terminate in a sensory receptor and a central branch that passes through the root of the nerve to terminate in the gray substance of the CNS.

Depending on their location and function, neurons are designated by different terms. An *afferent* neuron conducts a nervous impulse toward the CNS, whereas an *efferent* neuron conducts it peripherally. *Interneurons,* or *internuncial neurons,* lie wholly within the CNS. Sensory or receptor neurons, afferent in type, receive and convey impulses from receptor organs. The first sensory neuron is called the *primary* or *first-order* neuron. *Second-* and *third-order* sensory neurons are interneurons. *Motor* or *efferent* neurons convey nervous impulses to produce muscular or secretory effects. A *preganglionic neuron* is an autonomic efferent neuron whose nerve cell body is located in the CNS and terminates in an autonomic ganglion. A *postganglionic neuron* has its nerve cell body in the autonomic ganglion and terminates peripherally.

Nervous impulses are transmitted from one neuron to another only at a synaptic junction, or *synapse,* where the processes of two neurons are in close proximity. All afferent synapses are located within the gray substance of the CNS. It should be noted that the only synapses that normally occur outside the CNS are those of the efferent preganglionic and postganglionic autonomic fibers, and these are located in the autonomic ganglia. This indicates that there are no anatomic peripheral connections between sensory fibers. All connections are within the CNS, and the peripheral transmission of a sensory impulse from one fiber to another is abnormal. Any artificial or false peripheral synapse, called an *ephapse,* signifies an abnormal or pathologic change.[3]

Functional Neuroanatomy

Information from the tissues outside the CNS needs to be transferred into the CNS and on to the higher centers in the brainstem and cortex for interpretation and evaluation. Once this information is evaluated, appropriate action must be taken. The higher centers then send impulses down the spinal cord and back out to the periphery to an efferent organ for the desired action. The primary afferent neuron (first-order neuron) receives a stimulus from the sensory receptor. This impulse is carried by the primary afferent neuron into the CNS by way of the dorsal root to synapse in the dorsal horn of the spinal cord with a secondary (second-order) neuron. The cell bodies of all the primary afferent neurons are located in the dorsal root ganglia. The impulse is then carried by the second-order neuron across the spinal cord to the anterolateral spinothalamic pathway, which ascends to the higher centers. There may be multiple interneurons (third-order, fourth-order, etc) involved with the transfer of this impulse to the thalamus and cortex. There are also very small interneurons located in the dorsal horn that may become involved with the impulse as it synapses with the second-order neuron. Some of these neurons may directly synapse with efferent neurons that are directed back out the CNS by way of the ventral root to stimulate an efferent organ, such as a muscle (Fig 2-2).

Some neural circuits are simple. For example, an impulse from a sensory receptor is carried into the CNS by the primary af-

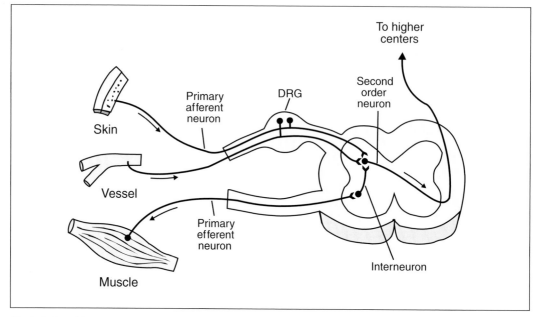

Fig 2-2 Graphic depiction of the peripheral nerve input into the spinal cord. Note that the first-order neurons (primary afferents) carry input into the dorsal horn to synapse with the second-order neurons. The second-order neuron then crosses over and ascends on to the higher centers. Small interneurons connect the primary afferent neuron with the primary motor (efferent) neuron, allowing reflex arc activity. The dorsal root ganglion (DRG) contains the cell bodies of the primary afferent neurons.

ferent neuron and synapses with an interneuron. This interneuron in turn synapses with an efferent motor neuron exiting back out the CNS to an efferent organ, such as a muscle. A circuit formed by a chain of neurons in such a way that stimulation is followed by an immediate and automatic response is called a *reflex arc*. As will be discussed, most reflex arcs or neural circuits are much more complex, involving several and sometimes vast numbers of interneurons, with many possible responses.

Sensory Receptors

At the distal terminals of afferent (sensory) nerves are specialized sensory receptors that respond to physical or chemical stimuli.

Once these receptors have been adequately stimulated, an impulse is generated in the primary afferent neuron that is carried centrally into the CNS. Sensory receptors are specific for certain types of stimuli. They can be classified into three main groups, namely, *exteroceptors, proprioceptors,* and *interoceptors.*[4]

Exteroceptors

Exteroceptors are sensory receptors that are stimulated by the immediate external environment and are appropriately fashioned and located so as to be exposed to the organism's environment. These receptors provide information from the skin and mucosa (the envelope). Most impulses arising from these receptors are sensed at conscious levels. Some examples of this type of receptor are:

1. Merkel's corpuscles: tactile receptors in the submucosa of the tongue and oral mucosa
2. Meissner's corpuscles: tactile receptors in skin
3. Ruffini's corpuscles: pressure and warmth receptors
4. Krause's corpuscles or end-bulbs: cold receptors
5. Free nerve endings: perceive superficial pain and touch

Proprioceptors

Proprioceptors are sensory receptors that provide information from the musculoskeletal structures concerning the presence, position, and movement of the body. They are involved chiefly with automatic functioning. For the most part, sensations conducted from proprioceptors are below conscious levels, although many such sensations can be brought into consciousness voluntarily. Some examples of this type of receptor are:

1. Muscle spindles: mechanoreceptors found between the skeletal muscle fibers that respond to passive stretch of the muscle, thus signaling muscle length. They are responsible in part for regulating and maintaining muscle tonicity by way of the myotatic reflex.
2. Golgi tendon organs: mechanoreceptors in the tendons of muscles that signal muscle tension in both contraction and stretching. These receptors act with the muscle spindles to regulate muscle tonicity, as well as the inverse stretch reflexes, and may even play a role in nociception.
3. Pacinian corpuscles: receptors concerned in the perception of pressure.
4. Periodontal mechanoreceptors: respond to biomechanical stimuli.
5. Free nerve endings: perceive deep somatic pain and other sensations.

Interoceptors

Interoceptors are sensory receptors that are located in and transmit impulses from the viscera (supply system) of the body. Sensation from these receptors for the most part is involved in the involuntary functioning of the body and as such is below conscious levels. Some examples of this type of receptor include the following:

1. Pacinian corpuscles: concerned in perception of pressure.
2. Free nerve endings: perceive visceral pain and other sensations.

Nociceptors

As described above, free nerve endings are found in almost all tissues. These receptors are responsible for identifying tissue injury and are therefore referred to as *nociceptors*. The tissue area for which the nociceptor is responsible is called its *receptive field*. Unlike the other types of cutaneous receptors, nociceptors may respond to multiple stimulus modalities, such as mechanical, heat, cold, and chemical stimuli.[5] Nociceptors are therefore considered to be polymodal. Early studies of nociceptors only investigated heat and mechanical stimuli, and therefore two types of nociceptors were identified: the C-fiber mechano/heat-sensitive nociceptors (CMH), and the A-fiber mechano/heat-sensitive nociceptors (AMH). The CMH nociceptor is commonly found in cutaneous tissues and when stimulated in sufficient magnitude is thought to evoke a burning pain sensation. The receptive field of the CMH in humans is about 100 mm.[6] However, many of these will overlap each other, giving a particular receptive field more than one nociceptor. CMH nociceptors also respond to chemical stimuli, making them polymodal.[7]

The AMH nociceptors are thought to evoke pricking pain, sharpness, and perhaps aching pain. As a general rule, the A-fiber nociceptors do what the C-fiber nociceptors do, but they do it more robustly. Although specific pain sensations have been described, further investigations reveal that it is not nearly this simple. Under certain conditions CMH and AMH nociceptors can provoke similar pain sensations.

It is now known that the nerve itself has its own nociceptors. The connective tissue sheath surrounding a peripheral nerve is innervated by primary afferents called the *nervi nervorum*. The nervi nervorum appear to enter the nerve trunk with the neurovascular bundle.[8,9] Because of the nervi nervorum, peripheral nerves can be a source of pain in a manner similar to joints, muscles, and ligaments. The role of the nervi nervorum in certain pain conditions will be discussed in later chapters.

Specialized Receptors and Reflexes

The more highly specialized receptor organs are complex and admirably designed to receive a particular type of stimulus. The neuromuscular receptors, or muscle spindles, have their own sensory and motor innervation comprising a monosynaptic reflex system known as the *myotatic* or *stretch reflex*. When muscle spindles are elongated due to passive stretching of the muscle, reflex contraction occurs. This appears to function not only to oppose the forces of gravity but also during reflex and voluntary contraction of muscles, both flexor and extensor.

It should be noted that the neurotendinous receptors called *Golgi tendon organs* respond to tendon stretch and muscle contraction. When these receptors are stimulated, an inhibitory reflex occurs that limits contraction and thus protects the muscle from disruption or detachment. The reflex

mechanism involved in this activity is called the *nociceptive reflex* and is a polysynaptic relay that involves concurrently the contraction of flexor muscles and the inhibition of extensor muscles, resulting in withdrawal of the part stimulated.[10,11]

When a muscle is maximally stretched, stimulation of Golgi tendon organs induces a reflex that causes contraction to cease and the muscle to relax. This reflex is called the *inverse stretch reflex*. It should be noted that occasional stretching of a muscle that induces this reflex activity is necessary for the muscle to maintain its normal resting length. If conditions prevent normal operation of this reflex, muscular contracture may occur, which causes the muscle to become functionally shortened.[12] For example, the simple act of yawning lengthens the masticatory elevator muscles, stimulating the inverse stretch reflex, which maintains the full range of mouth opening. If the mouth were wired closed because of a mandibular fracture, the elevator muscles would functionally shorten, disallowing full mouth opening at the time of fixation removal. However, as the individual attempted to open the mouth wider, the elevator muscle would be lengthened, stimulating the Golgi tendon organ. This excites the inverse stretch reflex and eventually allows a return of the original functional length of the muscle. This phenomenon is also seen with the lateral pterygoid muscles in edentulous patients. When an individual with complete natural dentition fully intercuspates the teeth, the inferior lateral pterygoid muscles lengthen completely, maintaining normal functional length. However, with artificial dentures the resiliency of the interposed underlying soft tissues may not allow full contraction, and therefore muscle contracture can occur in the inferior lateral pterygoid muscles. This can result in a progressive shift of the mandible into a more anterior position.

The simplest type of receptor is the nonencapsulated branching of the axon called

Table 2-1 General Classification of Neurons

Nerve fiber	Diameter	Velocity
Type A fibers		
Alpha fibers	13 to 20 µm	70 to 120 m/s
Beta fibers	6 to 13 µm	40 to 70 m/s
Gamma fibers	3 to 8 µm	15 to 40 m/s
Delta fibers	1 to 5 µm	5 to 15 m/s
Type C fibers	0.5 to 1 µm	0.5 to 2 m/s

the *free nerve ending*. These terminations are usually described as naked, and they form a network that is especially dense in the cutaneous layers, mucous membranes, and periodontium. In deeper tissues the network is neither as widely spread nor as dense. Simple free nerve endings are no doubt the receptors for nociception and pain, but they are not specific for pain only.

Stimulation of the free nerve ending receptors can occur as a result of mechanical stimulation (eg, pressure), thermal stimulation (eg, heat), or by chemical stimulation (eg, that produced by substances released following tissue damage).[13] It should be noted that free nerve endings are not required for the reception of noxious stimulation, since the nerve fiber itself has the same propensity and the evoked response is similar to that initiated by receptors.

Associated with all vascular tissue, including the endocardium, is a remarkable network of sensory receptors derived from myelinated nerve fibers called the *end-net*.[14] These receptors provide sensory information from the vessels.

The First-Order Neuron

Each sensory receptor is attached to an afferent neuron that carries the impulses to the CNS. Since these neurons are the first to carry the information into the CNS, they are called *first-order neurons* or *primary afferent neurons*. The axons of these first-order neurons are found to have varying thickness. It has long been known that a relationship exists between the diameter of nerve fibers and their conduction velocities.[15-17] The larger fibers conduct impulses more rapidly than the smaller ones. A general classification of neurons divides the larger fibers from the smaller ones; the larger fibers are called A fibers and the smaller fibers are called C fibers. The A fibers are further divided by diameter into alpha, beta, gamma, and delta. This relationship is summarized in Table 2-1.[18]

It is generally thought that there is a relationship between fiber size and the type of impulse transmitted. The fast conducting A-alpha, A-beta, and A-gamma fibers carry impulses that induce tactile and proprioceptive responses but not pain. It seems that pain is conducted by A-delta fibers and C fibers, but these are not specific for nociception only.

It is recognized that there are two types of cutaneous pain sensation: pricking pain, which is felt rapidly, and dull, aching, sometimes burning pain, which is slightly delayed. It is thought that these sensations are mediated by different fibers, the pricking sensation by A-delta fibers and the dull aching sensation by C fibers.[19] It is known, however, that A-delta fibers also conduct touch, warmth, and cold, whereas C fibers also conduct itch, warmth, and cold.[20-22]

There are three types of afferent neurons that can provide nociceptive input to the CNS:

1. Mechanothermal afferents are primarily A-delta fibers that conduct at a velocity of 12 to 15 m/s and respond to intense thermal and mechanical stimuli. They provide a high degree of discriminative information and are peculiar to primates.
2. High-threshold mechanoreceptive afferents are chiefly A-delta fibers and normally respond to intense mechanical stimuli in all mammals. They can, however, be sensitized by algogenic substances or repeated noxious stimulation to respond to noxious heat as well (see chapter 4).
3. Polymodal afferents are C fibers that conduct much more slowly, at a velocity of 0.5 m/s, and respond to mechanical, thermal, and chemical stimuli in all mammals. At this rate it takes an impulse 2 seconds to go from the big toe to the spinal cord.

Of these three afferent neurons, only the mechanothermal A-delta and C-fiber afferents normally respond to noxious heat.[23,24]

The Second-Order Neuron

The primary afferent neuron carries impulses into the CNS and synapses with the second-order neuron. This second-order neuron has been called a *transmission neuron*, since it transfers the impulse to the higher centers. The synapse of the primary afferent neuron and the second-order neuron occurs in the dorsal horn of the spinal cord (see Fig 2-2). The specific anatomy of the trigeminal system will be reviewed later in this chapter.

There appear to be three specific types of second-order neurons that transfer impulses to the higher centers.[13,25] These neurons are named according to the type of impulses they predominantly carry. The *low-threshold mechanosensitive neurons* (LTM neurons) transfer information of light touch, pressure, and proprioception. The *nociceptive-specific neurons* (NS neurons) exclusively carry impulses related to noxious stimulation. The third type of second-order neuron is called a *wide dynamic range neuron* (WDR neuron). This neuron is able to respond to a wide range of stimulus intensities from nonnoxious to noxious.

Recently an additional type of second-order neuron has been identified, called a *silent nociceptor*. The silent nociceptor is an afferent neuron that appears to remain inactive or "silent" to any mechanical stimulation. These neurons become active with tissue injury and add to the nociceptive input entering the CNS.[26]

Under normal conditions it is not believed that the LTM neurons are involved in the transfer of nociception. Nociception is primarily carried by the NS and WDR neurons.

The dorsal horn of the spinal cord is subdivided into different layers, or *laminae*.[27-29] These laminae are numbered according to their depth in the dorsal horn from I to VI, with the most superficial being I and the deepest being VI[13] (Fig 2-3). Studies suggest that nociceptive input enters the dorsal horn by way of the NS and WDR neurons in the area of laminae I, II, and V.[30,31] The LTM neurons that do not carry nociception seem to be more concentrated in laminae III and IV.

Within the dorsal horn there are interneurons that transfer impulses to other interneurons or to the ascending neurons. These neurons can be either *inhibitory* or *excitatory*. In other words, when some of the neurons are stimulated, they tend to reduce the activity of the neuron to which they synapse. These are called *inhibitory neurons*.

Fig 2-3 Cross section of the spinal cord showing the anatomic laminae I through X of the cord gray matter and the ascending sensory anterolateral spinothalamic tract (ALST tract) in the white columns. DR = Dorsal root; VR = ventral root.

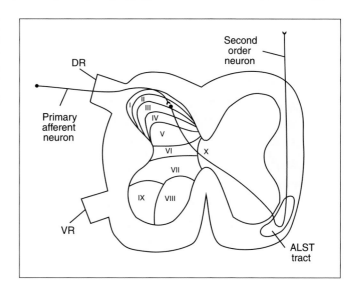

Other interneurons, when excited, increase the activity of the neurons on which they synapse. These are called *excitatory neurons.* There are a significant population of these interneurons in laminae II and III, and this region is collectively called the *substantia gelatinosa.*

Once the impulses have been transferred from the primary afferents, most of the second-order neurons cross to the opposite side of the spinal cord and enter the *anterolateral spinothalamic tract,* which ascends to the higher centers. Some of the second-order neurons remain on the same side of the dorsal column and ascend by way of the *lemniscal system.* These neurons cross over to the opposite side at the level of the medulla. The dorsal column lemniscal system is composed of large, myelinated nerve fibers that transmit signals to the brain at velocities of 30 to 110 m/s. The anterolateral system is composed of much smaller myelinated and unmyelinated fibers that transmit signals at velocities ranging from a few meters per second up to 40 m/s.

These differences immediately characterize the types of sensory information that can be transmitted by these two systems. The dorsal column lemniscal system rapidly transmits information regarding touch, pressure, vibration, and proprioception needed for immediate response of the musculoskeletal system to environmental changes. The anterolateral system transmits impulses at a slower rate but carries a much broader spectrum of sensory information, such as pain, warmth, cold, and crude tactile sensations.[32]

Nociceptive input is predominantly carried by the anterolateral system, which is divided into two tracts: the *neospinothalamic tract* and the *paleospinothalamic tract.* The neospinothalamic tract carries the A-delta nociceptive inputs directly to the higher centers. The paleospinothalamic tract predominantly carries the slower C-fiber nociception and travels through many other centers before reaching the brain. The significance of these two pathways with regard to "fast" and "slow" pain will be discussed in chapter 3.

Brainstem and Brain

Once the impulses have been passed to the second-order neurons, these neurons carry them to the higher centers for interpretation and evaluation. There are numerous centers in the brainstem and brain that help give meaning to the impulses. It should also be remembered that numerous interneurons may be involved in transmitting the impulses on to higher centers. In fact, attempting to follow an impulse through the brainstem on to the cortex is no simple task. To intelligently discuss pain in this text, certain functional regions of the brainstem and brain will need to be described. The reader should be reminded that the following description will merely be an overview of what are thought to be the most important functions of each area. The complexity of the organ we call the brain is beyond the scope of this text. In fact, it may be beyond the scope of the human mind itself. In a very thought-provoking statement, Thibodeau[33] wrote, "Perhaps the capacity of the human brain falls short of the ability to understand its own complexity."

The higher centers of the CNS can be subdivided into the following four regions, from the most inferior to the most superior:

1. The brainstem, which is made up of the medulla oblongata, the pons, and the midbrain (or mesencephalon)
2. The cerebellum
3. The diencephalon, which is made up of the thalamus and the hypothalamus
4. The cerebrum, which is made up of the cerebral cortex, the basal ganglia, and the limbic structures

The figures used throughout this text are graphic representations of the brain and brainstem. They are not meant to accurately depict the anatomy of each area but instead to give the reader an idea of the functional relationship so that pain processing can be better understood (Fig 2-4).

The brainstem

The brainstem is the most superior portion of the spinal cord that attaches to the brain structures. It is divided into three regions: the *medulla oblongata,* which forms the lowest part of the brainstem; the *midbrain,* which forms the uppermost part; and the *pons,* which lies between them.

The medulla oblongata

The medulla oblongata, often referred to as simply the medulla, is an enlarged extension of the spinal cord located just above the foramen magnum. It is composed of white matter, which makes up several projection tracts that route impulses directly to the higher centers (ie, the spinothalamic tract to the thalamus). The medulla also has a region made up of both white and gray matter called the *reticular formation.* Within the reticular formation are concentrations of cells, or *nuclei,* that represent "centers" for various functions. Some of the more important centers are the cardiac, respiratory, and vasomotor centers, which are often referred to as the vital centers. Some of the medullary nuclei bear individual names, such as the *nucleus gracilis,* the *nucleus cuneatus,* and the *olivary nuclei.* Within each nucleus are high concentrations of specific neurotransmitters; this will be discussed in chapter 3.

The reticular formation plays an extremely important role in monitoring the impulses that enter the brainstem. The reticular formation controls the overall activity of the brain, either by enhancing or inhibiting the impulses to the brain. As will be discussed in chapter 3, this portion of the brainstem has an extremely important impact on pain and other sensory input.

The pons

The pons is located just above the medulla and like the medulla is composed of both

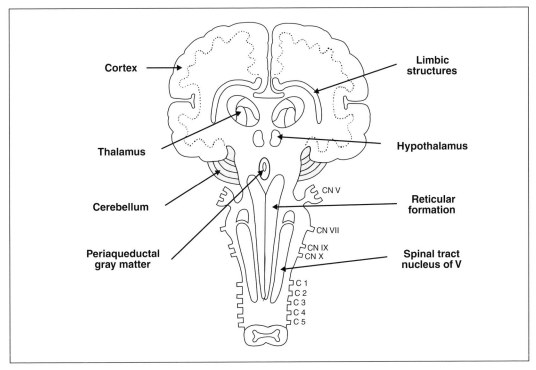

Fig 2-4 A graphic depiction of the brain and brainstem. This figure will be used throughout the text to demonstrate the neuroanatomy and neurophysiology of orofacial pain. CN = cranial nerve.

white matter and reticular formation. Fibers seem to run transversely across the pons into the cerebellum and likely act to communicate with these and other structures. The pons also has centers for reflexes that are mediated by the fifth, sixth, seventh, and eighth cranial nerves.

The midbrain

The midbrain is appropriately named, since it forms the midsection of the brain, lying above the pons and below the cerebrum. It is also referred to as the *mesencephalon.* The midbrain contains several tracts that relay impulses to the cerebrum. Two other important midbrain structures are the *red nucleus* and the *substantia nigra.* Each of these consists of clusters of cell bodies of neurons involved in muscular control.

The cerebellum

The cerebellum, the second largest part of the brain, is located just below the posterior portion of the cerebrum and is partially covered by it. The outer portion of the cerebellum is made up of gray matter, while the inner portion is predominantly white matter. The cerebellum functions to control skeletal muscles in three ways. First, it acts with the cerebral cortex to produce skilled movements by coordinating the activities of groups of muscles. It also controls skeletal muscles so as to maintain equilibrium and posture. Last, it functions below the level of consciousness to make movements smooth instead of jerky; steady instead of trembling; and coordinated instead of inefficient, awkward, and uncoordinated.

The diencephalon

The diencephalon has sometimes been referred to as the "between brain," since it links the brainstem with the cerebrum. The most important structures of the diencephalon are the *thalamus* and the *hypothalamus*. Both of these are composed of multiple nuclei that perform many different important functions. In addition to these areas of the diencephalon are two smaller nuclear areas located posterior and inferior to the thalamus: the *epithalamus* and the *subthalamus*.

The thalamus

The thalamus is located in the very center of the brain, with the cerebrum surrounding it from the top and sides and the midbrain below (see Fig 2-4). It is made up of numerous nuclei that function together to interrupt impulses. Almost all impulses from the midbrain and other lower regions of the brain, as well as those from the spinal cord, are relayed through synapses in the thalamus before proceeding to the cerebral cortex. The thalamus acts as a relay station for most of the communication between the brainstem, the cerebellum, and the cerebrum. As impulses arrive at the thalamus, the thalamus makes assessments and directs the impulses to appropriate regions in the higher centers for interpretation and response.

If one were to compare the human brain with a computer, the thalamus would represent the keyboard, which controls the functions and directs the signals. The thalamus drives the cortex to activity and enables the cortex to communicate with the other regions of the CNS. Without the thalamus, the cortex is useless.

The hypothalamus

The hypothalamus is a small structure in the middle of the base of the brain. Although it is small, its function is significant. The hypothalamus is the major center of the brain for controlling internal body functions (the supply system). There are numerous nuclei that make up the hypothalamus, with each predominantly controlling a separator function. The important ones include the *preoptic nucleus*, located anteriorly and primarily concerned with body temperature control. The *supraoptic nucleus* is located anteriorly and inferiorly and controls the secretion of antidiuretic hormone, which in turn controls the concentration of electrolytes in the body fluids. The *medial nucleus* of the hypothalamus, when stimulated, gives a person a sense of satisfaction especially associated with food. The *lateral regions* of the hypothalamus can cause a person to become very hungry, while the *anterior lateral region* will cause a person to become very thirsty. Stimulation of the *posterior hypothalamus* excites the sympathetic nervous system throughout the body, increasing the overall level of activity of many internal parts of the body, especially increasing heart rate and causing blood vessel constriction.

The hypothalamus has neurons that, when stimulated, can cause secretion of releasing hormones that are carried by the venous blood directly to the anterior pituitary gland, which in turn causes a release of some of the pituitary hormones. These pituitary hormones can cause changes in the body's metabolism of carbohydrates, proteins, and fats as well as alter other body functions. An important functional relationship exists between the hypothalamus, the pituitary gland, and the adrenal gland; this is known as the *hypothalamus-pituitary-adrenal* (HPA) axis. The HPA axis is extremely important in the body's response to environmental challenges such as stress. It is responsible for the fight-or-flight reaction and will be discussed more in later chapters.

Clearly, this small area of the brain has some powerful effects on the function of the individual. As will be discussed later, increased levels of emotional stress can stimulate the hypothalamus to up-regulate the sympathetic nervous system and greatly influence nociceptive impulses entering the brain. This simple statement should have great meaning to clinicians who manage pain.

The cerebrum

The cerebrum is the largest and uppermost division of the brain. It consists of two halves, the right and left cerebral hemispheres. Three major functional units make up the cerebrum: the *cerebral cortex,* the *basal ganglia*, and the *limbic structures*.

The cerebral cortex

The cerebral cortex represents the outer region of the cerebrum and is made up predominantly of gray matter. The cerebral cortex is the portion of the brain most frequently associated with the thinking process, even though it cannot provide thinking without the simultaneous action of deeper structures of the brain. The cerebral cortex is the portion of the brain in which essentially all memories are stored, and it is also the area most responsible for the ability to acquire muscle skills. We still do not know the basic physiologic mechanisms by which the cerebral cortex stores either memories or knowledge of muscle skills.

In most areas, the cerebral cortex is about 6 mm thick, and all together it contains an estimated 50 to 80 billion nerve cell bodies. Perhaps a billion nerve fibers lead away from the cortex, with comparable numbers leading into it, passing to other areas of the cortex, and passing to and from deeper structures of the brain, some all the way to the spinal cord.

The surface of the cerebral cortex looks like a group of small sausages, each of which is called a *convolution* or *gyrus.* In between each gyrus lies a shallow groove called a *sulci* or a deeper groove called a *fissure.* Fissures divide each cerebral hemisphere into five lobes. Four of them are named for the bones that lie over them: the *frontal lobe,* the *parietal lobe,* the *temporal lobe,* and the *occipital lobe.* A fifth lobe, the *insula* (island of Reil), lies hidden from view in the lateral fissure.

Different regions of the cerebral cortex have been identified to have different functions. There is a motor area, which is primarily involved with coordinating motor function. There is a sensory area, which receives somatosensory input for evaluation. There are also areas devoted to specific senses, such as a visual and auditory area.

Wernicke's area is a region of the cortex that is important for sensory integration. It is in this region that the meaning of the sensory input is interpreted. Wernicke's area interprets the ultimate meanings of almost all the different types of sensory information, such as the meanings of sentences and thoughts, whether they are heard, read, felt, or even generated within the brain itself. This area is well developed in only one of the cerebral hemispheres, usually in the left hemisphere. This unilateral development prevents confusion of thought processes between the two halves of the brain.

Deep within the gray matter of the cerebral cortex lie tracts made up of white matter. There are three types of tracts: *projection tracts, association tracts,* and *commissural tracts.* The projection tracts are extensions of the ascending or sensory spinothalamic tracts and descending or motor corticospinal tracts. The association tracts are the most numerous of the cerebral tracts and extend from one convolution to another in the same hemisphere. Commissural tracts extend from one convolution to a corresponding convolution in the other hemisphere. Commissural tracts compose the *corpus callosum,* by which all direct communication passes between hemispheres.

If one were to again compare the human brain with a computer, the cerebral cortex would represent the hard drive, which stores all information of memory and motor function. Once again, one should remember that the thalamus (the keyboard) is the necessary unit that calls the cortex to function.

The basal ganglia

Central to the cerebral cortex is a portion of gray matter called the *basal ganglia.* The basal ganglia are composed of several nuclei that appear to be intimately involved with coordinating cerebral activities with other brainstem functions. Some of the important nuclei are the *caudate nucleus,* the *putamen,* and the *globus pallidus.* The basal ganglia are important in controlling background gross body movements, whereas the cerebral cortex is necessary for performance of the more precise movements of arms, hands, fingers, and feet. When the hand is performing some precise activity that requires a background stance of the body, the basal ganglia provide the body movements, while the cerebral cortex provides the precise movements. The high degree of coordination among the muscles of the body that is needed for most motor functions requires a very complex circuitry of nerve fibers, not only between the cerebral cortex and the basal ganglia but also between these structures and the thalamus, cerebellum, red nucleus, and substantia nigra.

The limbic structures

The word *limbic* means border. The limbic system comprises the border structures of the cerebrum and the diencephalon. The limbic structures control emotional and behavioral activities. Within the limbic structures are centers or nuclei that are responsible for specific behaviors. There appears to be a pain/pleasure center that on an instinctive level drives the individual toward behaviors that stimulate the pleasure side of the center. These drives are not generally perceived at a conscious level but more as basic instincts. However, the instincts will bring certain behaviors to a conscious level. For example, when an individual experiences chronic pain, behavior will be oriented toward withdrawal from any stimulus that may increase the pain. Often the sufferer will withdraw from life itself, and mood alterations such as depression will

appear. The very important relationship between the limbic system and pain will be discussed in later chapters.

The limbic system is divided into the following functional structures, which will be discussed in this section: the *amygdala,* the *hippocampus,* the *mammillary bodies,* the *septum pellucidum,* the *cingulate gyrus,* the *cingulum,* the *insula,* and the *parahippocampal gyrus.* It should also be noted that many of the limbic structures function in close coordination with the hypothalamus. Some researchers consider the hypothalamus a limbic structure.

The *amygdala* is a small nuclear structure located deep inside each anterior temporal lobe of the cerebrum. It is believed that this structure functions with the hypothalamus to control the appropriate behavior of the person for each type of social situation.

The *hippocampus* is a primitive portion of the cerebral cortex that lies along the medialmost border of the temporal lobe. It is believed to interpret for the brain the importance of most of our sensory experiences. If the hippocampus determines that an experience is important enough, then the experience will be stored as a memory in the cerebral cortex. Without the hippocampus, a person's ability to store memories becomes very deficient.

The *mammillary bodies* lie immediately behind the hypothalamus and function in close association with the thalamus, hypothalamus, and brainstem to help control many behavioral functions, such as the degree of wakefulness and perhaps also feelings of well-being.

The *septum pellucidum* is located anterior to the thalamus, superior to the hypothalamus, and between the basal ganglia. Stimulation of this region can cause many different behavioral effects, such as anger and rage.

The *cingulate gyrus,* the *cingulum,* the *insula,* and the *parahippocampal gyrus* form a ring in each hemisphere of the cerebrum around the deeper structures of the limbic system. It is believed that these structures

Fig 2-5 The pathway of cerebrospinal fluid flow, from the choroid plexuses in the lateral ventricles to the arachnoidal villi that protrude into the dural sinuses. Note the lateral, third, and fourth ventricles. (From Guyton AC. Textbook of Medical Physiology, ed 8. Philadelphia: Saunders, 1991:681. Used with permission.)

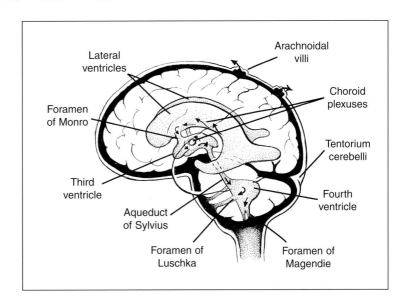

interact and develop associations between the limbic functions and the cerebral functions. This interaction coordinates the conscious cerebral behavioral functions with the subconscious behavioral functions of the deeper limbic system.

Impulses from the limbic system leading into the hypothalamus can modify any or all of the many internal bodily functions controlled by the hypothalamus. Impulses from the limbic system feeding into the midbrain and medulla can control such behavior as wakefulness, sleep, excitement, attentiveness, and even rage or docility. With this basic understanding of limbic function one can quickly understand the impact it can have on the overall function of the individual. The limbic system certainly plays a major role in chronic pain problems as will be discussed in later chapters.

Other important brainstem structures

This brief summary of brain and brainstem structures is by no means complete. It is presented so that future discussions regarding pain can have meaning. There are several other structures within the brainstem

that should be mentioned before this section is completed. These structures are the *ventricles,* the *periaqueductal gray area,* and the *nucleus raphes magnus.*

The ventricles

The entire brain, brainstem, and spinal cord are surrounded by cerebrospinal fluid, which is encapsulated by the meninges. This fluid acts as a cushion during trauma and also serves as a transport medium for neurotransmitters and other chemicals such as carbon dioxide. Carbon dioxide levels in the cerebrospinal fluid affect neurons of the respiratory center in the medulla and thereby help control respiration.

The cerebrospinal fluid is confined to certain spaces within the brain and brainstem. There are four of these spaces, which are called the *ventricles* (Fig 2-5). Two of the ventricles are called the *lateral ventricles;* one is located in each cerebral hemisphere. The third ventricle is little more than a lengthwise slit between the right and left thalamus. The fourth ventricle is a diamond-shaped space located between the cerebellum posteriorly and the medulla and pons anteriorly.

Formation of the cerebrospinal fluid occurs mainly by filtration from blood in the choroid plexuses. The choroid plexuses are networks of capillaries that project from the inner lining of the meninges (the pia mater) into the lateral ventricles and into the roofs of the third and fourth ventricles. The cerebrospinal fluid then passes from the third ventricle to the fourth by way of a narrow channel called the *aqueduct of Sylvius*.

The periaqueductal gray area

The *periaqueductal gray area* is a region of the mesencephalon and upper pons surrounding the aqueduct of Sylvius. This region of the brainstem has a high concentration of neurons that are capable of producing power neurotransmitters that can greatly modulate nociceptive impulses. The significance of this region will be discussed in chapter 4.

The nucleus raphes magnus

The *nucleus raphes magnus* is a midline nucleus located in the lower pons and upper medulla. Like the periaqueductal gray area, it functions to modulate nociceptive input ascending on to the thalamus. The importance of this nucleus will be discussed in chapter 4.

The Trigeminal System

The neural pathways that have been described so far are the common pathways that transmit somatic impulses into the spinal cord and on to the brain. Somatic input from the face and oral structures does not enter the spinal cord by way of spinal nerves (Fig 2-6). Instead, sensory input from the face and mouth is carried by way of the fifth cranial nerve, the trigeminal nerve. The cell bodies of the trigeminal afferent neurons are located in the large gasserian ganglion. The sensory distribution of this nerve will be discussed later in this chapter. Impulses carried by the trigeminal nerve enter directly into the brainstem in the region of the pons to synapse in the trigeminal spinal tract nucleus (Fig 2-7). This region of the brainstem is structurally very similar to the dorsal horn of the spinal cord. In fact, it may be considered an extension of the dorsal horn and is sometimes referred to as the medullary dorsal horn.

The brainstem trigeminal nucleus complex consists of the main sensory trigeminal nucleus, which is rostrally located and receives periodontal and some pulpal afferents, and the spinal tract of the trigeminal nucleus, which is more caudally located. The spinal tract is divided into three parts: *(1)* the subnucleus oralis, *(2)* the subnucleus interpolaris, and *(3)* the subnucleus caudalis, which corresponds to the medullary dorsal horn. Tooth pulp afferents go to all three subnuclei.[34] The subnucleus caudalis has especially been implicated in trigeminal nociceptive mechanisms on the basis of electrophysiologic observations of nociceptive neurons.[25,31,35] The subnucleus oralis appears to be a significant area of this trigeminal brainstem complex with regard to oral pain mechanisms.[35–37]

There is sufficient evidence that facial nociceptive afferents project to the subnucleus caudalis of the trigeminal spinal tract nucleus.[38] The current evidence supports the concept that the subnucleus caudalis is homologous to the substantia gelatinosa of the spinal dorsal horn.[39] Therefore, information concerning the dorsal horn structure can be safely extrapolated and applied to the subnucleus caudalis. The marginal rim of the nucleus corresponds to lamina I of the dorsal horn. The structure of laminae II and III, comprising the substantia gelatinosa of the dorsal horn, should represent the cellular arrangement that is present in the subnucleus caudalis. Although it is usually presumed that the subnucleus

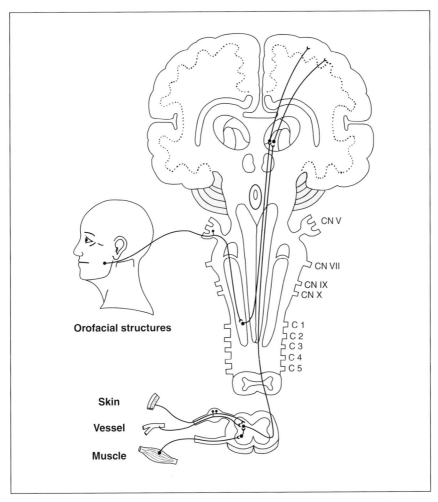

Fig 2-6 The relationship of the trigeminal nerve input and the spinal nerve input as impulses ascend to the higher centers.

caudalis predominates in trigeminal nociception, there is no doubt that the more rostrally located nuclei also play important roles in nociception.

Another component of the trigeminal brainstem complex is the motor nucleus of the trigeminal nerve. This area of the complex is involved with interpretation of impulses that demand motor responses. Motor reflex activities of the face are initiated from this area in a manner similar to the spinal reflex activities in the rest of the body.[40]

Second-order trigeminal neurons project to the thalamus from synaptic junctions with primary afferents in the subnucleus caudalis. As in the dorsal horn, these interneurons represent three types of transmission cells:

1. WDR neurons that respond to input from tactile and nociceptive fibers are ac-

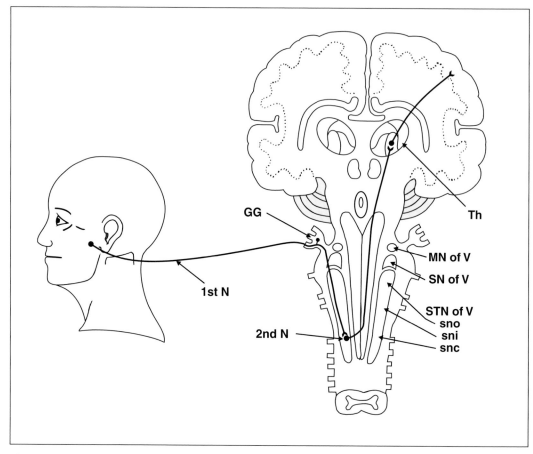

Fig 2-7 A graphic depiction of the trigeminal nerve entering the brainstem at the level of the pons. The primary afferent neuron (1st N) enters the brainstem to synapse with a second-order neuron (2nd N) in the trigeminal spinal tract nucleus (STN of V). The spinal tract nucleus is divided into three regions: the subnucleus oralis (sno), the subnucleus interpolaris (sni), and the subnucleus caudalis (snc). The trigeminal brainstem complex is also composed of the motor nucleus of V (MN of V) and the main sensory nucleus of V (SN of V). The cell bodies of the trigeminal nerve are located in the gasserian ganglion (GG). Once the second-order neuron receives the input it is carried on to the thalamus (Th) for interpretation.

tivated by weak and strong stimuli from both nociceptive and myelinated LTM afferents.

2. NS neurons that respond exclusively to input from thin nociceptive fibers are activated by intense noxious mechanical and thermal stimuli. The WDR and NS neurons predominate in laminae I, II V, and VI and compose the trigeminal noci-

ceptive pathways. They all receive input from cutaneous structures, and at least half of them receive input from deep structures of the mouth and face as well.

3. LTM neurons are normally nonnociceptive and respond to light tactile stimuli. They predominate in laminae III and IV but have been found in all the subdivisions of the trigeminal brainstem com-

plex and have especially been implicated in the relay of touch from the face and mouth. The LTM neurons appear to be excited by strong electrical stimulation of tooth pulps and may be involved in some painful pathological situations.[37]

Dubner[24] showed that pain is signaled by specialized central pathways that are exquisitely sensitive to stimulus features. He concluded that the idea that nociceptive pathways merely provide information about the threat of tissue damage should be discarded.

It is interesting to note that the trigeminal spinal tract nucleus also receives input from nerves other than the trigeminal. Cranial nerves IX and X as well as the upper cervical nerves supply input to the tract (see Fig 2-6). The importance of these multiple innervations will be discussed in chapter 4.

The Autonomic Nervous System

The visceral nervous system is composed of two divisions: the craniosacral portion, known as the *parasympathetics,* and the thoracolumbar portion, known as the *sympathetics.* The afferent elements of these nerves receive interoceptive stimuli that normally do not reach the level of consciousness. Under unusual or abnormal conditions, however, such stimuli may be perceived as pain. The efferent elements of these nerves constitute the *autonomic nervous system* (ANS), the activities of which are relatively independent of volition. The craniosacral visceral efferents constitute the parasympathetic autonomics, and the thoracolumbar visceral efferents constitute the sympathetic autonomics.

The ANS controls various internal functions that are vital to the individual. It helps control arterial blood pressure, gastrointestinal motility and secretion, urinary bladder emptying, sweating, body temperature, and many other activities that are controlled in conjunction with other systems. Most of the functions occur continuously and below the conscious level. When stimulated, the ANS can respond quickly to change body functions. For example, the heart rate can be doubled in 3 to 5 seconds and arterial pressure can be doubled in 10 to 15 seconds. On the other extreme, the blood pressure can be lowered enough to cause fainting in 4 to 5 seconds. Sweating can begin within seconds, and the bladder may empty involuntarily, also within seconds. It is these characteristics that allow the body to respond appropriately to environmental challenge.

Since this text is directed toward orofacial pains, only a brief description of the ANS will be presented. It is important, however, that the clinician have a basic understanding of this system, since some pain conditions are influenced and may even be maintained by the activity of the ANS (see chapter 17). Other texts should be consulted for a more thorough review of the ANS.

The ANS is activated mainly by centers located in the spinal cord, the brainstem, and the hypothalamus. Portions of the cortex and limbic system can also influence ANS activity. The efferent impulses are transmitted to various organs by two major subdivisions: the *sympathetic nervous system* and the *parasympathetic nervous system.*

The Sympathetic Nervous System

The sympathetic nerves originate in the spinal cord between segments T-1 and L-2 and pass first into the sympathetic chain and from there to the tissues and organs that are stimulated by the sympathetic

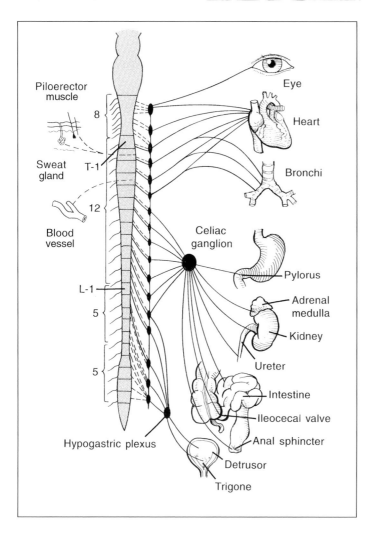

Fig 2-8 The sympathetic nervous system. Dashed lines represent postganglionic fibers in the gray rami leading into the spinal nerves for distribution to blood vessels, sweat glands, and piloerector muscles. (From Guyton AC. Textbook of Medical Physiology, ed 8. Philadelphia: Saunders, 1991:668. Used with permission.)

nerves (Fig 2-8). The *sympathetic chain* is a chain of ganglia that lies to each side of the spinal column. Each sympathetic pathway, therefore, is composed of two neurons: a preganglionic neuron and a postganglionic neuron. The cell body of each preganglionic neuron lies in the intermediolateral horn of the spinal cord, and its fiber passes through an anterior root of the cord into the corresponding spinal nerve. Immediately after the spinal nerve leaves the spinal column, the preganglionic sympathetic fiber leaves the nerve and passes through the white ramus into one of the ganglia of the sym-

pathetic chain. Once it reaches the ganglia, it may immediately synapse with a postganglionic neuron or it may travel up or down the sympathetic chain to synapse with another postganglionic neuron. The postganglionic neuron then transmits the impulse to the target organ.

Some of the postganglionic neurons pass back from the sympathetic chain into the spinal nerves through gray rami at all levels of the cord. These pathways are made up of C fibers that extend to all parts of the body in the skeletal nerves. They control the blood vessels, sweat glands, and pilo-

Fig 2-9 The parasympathetic nervous system. (From Guyton AC. Textbook of Medical Physiology, ed 8. Philadelphia: Saunders, 1991:669. Used with permission.)

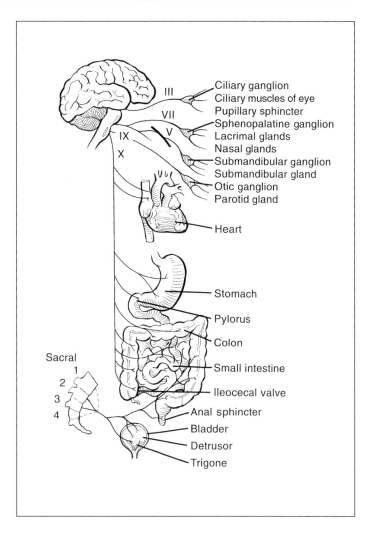

erector muscles of the hairs. Approximately 8% of the fibers in the average skeletal nerve are sympathetic fibers. This is a significant finding when considering muscle pain (see chapter 12).

It is worthwhile to note that some preganglionic sympathetic neurons pass without synapsing all the way from the intermediolateral horn cells of the spinal cord, through the sympathetic chain, through the splanchnic nerve, and finally into the adrenal medullae. There they end directly on modified neuronal cells that secrete epinephrine and norepinephrine into the bloodstream. The importance of these neurochemicals will be discussed in chapter 3.

The Parasympathetic Nervous System

The parasympathetic nervous system consists of fibers that leave the CNS through cranial nerves III, VII, IX, and X as well as through the second and third sacral spinal nerves and occasionally the first and fourth sacral nerves (Fig 2-9). About 75% of all parasympathetic nerve fibers are in the vagus nerves and pass to the entire thoracic and abdominal regions of the body. In the orofacial region, the parasympathetic nerve fibers travel with the third cranial nerve to the pupillary sphincters and ciliary muscles of the eye. Fibers from the seventh cranial nerve pass to the lacrimal, nasal, and sub-mandibular glands, and fibers from the ninth cranial nerve pass to the parotid gland.

Like the sympathetic nervous system, the parasympathetic system also has pre- and postganglionic neurons. The difference, however, lies in the location of the synapse. In the parasympathetic nervous system, the preganglionic fiber passes uninterrupted all the way to the organ that is to be con-trolled. The postganglionic neurons are located in the wall of the organ. The pre-ganglionic fibers synapse with these neu-rons, and short postganglionic fibers, 1 mm to several centimeters in length, leave and spread through the substance of the organ.

Functions of the ANS

As already mentioned, the ANS exists to maintain visceral activities of the body. These activities are constantly monitored and, when indicated, altered to maintain proper function of the body. To maintain this constant influence, both the sympa-thetic and parasympathetic systems remain constantly active at a low level. This base level of activity is called *sympathetic tone* or *parasympathetic tone*. The value of tone is that it allows a single nervous system to in-crease or decrease the activity of a stimu-lated organ. For example, sympathetic tone normally keeps almost all of the systemic arterioles constricted to approximately half their maximum diameter. If the degree of sympathetic stimulation is increased, these vessels can be constricted even more. On the other hand, when the normal tone is in-hibited, these same vessels can be dilated. If

not for this continual sympathetic tone, the sympathetic system could cause only vaso-constriction, never vasodilatation.

The sympathetic nervous system plays a very important role in immediately prepar-ing the individual for environmental chal-lenges. This is commonly called the *fight-or-flight reaction*. When the individual is physically or emotionally threatened a mass discharge of the sympathetic nervous sys-tem can occur. The result of this discharge permits the person to perform far more strenuous physical activity than would oth-erwise be possible. This sympathetic mass discharge is characterized by the following changes[41]:

1. Increased arterial pressure
2. Increased blood flow to muscles and away from other organs
3. Increased rates of cellular metabolism throughout the body
4. Increased blood glucose concentration
5. Increased glycolysis in the liver and in muscles
6. Increased muscle strength
7. Increased mental activity
8. Increased rate of blood coagulation

The importance of this response, especially in its relationship to pain, will be discussed in later chapters.

Peripheral Nociceptive Pathways

It is important for the clinician to have a sound understanding of the pathways by which nociception can arise. It is the basis for understanding somatic pain. Each of the nerves that innervate the face and oral structures will be reviewed in this section.

First, afferent or sensory pathways will be discussed (Fig 2-10). Next, the efferent or motor pathways will be reviewed (Fig 2-11). Last, the visceral pathways will be described (Fig 2-12).

Afferent (Sensory) Somatic Nerves

The trigeminal nerve

The chief mediator of somatic sensation from the mouth and face is the fifth cranial nerve, which innervates the face superficially in the region forward of a line drawn vertically from the ears across the top of the head and superior to the level of the lower border of the mandible (Fig 2-10). The ophthalmic division supplies the parietal and frontal areas as well as the upper eyelid and nasal bridge down to the tip of the nose. The maxillary division supplies the anterior portion of the temple, the malar, and the maxillary areas, including the lower eyelid, the ala of the nose, and the upper lip. The mandibular division supplies the posterior temple, the tragus, the preauricular area, the masseter area, and the mandibular region down to the lower border of the mandible, excluding the mandibular angle area. This includes the lower lip and a portion of the auricle and external auditory canal.

The deeper structures of the orofacial region are innervated by branches of the same cranial nerve. The ophthalmic division supplies the orbit and the upper part of the nasal cavity. The maxillary division supplies a major portion of the nasal cavity; the palate; the maxillary antrum; the maxillary alveolar process along with the teeth, periodontium, and overlying gingiva; and a small portion of the buccal mucosa in the posterior oral vestibule. The mandibular division supplies sensory innervation to the anterior two thirds of the tongue; the mandible along with the teeth, periodontium,

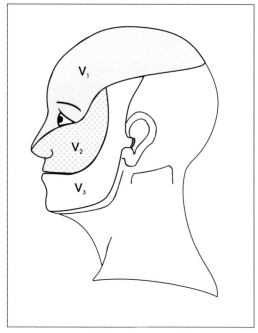

Fig 2-10 Diagrammatic representation of the superficial sensory distribution of the trigeminal nerve: the ophthalmic division (V_1), the maxillary division (V_2), and the mandibular division (V_3).

and overlying gingiva; the mucosa of the floor of the mouth; and most of the oral vestibule. This division also contains proprioceptive sensory fibers that serve the deep sensibility of the mandibular muscles (masseter, temporalis, medial pterygoid, lateral pterygoid, mylohyoid, anterior digastric) as well as the tensor muscles of the soft palate and the tympanic membrane. A branch of the mandibular division of the fifth cranial nerve, the auriculotemporal nerve, innervates the temporomandibular joint.

Each of the three divisions gives off sensory branches that pass intracranially to supply structures above the tentorium cerebelli.

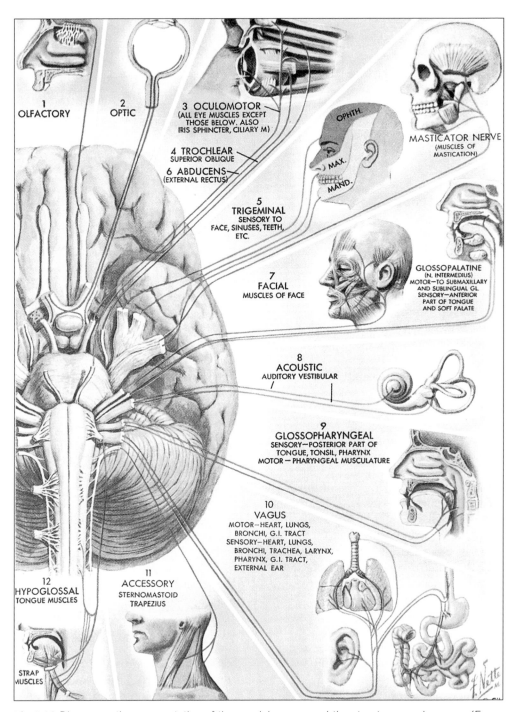

Fig 2-11 Diagrammatic representation of the cranial nerves and the structures each serves. (From Netter FH. The CIBA Collection of Medical Illustrations. Indianapolis: Curtis, 1953. Used with permission.)

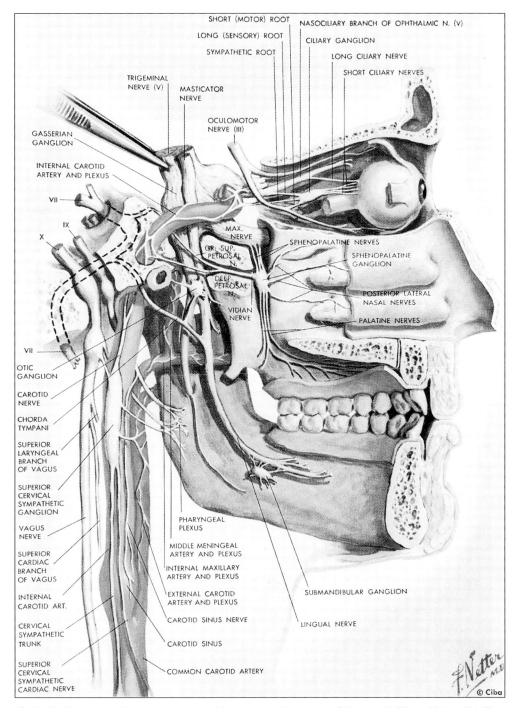

Fig 2-12 Diagrammatic representation of the autonomic nerves of the head. (From Netter FH. The CIBA Collection of Medical Illustrations. Indianapolis: Curtis, 1953. Used with permission.)

The facial nerve

The nervus intermedius contains proprioceptive sensory fibers that serve the deep sensibility of the face, except for the muscles innervated by the 5th cranial nerve and the 12th cranial nerve. These fibers also serve the deep sensibility of the platysma, stylohyoid, and posterior digastric muscles, which are innervated by the seventh nerve. According to Coffey and Rhoton[42] and Finneson,[43] this nerve contains sensory fibers that supply superficial sensation to the tympanic membrane and part of the external auditory canal.

The facial nerve contains taste fibers to the anterior two thirds of the tongue. These fibers form part of the chorda tympani nerve, which is carried in the terminal areas within the sheath of the lingual branch of the trigeminal nerve.

The glossopharyngeal nerve

Sensory fibers of the ninth cranial nerve innervate the base of the tongue, the pharynx, and most of the ear and tympanic membrane. There is considerable overlapping of trigeminal and glossopharyngeal terminal afferent fibers in the throat area, so that pain arising from the deeper recesses of the oral cavity may be mediated by either or both nerve trunks. This nerve also contains the taste fibers to the posterior third of the tongue. Some intracranial fibers of this nerve mediate sensation below the level of the tentorium cerebelli.

The glossopharyngeal nerve contains proprioceptive sensory fibers that serve the deep sensibility of the pharyngeal area.

The vagus nerve

Sensory fibers of the 10th cranial nerve innervate the lower part of the pharynx, the larynx, the posterior part of the external auditory canal, and the skin immediately behind the auricle. The vagus nerve also contains taste fibers to the region of the epiglottis.

The cervical spinal nerves

The upper three cervical spinal nerves mediate sensory impulses from the superficial structures of the head and face posterior to the trigeminal area and below the lower border of the mandible, including the mandibular angle. This includes most of the auricle as well as the postauricular region, except for the skin immediately posterior to the auricle, which is supplied by the vagus nerve. In about 8% of subjects, the sensory root of the first cervical nerve is missing.

The upper cervical spinal nerves contain proprioceptive sensory fibers that serve the deep sensibility of the cervical areas, except for those muscles innervated by other nerves (mylohyoid and anterior digastric by the 5th cranial nerve; platysma, stylohyoid, and posterior digastric by the 7th cranial nerve; tongue muscles by the 12th cranial nerve). Although parts of the sternocleidomastoid and trapezius muscles are innervated by the 11th cranial nerve, these fibers in fact arise from the upper cervical segments. These muscles may be considered to be innervated by cervical spinal nerves.

Efferent (Motor) Somatic Nerves

The oculomotor, trochlear, and abducent nerves

The third, fourth, and sixth cranial nerves contain somatic motor fibers to the ocular muscles and the levator muscle of the upper eyelid.

The trigeminal nerve

The fifth cranial nerve contains somatic motor fibers that innervate the masseter, temporalis, medial pterygoid, lateral pterygoid, mylohyoid, and anterior digastric muscles and the tensor muscles of the soft palate and tympanic membrane. All these motor fibers are part of the mandibular division of this nerve.

The facial nerve

The seventh cranial nerve contains somatic motor fibers that innervate the muscles of facial expression, including the occipitofrontal scalp muscles, the muscles of the auricle, and the platysma. They also supply the stapedius, stylohyoid, and posterior digastric muscles.

The glossopharyngeal nerve

The ninth cranial nerve contains somatic motor fibers that innervate the stylopharyngeal muscle, and, along with the vagus, it supplies the constrictor muscles of the pharynx and palatopharyngeal muscle.

The vagus nerve

The 10th cranial nerve contains somatic motor fibers that innervate the musculature of the pharynx and larynx.

The accessory nerve

The 11th cranial nerve contains somatic motor fibers of both cranial and cervical origin. Those of cranial origin innervate muscles of the larynx and pharynx as branches of the vagus nerve. Those of cervical origin arise from several of the upper cervical segments and innervate parts of the sternocleidomastoid and trapezius muscles.

The hypoglossal nerve

The 12th cranial nerve contains somatic motor fibers that innervate the intrinsic and extrinsic muscles of the tongue. This nerve also contains motor fibers of cervical origin that innervate some of the hyoid muscles, including the geniohyoid muscle.

The cervical spinal nerves

The upper cervical spinal nerves contain somatic motor fibers that supply the cervical and hyoid muscles directly as well as indirectly via the 11th and 12th cranial nerves, as noted earlier. It should be remembered that the mylohyoid and anterior digastric muscles are innervated by the fifth cranial nerve, and the platysma, posterior digastric, and stylohyoid muscles are innervated by the seventh cranial nerve.

Visceral (Autonomic) Nerves

Sympathetic nerves

The sympathetic afferents
The oral and facial structures are supplied with sympathetic visceral afferents[44-46] that are carried within the sheaths of the fifth, seventh, and ninth cranial nerves. All the sympathetic fibers leave these vehicular nerve trunks and pass to the cervical sympathetic chain, where they enter the CNS through the sensory roots of the upper thoracic spinal nerves.

The sympathetic efferents
The dilator of the pupil, the tarsal and orbital muscles, and the salivary glands, as well as the blood vessels and skin, receive sympathetic autonomic efferents. All sympathetic efferents to the head are postgan-

glionic. The preganglionic fibers are contained within the upper thoracic spinal nerves, from which they take leave to join the sympathetic chain at about the level of the stellate ganglion and synapse with the cranial postganglionic fibers in the superior cervical ganglion. These fibers follow the external and internal carotid arteries. Those that follow the internal carotid artery form the internal carotid nerve, which becomes a loose plexus from which fibers join several cranial nerves for terminal distribution to the pupil and orbital muscles as well as to the glands of the nasal cavity, palate, and pharynx. The fibers that follow the external carotid artery supply the smooth muscle of blood vessels and skin as well as the cutaneous glands and large salivary glands.

Parasympathetic nerves

The parasympathetic afferents
The oral and facial structures are supplied with parasympathetic visceral afferents that are carried within the trigeminal sheath but exit by way of the sensory roots of the seventh and ninth cranial nerves, rather than the fifth. The fibers from the lacrimal, submandibular, and sublingual glands leave the fifth nerve and join with the seventh, whereas those from the parotid gland leave the fifth and join with the ninth.

The parasympathetic efferents
The sphincter of the pupil, the ciliary muscle of accommodation, the lacrimal gland, and all the salivary glands receive parasympathetic autonomic efferent fibers that are incorporated in the oculomotor, facial, and glossopharyngeal nerves. The preganglionic fibers in the oculomotor nerve leave it to synapse with postganglionic fibers in the ciliary ganglion and henceforth are contained within the trigeminal sheath to supply the sphincter of the pupil and the ciliary muscle. The preganglionic fibers in the facial nerve leave it to synapse with postganglionic fibers in the pterygopalatine and submandibular ganglia and henceforth are contained within the trigeminal sheath. Those from the pterygopalatine ganglion supply the lacrimal gland, and those from the submandibular ganglion supply the submandibular and sublingual glands. The preganglionic fibers in the glossopharyngeal nerve leave it to synapse with postganglionic fibers in the otic ganglion and henceforth are contained within the trigeminal sheath to supply the parotid gland. None of the parasympathetic efferents of the vagus nerve supply structures in the masticatory area.

General Considerations of Peripheral Nociceptive Pathways

An understanding of the functional neuroanatomy involved in the sensory and motor innervation of structures of the mouth and face is essential for the effective management of nociceptive activity in this region. A somewhat wider area than just the face, however, is implicated in masticatory function.

Pains arising from peripheral sources are mediated by anatomic structures of the nervous system, namely, sensory receptors and primary sensory neurons. These structures constitute the peripheral pain pathways. In light of the currently held concepts regarding the mechanisms of pain, the clinician should be well informed concerning all the sensory pathways that exist. The brain is constantly receiving an enormous amount of sensory input initiated by stimulation of sensory receptors of all types: exteroceptive, proprioceptive, and interoceptive. Of this volume, only a fraction is ordinarily perceived at conscious levels. Most of this ongoing sensory input is for regulatory purposes to control automatic body functioning. Formerly, the significance of such sensation in pain processes appears not to have been fully appreciated. It is important to be aware of the various routes by which such sensation is conducted. This includes both the somatic and the visceral pathways that have just been reviewed.

Dental practitioners traditionally have received excellent instruction concerning the trigeminal pathways, which are of great significance in orofacial pain complaints. Unfortunately, the impression is sometimes gained that the trigeminal pathways are exclusively responsible for the mediation of painful sensation from this region. This impression is a fundamental error and may account for some of the confusion that exists in the clinical management of pain complaints. For example, it is a common notion that surgical interruption of the posterior root of the trigeminal nerve will assuredly arrest oral and facial pain, and great consternation may follow the failure of such an operation to be effective.

It should be noted that the oral and masticatory region is innervated by at least six major sensory somatic nerve trunks other than the trigeminal: the 7th, 9th, and 10th cranial nerves and the 1st, 2nd, and 3rd cervical spinal nerves. It should also be well understood that the visceral nerves actively participate in the mediation of painful sensations. It has been established that all sympathetic afferents and at least the sacral parasympathetic afferents mediate pain at conscious levels.[47] Hannington-Kiff[48] believed strongly that cranial parasympathetic afferent fibers mediate pain, especially that of neurovascular disorders. An understanding of the anatomy of these pathways is important in the management of orofacial pains. Vast numbers of impulses are conducted to the CNS by afferent visceral nerves. Such ongoing sensory input is normally below conscious levels.

It should be noted that all cranial parasympathetics, although carried in the sheaths of trigeminal branches for peripheral distribution, leave the trigeminal before entering the CNS, and none of them passes through the posterior root of the fifth cranial nerve. The parasympathetic afferents in the trigeminal region enter the CNS by way of the seventh and ninth cranial nerves. It should also be noted that all sympathetic afferents of the head regions, although carried in the sheaths of various cranial nerves including the trigeminal for peripheral distribution, leave these cranial nerves and join the cervical portion of the sympathetic chain and finally enter the spinal cord by way of the posterior roots of the upper thoracic spinal nerves.

It has long been known that the afferent as well as the efferent limb of the myotatic reflex is mediated by motor nerves.[49] Since there is ample evidence of the presence of many afferent fibers in the trigeminal motor root, the motor nerves should be included among nociceptive pathways. It is quite certain that motor nerves mediate normal sensory impulses from the skeletal musculature. This phenomenon may explain why noxious stimulation of motor trunks elicits deep somatic pain felt diffusely in the muscles innervated by those nerves.[50]

It should be evident that painful sensations from the mouth and face can be mediated by many pathways other than the familiar trigeminal route. For this reason, pain from the facial region may not necessarily be arrested by division of the trigeminal sensory root. Such an operation would not affect the mediation of nociceptive sensation conducted by afferents of the 7th, 9th, and 10th cranial nerves or the 1st, 2nd, and 3rd cervical nerves; afferent neurons carried by motor elements of the trigeminal as well as other cranial and upper cervical nerves; and afferent visceral nerves of the sympathetic and parasympathetic systems.

With this review it becomes obvious that the peripheral nociceptive input from the orofacial structures follows no simple pathway. This complexity certainly adds to the challenge of the clinician attempting to manage an orofacial pain disorder.

References

1. Kramer H, Schmidt W. Regional anesthesia of the maxillofacial region. In: Alling CC, Mahan P (eds). Facial Pain, ed 2. Philadelphia: Lea & Febiger, 1977:237–256.

2. Kerr F. Fine structure and functional characteristics of the primary trigeminal neuron. In: Hassler R, Walker A (eds). Trigeminal Neuralgia. Stuttgart: Thieme, 1970:11–21.

3. Gardner W. Trigeminal neuralgia. In: Hassler R, Walker A (eds). Trigeminal Neuralgia. Stuttgart: Thieme, 1970:153–174.

4. Guyton AC, Hall JE. Organization of the nervous system. In: Textbook of Medical Physiology, ed 10. Philadelphia: Saunders, 2000:512–527.

5. Van Hees J, Gybels J. C nociceptor activity in human nerve during painful and non-painful skin stimulation. J Neurol Neurosurg Psychiatry 1981;44:600–607.

6. Schmidt R, Schmelz M, Ringkamp M, Handwerker HO, Torebjork HE. Innervation territories of mechanically activated C nociceptor units in human skin. J Neurophysiol 1997;78:2641–2648.

7. Davis KD, Meyer RA, Turnquist JL, Filloon TG, Pappagallo M, Campbell JN. Cutaneous pretreatment with the capsaicin analog NE-21610 prevents the pain to a burn and subsequent hyperalgesia. Pain 1995;62:373–378.

8. Bahns E, Ernsberger U, Janig W, Nelke A. Discharge properties of mechanosensitive afferents supplying the retroperitoneal space. Pflugers Arch 1986;407:519–525.

9. Bove GM, Light AR. Unmyelinated nociceptors of rat paraspinal tissues. J Neurophysiol 1995;73:1752–1762.

10. Okeson JP. Functional neuroanatomy and physiology of the masticatory system. In: Management of Temporomandibular Disorders and Occlusion, ed 5. St Louis: Mosby, 2003:29–66.

11. Widmer C. Jaw-opening reflex activity in the inferior head of the lateral pterygoid muscle in man. Arch Oral Biol 1987;32:135–142.

12. Bechtol C. Muscle Physiology. The American Academy of Orthopedic Surgical Instructional Course Lectures. St Louis: Mosby, 1948.

13. Fields H. Pain. New York: McGraw-Hill, 1987:41–78.

14. Miller M. Pain: Morphologic aspects. In: Way E (ed). New Concepts in Pain. Philadelphia: Davis, 1967:7–12.

15. Clark D, Hughes JR, Gasser H. Afferent function in the group of nerves of slowest conduction velocity. Am J Physiol Renal Physiol 1935;114:69.

16. Gasser H, Erlanger J. The role played by sizes of constituent fibers of a nerve trunk in determining the form of its action potential wave. Am J Physiol Renal Physiol 1927;80:522.

17. Gasser H. Conduction in nerves and relation to fiber types. Assoc Res Nerv Dis Proc 1934;15:35.

18. Guyton AC, Hall JE. Sensory receptors. In: Textbook of Medical Physiology, ed 10. Philadelphia: Saunders, 2000:528–539.

19. Hallin R, Wiesenfeld Z, Persson A. Do large-diameter cutaneous afferents have a role in the transmission of nociceptive information? Pain 1981;11(suppl 1):90.

20. Bishop G. Neural mechanism of cutaneous nerves. Physiol Rev 1946;26.

21. Bishop G. The relationship between nerve fiber size and sensory modality: Phylogenetic implications of the afferent innervation of cortex. J Nerv Ment Dis 1959;128:89.

22. Bishop G. Fiber size and myelinization in afferent systems. In: Knighton R, Dumke P (eds). Pain. Boston: Little, Brown, 1966:83–89.

23. Sessle B. The neurobiology of facial and dental pain: Present knowledge, future directions. J Dent Res 1987;66:962–981.

24. Dubner R. Specialization of nociceptive pathways: Sensory discrimination, sensory modulation, and neural connectivity. In: Fields HL, Dubner R, Cervero F (eds). Proceedings of the Fourth World Congress on Pain: Seattle, vol 9, Advances in Pain Research and Therapy. New York: Raven Press, 1985:111–137.

25. Sessle BJ, Hu JW. Mechanisms of pain arising from articular tissues. Can J Physiol Pharmacol 1991;69:617–626.

26. Hiltunen K, Schmidt-Kaunisaho K, Nevalainen J, Narhi T, Ainamo A. Prevalence of signs of temporomandibular disorders among elderly inhabitants of Helsinki, Finland. Acta Odontol Scand 1995 Feb;53:20–23.

27. Rexed B. The cytoarchitectonic organization of the spinal cord in the cat. J Comp Neurol 1954:100–297.

28. Gobel S. Neural circuitry in the substantia gelatinosa of Rolands: Anatomical insight. In: Bonica JJ, Liebeskind JC, Albe-Fessard DG (eds). Proceedings of the Second World Congress on Pain, vol 3, Advances in Pain Research and Therapy. New York: Raven Press, 1979:175–195.

29. Kerr F. Neuroanatomical substrates of nociception in the spinal cord. Pain 1975;1:325–326.

30. Dubner R, Bennett GJ. Spinal and trigeminal mechanisms of nociception. Ann Rev Neurosci 1983;6:381–418.

31. Doubell T, Mannion R, Woolf C. The dorsal horn: State-dependent sensory processing, plasticity and the generation of pain. In: Wall P, Melzack R (eds). Textbook of Pain. London: Churchill-Livingstone, 2002:165–181.

32. Guyton AC, Hall JE. Somatic sensations. In: Textbook of Medical Physiology. Philadelphia: Saunders, 2000:540–551.

33. Thibodeau G. Anatomy and Physiology. St Louis: Times Mirror/Mosby College, 1987:327.

34. De Laat A. Reflexes excitable in the jaw muscles and their role during jaw function and dysfunction: A review of the literature. Part II. Central connections of orofacial afferent fibers. Cranio 1987;5:246–253.

35. Dubner R, Sessle B, Storey A. The Neural Basis of Oral and Facial Function. New York: Plenum Press, 1978.

36. Hu JW, Dostrovsky JO, Sessle BJ. Functional properties of neurons in cat trigeminal subnucleus caudalis (medullary dorsal horn). I. Responses to oral-facial noxious and nonnoxious stimuli and projections to thalamus and subnucleus oralis. J Neurophysiol 1981;45:173–192.

37. Sessle BJ. The neurobiology of facial and dental pain: Present knowledge, future directions. J Dent Res 1987;66:962-981.

38. Henry JL, Sessle BJ, Lucier GE, Hu JW. Effects of substance P on nociceptive and nonnociceptive trigeminal brain stem neurons. Pain 1980; 8:33–45.

39. Shigenaga Y, Nakatani J. Distribution of trigeminothalamic projection cells in the caudal medulla of the cat. In: Matthew B, Hill R (eds). Anatomical, Physiological and Pharmacological Aspects of Trigeminal Pain. Amsterdam: Elsevier, 1982:163–174.

40. Lund JP, Donga R, Widmer CG, Stohler CS. The pain-adaptation model: A discussion of the relationship between chronic musculoskeletal pain and motor activity. Can J Physiol Pharmacol 1991;69:683–694.

41. Guyton AC, Hall JE. The autonomic nervous system and the adrenal medulla. In: Textbook of Medical Physiology, ed 10. Philadelphia: Saunders, 2000:697–708.

42. Coffey RJ, Rhoton AL. Pain-sensitive cranial structures. In: Dalessio DJ, Silberstein SD (eds). Wolff's Headache and Other Head Pain, ed 6. New York: Oxford University Press, 1993:19–41.

43. Finneson BE. Diagnosis and Management of Pain Syndromes. Philadelphia: Saunders, 1969.

44. Procacci P, Maresca M. Reflex sympathetic dystrophies and algodystrophies: Historical and pathogenic considerations. Pain 1987;31: 137–140.

45. Paintal A. The visceral sensations: Some basic mechanisms. In: Cervero F, Morrison J (eds). Visceral Sensation, vol 67, Progress in Brain Research. Amsterdam: Elsevier, 1986:3–19.

46. Wildicombe J. Sensory innervation of the lungs and airways. In: Cervero F, Morrison J (eds). Visceral Sensation, vol 67, Progress in Brain Research. Amsterdam: Elsevier, 1986:49–64.

47. Wolff HG, Wolf S. Pain, ed 2. Springfield, IL: Thomas, 1958.

48. Hannington-Kiff J. Pain Relief. Philadelphia: Lippincott, 1974.

49. McIntyre AK. Afferent limb of the myotatic reflex arc. Nature 1951;168:168–169.

50. Cailliet R. Neck and Arm Pain. Philadelphia: Davis, 1964.

The Neurophysiology of Orofacial Pain

Now that the anatomy of the peripheral and central nervous systems has been reviewed, the manner by which neural impulses are transferred from one neuron to another will be discussed. This chapter will outline the actual mechanisms that allow for the transfer of impulses from the peripheral sensory receptor into the central nervous system (CNS) and back out again to receptor organs from appropriate action.

Nerve Action Potential

As discussed in chapter 2, the neuron is made up of the cell body, the dendrites, and the axon. The *cell body* provides nutrients to the cell. The *dendrites* are multiple branching outgrowths from the cell body and are the main receptors for the neuron. The dendrites provide for communication between adjacent neurons. The *axon* is a single fiber that leaves the cell body to communicate with another neuron at a distant site. The axon is also called the *nerve fiber* and may extend from a few millimeters to as

long as a meter. Impulses are carried from the dendrites down the axon by way of an *action potential*. The surface of the cell membrane is charged slightly negatively. An action potential begins with a sudden change from the normal resting negative potential to a positive membrane potential and then ends with an almost equally rapid change back to the negative potential. The action potential moves down the cell membrane until it reaches the end of the axon.

The resting state of the cell membrane is said to be *polarized* with a slight negative charge. This polarization is maintained by a balance between sodium ions on the outside and potassium ions on the inside. When the membrane becomes *depolarized,* there is a sudden permeability to sodium ions into the interior of the axon through specific channels in the cell membrane called *sodium channels.* At the same time, specific channels sensitive to potassium open, allowing a rapid outflow of potassium. After the membrane becomes highly permeable to sodium ions, the sodium channels begin to close and the potassium channels open more than usual. This causes a rapid diffusion of potassium ions back into the cell to re-establish the normal negative resting membrane potential. This is called *repolarization* of the membrane.

The depolarization and repolarization of the membrane are dependent on the action of a variety of ion channels, which are found mostly in the synapse.

The Synapse

Nerve signals are transmitted from one neuron to the next through interneuronal junctions called *synapses*. Synapses occur between different neurons, predominantly through contact with the dendrites. There are as many as 100,000 small knobs, called *presynaptic terminals,* that lie on the surfaces of the dendrites and some on the soma of the neuron. It is thought that in some parts of the brain a single neuron may have as many as 400,000 synaptic terminals.[1]

Impulses that cross these synapses create an action potential that is carried down to the terminal end of the axon to synapse with another neuron. Each presynaptic terminal is separated from its adjacent neuron by a small distance called the *synaptic cleft*. The synaptic clefts range in size from 200 to 300 Å. An understanding of the neurochemistry of the synapse is basic to controlling the neural pathway of nociception and eventually pain.

Humans have two types of synapses: the *chemical synapse* and the *electrical synapse*. Electrical synapses are found in some smooth and cardiac muscles and will not be discussed here. Almost all of the synapses in the CNS are chemical.

Within the presynaptic terminals are two important groups of structures: the *synaptic vesicles* and the *mitochondria* (Fig 3-1). The synaptic vesicles contain transmitter substances that, when released into the synaptic cleft, either excite or inhibit the postsynaptic neuron. In a similar sense, the postsynaptic neural membrane has both excitatory and inhibitory receptors. Therefore, if an excitatory transmitter is released in the presence of an excitatory receptor, the neuron is *excited*. If an inhibitory transmitter is released in the presence of inhibitory receptors, the neural activity is *inhibited*.

The second important structure in the terminal of the neuron is the mitochondron. Mitochondria provide the adenosine triphosphate (ATP) required to synthesize new transmitter substances.

At the synapse, the membrane of the postsynaptic neuron houses large numbers of receptor proteins (Fig 3-1). These receptor proteins project out into the synaptic cleft and extend into the interior of the postsynaptic neuron. The portion that protrudes into the cleft acts as a binding area for the released neurotransmitters. The portion that extends into the neuron is called the *ionophore component* and carries neurotransmitters into the neuron by way of channels that can influence cell activity. The characteristics of these channels will be discussed below.

The Dynamic Nerve Terminal

In the early studies of ion channels, terminal receptors, and the cell's production of specific neurotransmitters in the presynaptic vesicles, it was believed that all these components were fixed to specific types of afferent neurons. More recent studies have demonstrated that these terminals are much more dynamic. Although each nerve is genetically predetermined to carry out specific tasks and transmit needed impulses to the CNS, the neuron is actually quite dynamic. When a postsynaptic neuron is continuously excited with a particu-

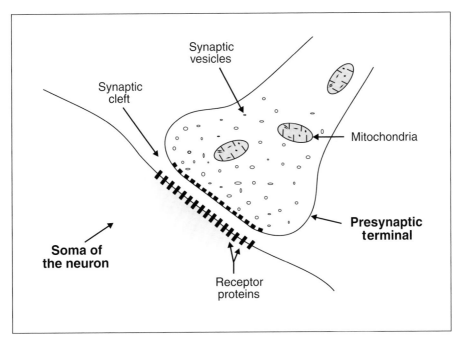

Fig 3-1 The physiologic anatomy of the synapse.

lar type of stimulation (ie, nociception) the cell itself can activate cellular genes that change its function to these demands. This induction of early gene expression causes the release of proto-oncogenes called *c-fos* and *c-jun*.[2] The release of these substances by the cell alters messenger RNA (mRNA), which in turn can change the type and number of receptors that are formed on the cell membrane. As the number and type of receptors change, so also is the cell's function changed. This process is called *neuroplasticity* and is nature's way to adapt to environmental demands. Changes such as these can alter the reactivity of the synapse for minutes, days, months, or even years. The importance of this feature will be discussed in future chapters.

The Ion Channels

The synaptic membrane of the presynaptic terminals contains large numbers of ion channels. There are three general types of ion channels that have been extensively studied: the *voltage-gated ion channel*, the *G-protein–linked ion channel*, and the *ligand-gated ion channel*. Each of these types will be briefly discussed so that the general relationship of the neurochemistry of nociception can be appreciated. There are many more types of channels that have been identified, but it is not within the scope of this text to elaborate on each of these. A more complete description can be found elsewhere.[3]

The Voltage-Gated Ion Channels

Voltage-gated ion channels are the basic functional component of the membrane's ability to depolarize. As has been stated, these channels allow the passing of positive and negative ions in and out of the cell.

The sodium ion channel

When the cell membrane depolarizes to −60 to −40 mV, the sodium ion channel opens rapidly, allowing sodium to enter the cell membrane. In most neurons the sodium channel is primarily responsible for the action potential generation and conduction. There appear to be several subtypes of sodium channels. Some of the channels are blocked by tetrodotoxin (TTX) and some are not.[4] The TTX-resistant sodium channel subtype (TTX-R) seems to be more common in C fibers, while the TTX-sensitive sodium channels (TTX-S) are found more often in the large A fibers. The TTX-R channels have a higher depolarization threshold for action potential generation and a faster recovery rate. This suggests that the C fibers are ideally suited to generate sustained bursts of action potentials in response to a prolonged depolarizing noxious stimulus.[5,6]

The potassium channel

In the presence of depolarization the potassium channel opens rapidly, allowing potassium to leave the cell. Immediately following this, the channel reverses, allowing the return of potassium back into the cell and causing the repolarization of the cell membrane. There are a variety of voltage-gated potassium channels found in sensory neurons.[7] These subtypes are responsible for the shifting of potassium in and out of the cell and are therefore important in determining the action potential.

Some potassium channels are activated by calcium. These calcium-activated potassium channels seem to affect the return of the action potential, thus reducing excitability after each action potential. Therefore, these channels are important in regulating the firing pattern of the neuron.[7]

The calcium channel

At least five major types of voltage-activated calcium channels have been identified on sensory neurons. They are labeled L, N, P/Q, T, and R. Each type is distinguished by the degree of membrane depolarization needed to activate it (activation threshold), its inactivation characteristics, and its pharmacologic properties. The T channels are known as the low voltage-activated (LVA) channels. The L, N, P/Q, and R channels are known as the high voltage-activated (HVA) channels. Activation of calcium channels can affect many cellular processes, including activation of other membrane channels, release of transmitters, and regulation of enzymes.

The G-Protein–Linked Channel

Ion channels can be opened by activation of what are called *G-protein–coupled receptors.* These receptors do not immediately cause the opening of an ion channel; instead, when they are activated by certain mediators, they stimulate the production of intracellular messengers. The messenger in turn activates a series of events that leads to the opening of the channel. This process is slower than the direct ion channel activation that has been described above. It may take minutes, in contrast to the rapid exchange when the ion channel is affected directly. Some of the mediators that are associated with G-protein–linked channels are bradykinin, 5-hydroxytryptamine (5HT; also known as serotonin), and prostaglandins.

The Ligand-Gated Channels

Ligands are mediators that when present can cause the opening of the channel. There are a great variety of substances that can activate these ion channels. Some of the most important are 5HT, ATP, acetylcholine glutamate, and gamma-aminobutyric acid (GABA).

Neurotransmitters

The neurochemicals that are released by the presynaptic neuron into the synaptic cleft and activate ion channels are called *neurotransmitters*. Neurotransmitters are either small rapid-acting molecules or larger slower-acting molecules. The smaller rapid-acting transmitters cause most of the acute responses of the nervous system, such as transmission of sensory signals to and inside the brain and motor signals back to the muscles. The larger molecules are the *neuropeptides* and represent a different group of chemicals. These are not manufactured in the presynaptic terminal but instead in the ribosomes of the neuronal body. The neuropeptides are then transported to the synapse for release in the cleft. These neurotransmitters are much slower acting than the smaller molecules, but when released they have a much longer effect on the postsynaptic neuron. Although this chapter has mainly discussed the peripheral nerve terminal, neurotransmitters are formed and released in all nerves, both peripherally and centrally. Since it is difficult to separate neurotransmitters by location, this discussion will include the common neurotransmitters and mention their more common locations and functions.

Rapid-Acting (Small-Molecule) Neurotransmitters

Some of the more common small-molecule neurotransmitters are listed here, with their common sites of location and effects on the postsynaptic neurons:

Acetylcholine

Acetylcholine is one of the most commonly found neurotransmitters in the human. It is secreted by neurons in many areas of the brain but specifically by the motor cortex and the basal ganglia and by the motor neurons that innervate the skeletal muscles. It is also secreted by the preganglionic neurons of the autonomic nervous system, the postganglionic neurons of the parasympathetic nervous system, and some of the postganglionic neurons of the sympathetic nervous system. In almost all instances, acetylcholine has an excitatory effect on the postsynaptic neuron.

Norepinephrine

Norepinephrine is secreted by many neurons whose cell bodies are in the brainstem and hypothalamus. The highest concentration of norepinephrine-secreting neurons is found in the locus ceruleus of the pons. From this region, norepinephrine-producing neurons extend to many other regions of the brain and brainstem, influencing the overall activity and mood of the mind. Norepinephrine is almost always an excitatory neurotransmitter.

Glutamate

Glutamate is an amino acid that is secreted by the presynaptic terminals in many of the sensory pathways, as well as in many areas of the cortex. It has been found in the spinal cord dorsal horn and is associated with noxious input.[8,9] It is thought to always cause excitation.

Aspartate

Like glutamate, aspartate is an amino acid that is secreted by the presynaptic terminals of many of the sensory pathways in the dorsal horn. It is thought to always cause excitation.

Serotonin

Serotonin (5HT) is secreted by nuclei that originate in the median raphe of the brainstem and project to many areas of the brain and down into the spinal dorsal horn. Serotonin is a monoamine that is also released by blood platelets. It is synthesized in the CNS from L-tryptophan, a dietary essential amino acid.[10] It is released when the nucleus raphes magnus in the brainstem is stimulated by sensory input.[11] Peripherally, serotonin is an algogenic agent[12] and is thought to relate especially to neurovascular pain syndromes (see chapter 16). In the CNS, serotonin is an important neurotransmitter in the endogenous antinociceptive mechanism.[13] Central serotonin is thought to potentiate endorphin analgesia.[10] It reduces stimulation-evoked excitation of nociceptive dorsal horn interneurons.[14] The activation of serotoninergic pathways in the brainstem by tricyclic antidepressants yields paralleling analgesic effects along with its action on depressive states.[15] Descending serotoninergic and norepinephrinergic neurons in the dorsal horn suggest that they provide global suppression or enhancement that enables nociceptive pathways to respond more effectively to incoming sensory information.[16]

GABA

GABA is secreted by neurons in the spinal cord, cerebellum, basal ganglia, and parts of the cortex. It is believed to always have an inhibitory effect on the postsynaptic neuron.

Glycine

Glycine is secreted in many areas of the spinal cord and is likely also secreted in the trigeminal spinal nucleus. It is probably always an inhibitory transmitter.

Dopamine

Dopamine is secreted by neurons that originate in the substantia nigra and extend into the basal ganglia. The normal effect of dopamine is inhibitory.

Histamine

Histamine is a vasoactive amine that derives from the amino acid histadine. Although histamine serves as a neurotransmitter in the CNS, it is probably best known as a vasodilator and for its action to increase small-vessel permeability. It also causes contraction of smooth muscle in the lungs.

Nitric Oxide

Nitric oxide (NO) is an important intercellular mediator and is produced by many cells that have a close physical association with sensory neurons. NO is formed from L-arginine following the activation of the enzyme nitric oxide synthase (NOS) by calcium and other cofactors.[17] The physiologic actions of NO in nociceptive neurons is still unclear, but there is strong evidence that it enhances nociceptive transmission in several ways.[18,19]

Slow-Acting (Large-Molecule) Neurotransmitters

The large-molecule neurotransmitters are the neuropeptides. The following is a short description of a few of the important neuropeptides that serve as neurotransmitters:

Substance P

Substance P is a polypeptide composed of 11 amino acids. It is released at the central terminals of primary nociceptive neurons and acts as a transport substance, since it is found at the distal terminals as well.[20] Centrally, it acts as an excitatory neurotransmitter for nociceptive impulses.[21,22] It is released from spinal cord cells by the stimulation of A-delta and C-fiber afferents and excites neurons in the dorsal horn that are activated by noxious stimuli.[23] Its modulating action on pain is both rapid and short-lived.[24] Substance P released from unmyelinated afferents is involved in neurogenic inflammation such as cutaneous wheal formation and the hyperemia of reflex axon flare. It is known that substance P content is highest in the most severely inflamed joints. When injected into a joint, substance P increases both the inflammation and destructive changes.[25]

Endorphins

The endorphins are polypeptides (ie, chains of amino acids). They are identical to portions of the pituitary hormone beta-lipotropin, which consists of 91 amino acids.[26-28] They behave like morphine and bind to morphine receptors to dull pain. Like morphine, they are displaced from these receptors by the morphine antagonist naloxone. Repeated injections of enkephalin and beta-endorphin will cause tolerance and physical dependence.[29]

The short-chain enkephalins appear to act chiefly in the cerebral spinal fluid. They have a short, rapid action and serve more to limit the experience of excessive, sudden pain than as an analgesic. The longer-chain beta-endorphin appears to be closely related to pituitary function and may act somewhat like a hormone. It is longer lasting, requires the passage of a latent period before it becomes active, and has high antinociceptive potency.[29-31] Evidence exists that the endogenous opiates may act more as neuromodulators of postsynaptic activity than as classic neurotransmitters.[28,32] It has been shown that endorphins are important contributors to pain threshold and pain tolerance.[33] There is considerable interneurotransmitter action associated with the antinociceptive system (see chapter 4). For example, endorphin is potentiated by serotonin that is released from serotoninergic neurons only in the presence of dopamine, while norepinephrine exerts a deterring effect.[34,35] It should be noted that Kosterlitz[36] remarked, "While it has been shown in many laboratories that the enkephalins and endorphins have antinociceptive effects, the underlying mechanisms have not been fully analyzed, and, in particular, the conditions controlling the release of opioid peptides are still not understood."

It should be noted that beta-endorphin is appreciably released in long-distance runners.[37] It is also significant that placebo analgesia is endorphin-mediated and reversible by naloxone.[38,39] Analgesia produced by hypnosis, however, is not reversed by naloxone.[40,41] Hypnoanalgesia no doubt is based on other mechanisms.

Bradykinin

Bradykinin is an endogenous polypeptide consisting of a chain of nine amino acids. Released as part of an inflammatory reaction, it is a powerful vasodilator and causes increased capillary permeability. With few exceptions, bradykinin acts as an algogenic agent that excites all types of receptors. It sensitizes some high-threshold receptors so that they respond to otherwise innocuous stimuli such as those that occur during normal activities.[42] Bradykinin requires the presence of prostaglandins to act.[43] It is also released during ischemic episodes.[44]

Elimination of the Transmitter from the Synapse

Once the transmitter has been released into the synapse, a mechanism must be present to remove the transmitter. If this does not occur, the transmitter's effect on the postsynaptic neuron is prolonged. In most instances the transmitter is removed immediately, which enables the postsynaptic neuron to return to its normal membrane resting potential. The elimination of the neurotransmitter can occur by one of three methods: diffusion, enzymatic destruction, or reuptake.

In some instances a released neurotransmitter will merely diffuse out of the synaptic cleft. As the transmitter leaves the synapse, its effect on the postsynaptic neuron is eliminated. This process is called *diffusion*.

Some neurotransmitters are immediately destroyed by enzymes that are either released or already present in the synaptic cleft. This process of eliminating the transmitter is called *enzymatic destruction*. For example, when acetylcholine is released, the enzyme cholinesterase is present in the cleft, bound in the proteoglycan matrix that fills the space. This enzyme can very rapidly split the acetylcholine, rendering it immediately inactive.

A third method of eliminating the neurotransmitter from the synapse is by neurotransmitter *re-uptake*. Some neurotransmitters are actively transported back into the presynaptic terminal itself for reuse. This occurs in the presynaptic terminals of the sympathetic nervous system with the reuptake of norepinephrine.

The Neurochemistry of Nociception

The peripheral nociceptor can be activated by thermal, mechanical, and chemical stimulation. When thermal and mechanical stimulation produce nociceptive input, the reason for the pain is usually apparent. Chemical stimulation of the nociceptor, on the other hand, may be less apparent to the sufferer. In fact, once the mechanical or thermal stimulation has terminated, the reason for continued nociceptive input is likely to be neurochemical. There are a variety of compounds that can accumulate near the nociceptor following tissue injury that can be responsible for maintaining nociceptive input. There are at least three sources of these compounds: the damaged cell itself, the secondary effects of plasma extravasation and lymphocyte migration, or the nociceptor itself.

Damage to tissue cells produces leakage of intracellular contents. Among the substances released by tissue damage are potassium and histamine, both of which either activate or sensitize the nociceptor.[45] These substances have been documented to excite polymodal nociceptors and produce pain when injected into skin.[46,47] Other compounds, such as acetylcholine, 5HT, and ATP, may be released by tissue damage and are known to either activate or sensitize nociceptors. In fact, there is evidence that several of these compounds can act in combination to sensitize nociceptors.[48]

One of the most potent pain-producing substances that appear in injured tissue is bradykinin. Polymodal nociceptors can be activated by bradykinin[49] and they then can

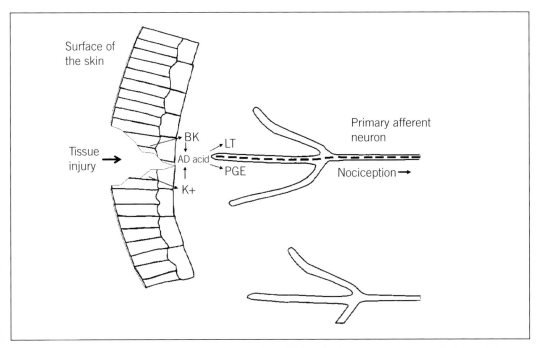

Fig 3-2a Tissue injury causes the release of potassium (K+) and other potent pain-producing substances such as bradykinin (BK) and arachidonic acid (AD). Arachidonic acid is further broken down to prostaglandins (PGE) and leukotrienes (LT), which are the primary initiators of inflammation. The presence of these neurochemicals at the free nerve ending initiates a nociceptive response in the primary afferent neuron.

become sensitized to thermal stimuli (Fig 3-2a).

Another group of compounds that are synthesized in the regions of tissue damage are the metabolic products of arachidonic acid. These compounds are considered inflammatory mediators and include both prostaglandins and leukotrienes. These compounds appear whenever animal cells are damaged and are present in increased concentration in inflammatory exudates. The prostaglandins are a group of chemically related long-chain hydroxy fatty acids. There are six types, each designated by a suffix letter. (Subscript numerals indicate the degree of saturation of the side chain.) Prostaglandin E_2 is metabolized from arachidonic acid through action of an en-

zyme cyclooxygenase (COX). There are two identified isomers of COX: COX_1 and COX_2. The action of COX_1 produces prostaglandins that play a physiologic housekeeping role in renal parenchyma, gastric mucosa, platelets, and other tissues. It aids in maintaining normal function. Inhibition of COX_1 is responsible for gastrointestinal toxicity. COX_2 is present in most tissues in small amounts. It is expressed primarily in sites of inflammation and produces prostaglandins that are involved in inflammation and mitogenesis. Therefore, if COX_2 is inhibited, there is a reduction of the inflammatory response, resulting in less nociception and pain. In recent years there has been a strong interest in the "COX_2 inhibitor" drugs, so that pain

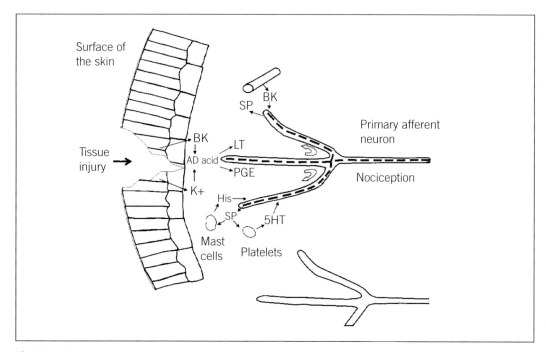

Fig 3-2b Once the primary afferent is activated, the nociceptive response causes an antidromic release of substance P in another branch of the same afferent neuron. The presence of substance P causes the release of histamine (His) from mast cells and serotonin (5HT) from platelets. Substance P also causes the release of bradykinin from neighboring blood vessels, furthering the nociceptive response. This neurogenic inflammation expands the pain at the site. Now not only the cut tissue is painful, but also a broader area around the injury.

may be reduced without the adverse side effects of gastrointestinal irritation. Interestingly, COX_2 may also play a role in pain inhibition in the CNS.[50,51]

Prostaglandins do not seem to be algogenic substances per se. They sensitize nociceptive nerve endings to different types of stimuli, thus lowering their pain thresholds to all kinds of stimulation.[52] Prostaglandins are required for bradykinin to act[43]; bradykinin in turn stimulates the release of prostaglandins.[53] The two therefore are mutually potentiating. Prostaglandin E also increases the response of slowly adapting A-delta mechanoreceptors to nonnoxious stimuli.[54] There is evidence that a prostaglandin-like substance is released in the CNS during an inflammatory reaction that induces prostaglandin hyperalgesia.[55]

Another important metabolic pathway of arachidonic acid is the lipoxygenase pathway, which produces the leukotrienes. Leukotrienes produce hyperalgesia in animal models and in humans.[56] The hyperalgesia produced by leukotriene B_4 is not blocked by COX inhibitors but is blocked by depletion of polymorphonuclear leukocytes.[57] This suggests that leukocytes may contribute to nociceptor activation, but this has yet to be documented.

In addition to the chemical mediators that are released from damaged cells or synthesized in the region of damage, the nociceptors themselves can release substances

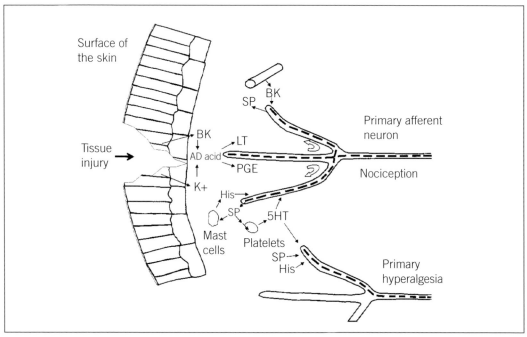

Fig 3-2c The release of substance P, histamine, and serotonin can now influence another primary afferent neuron in the region, which initiates more nociception. This broadening of the painful area is known as *primary hyperalgesia*.

that enhance nociception. One such substance is substance P. Unmyelinated primary afferent neurons seem to produce substance P and, when stimulated, can release this potent excitatory neurotransmitter into the extracellular space.[58] Substance P is a very strong vasodilator and produces edema. Substance P also causes release of histamine from mast cells; histamine is itself an excitatory neurotransmitter and also causes vasodilation and edema.[59]

Neuronal Sensitization

When excitatory neurotransmitters are released in the synaptic cleft, the postsynaptic neuron is excited and an impulse is started and carried down the axon. If excitatory neurochemicals remain in the region of the synapse, the neuron can be depolarized more quickly with the next release of a neurotransmitter. This process is called *sensitization*. Sensitization is the result of a lowering of the threshold that causes the depolarization of the primary afferent neuron. It is one explanation for the hyperalgesic state that is commonly associated with inflammatory tissues. For example, several hours after receiving a small cut, an individual will develop a region around the injured tissue that is quite sensitive, even to light touch. This increased sensitivity of local tissues is a result of the neurochemicals that sensitize nearby primary afferent neurons, so that even light mechanical stimulation creates depolarization and nociceptive input. This type of sensitization is called *peripheral sensitization* (see Figs 3-2b and 3-2c on pages 54 and 55). As will be discussed later, sensitization of neurons can also occur within the CNS.

The Axon Transport System

The nerve cell body (soma) of the primary trigeminal neuron located in the gasserian ganglion produces peptides and proteins that are moved to the central terminal by an *axon transport system*, it is believed via microtubules or microfilaments in the axon. The velocity of this transport system does not seem to vary appreciably between myelinated and nonmyelinated fibers. Some transport substances likely serve as primary afferent neurotransmitters and therefore are essential to the transmission of pain information. It is likely that the axon transport system is involved in this complex neurochemical process. Substance P is thought to be one neurotransmitter released at the central terminal of nociceptive primary neurons. This substance also is found at the distal terminals, having reached these no doubt by way of the axon transport system.[20] Thus, sensory information may be signaled very rapidly to the CNS by transmission of nerve impulses—or more slowly, by way of neurochemical substances conducted through the axon transport system.[60]

There is evidence that the axon transport system can move neurotransmitters in the primary afferent neurons both centrally (orthodromically, in the normal direction of impulses) as well as peripherally (antidromically, in the opposite direction of normal impulses). Antidromic activity of the primary afferent neuron results in the release of neurotransmitters into the pe-

ripheral terminals, leading to sensitization of other neurons in the adjacent area. This process is called *neurogenic inflammation*. Neurogenic inflammation not only results in peripheral sensitization (hyperalgesia) but can also cause local vasodilation and edema. Local vasodilation caused by neurogenic inflammation is called *flare*, while local edema is called *wheal*.

The sympathetic efferents may also produce neurogenic inflammation, as indicated by the fact that sympathetic blockade reduces the inflammation of sympathetically maintained pain as well as that of inflammatory arthritis.[25]

Transmission of Afferent Impulses to the Cortex

When a peripheral nociceptor is stimulated, a series of events occurs that carries that impulse into the CNS and on to the higher centers for interpretation and evaluation. If the impulse has significance, the higher centers may pass it on to the cortex, where it is then perceived as pain. This series of events is by no means simple. In fact, most of the impulses that enter the CNS never reach the cortex. To better understand orofacial pains, we will now follow the pathway of a nociceptive impulse from the peripheral receptor to the cortex.

It would be easy to believe that orofacial nociception begins with a trigeminal nerve pathway. Although this is commonly true, it is only one of many pathways that carry orofacial nociception to the brain. Nociceptive impulses from the face and mouth may be mediated centrally by way of afferent primary neurons that pass through the 5th, 7th, 9th, and 10th cranial nerves as well as the 1st, 2nd, and 3rd cervical spinal nerves and by way of visceral afferents that descend through the cervical sympathetic chain to pass through the posterior roots of the upper thoracic spinal nerves. The nerve cell bodies of the primary sensory neurons are located in the posterior root ganglion of the nerve through which they pass, except for the proprioceptive fibers of the fifth cranial nerve, which are located in the mesencephalic nucleus in the midbrain.[61]

To simplify our discussion, we will only discuss the pathway of a single trigeminal primary afferent neuron, for example, coming from the pulp of a mandibular molar. Once the nociceptor located in the pulp is activated, the impulse is carried into the CNS by a primary afferent neuron in the mandibular branch of the fifth cranial nerve (Fig 3-3). The cell body of this neuron is located in the gasserian or trigeminal ganglia. This primary afferent neuron enters the brainstem and synapses with a second-order neuron in the subnucleus caudalis of the trigeminal spinal tract nucleus. Although the subnucleus caudalis has been well implicated as the primary location of nociceptive input for the face, recent information suggests that the subnucleus oralis may play an important role in nociception of the intraoral structures.[62] For this discussion, we will continue to use the subnucleus caudalis. The primary neuron will synapse in this subnucleus with one of the three types of second-order neurons. Since our discussion is with nociception, let us assume that the second-order neuron is a nociceptive-specific (NS) neuron. This NS neuron will then be activated and the impulse will be carried to the higher centers by this second-order neuron. In some instances the neuron may carry the impulse directly higher on the same side of the brain (see chapter 2). This is not usually the case with nociception. In most instances, the NS neuron will cross the brainstem and ascend in the anterolateral tract on the opposite side. At this point nociceptive input can be carried by one of two tracts. Nociceptive impulses that have been carried by the

faster A-delta primary fibers synapse mainly in lamina I of the subnucleus caudalis. These NS neurons carry the impulses by way of the neospinothalamic tract directly to the thalamus. These fibers are mainly carrying mechanical and thermal pain. Since this pathway ascends directly to the thalamus, it is said to carry *fast pain*.

Nociceptive impulses carried by primary afferent C fibers synapse in laminae II, III (substantia gelatinosa), and V. The NS neurons that synapse with these fibers carry impulses by way of the paleospinothalamic tract. This tract does not ascend directly to the thalamus but instead projects numerous interneurons into the reticular formation of the brainstem. The impulses are then carried by way of many interneurons through the reticular formation and on to the thalamus. The nociceptive impulse can be therefore be changed or modulated by the reticular formation before it ascends to the thalamus. Since the impulse takes longer to reach the thalamus, this type of pain is called *slow pain*.

There are significant functional differences between fast pain and slow pain. Fast pain can be easily localized as to the exact location of its origin. It is likely to be perceived by the individual as sharp pain. It is important that the individual perceive this pain quickly and react in an appropriate manner. Slow pain, in contrast, is much more difficult to locate and is felt as a deep, dull, aching sensation. This type of pain is likely to be responsible for suffering. Since this type of nociception is thought to be primarily carried by C fibers, substance P is likely to be a major neurotransmitter. Substance P is slow to build up at the synapse and slow to be destroyed. Therefore, its concentration at the synapse is believed to increase for at least several seconds, and perhaps much longer, after nociceptive stimulation begins. After the impulse is over, substance P probably persists for many more seconds or perhaps even minutes. This might explain the progressive increase

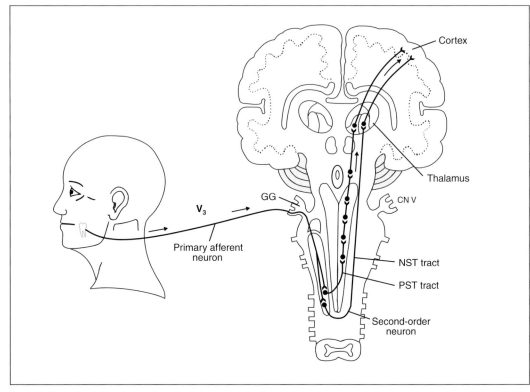

Fig 3-3 A graphic depiction following an impulse arising from a molar on to interpretation in the higher centers. The impulse is carried by the primary afferent neuron of the mandibular division of the trigeminal nerve (V_3) through the gasserian ganglion (GG) into the subnucleus caudalis region of the trigeminal spinal tract. At that point, it synapses with a second-order neuron to be transferred on to the higher centers for evaluation. If the input is carried by an A-delta fiber, it may synapse with a wide dynamic range neuron and be carried to the higher centers by way of the neospinothalmic tract (NST tract). This input is carried quickly to the higher centers and is therefore referred to as *fast pain*. If the primary afferent input is carried by a C fiber, it may synapse with a nociceptive-specific neuron and be carried up the paleo-spinothalamic tract (PST tract). This tract passes through the reticular formation and may therefore be influenced by many modulating interneurons. Nociception carried on this tract is called *slow pain*.

in intensity of slow-chronic pain with time. It might also explain, at least partially, the persistence of this type of pain even after the painful stimulus has been removed.

If the nociceptive impulse we are following enters the fast pain tract, the thalamus would immediately receive the information and send it on to the cortex for evaluation and response. The motor cortex would quickly coordinate a response with the basal ganglia and cerebellum, producing a descending impulse to a motor neuron and

creating a muscle action. This response may even be a reflex.

If, however, the nociceptive impulse that we are following enters the slow pain tract, a different series of events would occur. As discussed in chapter 2, the reticular formation is a portion of the brainstem that contains a number of nuclei that can either excite or inhibit the incoming impulses. The reticular formation therefore controls the overall activity of the brain. The area of the reticular formation that seems to increase or excite incoming impulses is called the *bulboreticular facilitory area.* This region contains a group of neurons that secrete acetylcholine, an excitatory transmitter. Fibers passing through this region of the reticular formation travel on to the intralaminar nuclei of the thalamus. The level of activity of the brainstem bulboreticular facilitory area (and therefore the level of activity of the entire brain) is determined to a great extent by the sensory signals that enter this area from the periphery. Pain signals, in particular, increase the activity in this area and strongly excite the brain to attention.[63]

Not only does an excited bulboreticular facilitory area send impulses quickly to the thalamus and cortex, but return impulses are also influenced. In other words, impulses leaving the cortex travel down to the thalamus and on through this facilitory area. When this area is activated, these descending impulses are enhanced. Therefore, any time the cerebral cortex becomes activated by either thinking or motor processes, reverse signals are sent back to the brainstem excitatory area, increasing the impulses. This generally provides a positive feedback system that allows any beginning activity in the cerebrum to support still more activity, thus leading to an awake mind. Perhaps it is this mechanism that is responsible for sleep disruption in individuals suffering with chronic pain.

Another important area in the reticular formation that controls brain activity is the *reticular inhibitory area.* This area is located medially and ventrally in the medulla and can reduce the tonic nerve signals transmitted through the spinal cord and trigeminal brainstem complex. This region of the reticular formation has a high concentration of neurons that secrete 5HT (serotonin), an inhibitory transmitter. This area will be discussed in chapter 4.

Now let us continue to follow our nociceptive impulse and assume that the excitatory area of the reticular formation enhanced it and sent it on to the thalamus.

(In many instances the impulse may have been terminated in the reticular formation.) Once the impulse reaches the thalamus it is sent not only to the sensory cortex, but signals are simultaneously sent to the limbic structures and hypothalamus. The sensory cortex now recognizes the nociceptive impulse as pain. Along with this recognition comes evaluation of the meaning of this sensation. The cortex may reach back into memory for assistance in evaluating this unpleasant sensation. It is at this point that prior experiences of pain and suffering begin to give meaning to the sensation. If the individual has experienced this sensation before and learned it was of little consequence, the pain may be totally ignored. On the other hand, if this same pain sensation has previously caused considerable alteration in the quality of life, much attention will be drawn to the sensation.

In addition to these responses, there are still other responses influenced by the limbic system and hypothalamus. As discussed in chapter 2, the limbic system is responsible for basic instincts and behavior. Within the limbic system are certain centers that determine behavior. These centers influence the *affective nature* of sensory sensation— that is, whether the sensory sensations are pleasant or unpleasant. The centers have been described in terms of pain/pleasure, reward/punishment, and satisfaction/aversion centers. Electrical stimulation of certain regions pleases or satisfies the animal, whereas electrical stimulation of other regions causes terror, pain, fear, rage, defense, and escape reactions. Painful or other negative sensations (ie, hunger, thirst) will drive the individual toward behavior that will eliminate or terminate the unpleasant sensation. This behavioral response is instinctive; however, it can be influenced by the cortex. Therefore the present level of activity of the limbic system (ie, mood, anger, rage) can greatly influence the individual's response to pain.

Summary

Following the transmission of a single impulse from a receptor to the brain and back out as a response can help in understanding the neuroanatomy and physiology of pain. Yet even this simple example becomes complex when one examines the many factors that can alter the impulse as it travels. From the moment the sensory receptor is activated (transduction), the impulse can be altered, for example, with peripheral sensitization. Depending on the type of nerve fiber that carries the impulse, different tracts are taken, which influences transmission. Then, as the impulse travels, it may be significantly modulated before even reaching the cortex. When the cortex finally receives the impulse, perception is determined by interaction of the cortex, thalamus, and limbic structures.

The clinician can appreciate the reason for so much variation in pain and suffering between different individuals. Yet as will be discussed in the next chapter, the complexity is far greater than what has been presented in this chapter.

References

1. Melzack R. Neuropsychological basis of pain measurement. In: Kruger L, Liebeskind JC (eds). Neural Mechanisms of Pain, vol 6, Advances in Pain Research and Therapy. New York: Raven Press, 1984:323–339.
2. Abbadie C, Besson JM, Calvino B. c-Fos expression in the spinal cord and pain-related symptoms induced by chronic arthritis in the rat are prevented by pretreatment with Freund adjuvant. J Neurosci 1994;14:5865–5871.
3. Wall PD, Melzack R. Textbook of Pain, ed 4. Edinburgh: Churchill Livingstone, 1999.
4. Koerber H, Mendell L. Functional heterogeneity of dorsal root ganglion cells. In: Scott S (ed). Sensory Neurons: Diversity, Development and Plasticity. New York: Oxford University Press, 1992:77–96.
5. Elliott AA, Elliott JR. Characterization of TTX-sensitive and TTX-resistant sodium currents in small cells from adult rat dorsal root ganglia. J Physiol 1993;463:39–56.
6. Elliott JR. Slow Na+ channel inactivation and bursting discharge in a simple model axon: Implications for neuropathic pain. Brain Res 1997;754:221–226.
7. Bevan S. Nociceptive peripheral neurons: Cellular properties. In: Wall PD, Melzack R (eds). Textbook of Pain, ed 4. Edinburgh: Churchill Livingstone, 1999:85–102.
8. Skilling S, Smullin D, Larson A. Extracellular amino acid concentrations in the dorsal spinal cord of freely moving rats following veratridine and nociceptive stimulation. J Neurochem 1988;51:127–132.
9. Sorkin L, Westlund K, Sluks K, Dougherty P, Willis W. Neural changes in acute arthritis in monkeys. IV. Time course of amino acid release into the lumbar dorsal horn. Brain Res Rev 1992;17:39–50.
10. Seltzer S, Marcus R, Stoch R. Perspectives in the control of chronic pain by nutritional manipulation. Pain 1981;11:141–148.
11. Basbaum AT. Brainstem control of nociception: The contribution of the monoamines. Pain 1981;11(suppl 1):231–239.
12. Beck P, Handwerker H. Bradykinin and serotonin effects on various types of cutaneous nerve fibers. Pflugers Arch 1974;347:209–222.
13. Messing R, Lytle L. Serotonin-containing neurons: Their possible role in pain and analgesia. Pain 1977;4:1–21.
14. Belcher G, Ryall R, Schaffner R. The differential effects of 5-hydroxytryptamine, noradrenalin, and raphe stimulation on nociceptive and non-nociceptive dorsal horn interneurons in the cat. Brain Res 1978;151:307–321.
15. Ward N, Bloom V, Friedel R. The effectiveness of tricyclic antidepressants in the treatment of coexisting pain and depression. Pain 1979;7:331–341.
16. Dubner R. Specialization of nociceptive pathways: Sensory discrimination, sensory modulation, and neural connectivity. In: Fields HL, Dubner R, Cervero F (eds). Proceedings of the Fourth World Congress on Pain: Seattle, vol 9, Advances in Pain Research and Therapy. New York: Raven Press, 1985:111–137.

17. Bredt DS, Snyder SH. Nitric oxide: A physiologic messenger molecule. Ann Rev Biochem 1994;63:175–195.

18. Hoheisel U, Mense S. The role of spinal nitric oxide in the control of spontaneous pain following nociceptive input. Prog Brain Res 2000; 129:163–172.

19. Hoheisel U, Unger T, Mense S. A block of spinal nitric oxide synthesis leads to increased background activity predominantly in nociceptive dorsal horn neurones in the rat. Pain 2000;88:249–257.

20. Yaksh T, Hammond D. Peripheral and central substrates involved in the rostral transmission of nociceptive information. Pain 1982;13:1–85.

21. Zimmerman M. Peripheral and central nervous mechanisms of nociception, pain, and pain therapy: Facts and hypotheses. In: Bonica JJ, Liebeskind JC, Albe-Fessard DG (eds). Proceedings of the Second World Congress on Pain, vol 3, Advances in Pain Research and Therapy. New York: Raven Press, 1979:3–32.

22. Hosobuchi Y. Emson PC, Iversen LL. Elevated cerebrospinal fluid substance P in arachnoiditis is reduced by systemic administration of morphine. Adv Biochem Psychopharmacol 1982: 33;497–500.

23. Bucsics A, Lembeck F. In vitro release of substance P from spinal cord slices by capsaicin congeners. Eur J Pharmacol 1981;71:71–77.

24. Yasphal K, Wright D, Henry J. Substance P reduces tail-flick latency: Implications for chronic pain syndromes. Pain 1982;14:155–167.

25. Basbaum AI, Levine JD. The contribution of the nervous system to inflammation and inflammatory disease. Can J Physiol Pharmacol 1991;69:647–651.

26. Allen G. Dental Anesthesia and Analgesia. Baltimore: Williams & Wilkins, 1979.

27. Kroening R, Donaldson D. Proposed mechanism of acupuncture. SAAD Dig 1979;4:28–32.

28. Watkins L, Mayer D. Organization of endogenous opiate and nonopiate pain control systems. Science 1982;216:1185–1192.

29. Synder S. Opiate receptors and internal opiates. Sci Am 1977;236:44–56.

30. Kosterlitz H. Interaction of endogenous opioid peptides and their analogs with opiate receptors. In: Bonica JJ, Liebeskind JC, Albe-Fessard DG (eds). Proceedings of the Second World Congress on Pain, vol 3, Advances in Pain Research and Therapy. New York: Raven Press, 1979: 377–384.

31. Stacher G, Bauer P, Steinringer H. Effects of the synthetic enkephalin analogue K33-824 on pain threshold and pain tolerance in man. Pain 1979;7:159–172.

32. Gutstein H, Bronstein D, Huda A. Beta endorphin processing and cellular origins in rat spinal cord. Pain 1992;51:241–247.

33. Von Knorring L, Almay B, Johansson F. Pain perception and endorphin levels in cerebrospinal fluid. Pain 1978;5:359–365.

34. Mayer D, Price D. Central nervous system mechanisms of analgesia. Pain 1976;2:379–404.

35. Akil H, Liebeskind J. Monoaminergic mechanisms of stimulation-produced analgesia. Brain Res 1975;94:279–296.

36. Kosterlitz H. Opioid peptides and pain: An update. In: Bonica J, Lindblom U, Iggo A (eds). Proceedings of the Third World Congress on Pain, vol 5, Advances in Pain Research and Therapy. New York: Raven Press, 1983:199–208.

37. Colt E, Wardlaw S, Frantz A. The effect of running on plasma endorphin. Life Sci 1981; 28:1637–1640.

38. Levine J, Gordon N, Fields H. The role of endorphins in placebo analgesia. In: Bonica JJ Liebeskind JC, Albe-Fessard DG (eds). Proceedings of the Second World Congress on Pain, vol 3, Advances in Pain Research and Therapy. New York: Raven Press, 1979:547–551.

39. Grevert P, Albert L, Goldstein A. Partial antagonism of placebo analgesia by naloxone. Pain 1983;16:129–143.

40. Barber J, Mayer D. Evaluation of the efficacy and neural mechanism of a hypnotic analgesia procedure in experimental and clinical dental pain. Pain 1977;4:41–48.

41. Mayer D. Endogenous analgesia systems: Neural and behavioral mechanisms. In: Bonica JJ, Liebeskind JC, Albe-Fessard DG (eds). Proceedings of the Second World Congress on Pain, vol 3, Advances in Pain Research and Therapy. New York: Raven Press, 1979:385–410.

42. Mense S, Meyer H. Bradykinin-induced modulation of the response behaviour of different types of feline group III and IV muscle receptors. J Physiol 1988;398:49–63.

43. Chahl L, Iggo A. The effects of bradykinin and prostaglandin E1 on rat cutaneous afferent nerve activity. Br J Pharmacol 1977;59:343–347.

44. Blair RW, Weber RN, Foreman RD. Responses of thoracic spinoreticular and spinothalamic cells to intracardiac bradykinin. Am J Physiol 1984;246:H500–H507.

45. Keele K. A physician looks at pain. In: Weisenberg M (ed). Pain: Clinical and Experimental Perspectives. St Louis: Mosby, 1975:45–55.

46. Juan H, Lembeck F. Action of peptides and other algesic agents on paravascular pain receptors of the isolated perfused rabbit ear. Naunyn Schmiedebergs Arch Pharmacol 1974;283:151–164.

47. Armstrong D. Bradykinin, kallidin and kallikrein. In: Erdos EG (ed). Handbook of Experimental Pharmacology, vol 25. Berlin: Springer, 1970:434–481.

48. Perl E. Sensitization of nociceptors and its relation to sensation. In: Bonica J (eds). Introduction to the First World Congress on Pain: Goals of the IASP and the World Congress, vol 1, Advances in Pain Research and Therapy. New York: Raven Press, 1976:17–28.

49. Beck P, Handwerker H. Bradykinin and serotonin effects on various types of cutaneous nerve fibres. Pflugers Arch 1974;347:209–222.

50. Cashman J, McAnulty G. Nonsteroidal anti-inflammatory drugs in perisurgical pain management. Mechanisms of action and rationale for optimum use. Drugs 1995;49:51–70.

51. Seibert K, Masferrer J, Zhang Y, et al. Mediation of inflammation by cyclooxygenase-2. Agents Actions Suppl 1995;46:41–50.

52. Higgs G, Moncada S. Interactions of arachidonate products with other pain mediators. In: Bonica J, Lindblom U, Iggo A (eds). Proceedings of the Third World Congress on Pain, vol 5, Advances in Pain Research and Therapy. New York: Raven Press, 1983:617–626.

53. Greenberg S, Palmer G. Biochemical basis of analgesia: Metabolism, storage, regulation, and actions. Dent Clin North Am 1978;22:31–46.

54. Pateromichelakis S, Rood JP. Prostaglandin E1-induced sensitization of A delta moderate pressure mechanoreceptors. Brain Res 1982;232:89–96.

55. Ferreira S. Prostaglandins: Peripheral and central analgesia. In: Bonica J, Lindblom U, Iggo A (eds). Proceedings of the Third World Congress on Pain, vol 5, Advances in Pain Research and Therapy. New York: Raven Press, 1983:627–634.

56. Bisgaard H, Kristensen J. Leukotriene B4 produces hyperalgesia in humans. Prostaglandins 1985;30:791–797.

57. Levine J, Lau W, Kwiat G, Goetzl E. Leukotriene B4 produces hyperalgesia that is dependent on polymorphonuclear leukocytes. Science 1984;225:743–745.

58. Otsuka M, Konishi S, Yanagisawa M, Tsunoo A, Takagi H. Role of substance P as a sensory transmitter in spinal cord and sympathetic ganglia. Ciba Found Symp 1982;91:13–34.

59. LaMotte R, Thalhammer J, Robinson C. Peripheral neural correlates of magnitude of cutaneous pain and hyperalgesia: A comparison of neural events in monkey with sensory judgments in human. J Neurophysiol 1983;50:1–26.

60. Wall P. Mechanisms of acute and chronic pain. In: Kruger L, Liebeskind JC (eds). Neural Mechanisms of Pain, vol 6, Advances in Pain Research and Therapy. New York: Raven Press, 1984:95–104.

61. DuBrul E. Sicher's Oral Anatomy. St Louis: Mosby, 1980:391–414.

62. Sessle B. Anatomy, physiology and pathophysiology of orofacial pain. In: Jacobson A, Donlon W (eds). Headache and Facial Pain. New York: Raven Press, 1990:1–24.

63. Bowsher D. Role of the reticular formation in responses to noxious stimulation. Pain 1976;2:361–378.

chapter 4

The Processing of Pain at the Brainstem Level

Now that the normal anatomy and physiology of the peripheral and central nervous systems (CNS) have been described, a more thorough description of the manner by which pain is initiated and processed can be reviewed. An understanding of how noxious impulses are credited in the periphery and are processed by the CNS is essential for the clinician who wishes to manage pain disorders.

The Initiation of Nociception in the Peripheral Tissues

When tissue is injured, the damaged cells release potassium (K+), which initiates the synthesis and release of bradykinin, a nine-amino acid peptide, from large plasma proteins. Bradykinin is a very potent pain-producing substance. Tissue injury also causes the breakdown of arachidonic acid into prostaglandins by the enzymatic action of cyclooxygenase (COX). Arachidonic acid is also converted to leukotrienes by the enzy-

matic action of 5-lipoxygenase (see chapter 2). The presence of these substances activates the A-delta and C fibers in the immediate region of the injury. The initial activation of the A-delta fiber produces a quick volley of afferent nociceptive input into the CNS, signaling a sharp, acute pain. Prostaglandins also sensitize the nociceptors to bradykinin, substance P (SP), and other algesic substances, which now begin to discharge, causing sensitization of the slower conducting C fibers. The pain experience now becomes more of a dull, aching, sometimes burning sensation.

Although the tissue injury may only originally affect one portion of the primary afferent neuron, a series of events often takes place that leads to an expansion of the involved area. This occurs through the antidromic release of algesic substances. When an afferent nerve pathway is discussed, the term *orthodromic* means that the transmission of impulses is passing from the periphery into the CNS. The term *antidromic* means that the pathway of transmission is actually reversed, so that an afferent neuron is functioning in reverse, causing changes to occur in the periphery. This is precisely what occurs at the

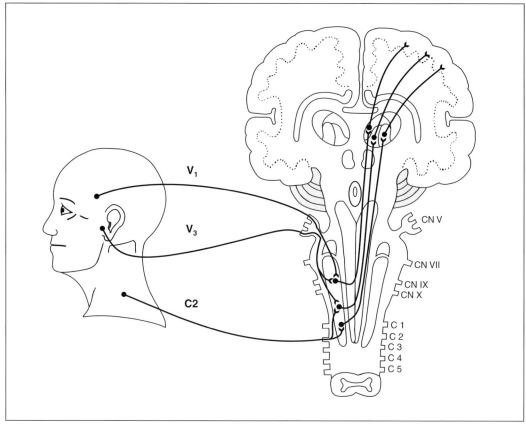

Fig 4-1 A simplified graphic depiction of convergence of the primary neurons in the nucleus caudalis region of the trigeminal spinal tract nucleus. The neuron representing the ophthalmic division (V_1) and the neuron representing the mandibular division (V_3) of the trigeminal nerve converge on the same second-order neuron. The trigeminal spinal tract nucleus extends caudally to the region of the entrance zone of upper cervical nerves. The second cervical nerve (C2) enters this region of the brainstem and converges on both a cervical-input, second-order neuron as well as a second-order neuron that is also receiving trigeminal input.

branches of a primary afferent neuron when a single branch is injured. With injury, SP and calcitonin gene-related peptide (CGRP) are antidromically released in the other peripheral branches of the same afferent neuron (Fig 4-1). SP then causes mast cells in the area to release histamine and the platelets to release serotonin (5-hydoxytryptamine [5HT]). Histamine, CGRP, and 5HT mediate swelling, redness, and heat and increase peripheral sensitivity to further stimulation.[1] This leads to *hyperalgesia* (increased sensitivity to stimulation-evoked pain). As the level of histamine and 5HT increases in the extracellular space, there is more sensitization of neighboring nociceptors, leading to a spreading of the hyperalgesic area.[2] Additionally, SP causes the blood vessels in the area to release more bradykinin into the site of injury, leading to further sensitization. This spreading of the painful area beyond the site of the actual injury is called *primary hyperalgesia.*

The Central Processing of Nociception

Convergence

It has been known for many years that there are more primary afferent neurons entering the CNS than there are second-order neurons to carry the impulses on to the higher centers.[3] It therefore follows that several primary sensory neurons must synapse with a single second-order neuron. The synapsing of several primary afferent neurons with one second-order neuron is known as *convergence*. In the same sense, a single primary afferent neuron can also enter the CNS and synapse with more than one second-order neuron. This condition is called *divergence*. Activity at the synapse may be a cumulative effect, called *summation*. When several afferent neurons simultaneously stimulate the same second-order neuron, the summation is called *spatial*. Summation can also occur when a single neuron stimulates a second-order neuron in rapid succession. This is known as *temporal summation*. Intensification of response is known as *facilitation;* suppression of response is called *inhibition*.

Convergence has been well documented in the trigeminal brainstem sensory nuclear complex. The subnucleus oralis and interpolaris receive extensive convergence of orofacial and muscle afferent inputs[4-13] (Fig 4-2). The same convergence has been shown in the subnucleus caudalis. In fact, in one study[14] of the cat brain, almost all of the neurons with input from the temporomandibular joint (TMJ) received additional afferent input, predominantly from facial skin or intraoral sites. In this same study, 74% of the neurons tested in the subnucleus caudalis showed convergence of tooth pulp and/or hypoglossal nerve afferent inputs. In another study,[15] afferent input from the TMJ and masseter muscle converged on the same second-order neuron in 80% of the nerves that were tested in the subnucleus caudalis. It appears that afferent inputs from deep structures converge to a greater degree than do afferents from cutaneous structures.[16,17] Perhaps this is why pain from deep structures is felt to be more diffuse and less localized than the more localized pain that is felt from cutaneous structures. In fact, deep pains are often very difficult for the patient to locate. As will be discussed in the next section, convergence of nociceptive input can lead to a confusing diagnostic clinical presentation.

Site of Pain Versus Source of Pain

For the clinician to successfully evaluate pain disorders, he or she must appreciate the difference between the site and the source of pain. Although these words are often used interchangeably, they have significantly different meanings. The *site of pain* is the location that the patient feels the pain. The site of pain is easily located by merely asking the patient to point out the region of the body that is painful. The *source of pain* is that area of the body from which the pain actually originates. When the site and the source of pain are in the same location, it is called *primary pain*. Primary pains are very common and likely to be the only type of pain familiar to the patient. When one cuts a finger, the area of tissue damage is also the location of the pain. This is an example of primary pain, since the site of pain (where it hurts) and the source of pain (where it originates) are in the same location. This type of pain makes sense to the patient and the clinician, and therefore therapy is obvious.

There are pains, however, in which the site of the pain is not in the same location as the source of the pain. This type of pain

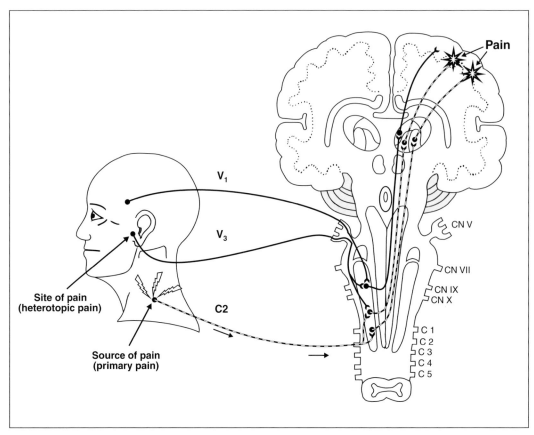

Pain

V₁

V₃

Site of pain
(heterotopic pain)

C2

Source of pain
(primary pain)

CN V

CN VII

CN IX
CN X

C 1
C 2
C 3
C 4
C 5

Fig 4-2 Injury to the trapezius muscle results in tissue damage. Nociception arising in this cervical region is transmitted to the second-order neuron and relayed on to the higher centers for interruption. As this input becomes protracted, note that the adjacent converging neuron is also centrally excited, which relays additional nociception on to the higher centers. The sensory cortex now perceives two locations of pain. One area is the trapezius region, which represents a true source of nociception (primary pain). The second area of perceived pain is felt in the temporomandibular joint area, which is only a site of pain, not a source of pain. This pain is heterotopic (referred).

is called *heterotopic pain.* Heterotopic pains can be quite confusing to both the patient and the clinician. A commonly known heterotopic pain is cardiac pain. When an individual experiences myocardial ischemia, the site of pain is frequently felt in the mandible, in the shoulder, or radiating down the left arm. The source of pain is the myocardial tissues, yet the site of pain is distant from the site. Heterotopic pains pose a significant problem for the clinician. A basic cardinal rule in therapy is that treatment

must be directed toward the source of pain, not the site of pain. Treatments directed toward the site of pain will have little to no effect on the pain. The clinician must therefore be able to first recognize heterotopic pains and then differentiate the site from the source of pain. This is basic to orofacial pain therapy, since heterotopic pains are extremely common in the head and neck regions. Other common examples of heterotopic pain in the head and neck are frontal and temporal headaches from the neck, and ear and temporomandibular joint pain produced from the sternocleidomastoid muscle. Sooner or later, every dental practitioner is confronted with a patient who complains of tooth pain but may not present any objective findings. As will be discussed later, many toothaches do not arise from the teeth at all.

Each clinician must be prepared to accept the fact that pain, especially from deep sources, is frequently felt in structures that are normal. The clinician must therefore guard against extending treatment to such structures in an attempt to control pain until an accurate diagnosis has been made.

Types of Heterotopic Pains

The term *heterotopic pain* refers to any pain that is felt in an area other than its true source. Although the terms *referred* and *heterotopic* are frequently used interchangeably, a more restricted usage of the term referred is advocated. There are three general types of heterotopic pain: *(1)* central pain, *(2)* projected pain, and *(3)* referred pain.

Central pain

Pain that emanates from structures of the CNS is felt peripherally as heterotopic pain. This is especially true of intracranial structures that are insensitive to pain. When a tumor or other disturbance is present in the CNS, the pain is often felt not in the CNS but in peripheral structures. Pain emanating from pain-sensitive intracranial structures on or above the tentorium cerebelli (ie, cerebral vessels) is felt in the peripheral distribution of the trigeminal nerve (ie, migraine).

Projected pain

Projected pain is felt in the peripheral distribution of the same nerve that mediates the primary nociceptive input. Pain resulting from noxious stimulation of a sensory root or a major nerve trunk is felt in the exact anatomic distribution of that nerve. An example is the radicular pain of posterior root compression. It has been assumed that compression due to herniation of an intervertebral disc produces prolonged firing in the injured sensory fibers. It should be noted, however, that acute peripheral nerve compression is usually painless and rarely lasts more than a few seconds. It is likely, therefore, that radicular pain is felt in the peripheral structures through activation of deeper interneurons.[18] The mechanism, however, seems to be different from that of central excitation, in that projected pain follows a more precise anatomic pattern relative to the peripheral distribution, while central excitation pain is felt in a reference zone that is only segmentally related to the primary pain source. Projected sensory nerve pain is primarily neurogenous and follows dermatome mapping faithfully. Examples of projected pain include paroxysmal neuralgia, peripheral neuritis, herpes zoster, and postherpetic neuralgia.

It has long been known that noxious stimulation of a motor root or major motor nerve also induces pain, but of a different type that is felt in different areas. Rather than the bright, burning, neuropathic pain felt in the dermatome distribution, motor nerve pain is sensed as dull, deep somatic pain diffusely located in the muscles innervated by that nerve.[19] Such pain is now explicable on the basis of afferent neurons that are present in the motor nerves. Undoubtedly, such pain should be classified as projected pain, even though it displays a deep somatic rather than neuropathic quality and follows a motor nerve route rather than a dermatome field. Although the neural mechanisms have not been identified, it is likely that interneurons are involved in a manner similar to that for projected sensory nerve pain. It likewise differs from the heterotopic pain of referred pain.

Projected pains may be accompanied by areas of secondary hyperalgesia that are hypersensitive to stimulation without an appreciable reduction in the local pain threshold. Whatever the mechanism responsible for this phenomenon, it is likely similar to that of secondary hyperalgesia of central hyperexcitability, as described in the next section.

Referred pain

Referred pain is a spontaneous heterotopic pain that is felt in an area innervated by a different nerve than the one that mediates the primary pain. Since it is spontaneous, referred pain occurs without provocation at the site of pain and is wholly dependent upon the original source of pain. The reason for this dependence is because the original source of nociceptive input produces a sensitization of interneurons that is responsible for this type of heterotopic pain.[20-25] Since the sensitization of interneurons (also called *central excitatory effects*) is very important in understanding heterotopic pains, it is worthwhile to discuss this phenomenon at this time.

Central Sensitization

The diagnostic differentiation between true primary pain and symptoms that occur as secondary effects of that pain is essential. Such manifestations are usually referred to as *central excitatory effects,* on the assumption that they result from hyperexcitability of CNS interneurons.

The neurologic mechanisms involved in the secondary effects of pain are not fully understood. Some researchers think that reflex activity is involved.[26] There seems to be little doubt that convergence of afferent impulses among CNS interneurons takes place.[9,27,28] However, the factors that control the mechanisms involved have not

been elucidated. Sessle et al[29] have shown that, while primary trigeminal neurons normally respond only to stimuli located within their respective receptive fields, at least half of the second-order nociceptive neurons (ie, wide dynamic range and nociceptive-specific neurons) are activated by electric stimulation applied outside the normal receptive fields of the corresponding primary neurons. The neurons thus activated are presumed to be those that respond to input from deep structures of the mouth and face. This is taken as evidence that the reference of pain occurs in conjunction with deep pain input, rather than a superficial one.[30] It suggests that under certain conditions, trigeminal nociceptive interneurons are subject to subliminal stimulation from structures other than those located in the normal receptive fields. Such evidence supports the convergence theory of pain reference. Gross[31] reported that referred pain due to visceral disease followed known dermatomes, but referred pain from deep somatic structures did not.

Studies[32] demonstrate that the function of a second-order neuron can actually change according to the type and intensity of input that the neuron receives. As discussed in the previous chapter, when a second-order neuron receives a constant barrage of nociceptive input, the cell itself activates cellular genes that change its function to these demands. This induction of early gene expression causes the release of proto-oncogenes called *c-fos* and *c-jun*.[33] The release of these substances by the cell alters messenger RNA (mRNA), which in turn can change the type and number of receptors that are formed on the cell membrane. As the number and type of receptors change, so also does the cell's function. These changes can result in a lowering of the firing threshold of the cell, thus sensitizing it to future stimulation. This is known as *sensitization,* and since the neurons being discussed here are in the CNS, this is referred to as *central sensitization*. The fact that a neuron can react and change function according to its input has only recently been appreciated. This process is called *neuroplasticity* and is nature's way to adapt to environmental demands. Changes such as these can alter the reactivity of the neuron for minutes, days, months, or even years.

Some of the receptors that become involved when sensitization is prolonged are the N-methyl-D-aspartate (NMDA) receptors.[23,34–37] Stimulation of these receptors by excitatory amino acids, such as aspartate and glutamate, further increases the sensitization of the neurons. This increased sensitization can alter neural impulses as they are processed on the way to the higher centers. This is referred to as *central excitatory effects*. When this occurs, even normally nonnoxious input may be misinterpreted at the higher centers.

Clinically, sensitization and central excitatory effects are induced by more or less continuous barrages of noxious sensation emanating from deep somatic structures. If the input is not continuous, these secondary effects are less likely to occur. Increased intensity and duration of the deep pain input enhances the secondary effects. Initially, these changes in neural sensitization are usual and reversible. With chronicity, however, changes may occur that alter the neural processing more permanently. Permanent alterations can lead to chronic neuropathic pain, as will be discussed in chapter 17. The symptoms of central sensitization complicate continuous deep somatic pains, since they increase with the intensity and duration of the primary pain. Such symptoms can occur in otherwise normal structures, and therefore treatment can be misdirected.

The central excitatory effects produced by deep pain input may involve afferent (sensory) neurons, efferent (motor) neurons, and/or autonomic neurons. Each of these effects will now be discussed.

Afferent (sensory) neuron effects

When central excitatory effects are produced in a sensory neuron, the most common clinical finding is pain. The type of pain complaint is either referred pain or secondary hyperalgesia.

Referred pain

Referred pain due to central sensitization is initially wholly spontaneous as far as the site of pain is concerned. It is not accentuated by provocation of the site where the pain is felt; it is accentuated only by manipulation of the primary pain source (see Fig 4-2). It is dependent on continuation of the primary initiating pain and ceases immediately if the primary pain is arrested or interrupted. Anesthesia of the structure where the referred pain is felt does not arrest the pain.[38] Only by anesthesia of the neural pathway that mediates the primary pain can the referred pain be arrested.[39]

It should be noted that although the primary initiating pain is of the deep somatic type, the secondary referred pain may be felt in either deep or superficial structures. This may present a bizarre clinical picture. When reference is felt superficially, it must be differentiated from superficial somatic pain and from projected neuropathic pain. When it is felt deeply, it must be differentiated from other deep somatic pains.

Referred pain does not occur haphazardly, but in fact follows three clinical rules. Referred pain most frequently occurs within a single nerve root, passing from one branch to another. The trigeminal nerve is a good illustration, since it has three major branches. For example, when a mandibular molar presents with a source of pain (eg, caries) it is not uncommon to have the patient report that a maxillary molar is also painful. In this case, the mandibular branch of the trigeminal nerve is referring pain to the maxillary branch of the same nerve.

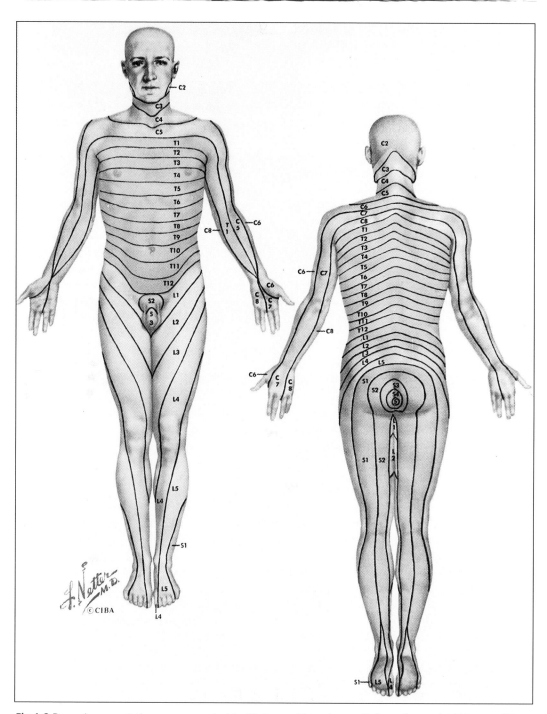

Fig 4-3 Dermal segmentation as represented by Netter and based essentially on the work of Keegan. (From Netter FH. The CIBA Collection of Medical Illustrations. Indianapolis: Curtis, 1953. Used with permission.)

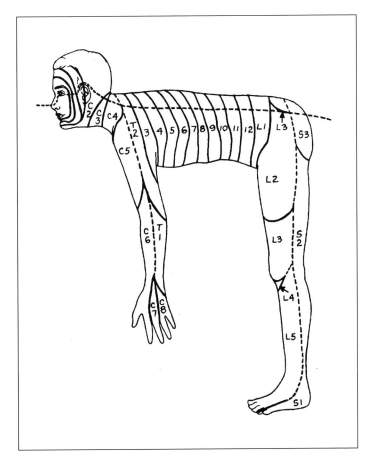

Fig 4-4 The orderly metameric arrangement of dermatomes becomes apparent if we visualize a man in the quadruped position. (From Finneson BE. Diagnosis and Management of Pain Syndromes, ed 2. Philadelphia: Saunders, 1969. Used with permission.)

This is a fairly common occurrence with dental pain. Generally, if the pain is referred to another distribution of the same nerve, it does so in a "laminated" manner. This lamination follows the pattern of the *dermatomes*. A dermatome is a sensory root field on the skin where pain is felt when a particular neural segment mediates a painful sensation. These have been well charted (Fig 4-3). Each nerve has a corresponding dermatome, but there is considerable overlapping. The upright posture of humans causes some confusion in dermatome arrangement, especially in the extremities. They are better visualized with the subject in the quadruped position (Fig 4-4). This places them in a more logical metameric arrangement and helps considerably to identify the proper segmental relationships.[40]

Trigeminal lamination patterns are determined by the manner in which the primary afferent neurons enter in the spinal tract nucleus. According to Kunc,[41,42] the location of trigeminal nociceptive terminals within the nucleus caudalis is as follows:

1. The fibers from tissues near the sagittal midline of the face terminate highest in the nucleus (cephalic).
2. The fibers from tissues located more laterally terminate lowest in the nucleus (caudal).

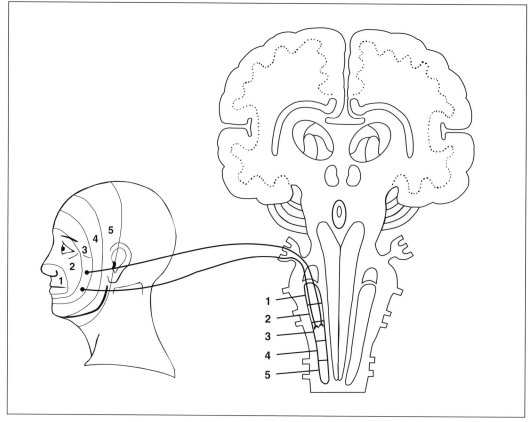

Fig 4-5 Graphic depiction of the spinal trigeminal nucleus and its relationship with incoming sensory input. Note the laminated pattern of innervation from the facial structures into the spinal tract nucleus. These laminated patterns reflect the patterns of referred pain commonly felt in the orofacial structures.

3. The intermediate fibers terminate intermediately in the nucleus (Fig 4-5). This laminated arrangement of facial innervation appears to coincide with Finneson's metameric arrangement of the dermatomes in the quadruped position.[40]

This grouping of the terminals of the primary trigeminal neurons should influence the location of clinical effects of central excitation, especially with regard to referred pain. It probably accounts for some effects not otherwise readily explained. Kawamura and Nishiyama showed that a molar tooth can project pain to a canine, and a canine can project to an incisor, which confirms the vertical lamination just cited.[43]

Simply speaking, this means that incisors refer to incisors, premolars to premolars, and molars to molars on the same side of the mouth. In other words, molars do not refer pain to incisors or incisors to molars.

The second clinical rule is that referred pain in the trigeminal area rarely crosses the midline unless it originates at the midline. For example, pain in the right temporomandibular joint will not likely cross over to the left side of the face, nor will right molar referred pain cross to a left molar. However, this is not true in the cervical region or below. Cervicospinal pain can be referred across the midline, although it most commonly stays on the same side as the source.

A third clinical rule of referred pain is that if the referred pain is felt outside the nerve that mediates the pain, it is generally felt cephalic to the nerve (upward, toward the head) and not caudally. Clinically, this means that deep pain felt in the sacral area maybe be referred to the lumbar area, as well as lumbar to thoracic, thoracic to cervical, and cervical to trigeminal. Rarely will trigeminal pain refer to the cervical region. Only very intense primary pain causes excitatory effects in a segment caudal to the site of initiating input.[44,45]

Secondary hyperalgesia

Hyperalgesia is defined as increased sensitivity to stimulation at the site of pain. Primary hyperalgesia occurs as the result of a lowered pain threshold (sensitization) in the peripheral structures, resulting presumably from the presence of algogenic substances such as bradykinin, potassium, histamine, and 5HT (see chapter 3). Secondary hyperalgesia is different. It is an increased response to stimulation at the site of pain in the absence of any local cause.[46] It may occur with or without accompanying referred pain.

Secondary hyperalgesia is also different from referred pain in that it occurs in response to stimulation (provocation) at the site of pain, while referred pain cannot be increased at the site of pain. It is wholly dependent on the source of pain. Both referred pain and secondary hyperalgesia are initiated by deep pain input and remain dependent upon the continuation of such input. They differ, however, in that secondary hyperalgesia persists for a while

after the primary pain ceases. Thus, analgesic blocking of the primary pain site does not immediately arrest the hyperalgesia as it does referred pain.

As with referred pain, secondary hyperalgesia may be felt in either superficial or deep structures. Superficial secondary hyperalgesia is felt as sensitive skin, scalp, hair, or gingiva. Deep secondary hyperalgesia is sensed as an area of palpable tenderness, discomfort due to functional manipulation, or hypersensitive or tender teeth.

There are two explanations for the occurrence of secondary hyperalgesia. The first is that related to the sensitization of the second-order neuron. As central sensitization occurs, even normal input can be misinterpreted as noxious.[47,48] Therefore, even input carried by the nonnoxious A-beta fibers can be felt as pain. When this occurs, even light touch to the face becomes painful. Pain produced by normally nonpainful stimuli is called *allodynia*.

A second explanation for secondary hyperalgesia is one that addresses a local cause produced by neurogenic inflammation. As discussed in the last chapter, tissue injury initiates the inflammatory process, which in turn sensitizes neighboring neurons. This is called primary hyperalgesia. With central sensitization, the primary afferent neuron can antidromically release excitatory neurotransmitters (eg, SP) into peripheral tissues, increasing the sensitivity of the primary nociceptors (neurogenic inflammation). When this occurs there can be a small central area of hyperemia, indicating some local tissue reaction. In this flare area of an axon reflex, the pain threshold is lowered, thus indicating that this portion of the hyperalgesic area reflects local tissue change. The entire area of sensitivity, however, extends far beyond the hyperemic zone. The wider area represents true secondary hyperalgesia that is dependent on the continuation of primary deep pain impulses.[45] Analgesic blocking of the source of deep pain that is creating the secondary hyperalgesia does not in fact immediately decrease the total discomfort, presumably because of the flare area that is present.[49,50] Anesthetic blocking of the region of primary hyperalgesia will immediately eliminate the pain since the cause is local.

At a clinical level, superficial secondary hyperalgesia usually presents no great problem because there is an obvious lack of local cause. Deep secondary hyperalgesia, however, cannot be distinguished from primary hyperalgesia on the basis of manual palpation or functional manipulation (see chapter 8). Special diagnostic effort is required to make this judgment, which is important therapeutically. It should be noted that palpable tenderness or deep discomfort from functional manipulation identifies only a site of pain, not a source of pain. Whether such an identified site of pain is primary hyperalgesia from a local cause such as inflammation or a heterotopic manifestation of deep pain input located elsewhere is a judgment that must precede definitive therapy.

Efferent (motor) neuron effects

When central excitatory effects alter the function of an efferent neuron, the influence is seen in the muscle innervated by that neuron. There are two effects that may result: muscle co-contraction and the development of myofascial trigger points.

Muscle co-contraction

A common efferent effect secondary to constant deep pain is a reflex excitation of the muscle, which slightly modifies its functional activity[51](Fig 4-6). Deep pain input seems to activate a protective response of muscle to limit the movement of the painful part. This response is normal and likely protective in nature. It does not represent pathology. It is interesting to note that, in the presence of deep pain, the antagonist muscles appear to become activated in an attempt to limit activity of the

agonist muscle.[52,53] This phenomenon is called *co-contraction*[54] and has previously been referred to as *protective muscle splinting.* The exact mechanisms involved will be discussed in later chapters. It is sufficient to say at this time that deep pains that produce central excitatory effects can influence muscle activity.[55]

Myofascial trigger points

Another motor effect of central excitation is the development of *myofascial trigger points*. Myofascial trigger points are characterized by localized areas of hypersensitive bands of muscle tissues found within the body of a muscle. The presence of these trigger points is paramount in the muscle pain condition called *myofascial pain*.[56-58] Continued deep pain of significant intensity can induce the development of myofascial trigger points. The mechanism involved seems to be segmentally related to the site of primary pain. The masseter and temporalis are the masticatory muscles most frequently affected. The trigger point, in turn, refers pain that is frequently felt at or near the site of the initiating primary pain. The trigger itself, however, is usually silent unless manually palpated; then local muscle pain is felt. Although this mechanism may be initiated by pain, once trigger points become established, they remain active or latent until eliminated by therapeutic effort.[57,58] Thus, pain at or near the initial site of primary pain may persist as a continuing or recurrent heterotopic manifestation long after the original pain has ceased. The complexity of such pain problems makes accurate diagnosis all the more necessary for effective management of the patient's complaint. Myofascial trigger point pain will be discussed in more detail in chapter 12.

The muscles that are affected by central sensitization are usually those innervated by the same major nerve that mediates deep pain input, thus establishing a segmental relationship. If the primary pain is medi-

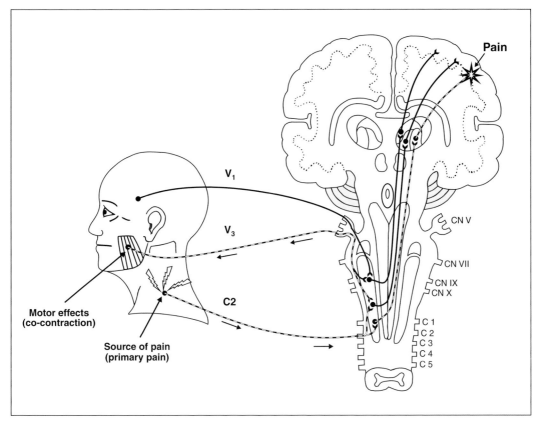

Fig 4-6 Constant afferent nociceptive input can centrally excite efferent (motor) neurons, resulting in co-contraction of associated muscle or the development of myofascial trigger points.

ated by the trigeminal nerve, the muscles most likely to be affected are those innervated by the trigeminal nerve. Eight muscles are innervated by the trigeminal nerve: the masseter, the temporalis, the medial pterygoid, the lateral pterygoid, the mylohyoid, the anterior belly of the digastric, and the tensor muscles of the soft palate and tympanic membrane.

Autonomic neuron effects

Deep somatic pain may induce autonomic effects in an area segmentally related to the site of primary pain. Vasomotor and glandular effects may occur. The symptoms may include temperature and color changes in the skin (flushing, blanching), puffy swelling of the eyelids and other loose cutaneous tissue, injection of the conjunctiva, lacrimation, nasal secretion, and nasal congestion. Such symptoms may simulate allergic rhinitis or maxillary sinusitis.

The autonomic changes induced by deep pain are thought to be central excitatory effects. Their behavior is similar to other such effects and remains dependent upon deep pain input. There is a recovery time lag, however, when the primary pain ceases; the autonomic symptoms may persist for a day or so.

It is believed that the secondary effects caused by central sensitization are the result of a barrage of continuous, deep nociceptive input entering the CNS. It is felt that these changes are all reversible once the source of deep pain is eliminated. On an acute basis, this is certainly true. However, when the duration is prolonged, these neuroplastic changes may not always be reversible. When these changes do not revert to normal, neuropathic pains are experienced. These pains will be discussed in chapter 17.

The Experience of Pain

Until recently, human pain was considered a sensory experience evoked by noxious stimulation of neural structures. The impulses thus generated were thought to be transmitted to the CNS, where they were perceived as pain and reacted to. The reaction was thought to comprise extensive behavior on the part of many body systems. The dominant factors in pain reaction were thought to be on a mental level, such as prior conditioning, evaluative significance of the pain, memory, and emotional response. This perception-reaction hypothesis was originated in the 19th century by Marshall[59] and Strong.[60] It was recognized that great difference in pain reaction was commonplace. Maurice concluded: "The exaggerated reaction is due to psychic factors and is termed psychoneurotic pain."[61] It became popular to think in terms of human discomfort as being organic or psychogenic. Organic pain constituted pain behavior that could be accounted for on the basis of structural conditions. When no structural condition could be found to explain the pain, the clinician labeled it *psychogenic pain.*

During the second half of the 20th century, there was an increased effort by researchers and clinicians to better under-

stand pain. New experiments and observations gave reason to question the validity of the perception-reaction concept of pain. Thus, the currently held concept of pain modulation evolved.

The Modulation Concept

We now appreciate that pain is much more than noxious stimulation of neural structures. It is more than a systemic reaction to unpleasant signals received by the brain. It is more than a choice between organic and psychogenic. Pain comprises all these features in a unified sensory and emotional experience. The concept of pain modulation is based on documented experimental evidence that neural impulses are altered, changed, or modulated as they travel up the neural axis to the higher centers. Excitatory and inhibitory influences bear on the impulses at various levels in the CNS so that perception and reaction become merely facets of the same mechanism rather than separate components of it.

Whether pain is generated by noxious stimulation of tissues or occurs spontaneously is no longer of great concern. Whether pain is the result of injury or of mental processes is of little significance. It is more important to consider the various factors that influence the inhibition and excitation of painful experience. In recent years, worldwide research into pain mechanisms has brought to light much information relative to these factors.

In 1965 Melzack and Wall[62] proposed a new theory to help explain and serve as a model to visualize pain modulation. This they termed the *gate control theory* (Fig 4-7). They brought to the scientific community the first explanation of how neural impulses can be altered or modulated as they

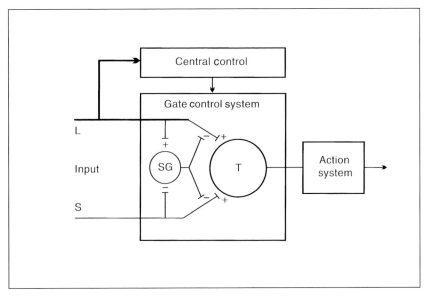

Fig 4-7 Schematic diagram of the gate control theory of pain mechanisms. The fibers (L = large-diameter fibers, S = small-diameter fibers) project to the substantia gelatinosa (SG) and first central transmission (T) cells. The inhibitory effect exerted by SG on the afferent fiber terminals is increased by activity in L fibers and decreased by activity in S fibers. The central control trigger is represented by a line running from the large-fiber system to the central control mechanisms; these mechanisms, in turn, project back to the gate control system. The T cells (second-order neurons) project to the entry cells of the action system. + = excitation; – = inhibition. (From Melzack R, Wall PD. Pain mechanisms: A new theory. Science 1965;150:971–979. Used with permission.)

ascend to the higher center. (Details of the gate control theory will be presented in the next section.) This paper was a landmark article that revolutionized how we look at pain. Although the neurophysiologic mechanisms are still under debate and many uncertainties remain, the theory served to move us from the former perception-reaction concept to the concept of pain modulation. The gate control theory as initially presented was subjected to further elaboration[63] (Fig 4-8). This combined the more obvious sensory-discriminative component of pain with a motivational-affective dimension as an integral part of the pain experience on an anatomic and physiologic

basis. In 1978, Wall[64] reexamined the gate control theory in the light of 13 years of additional neurophysiologic investigation. He confirmed that the substantia gelatinosa did play an important role in organizing the nociceptive input. However, he noted that all nociceptive neurons of the dorsal horn received inhibitory impulses from regions of the brain. He concluded that the theory in its original detail could no longer be sustained, but that the underlying concepts were still valid when restated in a more basic form.

It is now generally agreed that the experience of pain is much more complex than a simple perception-reaction mechanism.

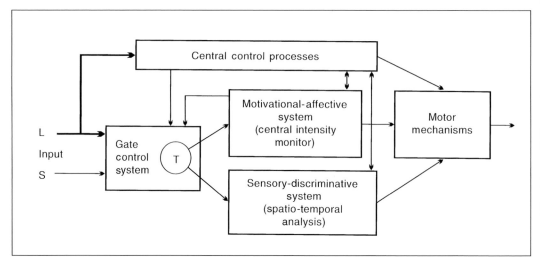

Fig 4-8 Conceptual model of the sensory, motivational, and central control determinants of pain. The output of the transmission (T) cells of the gate control system projects to the sensory-discriminative system (via neospinothalamic fibers) and the motivational-affective system (via the paramedial ascending system). The central control trigger (comprising the dorsal-column and dorsolateral projection systems) is represented by a line running from the large-fiber system to the central control processes; these, in turn, project back to the gate control system and to the sensory-discriminative and motivational-affective systems. All three systems interact with one another and project to the motor system. (From Casey KL, Melzack R. Neural mechanisms of pain: A conceptual model. In: Way EL (ed). New Concepts in Pain and Its Clinical Management. Philadelphia: Davis, 1967:13–31. Used with permission.)

Nor is pain variability explicable on the basis of conduction velocity and other structural features as embodied in the gate control theory, although such factors do, no doubt, have an effect. Perl[65] noted that all somatic sensation is subject to modulation by activity descending from rostral levels and, no doubt, by other factors. For example, it is known that fear augments suffering, as does anxiety or the attention that is directed toward discomfort. It has been demonstrated that the pain threshold is lowered by simply increasing the frequency of stimulation without altering its intensity.[66] Also, myelinated and unmyelinated fibers react differently to temperature change. Within the range of 14°C and 43°C, the firing rate of all myelinated fibers decreases with cooling, while unmyelinated fibers either show no change or actually increase in firing rate.[67] Ernst et al[68] demonstrated that the repetition of dental stimuli significantly increased pain sensitivity. All such evidence confirms that pain is more than a measure of noxious stimulation or threat. Indeed, much if not most pain arises in the absence of noxious stimulation or other identifiable local cause.

The concept of modulation is extremely important in understanding the patient's experience of pain. It is based on the premise that neural impulses rising to the higher centers that are termed "painful" can be altered en route. These impulses can be increased or enhanced, which can accentuate the pain experience. The process of increasing the impulse is called *facilitation*. Under other conditions, the impulses can be reduced or obtunded, which will lessen the pain experience. The process of decreasing noxious impulses is called *inhibition*. Pain modulation explains why in some instances a painful experience may occur without any apparent cause, while in other instances significant tissue damage may produce no pain at all. Presently much research is being directed toward gaining a better understanding of pain modulation, since this may provide valuable insight on therapy.

At this time it is known that pain modulation can occur at various levels of the CNS. The following areas of orofacial pain modulation will be discussed in the following section: the trigeminal spinal tract nucleus, the reticular formation, the descending inhibitory system, and psychologic modulating factors.

Pain Modulation in the Trigeminal Spinal Tract Nucleus

Melzack and Wall's original paper[62] described how nociceptive impulses could be altered in the dorsal horn of the spinal cord. Since the trigeminal spinal tract nucleus is the brainstem extension of the spinal dorsal horn (see chapter 2), it is assumed that the same discussion is true for trigeminal nerve input. The gate control theory suggested that both myelinated and unmyelinated primary afferent neurons converge to synapse with both second-order neurons as well as interneurons in the substantia gelatinosa (lamina II) (Fig 4-9). Both myelinated and unmyelinated primary afferents were proposed to have a direct excitatory effect on the second-order neuron, which they called the *transmission cell* (T cell). Since these T cells carry nociceptive impulses, we now know that they are either a nociceptive-specific neuron or a wide dynamic range neuron. The substantia gelatinosa neurons were proposed to inhibit neurotransmitter release from both primary afferent neurons, thus inhibiting

the impulse carried by the primary afferent neuron. The myelinated afferents were proposed to excite the inhibitory interneurons, which in turn would reduce the activity of the pain transmission neuron. This point is supported by the clinical observation that selective stimulation of large-diameter myelinated fibers produces analgesia. In contrast, activity of the unmyelinated nociceptive neurons was proposed to inhibit the inhibitory substantia gelatinosa cells, resulting in an enhancement of transmission from the primary afferents to the T cell. The result of this action is to increase the nociceptive impulses sent to the higher centers. This action would therefore increase nociceptive transmission to the higher centers.

The clinical relevance of the gate control theory can be demonstrated by a simple injury to the peripheral tissues. If an individual touches a hot stove, the nociceptive reflex immediately withdraws the hand. The nociceptive input caused by the tissue injury ascends to the higher center and pain is perceived. If, however, the individual begins rapidly waving the hand from side to side the pain is reduced or even eliminated. The C-fiber input carrying the nociception is inhibited ("gated out") by the A-beta fiber input associated with the motion. When the individual stops the movement, the pain associated with the burn returns. It is interesting to note that we humans know even instinctively to counterstimulate the injured area to reduce pain. We do this all the time. Melzack and Wall merely verbalized and explained a common human behavior, but they revolutionized the study of pain.

Transcutaneous Electrical Nerve Stimulation

One byproduct of the gate control theory was the introduction of transcutaneous electrical nerve stimulation (TENS) as a thera-

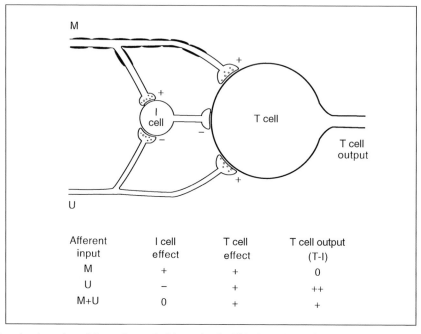

Afferent input	I cell effect	T cell effect	T cell output (T-I)
M	+	+	0
U	−	+	++
M+U	0	+	+

Fig 4-9 A revised version of the gate control hypothesis. This hypothesis focuses upon interactions in the dorsal horn of the spinal cord. *Top:* The four important types of neural elements: the unmyelinated nociceptive primary afferent (U); the myelinated nonnociceptive primary afferent (M); the transmission cell (T cell), whose activity usually results in the sensation of pain; and the inhibitory interneuron (I), which is spontaneously active and whose activity inhibits the T cell, thus reducing perceived pain intensity. The inhibitory interneuron is excited by the myelinated nonnociceptive afferent. The other crucial point is that the unmyelinated nociceptor inhibits the inhibitory interneuron, secondarily exciting the T cell. The unmyelinated primary afferent thus has both direct and indirect excitatory effects on the T cell. *Bottom:* The table shows how perceived pain (T cell output) is the result of a balance of input from myelinated (M) and unmyelinated (U) primary afferents. For example, a stimulus that activates only the M afferents has both a direct excitatory and an indirect inhibitory effect on the T cell. There is no net increase in T cell activity and no pain. A stimulus that activates only the U afferents produces a very large increase in T cell firing because there are both direct and indirect excitatory actions and no inhibition. Most stimuli activate both M and U afferents, producing intermediate levels of pain intensity. (From Fields HL. Pain. New York: McGraw-Hill, 1987:139. Used with permission.)

peutic modality. The mechanisms involved gave considerable insight into pain modulation. Kane and Taub[69] reviewed the history of local electrical analgesia from the time the early Egyptians used electric fish to minimize pain. They related that in 1858, Francis used forceps charged with electricity to extract teeth with less pain. The use of electricity to reduce pain has been "discovered and rediscovered" many times down

through the years. It lay dormant until resurrected by Wall and Sweet[70] in 1967. In 1975, Long and Hagfors[71] reviewed the resurgent use of electricity in various forms in treating some 3,000 patients.

The rationale of TENS is based on the antinociceptive effect of stimulating cutaneous sensory nerves. An interrupted faradic current of very low intensity at a frequency of 50 to 100 Hz is used.[72] The stimulation is usually below what is required to activate A-delta and C nociceptive fibers,[73] and only a tingling or vibratory sensation is felt. Although the antinociceptive effect results from stimulation of thick A-beta fibers,[74] stimulation of A-delta and C fibers also yields the same effect as long as it does not reach noxious levels.[75] The effect is immediate and usually disappears rapidly. Pain relief is localized to the segment stimulated.[72] The effect is not reversed by naloxone, thus indicating that it is not dependent upon the release of endorphins[76-81] (which will be discussed later in this section). Both 5HT and dynorphin are released when superficial cutaneous nerves are stimulated. About one third of all people are nonresponders to TENS.

At a clinical level, the modulating effect of cutaneous stimulation has been known for ages. The almost instinctive act of grabbing, holding, pressing, or rubbing a painful site exemplifies this effect. Many useful pain-reducing remedies are of this category. Massage, analgesic balms, counterirritants, mustard plasters, hot and cold compresses, vibration, hydrotherapy, and vapocoolant therapy are examples.[81,82]

Pain Modulation in the Reticular Formation

As discussed in chapter 2, the reticular formation is a portion of the brainstem that contains a number of nuclei that can either excite or inhibit incoming impulses. The reticular formation therefore controls the overall activity of the brain. Fibers passing through this region of the reticular formation travel on to the intralaminar nuclei of the thalamus. The level of activity of the reticular formation is determined to a great extent by the sensory signals that enter this area from the periphery. Pain signals, in particular, increase the activity in this area and strongly excite the brain to attention.[83]

Activity of the reticular formation is influenced by many brainstem structures as well as incoming impulses. Although many of these influences are not well known, the modulating effect of the reticular formation is likely to be great. There are certain areas of the reticular formation that have concentrated cells (nuclei) that produce certain neurotransmitters. When these neurotransmitters are released, they influence the neural activity in the area. Some neurotransmitters are excitatory and therefore enhance the ascending neural input, while other neurotransmitters are inhibitory, blocking the ascending input. Sometimes these neurotransmitters are quickly released and then quickly destroyed or experience re-uptake by the neuron. When this occurs, the effect of the nucleus is fast acting. Other neurotransmitters are more slowly released and remain in the synapse for long periods of time, which means their actions are long lasting. One can see that the release of neurotransmitters in the reticular formation greatly influence the ascending neural input to the higher centers.

There are several nuclei located in the reticular formation. One such nucleus is the *locus ceruleus*. This area contains a high concentration of cells that produce norepinephrine and is generally thought to excite brain activity. Another area is the *nucleus raphe*, which predominately produces serotonin. This area of the reticular formation usually inhibits brain activity. The *substantia nigra* is another area that produces high concentrations of dopamine. Dopamine seems to play a dual role; in some areas it inhibits brain activity, and in other areas it excites brain activity. The *gigantocellular nucleus* produces high levels of acetylcholine. This area seems to generally excite neural activity. These are only four examples of the many nuclei located in the reticular formation that regulate its function and ultimately brain activity.

Not only does the reticular formation influence ascending impulses on to the thalamus and cortex, but return impulses are also influenced. In other words, impulses leaving the cortex travel down to the thalamus and on through this facilitory area. When this area is activated, these descending impulses are enhanced. Therefore, any time the cerebral cortex becomes activated by either thinking or motor processes, reverse signals are sent back to the brainstem excitatory area, increasing the impulses. This generally provides a positive feedback system that allows any beginning activity in the cerebrum to support still more activity, thus leading to an awake mind.

Pain Modulation of the Descending Inhibitory System

In 1983, while studying nerve injuries in rats, Wall and Devor[84] made a significant discovery. They determined that the peripheral receptor is not the only region of the neuron that can initiate afferent impulses. The dorsal root ganglion cells also initiate sensory impulses. These cells initiate a tonic, low-level, spontaneous background discharge that is propagated orthodromically into the root and antidromically into the peripheral nerve. This source of afferent input may account for nociceptive impulses that persist after peripheral anesthesia. More importantly, this ongoing sensory input from the dorsal ganglia (assumed also to be true of the trigeminal gasserian ganglia) participates in the arousal system, which, if not countermanded, would tend to prevent sleep and perhaps even induce a continuous state of pain. The neural mechanism in the brainstem that appears to balance this continuous barrage of sensory input is called the *descending inhibitory system*. A suitable balance between the ongoing sensory barrage and the descending inhibitory system needs to be maintained for normal functional activities, allowing for adequate provision for periods of rest and

sleep. Should the balance be tilted in favor of increased excitation, the normal background barrage of sensory input would be facilitated, exciting the reticular formation, increasing the level of brain activity. Spontaneous firing may then occur, leading to ongoing activity.[85] Several neurotransmitters are important in the descending inhibitory system, one of the more important being 5HT. As the relationship between the brainstem descending inhibitory mechanism and the ongoing generation of sensory neural impulses by the dorsal ganglia becomes better understood, a more plausible explanation of the intimate pain-insomnia phenomenon may be forthcoming.

The descending inhibitory system is generally thought to affect all sensory input ascending into the brainstem. The portion of this system that affects nociceptive input has been referred to as the *analgesic system*. The analgesic system consists of three major components: the periaqueductal gray matter (PAG), the nucleus raphes magnus (NRM), and a group of descending neurons that terminate in the substantia gelatinosa of the spinal tract nucleus and dorsal horn (see chapter 2) (Fig 4-10). Electrical stimulation in either the PAG or the NRM can almost completely suppress strong nociceptive impulses. Several different transmitter substances are involved in the analgesia system, especially serotonin and the endorphins.

Recent studies have demonstrated that a pain-provoked stimulus in one area of the body can actually raise the pain threshold in another part of the body. Kakigi[86] demonstrated that application of a painful carbon dioxide laser stimulus to the left knee raises the threshold of a noxious thermal stimuli applied to the right hand. The term used to explain this phenomenon is called the *diffuse noxious inhibitory control*. This concept suggests that when a painful stimulus is felt in one portion of the body, the CNS activates a widespread or diffuse system that seems to reduce the transmis-

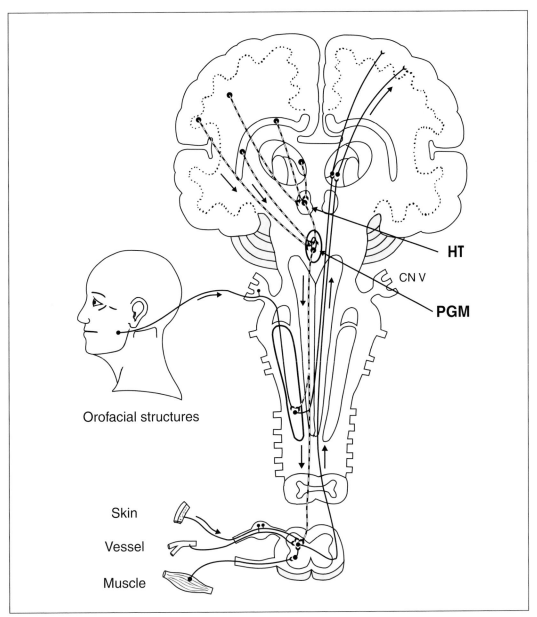

Fig 4-10 A graphic depiction of the descending inhibitory mechanism. Normal afferent input enters the trigeminal spinal tract nucleus from the orofacial structures and the dorsal horn from the rest of the body. The descending inhibitory mechanism *(dashed lines)* descends from the higher centers to the hypothalamus (HT) and periaqueductal gray matter (PGM), which then suppresses ascending input. The inhibition of ascending impulses can occur at the region of the PGM, at the nucleus raphes magnus, or at the synapse of the primary afferent in the substantia gelatinosa of the dorsal horn and the trigeminal tract nucleus.

sion of noxious input from other areas of the body. Perhaps this represents a protective control of the human that enables the individual to focus and respond to one important area of tissue injury, even when multiple sites exist.

The discovery of endorphins in 1975 opened a new avenue in pain research. This knowledge brought considerable insight to the mechanisms of pain modulation. Endorphins were discovered in connection with research seeking an answer to why we have "morphine receptors" in the CNS. The term endorphin is a contraction of the words "endogenous morphine." There are several endorphins, namely, methionine-enkephalin, leucine-enkephalin, alpha-endorphin, beta-endorphin, and gamma-endorphin. The enkephalins and beta-endorphin are particularly associated with antinociceptive mechanisms. No doubt these substances have other functions as well.[87]

Although what is presently known about the endogenous opioid system may be somewhat hypothetic, it appears that there are three families of peptides that bind to three different opioid receptors in the brain and spinal cord, namely, the mu, the delta, and the kappa receptors. The pro-opiomelanocortin (POMC) family includes beta-endorphin and corticotrophin, which bind to mu and delta receptors.[88] The pro-enkephalin A group includes four met-enkephalins, one leu-enkephalin, one heptapeptide, one octapeptide, and several large peptides. These opioids bind to all three receptors. The pro-dynorphin group (pro-enkephalin B group) includes dynorphin, three leu-enkephalins, and several large peptides. These opioids bind to delta and kappa receptors.[89,90] Endogenous opioids are released during highly threatening circumstances. This has been postulated to indicate that the body is able to defensively minimize the distracting effect of pain to facilitate the coping process. Blood levels of beta-endorphin increase following noxious stimulation. Acute pain and relatively se-

vere pain release POMC and pro-enkephalin A peptides in the brain, while dynorphin is released in the spinal cord. Although naloxone blocks the effect of the opioid peptides that bind to the receptors in the brain, which is the site of emotional and conscious sensation, it does not seem to block the action of dynorphin, which binds to the kappa receptors in the spinal cord, where reflex activity takes place. There is considerable multiplicative interaction between the brain and cord opioid receptors and ligands that make up the endogenous opioid system.[89]

The analgesic system appears to be dominant in the modulating effect of nonpainful cutaneous stimulation. Since direct stimulation of the PAG inhibits nociceptive neurons in the nucleus caudalis, and since stimulation of low-threshold mechanoreceptors in the peripheral field also inhibits the response of nociceptive-specific and wide dynamic range caudalis neurons, it is concluded that pain modulation may result from stimulation of the nonnociceptive peripheral sensory fibers and central regions of the brain.[91,92] The nonnoxious stimulation of cutaneous afferents activates neurons of the descending inhibitory system, particularly those of the NRM in the brainstem and the PAG in the midbrain.[93] The stimulation of serotoninergic neurons in the NRM releases serotonin, which reduces stimulation-evoked excitation of nociceptive dorsal horn neurons.[94] In other words, the inhibitory effects at the substantia gelatinosa occur not only by local effects of the primary afferent neurons but also by this descending inhibitory mechanism of the analgesic system.

Sensory responses from tooth pulp stimulation are readily suppressed for 250 to 1,000 ms by stimulation of the PAG and RMN.[95] Stimulation of the RMN reduces or abolishes neuronal responses in the subnucleus oralis and caudalis to nociceptive stimulation of the tooth pulp or cornea.[96] Serotonin appears to be the chief neurotransmitter active in this inhibitory mechanism. In rats, stimulation of the PAG reduces the aversive reaction to pain.[75]

Thus, this analgesic system can block nociception at the initial entry point as well as at other areas in the brainstem as the nociceptive input ascends.

Modulating Effects of Endorphins

The discovery of endorphins revealed the inherent presence of an endogenous antinociceptive system that normally modulates pain. Like the brainstem descending inhibitory mechanism, this endogenous system likely serves other important body functions. Its pain-modulating action may be little more than a spin-off from its other functions. For example, it is known that endorphins play a part in emotional states such as schizophrenia, in matters of addiction, in childbirth,[97] and in sustained physical activities.

Acute pain causes the release of endogenous opioids into the cerebrospinal fluid (CSF) and into the bloodstream. The action of enkephalin is very short, lasting only a few seconds. The action of bloodstream beta-endorphin is delayed by several minutes and lasts for longer periods. Although these actions, no doubt, do have some modulating effect on the pain experience, a sustained clinical analgesic effect requires slow but distinctly intermittent repetition of the pain input at a frequency of 1 to 3 Hz. Continuity of input soon nullifies the antinociceptive effect. The action of endorphins is partially if not completely arrested by the morphine antagonist naloxone.[98] Therefore, any modulating action that is significantly inhibited or arrested by naloxone is presumed to involve the endorphin antinociceptive system. Doubtless there is interaction between the brainstem descending inhibitory mechanism and the endogenous antinociceptive system. Enkephalin is known to inhibit the activity of thalamic projection neurons at postsynaptic sites.[99] Ward et al[100] reported that serotonin has a role in modulating chronic pain only, while beta-endorphin has a role in modulating acute pain only.

Acupuncture and Electroacupuncture

Although acupuncture has been used in Chinese medicine for centuries, it came to public notice in the United States in 1972. Since then, much research has been directed toward this ancient modality of pain control. Needle acupuncture and electroacupuncture, which employs an electric current applied to the skin over acupoints, appear to work in the same general way; both depend on noxious stimulation of specific sites. Both induce the release of beta-endorphin into the peripheral circulation.[89,101-108] Animal studies indicate a similar mechanism.[109,110] Some investigators believe, however, that acupuncture analgesia involves other mechanisms than the release of endorphin.[111,112]

Electroacupuncture differs from TENS in that electroacupuncture requires a current of sufficient intensity to cause pain and phasic muscle contractions, but at a very low frequency (2 Hz). The current must also be applied at specific sites where electrical impedance is low and where deeper nociceptors are available to be stimulated.[72] After an active induction period of about 20 to 30 minutes, the profound analgesic effect of acupuncture can be maintained for an hour or so by intermittent stimulation. After about 4 hours, it drops off substantially and is not truly effective again for 18 to 24 hours. When active stimulation is stopped, the residual analgesic effect drops 50% for each 15- to 17-minute interval.[113] Acupuncture nonresponders include about

15% to 20% of the population. Elsharkawy and Ali[108] demonstrated that acupuncture is as successful as an occlusal appliance in managing symptoms of temporomandibular disorders; however, critical reviews of the literature on acupuncture in dentistry reveal many inconsistencies.[114,115] Further studies are needed to better understand which diagnoses and which patients are the best responders.

Although unrelated to acupuncture, it should be noted that other deep noxious stimulation, such as strong visceral pain, may activate a similar antinociceptive effect.[116] Stimulation of the thalamus also exerts a powerful antinociceptive effect, presumably by way of activated raphe neurons.[117] Other antinociceptive amines, such as gamma-aminobutyric acid (GABA) and glycine, act as inhibitory neurotransmitters and likely are involved in the mechanism of stimulation-produced analgesia.[118]

TENS Versus Acupuncture

Conventional TENS and classic acupuncture are antinociceptive procedures that are mediated by clearly different neural mechanisms. TENS relates to the brainstem analgesic system associated with the descending inhibitory system that releases serotonin, while acupuncture activates the endogenous antinociceptive system that releases endorphins.[119] At the clinical level, however, the two methods of pain control have much in common. Conflicting research reports relative to the action of endorphins in the two methods abound.[107,120–123]

It is true that very low frequency stimulation (2 Hz) causes the release of enkephalins into the CSF and beta-endorphin into the bloodstream. Stimulation at 15 Hz or more causes the release of serotonin in the brain and dynorphin in the spinal cord, but enkephalin is not released. Local anes-

thesia of only the skin arrests TENS but not acupuncture. Only when the more deeply located nociceptive neurons are anesthetized are the effects of acupuncture arrested. Naloxone offsets only about half the analgesic effect of acupuncture, which indicates that more than just endorphins are involved.[109] Acupuncture therapy equals in effectiveness the tricyclic antidepressants for the treatment of depression, thus indicating that it does release serotonin into the CSF in substantial amounts. Taken together, there is adequate evidence that, at least some of the time, acupuncture activates the brainstem descending inhibitory mechanism as well as the endogenous antinociceptive system. The conclusion that should be drawn is that the acupuncture method stimulates superficial cutaneous nonnociceptive neurons at least some of the time, along with the deeper nociceptors located in muscle tissue. Techniques that take this into account should prove superior in clinical value.

Pain Modulation by Psychologic Factors

Some factors that modulate pain fit in a group considered to be psychologic. These factors will be briefly considered here, but a more detailed description can be found in chapter 5. Most psychologic factors are either excitatory or inhibitory.

Excitatory modulating factors

As a rule of thumb, egocentric psychologic conditions that center the subject's attention toward oneself have an excitatory effect on pain. This is borne out especially in the matter of attention. Wall[124] and Melzack et al[125] determined that the level of pain due to injury was directly related to the degree of attention directed toward the injury at the time. This appears to be true for all pains. The more one is absorbed with one's suffering, the more intense it becomes.

Expectancy is another important factor.[126] Whether due to memory, anticipation, or prior conditioning, whatever one expects in the way of pain is likely to be what one experiences.[127,128]

The really potent excitatory modulators, however, are anxiety and fear, products of the consequences of the pain experience. Then, as maladaptive behavior ensues, depression and despair flourish, and chronicity associated with the depletion of endorphins sets in.[129] Problems of neuroticism[130] and secondary gain[126,131] that sometimes accompany suffering may further modulate the pain.

Inhibitory modulating factors

Generally, outgoing psychologic conditions that direct one's attention to energies away from the self have a favorable modulating effect on pain. A feeling of serenity born of confidence and assurance has a marked inhibitory influence. Distraction is particularly inhibitory, as demonstrated by the effect of extraneous sounds,[132] suggestion and hypnosis,[133] mental absorption, and physical activities of different kinds.[134] Overcoming maladaptive behavior by constructively coping with the painful situation has a very favorable modulating influence.

Other Modulating Factors

There are still other factors that can alter the noxious stimulus and ultimately the experience of pain. Factors such as the modality, location, intensity, and duration of the physical characteristics of the stimulus itself have bearing on the discomfort that occurs. This implies that the higher centers receive accurate information concerning the stimulus and act on it by way of efferent

neural circuits. This phenomenon presupposes the organic presence of bypass circuits in the brainstem that permit direct cerebral evaluation of the impulse before it arrives at the nucleus caudalis. Such circuits involving the lemniscal system have been identified.[135]

State-Dependent Sensory Processing

As has been presented in this chapter, the manner by which the CNS receives, modulates, and eventually interprets neural impulses from the peripheral tissues is a highly complicated process. Not only is this complex, but it is also very dynamic, changing according to many factors. Doubell et al[136] have suggested that processing of peripheral input is influenced by the state or mode of the dorsal horn (or spinal tract nucleus) at the moment the input arrives. They summarize the state of the dorsal horn into four modes: normal, suppressed, sensitized, and reorganized. A general understanding of these modes can help one appreciate the dynamic processing of nociceptive input.

Mode 1: Normal

Mode 1 represents the normal state or sensibility of the spinal tract nucleus (dorsal horn), and the processing of input follows the description presented in this chapter. A low-intensity stimulus of sufficient energy to only activate low-threshold primary afferent neurons will produce a sensation that is always interpreted as innocuous. Also, a high-intensity stimulus sufficient to activate high-threshold primary afferent nociceptors but not to produce tissue injury produces a transient localized pain. In mode 1, low-intensity stimuli evoke innocuous sensations such as touch, vibration, pressure, warmth and cool, and high-intensity stimulus pain. This mode operates in healthy individuals and enables a clear distinction to be made between damaging and nondamaging stimuli. The reaction to noxious stimulation, including the elicitation of an unpleasant sensation, is a key physiologic protective mechanism warning of impending tissue damage and eliciting reflex and behavioral avoidance responses.

Mode 2: Suppressed

Mode 2 represents a reduced sensibility of the cells in the spinal tract nucleus. During this state, the processing of somatosensory input from the peripheral tissues is suppressed as a result of the activation of segmental and descending inhibitory mechanisms operating in the spinal cord and brainstem. Under these conditions, a high-intensity stimulus, although it activates nociceptors, fails to result in the sensation of pain. This hyposensibility can have a tremendous survival value, enabling the fight-or-flight reaction in the presence of substantial injury. These inhibitory mechanisms seem to reduce the amount of neurotransmitters released in the synapse, thereby reducing the activation of the second-order neuron. The source of inhibition may be peripheral, such as with TENS or counterstimulation, or may come from higher brain functions such as placebo, suggestion, hypnosis, distraction (ie, descending inhibitory mechanisms). Endogenous opioids likely play an important role in maintaining this mode. Mode 2 can be activated relatively quickly as environmental challenges demand. However, this state is not normally maintained on a chronic basis.

Mode 3: Sensitized

Mode 3 represents a state in which the excitability of the cells in the spinal tract nucleus is markedly increased. In this state, somatosensory input is facilitated or sensitized. A low-intensity stimulus acting via low-threshold afferents now generates pain (allodynia), and noxious input results in a pain response that is augmented in amplitude and duration (secondary hyperalgesia). This mode represents the state of the spinal tract nucleus associated with central sensitization, which was described earlier in this chapter. Mode 3 essentially represents an increase in the gain of the spinal tract nucleus, exaggerating pain responses, in contrast to mode 2, which reflects a decrease in gain, diminishing pain. As with mode 2, mode 3 may also have survival value. An excessive sensitivity, such that low-intensity stimuli begin to initiate pain, can potentially help the individual protect the injured body part from further injury when recuperating from the injury.

It is important to recognize that modes 1, 2, and 3 represent normal functioning of the spinal tract nucleus and dorsal horn. The variation of these modes demonstrates the functional plasticity of the CNS and does not represent disease. Transitions between these three modes occur as a response to the type, intensity, quality, and duration of the peripheral input. The mode by which the spinal tract nucleus processes the input determines how the input is passed on to the higher centers for supraspinal processing.

Mode 4: Reorganized

Mode 4 represents a very different state of neural processing. In this mode there is an actual structural reorganization of the synaptic circuitry in the spinal tract nucleus, which significantly alters the processing of neural input. Axon terminals can degenerate or atrophy, cells can die, new axon terminals can appear, and the structural contact between cells at the synapses may be modified considerably. Such changes occur after injury to the nervous system, both peripheral and central, and contribute to a range of sensory abnormalities, including neuropathic pain. Unlike modes 2 and 3, which tend to be transient, the structural reorganization of mode 4 has functional sequelae that can last long after the initial injury has healed, representing a persistent change in the neural processing of the spinal tract nucleus. As will be discussed more thoroughly in later chapters, neuropathic pains represent a group of orofacial pain disorders that are very resistant to therapies. This is a result in part of our considerable lack of knowledge about how to reverse the processing of input in mode 4 back to mode 1.

Summary

A prerequisite to the perception of orofacial pain sensation is the convergence of peripheral nociceptive impulses, other somatosensory inputs, and especially impulses descending from cortical structures that inhibit the sensory afferents.[137] It should be noted that pain is not a simple conduction of noxious impulses from the receptor through the primary peripheral neuron to synapse in the nucleus caudalis with the secondary medullary neuron, which in turn synapses in a thalamic nucleus with a third neuron that projects to the cerebral cortex, where the impulse is sensed and acted upon. What is sensed as pain may not necessarily arise from noxious stimulation of peripheral receptors or fibers. Normal ongoing somatosensory input that ordinarily would not be perceived at all—or at least not as painful sensation—may be sensed as pain if certain centrally initiated inhibitory influences are not effective. Conversely, the overactivity of such inhibitory influence may cause the subject not to perceive noxious stimulation as pain, even though under normal circumstances the input would unquestionably cause pain. Also, the general intensity of suffering relates to the preconditioning experience, attention, attitude, and temperament of the subject. This phenomenon of central pain modulation requires the organic presence of efferent neural circuits extending from the higher centers. Such circuits have been identified.[138] The central inhibitory mechanism is extremely complex.

Not only does knowledge of modulation of nociceptive impulses help us understand pain better, it also gives important clues that can be useful in the treatment of individuals who suffer with pain.

References

1. Lynn B. Efferent function of nociceptors. In: Belmonte C, Cervero F (eds). Neurobiology of Nociceptors. Oxford, UK: Oxford University Press, 1996:418–438.
2. Reeh PW, Bayer J, Kocher L, Handwerker HO. Sensitization of nociceptive cutaneous nerve fibers from the rat's tail by noxious mechanical stimulation. Exp Brain Res 1987;65:505–512.
3. Ruch T. Visceral sensation and referred pain. In: Fulton J (ed). A Textbook of Physiology. Philadelphia: Saunders, 1947.
4. Sessle B, Greenwood L. Inputs to trigeminal brain stem neurons from facial, oral, tooth pulp and pharyngolaryngeal tissues: I. Responses to innocuous and noxious stimuli. Brain Res 1976;117:211–226.
5. Hayashi H, Sumino R, Sessle B. Functional organization of trigeminal subnucleus interpolaris: Nociceptive and innocuous afferent inputs. Projections to thalamus, cerebellum, and spinal cord, and descending modulation from periaqueductal gray. J Neurophysiol 1984;51: 890–905.

6. Olsen K, Landgren S, Westberg K. Location of, and peripheral convergence on, the interneuron in the disynaptic path from the coronal gyrus of the cerebral cortex to the trigeminal motonerones in the cat. Exp Brain Res 1986; 65:83–97.

7. Olsen K, Westberg K. Interneurons in the trigeminal motor system. In: Steenberghe DV, De Laat A (eds). Electromyography of Jaw Reflexes in Man. Leuven, Belgium: Leuven University Press, 1989:19–50.

8. Sessle BJ, Hu JW. Mechanisms of pain arising from articular tissues. Can J Physiol Pharmacol 1991;69:617–626.

9. Chandler MJ, Qin C, Yuan Y, Foreman RD. Convergence of trigeminal input with visceral and phrenic inputs on primate C1-C2 spinothalamic tract neurons. Brain Res 1999;829: 204–208.

10. Kojima Y. Convergence patterns of afferent information from the temporomandibular joint and masseter muscle in the trigeminal subnucleus caudalis. Brain Res Bull 1990;24:609–616.

11. Dostrovsky JO. An electrophysiological study of canine, premolar and molar tooth pulp afferents and their convergence on medullary trigeminal neurons. Pain 1984;19:1–12.

12. Richardson HC, Cody FW, Paul VE, Thomas AG. Convergence of trigeminal and limb inputs onto cerebellar interpositus nuclear neurones in the cat. Brain Res 1978;156:355–359.

13. Piovesan EJ, Kowacs PA, Tatsui CE, Lange MC, Ribas LC, Werneck LC. Referred pain after painful stimulation of the greater occipital nerve in humans: Evidence of convergence of cervical afferences on trigeminal nuclei. Cephalalgia 2001;21:107–109.

14. Broton JG, Hu JW, Sessle BJ. Effects of temporomandibular joint stimulation on nociceptive and nonnociceptive neurons of the cat's trigeminal subnucleus caudalis (medullary dorsal horn). J Neurophysiol 1988;59:1575–1589.

15. Kojima Y. Convergence patterns of afferent information from the temporomandibular joint and masseter muscle in the trigeminal subnucleus caudalis. Brain Res Bull 1990;24:609–616.

16. Imbe H, Iwata K, Zhou QQ, Zou S, Dubner R, Ren K. Orofacial deep and cutaneous tissue inflammation and trigeminal neuronal activation. Implications for persistent temporomandibular pain. Cells Tissues Organs 2001; 169:238–247.

17. Keay KA, Clement CI, Owler B, Depaulis A, Bandler R. Convergence of deep somatic and visceral nociceptive information onto a discrete ventrolateral midbrain periaqueductal gray region. Neuroscience 1994;61:727–732.

18. Howe JF, Loeser JD, Calvin WH. Mechanosensitivity of dorsal root ganglia and chronically injured axons: A physiological basis for the radicular pain of nerve root compression. Pain 1977;3:25–41.

19. Maeda S, Miyawaki T, Kuboki T, Shimada M. A trigeminal neuralgia-like paroxysmal pain condition presumably due to buccal nerve compression in the temporalis muscle. Cranio 2001;19:56–60.

20. Sessle BJ. Acute and chronic craniofacial pain: Brainstem mechanisms of nociceptive transmission and neuroplasticity, and their clinical correlates. Crit Rev Oral Biol Med 2000;11: 57–91.

21. Kaube H, Katsarava Z, Przywara S, Drepper J, Ellrich J, Diener HC. Acute migraine headache: Possible sensitization of neurons in the spinal trigeminal nucleus? Neurology 2002;58:1234–1238.

22. Eide PK, Rabben T. Trigeminal neuropathic pain: Pathophysiological mechanisms examined by quantitative assessment of abnormal pain and sensory perception. Neurosurgery 1998;43:1103–1110.

23. Ren K, Dubner R. Central nervous system plasticity and persistent pain. J Orofac Pain 1999;13:155–163; discussion 164–171.

24. Bendtsen L. Central sensitization in tension-type headache—Possible pathophysiological mechanisms. Cephalalgia 2000;20:486–508.

25. Graven-Nielsen T, Babenko V, Svensson P, Arendt-Nielsen L. Experimentally induced muscle pain induces hypoalgesia in heterotopic deep tissues, but not in homotopic deep tissues. Brain Res 1998;787:203–210.

26. Procacci P, Zoppi M. Pathophysiology and clinical aspects of visceral and referred pain. In: Bonica JJ, Lindblom U, Iggo A (eds). Proceedings of the Third World Congress on Pain, vol 5, Advances in Pain Research and Therapy. New York: Raven Press, 1983:643–658.

27. Milne RJ, Foreman RD, Giesler GJ. Viscerosomatic convergence into primate spinothalamic neurons: An explanation for referral of pelvic visceral pain. In: Bonica JJ, Lindblom U, Iggo A (eds). Proceedings of the Third World Congress on Pain, vol 5, Advances in Pain Research and Therapy. New York: Raven Press, 1983:131–137.

28. Sessle BJ. Neural mechanisms and pathways in craniofacial pain. Can J Neurol Sci 1999;26 (suppl 3):S7–S11.

29. Sessle BJ, Hu JW, Amano N. Convergence of cutaneous, tooth pulp, visceral, neck and muscle afferents onto nociceptive and nonnociceptive neurons in trigeminal subnucleus caudalis (medullary dorsal horn) and its implications for referred pain. Pain 1986;27:219–235.

30. Cervero F, Laird JMA, Pozo MA. Selective changes of receptive field properties of spinal nociceptive neurons induced by noxious visceral stimulation in the cat. Pain 1992;51: 335–342.

31. Gross D. Pain and autonomic nervous system. In: Bonica JJ (ed). International Symposium on Pain, vol 4, Advances in Neurology. New York: Raven Press, 1974:93–103.

32. Coderre TJ, Katz J, Vaccarino AL, Melzack R. Contribution of central neuroplasticity to pathological pain: Review of clinical and experimental evidence. Pain 1993;52:259–285.

33. Abbadie C, Besson JM, Calvino B. c-Fos expression in the spinal cord and pain-related symptoms induced by chronic arthritis in the rat are prevented by pretreatment with Freund adjuvant. J Neurosci 1994;14:5865–5871.

34. Woolf CJ, Thompson SWN. The induction and maintenance of central sensitization is dependent on N-methyl-D-aspartic acid receptor activation: Implications for the treatment of postinjury pain hypersensitivity. Pain 1991;44: 293–300.

35. Coderre TJ, Melzack R. The role of NMDA receptor-operated calcium channels in persistent nociception after formalin-induced tissue injury. J Neurosci 1992;12:3671–3675.

36. Yu XM, Sessle BJ, Haas DA, Izzo A, Vernon H, Hu JW. Involvement of NMDA receptor mechanisms in jaw electromyographic activity and plasma extravasation induced by inflammatory irritant application to temporomandibular joint region of rats. Pain 1996;68:169–178.

37. Cairns BE, Sessle BJ, Hu JW. Temporomandibular-evoked jaw muscle reflex: Role of brain stem NMDA and non-NMDA receptors. Neuroreport 2001;12:1875–1878.

38. Wolff HG, Hardy JD. On the nature of pain. Pain Res 1947;27:167–179.

39. Kunkle EC, Kibler RF, Armstead GC. Central sensory excitation and inhibition in response to induced pain. Trans Am Neurol Assoc 1949;74:64–74.

40. Finneson BE. Diagnosis and Management of Pain Syndromes, ed 2. Philadelphia: Saunders, 1969.

41. Kunc Z. Significance of fresh anatomic data on spinal trigeminal tract for possibility of selective tractotomies. In: Knighton RS, Dumke PR (ed). Pain. Boston: Little, Brown, 1966:351–363.

42. Kunc Z. Significant factors pertaining to the results of trigeminal tractotomy. In: Hassler R, Albe-Fessard DG, Walker AE (eds). Trigeminal Neuralgia. Stuttgart: Thieme, 1970:90–100.

43. Kawamura Y, Nishiyama T. Projection of dental afferent impulses to the trigeminal nuclei. Jpn J Physiol 1966;16:584–597.

44. Dalessio DJ, Silberstein SD. Wolff's Headache and Other Head Pain, ed 6. New York: Oxford University Press, 1993.

45. Wolff HG. Headache and Other Head Pain, ed 2. New York: Oxford University Press, 1963: 35–47.

46. Treede RD, Cole JD. Dissociated secondary hyperalgesia in a subject with a large-fibre sensory neuropathy. Pain 1993;53:169–174.

47. Cervero F, Meyer RA, Campbell JN. A psychophysical study of secondary hyperalgesia: Evidence of increased pain to input from nociceptors. Pain 1994;58:21–28.

48. Tal M, Bennett GJ. Extra-territorial pain in rats with a peripheral mononeuropathy: Mechanohyperalgesia and mechano-allodynia in the territory of an uninjured nerve. Pain 1994;57: 375–382.

49. Wolff HG, Wolf S. Pain. Springfield, IL: Thomas, 1958.

50. Fields HL. Pain. New York: McGraw-Hill, 1987: 28–40.

51. Broton JG, Sessle BJ. Reflex excitation of masticatory muscles induced by algesic chemicals applied to the temporomandibular joint of the cat. Arch Oral Biol 1988;37:741–747.

52. Stohler CS, Wang JS, Veerasarn P. Motor unit behavior in response to experimental muscle pain [abstract]. J Dent Res 1990;69:273.

53. Stohler C, Yamada Y, Ash MM. Antagonistic muscle stiffness and associated reflex behaviour in the pain-dysfunctional state. Helv Odont Acta 1985;29:719–726.

54. Lund JP, Donga R, Widmer CG, Stohler CS. The pain-adaptation model: A discussion of the relationship between chronic musculoskeletal pain and motor activity. Can J Pharmacol 1991;69:683–694.

55. Carlson CR, Okeson JP, Falace DA, Nitz AJ, Curran SL, Anderson DT. Comparison of psychologic and physiologic functioning between patients with masticatory muscle pain and matched controls. J Orofac Pain 1993;7:15–22.

56. Travell JG, Rinzler SH. The myofascial genesis of pain. Postgrad Med 1952;11:425–434.

57. Travell JG, Simons DG. Myofascial Pain and Dysfunction: The Trigger Point Manual. Baltimore: Williams & Wilkins, 1983.

58. Simons DG, Travell JG, Simons LS. Travell & Simons' Myofascial Pain and Dysfunction: The Trigger Point Manual. Baltimore: Williams & Wilkins, 1999.

59. Marshall HR. Pain, Pleasure and Anesthesia. London: Macmillan, 1894.

60. Strong CA. The psychology of pain. Psychol Res 1895;2:329.

61. Maurice CG. Differential diagnosis of dental pain. J Am Dent Assoc 1955;50:316–327.

62. Melzack R, Wall PD. Pain mechanisms: A new theory. Science 1965;150:971–979.

63. Casey KL, Melzack R. Neural mechanisms of pain: A conceptual model. In: Way EL (ed). New Concepts in Pain and Its Clinical Management. Philadelphia: Davis, 1967:13–31.

64. Wall PD. The gate control theory of pain mechanisms: A reexamination and restatement. Brain 1978;101:1–18.

65. Perl ER. Unraveling the story of pain. In: Fields HL, Dubner R, Cervero F (eds). Proceedings of the Fourth World Congress on Pain: Seattle, vol 9, Advances in Pain Research and Therapy. New York: Raven Press, 1985:1–29.

66. Virtanen ASJ, Huopaniemi T, Narhi MVO. The effect of temporal parameters on subjective sensation evoked by electrical tooth stimulation. Pain 1987;30:361–371.

67. Matzner, Devor M. Contrasting thermal sensitivity of spontaneously active A- and C-fibers in experimental nerve-end neuromas. Pain 1987;30:373–384.

68. Ernst M, Lee MHM, Dworkin BR. Pain perception decrement produced through repeated stimulation. Pain 1986;26:221–231.

69. Kane K, Taub A. A history of local electrical analgesia. Pain 1975;1:125–138.

70. Wall PD, Sweet WH. Temporary abolition of pain in man. Science 1967;155:108–109.

71. Long DM, Hagfors N. Electrical stimulation in the nervous system: The current status of electrical stimulation of the nervous system for relief of pain. Pain 1975;1:109–123.

72. Andersson SA. Pain control by sensory stimulation. In: Bonica JJ, Liebeskind JC, Albe-Fessard DG (eds). Proceedings of the Second World Congress on Pain, vol 3, Advances in Pain Research and Therapy. New York: Raven Press, 1979:569–585.

73. Swett JE, Law JD. Analgesia with peripheral nerve stimulation: Absence of a peripheral mechanism. Pain 1983;15:55–70.

74. Zimmerman M. Peripheral and central nervous mechanisms of nociception, pain, and pain therapy: Facts and hypotheses. In: Bonica JJ, Liebeskind JC, Albe-Fessard DG (eds). Proceedings of the Second World Congress on Pain, vol 3, Advances in Pain Research and Therapy. New York: Raven Press, 1979:3–32.

75. Bowsher D. Role of the reticular formation in response to noxious stimulation. Pain 1976;2:361–378.

76. Sjolund BH, Eriksson MBF. Endorphins and analgesia produced by peripheral conditioning stimulation. In: Bonica JJ, Liebeskind JC, Albe-Fessard DG (eds). Proceedings of the Second World Congress on Pain, vol 3, Advances in Pain Research and Therapy. New York: Raven Press, 1979:587–592.

77. Walker JB, Katz RL. Non-opioid pathways suppress pain in humans. Pain 1981;11:347–354.

78. Freeman TB, Campbell JN, Long DM. Naloxone does not affect pain relief induced by electrical stimulation in man. Pain 1983;17:189–195.

79. Pertovaara A, Kemppainen P, Johansson G. Dental analgesia produced by nonpainful, low-frequency stimulation is not influenced by stress or reversed by naloxone. Pain 1982;13:379–384.

80. Wiler J, Roby A, Boulu P. Comparative effects of electroacupuncture and transcutaneous nerve stimulation on the human blink reflex. Pain 1982;14:267–278.

81. Ellis M. The relief of pain by cooling of the skin. Br Med J 1961:250–252.

82. Steinman JL, Komisaruk BR, Yaksh TL. Spinal cord monoamines modulate the antinociceptive effects of vaginal stimulation in rats. Pain 1983;16:155–166.

83. Bowsher D. Role of the reticular formation in responses to noxious stimulation. Pain 1976;2:361–378.

84. Wall PD, Devor M. Sensory afferent impulses originate from dorsal root ganglia as well as from the periphery in normal and nerve injured rats. Pain 1983;17:321–339.

85. Wall PD. Central control system syndromes: Disorder of sensory systems when the hemostatic set point may be changed [abstract]. Pain 1987;31(suppl 4):217.

86. Kakigi R. Diffuse noxious inhibitory control. Reappraisal by pain-related somatosensory evoked potentials following CO2 laser stimulation. J Neurol Sci 1994;125:198–205.

87. Snyder SH. Opiate receptors and internal opiates. Sci Am 1977;236:44–56.

88. Carr JA, Lovering AT. Mu and delta opioid receptor regulation of pro-opiomelanocortin peptide secretion from the rat neurointermediate pituitary in vitro. Neuropeptides 2000;34:69–75.

89. Kosten TR, Kieber HD. Control of nociception by endogenous opioids. Mediguide Pain 1987;8:1–5.

90. Qiu C, Sora I, Ren K, Uhl G, Dubner R. Enhanced delta-opioid receptor-mediated antinociception in mu-opioid receptor-deficient mice. Eur J Pharmacol 2000;387:163–169.

91. Bradley RM. Basic Oral Physiology. Chicago: Year Book, 1981.

92. Fields HL. Pain. New York: McGraw-Hill, 1987:99–125.

93. Basbaum AT. Brainstem control of nociception: The contribution of the monoamines [abstract]. Pain 1981;11(suppl 1):231.

94. Belcher G, Ryall RW, Schaffner R. The differential effects of 5-hydroxytryptamine, noradrenalin, and raphe stimulation on nociceptive and nonnociceptive dorsal horn interneurons in the cat. Brain Res 1978;151:307–321.

95. Sessle BJ, Hu JW. Raphe-induced suppression of the jaw-opening reflex and single neurons in trigeminal subnucleus oralis, and influence of naloxone and subnucleus caudalis. Pain 1981;10:19–36.

96. Lovick TA, Wolstencroft JH. Inhibitory effects of nucleus raphe magnus on neuronal responses in the spinal trigeminal nucleus to nociceptive compared with nonnociceptive inputs. Pain 1979;7:135–145.

97. Goolkasian P, Rimer BA. Pain reactions in pregnant women. Pain 1984;29:87–95.

98. Seltzer S. Pain Control in Dentistry. Philadelphia: Lippincott, 1978.

99. Dubner R. Specialization of nociceptive pathways: Sensory discrimination, sensory modulation, and neural connectivity. In: Fields HL, Dubner R, Cervero F (eds). Proceedings of the Fourth World Congress on Pain: Seattle, vol 9, Advances in Pain Research and Therapy. New York: Raven Press, 1985:111-137.

100. Ward NB, Bokan JA, Aug J. Differential effects of fenfluramine and dextroamphetamine on acute and chronic pain. In: Fields HL, Dubner R, Cervero F (eds). Proceedings of the Fourth World Congress on Pain: Seattle, vol 9, Advances in Pain Research and Therapy. New York: Raven Press, 1985:753–760.

101. Sjolund BH, Terenius L, Eriksson MBF. Increased cerebrospinal fluid levels of endorphins after electroacupuncture. Acta Physiol Scand 1977;100:382–384.

102. Pomeranz B, Cheng R. Suppression of noxious responses in single neurons of cat spinal cord by electroacupuncture and its reversal by the opiate antagonist naloxone. Exp Neurol 1979;64:327–341.

103. Cheng RSS, Pomeranz BH. Electroacupuncture analgesia is mediated by stereospecific opiate receptors and is reversed by antagonists of type I receptors. Life Sci 1980;26:631–638.

104. Salar G, Job I, Mingrino S. Effect of transcutaneous electrotherapy on CSF beta-endorphin content in patients without pain problems. Pain 1981;10:169–172.

105. Stratton SA. Role of endorphins in pain modulation. J Orthoped Sports Phys Ther 1982;3:200–211.

106. He L. Involvement of endogenous opioids in acupuncture analgesia. Pain 1987;31:99–121.

107. Lee JH, Beitz AJ. The distribution of brain-stem and spinal cord nuclei associated with different frequencies of electroacupuncture analgesia. Pain 1993;52:11–28.

108. Elsharkawy TM, Ali NM. Evaluation of acupuncture and occlusal splint therapy in the treatment of temporomandibular joint disorders. Egypt Dent J 1995;41:1227–1232.

109. Han J, Zhou Z, Xuan Y. Acupuncture has an analgesic effect in rabbits. Pain 1983;15:83–91.

110. Petti F, Bangrazi A, Liguori A, Reale G, Ippoliti F. Effects of acupuncture on immune response related to opioid-like peptides. J Tradit Chin Med 1998;18:55–63.

111. Chapman CR, Benedetti C, Colpitts YH. Naloxone fails to reverse pain thresholds elevated by acupuncture: Acupuncture analgesia reconsidered. Pain 1983;16:13–31.

112. Hsu DT. Acupuncture. A review. Reg Anesth 1996;21:361–370.

113. Research Group of Acupuncture Anesthesia PMC. Effect of acupuncture on the pain threshold of human skin. Natl Med J Chin 1973;3:151–157.

114. Rosted P. The use of acupuncture in dentistry: A review of the scientific validity of published papers. Oral Dis 1998;4:100–104.

115. Ernst E, White AR. Acupuncture as a treatment for temporomandibular joint dysfunction: A systematic review of randomized trials. Arch Otolaryngol Head Neck Surg 1999;125:269–272.

116. Kraus EE, LeBars L, Besson JM. Behavioral confirmation of diffuse noxious inhibitory controls (DNIC) and evidence for a role of endogenous opiates. Brain Res 1981;206:495–499.

117. Dickenson A. The inhibitory effects of thalamic stimulation on spinal transmission of nociceptive information in the cat. Pain 1983;17:213–224.

118. Lovick TA, Wolstencroft JH. Actions of GABA, glycine, methionine-enkephalin, and beta-endorphin compared with electrical stimulation of nucleus raphe magnus on responses evoked by tooth pulp stimulation in the medial reticular formation in the cat. Pain 1983;15:131–144.

119. Chen XH, Geller EB, Adler MW. Electrical stimulation at traditional acupuncture sites in periphery produces brain opioid-receptor-mediated antinociception in rats. J Pharmacol Exp Ther 1996;277:654–660.

120. Boureau F, Luu M, Kisielnicki E. Effects of transcutaneous nerve stimulation (TNS), electrotherapy (ET), and electroacupuncture (EA) on chronic pain: A comparative study. Pain 1981;11(suppl 1):277.

121. Chapman CR, Colpitts YM, Benedetti C. Evoked potential assessment of acupuncture analgesia: Attempted reversal with naloxone. Pain 1980;9:183–197.

122. Peets JM, Pomeranz B. Intrathecal or systemic naloxone antagonizes TNS analgesia [abstract]. Pain 1981;11(suppl 1):179.

123. Takagi J, Sawada T, Yonehara N. A possible involvement of monoaminergic and opioidergic systems in the analgesia induced by electroacupuncture in rabbits. Jpn J Pharmacol 1996;70:73–80.

124. Wall PD. On the relation of injury to pain. Pain 1979;6:253–264.

125. Melzack R, Wall PD, Ty TC. Acute pain in an emergency clinic: Latency of onset and descriptor patterns related to different injuries. Pain 1982;14:33–43.

126. Price DD, Barren JJ, Gracely RH. A psychophysical analysis of experimental factors that selectively influence the affective dimension of pain. Pain 1980;8:137–149.

127. Dworkin SF, Schubert M, Chen AC, Clark DW. Psychological preparation influences nitrous oxide analgesia: Replication of laboratory findings in a clinical setting. Oral Surg Oral Med Oral Pathol 1986;61:108–112.

128. Fordyce WE. Behavioral conditioning concepts in chronic pain. In: Bonica JJ, Lindblom U, Iggo A (eds). Proceedings of the Third World Congress on Pain, vol 5, Advances in Pain Research and Therapy. New York: Raven Press, 1983:781–788.

129. Lindblom U, Tegner R. Are the endorphins active in clinical pain states? Narcotic antagonism in chronic pain patients. Pain 1979;7:65–68.

130. Sternbach RA, Timmermans G. Personality changes associated with reduction of pain. Pain 1975;1:177–181.

131. Sternbach RA. Varieties of pain games. In: Bonica JJ (ed). International Symposium on Pain, vol 4, Advances in Neurology. New York: Raven Press, 1974:423–430.

132. Gardner WJ, Licklider JCR. Auditory analgesia in dental operations. J Am Dent Assoc 1959;59:1144–1149.

133. Orne MT. Hypnotic methods for managing pain. In: Bonica JJ, Lindblom U, Iggo A (eds). Proceedings of the Third World Congress on Pain, vol 5, Advances in Pain Research and Therapy. New York: Raven Press, 1983:847–856.

134. Szechtman FI, Hershkowitz M, Simantov R. Sexual behavior decreases pain sensitivity and stimulates endogenous opioids in male rats. Eur J Pharmacol 1981;70:279–285.

135. Darian-Smith I. The neural coding of tactile stimulus parameters in different trigeminal nuclei. In: Hassler R, Walker AE (eds). Trigeminal Neuralgia. Stuttgart: Thieme, 1970:59–72.

136. Doubell T, Mannion R, Woolf C. The dorsal horn: State-dependent sensory processing, plasticity and the generation of pain. In: Wall P, Melzack R (eds). Textbook of Pain. London: Churchill-Livingstone, 2002:165–181.

137. Hassler R. Dichotomy of facial pain conduction in the diencephalon. In: Hassler R, Walker AE (eds). Trigeminal Neuralgia. Stuttgart: Thieme, 1970:123–138.

138. Wiesendanger M, Hammer B, Hepp-Reymond MC. Corticofugal control mechanisms of somatosensory transmission in the spinal trigeminal nucleus of the cat. In: Hassler R, Walker AE (eds). Trigeminal Neuralgia. Stuttgart: Thieme, 1970:86–89.

chapter 5

The Processing of Pain at the Supraspinal Level

The pathways that carry nociceptive impulses have been mapped out in detail in previous chapters. Factors that influence these incoming and outgoing impulses have also been described (pain modulation). What now needs to be discussed is the effect of nociceptive impulses on the higher brain centers. Remember that nociception is not pain until it reaches and is processed by the higher brain centers. These higher centers are generally known as the *supraspinal structures* (above the spinal cord and brainstem). The significant supraspinal structures that will be considered in this text are the thalamus, the cortex, and the limbic structures (including the hypothalamus). It is only through interaction of these areas of the brain (and many more) that the patient begins to ascribe meaning to the nociceptive impulses. It is the interruption provided by these supraspinal structures that separates us from the lower animals. It is at this level that suffering and pain behavior begin.

Factors That Influence the Pain Experience

Once nociceptive impulses reach the higher centers, the patient judges the pain experience according to at least the following four factors or conditions: *(1)* the level of arousal of the brainstem, *(2)* prior experiences, *(3)* the emotional state, and *(4)* certain behavioral traits. Each of these factors will now be discussed.

Level of Arousal of the Brainstem

As mentioned in chapter 4, the dorsal root ganglion continuously generates an ongoing barrage of sensory impulses that are poured into the central nervous system

(CNS).[1] This constant flow of sensory input can be enhanced by the reticular formation and countered by the descending inhibitory system. This means that there is at all times a ready source of potentially painful neural impulses just waiting for a decrease in the level of systemic inhibitory influence. When inadequately inhibited, these neural impulses are felt as pain, even when there is no peripheral local cause. The ongoing neocortical evaluation of our sensibilities may alter the regulating influence of the brainstem descending inhibitory mechanism so that all shades of modulation, both excitatory and inhibitory, may occur. In other words, if a nociceptive impulse enters a normally calm, well-functioning brainstem, the impulse may never reach the higher centers, and if it did it would not likely initiate a significant response. If, however, the same impulse enters a brainstem with an up-regulated reticular formation and little descending inhibition, the impulse could greatly affect the supraspinal response. This is seen clinically in patients who have suffered with pain for a prolonged period of time. In these individuals, the brainstem is up-regulated, and even seemingly small levels of nociception often produce significant pain responses.

Prior Experiences

Once the nociceptive impulses pass through the brainstem, they move on to the thalamus. The thalamus recognizes these sensory impulses as important and directs them on to the sensory cortex and limbic structures for interpretation. The cortex is responsible for storing all memory of past experiences. It has long been recognized that one's previous pain experience may profoundly influence, if not actually generate, clinical pain. All mammals appear to demonstrate these conditioning effects. Humans are no exception. In fact, humans are subject to auto-conditioning, which can greatly affect their response to pain. The repetition of similar circumstances can generate clinical pain like that associated with a former traumatic experience, even though no actual noxious stimulation occurs. In lesser ways, prior conditioning can influence a wide variety of acute pain complaints. It perhaps forms the basis for *expectancy*, which is an important psychologic modulating factor. Prior conditioning, expectancy, and memory may bear on the peculiar tendency of some pain syndromes to cycle, a phenomenon that is very poorly understood. It is important to recognize such conditions if management is to be effective. It is the cortex that assigns meaning and consequence to the painful experience.

Emotional State

When the nociceptive impulses reach the thalamus, they are directed not only to the cortex but also to the limbic structures. It is at these sites that the pain experience is evaluated on an entirely different level: an emotional level. As discussed in chapter 2, the limbic structures are a group of structures that border the cerebrum and diencephalon. These structures contain certain centers or nuclei that are responsible for specific emotions and behaviors. When pain is perceived by the limbic system, certain emotions can be precipitated. Early on, these emotions may be fear or rage, which represent protective actions in an attempt to move the individual away from the source of nociception. Later, if the pain experience is prolonged, the emotion may change to helplessness, sadness, or depression.[2-6] The emotional state of the individual at the time of pain initiation can greatly influence the pain experience. If the patient is calm, comfortable, and has a sense of well-being, the pain experience is minimized. If, however, the patient is excited, angry, or agitated, the pain experience is enhanced.

Another significant influencing factor is stress. Stress can be thought of as the individual's response to environmental challenges. These challenges may be physical, for example, an automobile that is rapidly approaching while a person is crossing the street. In this situation the individual responds to the challenge with the *alarm* or *stress response*. As discussed in chapter 2, this response is driven by the sympathetic portion of the autonomic nervous system. To rapidly respond to this threat, the sympathetic nervous system quickly increases the blood pressure, blood flow to muscles, and muscle strength. In addition, the sympathetic activity increases certain cellular metabolism and generally increases mental activity. These rapid changes in body functions allow the individual to carry out important tasks—in this example, quickly crossing the street to avoid the oncoming automobile. This response is called the *fight-or-flight reaction*. The body is built to respond to these types of challenges and then return to normal functioning. This response is basic to survival.

Unfortunately, there are some challenges or stressors that are not momentary and therefore continue to elicit a fight-or-flight reaction over time. These prolonged challenges can have a great impact on the functions of the brainstem and higher centers. Many of these challenges are not physical but represent a continued emotional challenge that is present in an environmental situation. For example, an individual is employed in a position associated with significant responsibilities, deadlines, and unhappy coworkers. Although there does not appear to be any immediate physical threat to the individual, these conditions are likely to significantly increase sympathetic nervous system activity. This type of threat is often referred to as *emotional stress*. There is a strong relationship between pain and emotional stress. Sternbach[7] reports that

the greater the stress, the greater the frequency and severity of pain. He reports that stress is a major cause of headaches, backaches, stomach pains, and menstrual pain. The effect of emotional stress on pain, suffering, and pain behavior is enormous and must be considered when evaluating or managing any pain condition.[6,8-12]

Carlson et al[13] and Curran et al[14] have demonstrated that the major difference between patients with masticatory muscle pain and a control group was the patients' sympathetic responses to psychologic stressors. It would appear that these muscle pain patients had up-regulated their sympathetic nervous system so that it reacted more quickly to stressors. This alteration in sympathetic responsiveness is likely to be a significant factor in some chronic pain disorders. The importance of this concept will be discussed in later chapters.

Behavioral Traits

As previously discussed, once nociceptive impulses reach the thalamus, they are directed on to the cortex and limbic structures for interruption. Past experiences stored in the cortex, as well as the present emotional state, will influence the pain experience. However, there is still another dimension to the pain experience that represents direct interaction between the cortex and the limbic structures. This interaction relates to behavior. As mentioned in chapter 2, the limbic structures contain certain centers of neural activities. Among these centers is the pain/pleasure center, which drives the individual toward behaviors that stimulate the pleasure side of the center. These drives are not generally perceived at a conscious level but more as a basic instinct. These instinctive responses result in certain behaviors that present at a clinical level. For example, when an individual experiences chronic pain, behavior will be oriented toward withdrawal from any stimulus that may increase the pain. Often the sufferer will withdraw from life itself, and mood alterations such as depression will appear.

Once the limbic system has emotionally labeled the pain and the cortex has placed meaning and consequence according to past experiences, the individual reacts with a certain behavior. Some individuals may ascribe significant meaning and emotion to the pain and suffer greatly. Others, experiencing the exact same level of pain, may give it little meaning and emotion and not suffer at all.

The four factors that have just been discussed determine the response of the individual to nociceptive impulses. One can quickly understand that the experience of pain is the result of complex interactions in the higher centers. This helps explain why the experience of pain is as individual as people are individual. These functions separate us from the lower animals. In many lower animals, fast pain is the predominant drive for behavior and is heavily related to reflex responses. In the higher animals, slow pain is common, resulting in intense processing of impulses, which gives the pain meaning and consequence and eventually leads to suffering. We do not have evidence that lower animals suffer.

The influence of the higher centers on nociception is commonly referred to as the *psychologic aspect of pain*. These processes have not been well studied, yet they play an extremely important role in clinical pain. Unfortunately the idea is often used as an excuse or avenue of escape by the inexperienced clinician. In other words, all too often when the clinician finds no somatic reason for pain, the patient is believed to have a psychologic problem. I will always remember sitting in a lecture given by Dr Welden Bell when he reported that early in his career he saw many patients with psychogenic pains (personal communication, 1982). Yet at the time of his retirement from practice, some 56 years later, he rarely saw psychogenic pains. This was his way of saying that as a clinician becomes more experienced, he or she begins to understand the many possible diagnoses that exist, and pain disorders begin to make more sense. The inexperienced clinician will often have the tendency to label unknown pains as psychogenic. This leads to inappropriate patient management and can be improved only by educating the clinician.

Psychologic Factors Influence All Pains

Each time nociceptive impulses reach the thalamus, the cortex, and the limbic structures, psychologic factors influence the processing of pain. The clinician must appreciate that all pains, whether brief or long-term, whether somatic or neuropathic, whether slow or fast, are influenced by psychologic factors. Some types of pains are influenced more than others (as will be discussed), but all pains are affected. For the clinician to better understand the patient's pain disorder, one must first begin with an understanding and acknowledgment of the disease model on which he or she is basing therapy. There are two basic medical disease models that are commonly used today: the mechanistic model and the biopsychosocial model.

The Mechanistic Model Versus the Biopsychosocial Model

Most clinicians and patients have been trained to believe that all pains arise from somatic disease or structural damage. This concept makes clinical sense and is reinforced, for example, when one falls and injuries a knee. The damaged tissue causes pain, and once the tissue heals, the pain resolves. This same concept is reinforced in the dental office when a patient reports with a toothache; after the offending tissue (pulp) is removed, the pain is eliminated. This model is known as the *mechanistic model* of disease and implies that when pain is present there is always something wrong with a part of the body (somatic pain). According to this model, all the clinician needs to do to resolve the pain is to find the offending part and repair it. Although this may be appropriate for some somatic pains, it certainly does not represent all pains.

A more accurate way to understand the experience of pain is through the *biopsychosocial model* of disease. This model suggests that the person is a complex unit and that one cannot separate the mind from the body, especially when nociception is being experienced. As nociception enters the CNS from the somatic structures (bio), it passes through the reticular formation and up to the higher centers. The interaction between the higher centers can be thought of as the psychosocial influence on the pain experience. As an example, consider two individuals who both awake one morning with identical pains in the masseter muscles secondary to bruxism. The first individual feels the pain, acknowledges it as soreness from muscle overuse, and goes on with his daily activities. The threat of this pain is minimal and the consequence insignificant. The other individual, however, awakes and feels the pain but has no appreciation of its origin. In considering this pain he remembers that his aunt died 2 years ago from cancer of the jaw. Suddenly the meaning and consequence of this pain become enormous. This individual will begin to suffer, and his pain behavior will quickly drive him to seek care. It is important to recognize that these two individuals are experiencing the same amount of nociception (bio), yet their pain, suffering, and pain behavior (psychosocial) are quite different. It is also important to recognize that the validity of

the belief does not influence the amount of pain and suffering. In other words, it does not matter if the individual actually has cancer; if the individual believes he has cancer, the suffering begins. The biopsychosocial model reflects this pain experience and represents the best model for the clinician who manages pain disorders. This model is especially important when one considers chronic pain (as will soon be discussed).

Figure 5-1 attempts to graphically depict the biopsychosocial model of disease. The "bio" represents the nociceptive input arising from the somatic tissues, and the "psychosocial" component arises from interaction between the thalamus, the cortex, and the limbic structures (supraspinal structures). It is interesting to note that the neurotransmission of impulses between all these higher centers is responsible for what we call the psychologic aspects of pain. In fact, like all neural functions, psychologic factors and moods are based on neurotransmitter activity. Although some cling to the notion that psychologic activity somehow operates independent of somatic structures, there is a preponderance of evidence that points to an organic neural basis for all such activity. Receptors, neurons, synapses, electrical charges, and neurochemicals are the structural elements that underlie all functional activities, psychologic as well as physiologic. Neurochemistry seems to be the key to such mechanisms. One day in a seminar, one of my residents made the following statement: "Psychology is really neurology not yet understood" (P. Bertrand, personal communication, 1993). I believe this is a very profound statement, revealing great insight. Knowledge of neurotransmitter activity is a key in pain management and, in fact, all body functions. Additional neurochemicals are being identified almost daily. No doubt, as these mechanisms are better understood, we will know a great deal more about psychologic behavior and pain.

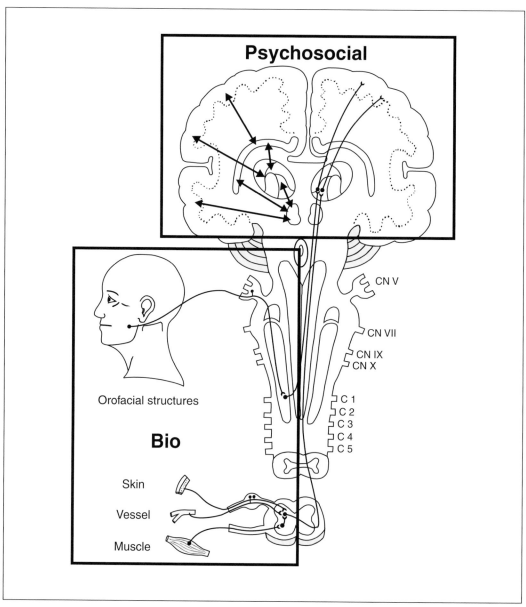

Fig 5-1 A graphic depiction of the biopsychosocial model of disease. The *Bio* is represented by the somatosensory nociceptive input, which arises in the peripheral structures. The *Psychosocial* factors are represented by the interaction of the thalamus, cortex, hypothalamus, and other limbic structures as the nociceptive input enters the higher centers. No pain is perceived without some influence of the psychosocial factors. CN = cranial nerve.

Acute Pain Versus Chronic Pain

Acute pain refers to pains that are of short duration. They are often closely related to somatic tissue changes, such as those produced by trauma or disease. *Chronic pain* refers to pains of long duration, and these pains take on a different therapeutic meaning. Most clinicians use the term to depict any pain that has lasted longer than 6 months, regardless of its origin. Although this is the classic definition, perhaps a better concept of chronic pain would be pains that last longer than a normal healing time. It is expected that tissue damage will produce nociception and pain, but when healing is complete, pain should subside. If pain continues after a normal healing time, the origin of the pain is in doubt. One reason for continued pain is the influence of psychologic factors. As pain becomes protracted, a shift in the origin of the pain can be expected from primary somatosensory input to the affective, cognitive, and behavioral origins of pain. As the duration of pain input continues, the level of suffering increases, even when the intensity of somatosensory input remains the same. In fact, chronic pain can sustain a high level of discomfort, although the intensity of the somatosensory input may decrease or the input may disappear altogether. It follows that a sustained level of discomfort may remain even after the initiating cause has resolved. With chronicity, all pains, regardless of initial type or origin, seem to take on the clinical characteristics of psychogenic intensification. *Psychogenic intensification* refers to the clinical finding that as pains become chronic, the pain experience can intensify, even as the somatosensory input decreases. As such, some chronic orofacial pain disorders display features suggestive of depressive illness. Treatment measures effective for alleviating acute pain may no longer be applicable. As pain becomes chronic, management options shift from local to systemic and central modalities. Pain that initially could be managed on a purely dental level may require extensive and coordinated interdisciplinary therapy when it becomes chronic.

When considering the effects of acute and chronic pains on the biopsychosocial model, the clinician should realize that, early in the pain experience, the somatosensory input (bio) has the greatest influence on the pain experience. As pain becomes protracted, the influence from the higher centers (psychosocial) will likely dominate (Fig 5-2). As already stated, this has therapeutic significance.

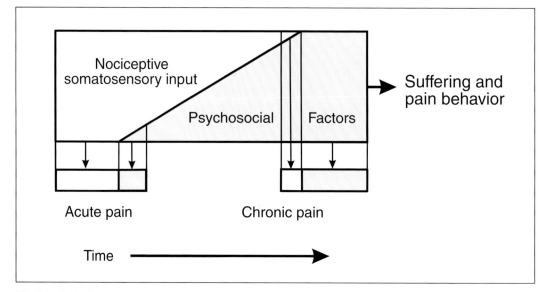

Fig 5-2 Suffering and pain behavior are determined by the interaction of the ascending somatosensory (bio) input with the input from the thalamus, cortex, and limbic structures (psychosocial factors). The longer the pain is present, the greater the influence of psychosocial factors. Acute pain is predominantly influenced by somatosensory input. As pain becomes chronic, suffering and pain behavior are influenced more by psychosocial factors. An understanding of this relationship will greatly improve the selection of effective therapy.

The Emotional Significance of Orofacial Pains

Historically, considerable emotional significance has been attached to pain in that it was once thought to have a beneficial effect on the person who suffered. In the sense that pain represented a penalty or punishment, it served the purpose of a guilt-canceling device and as such was thought to "cleanse the soul."[15] Painful experience therefore has deep religious and moral roots that affect human attitudes even today.

The emotional significance of orofacial pain has important implications, especially in relation to concepts of body image. As therapists, we must never lose sight of the emotional significance of the orofacial structures. The face is the major source of expression, communication, and gratification. We depend on these structures for both physical and emotional survival in our environment. We use these structures to express our feelings to others, providing gratification and satisfaction. We also depend on these structures to bring in nutrients that allow us to exist. Distortion of this image due to abuse, injury, or surgery may initiate a pain experience that has meaning far beyond somatic tissue damage. It is important for the clinician to keep this in mind when approaching a patient with orofacial pain. If the clinician approaches the orofacial structures aggressively, the patients may feel threatened and the pain experience may be heightened. It is best to first establish a rapport with and gain the confidence of the patient and then, with a degree of respect, begin to examine the orofacial structures.

Depending on past emotional experiences, especially those from childhood, one may use pain to gain attention, as a substitute for other forms of aggression, or to express grief.[16] Pain may even be used by the sufferer to gain certain benefits. It commonly excuses one from carrying out an unpleasant task. Headaches, for example, have been used frequently as socially acceptable excuses. Pain may serve as a means of avoiding responsibilities, with the actual physical pain being the lesser of the two forms of suffering. To be the "center of attention" may in some cases be ego-building.[17] Pain, as with other illness, can be used as a weapon or threat against those over whom the subject would have his way. Thus the "victim" not only becomes defenseless against his pain-ridden aggressor but frequently is made to suffer with him. When a patient benefits from his or her pain experience, the patient is said to receive *secondary gains*. Secondary gains can have a significant impact on the effectiveness of therapy.[17] Often patients who receive secondary gains will not relinquish their pain even to what appear to be appropriate therapies until these beneficial issues are addressed.

Pain may also become a dependable crutch to sustain the subject in a variety of emotional situations. In some instances the patient may not even be aware of this emotional crutch (wholly subconscious). It may be a form of malingering to avoid duty. Sometimes it may even represent justification for addiction to narcotic drugs.

Psychologic Considerations of Orofacial Pains

Orofacial pain disorders can be influenced by a variety of psychologic conditions. Sometimes the psychologic factors directly affect an existing physical condition. For example, a patient may be suffering with masseter muscle pain but reports that the pain is much greater on days when things are not going well at work. The physical condition is the muscle pain but when the psychologic factor of emotional stress is increased, the pain experience is intensified. In this instance, the physical condition is the predominant source of nociception, and the psychologic factor is merely a contributor to the pain experience. Other influencing psychologic factors may be anxiety, fear, rage, or certain moods such as depression.[3]

In other patients these psychologic factors may represent significant mental disorders[18] that may actually be the major contributing factor to the pain condition. For example, there are significant mood disorders and anxiety disorders that may present themselves with certain physical conditions (ie, pain). It is important for the clinician to appreciate this, since the therapeutic approach is quite different.

Another mental disorder that needs to be appreciated is *somatization*. With somatoform disorders, an individual may report physical complaints with no evidence of any physical condition. If pain is the chief complaint, the condition is called a *somatoform pain disorder*. Other types of somatoform disorders are conversion disorders and hypochondriasis. Clinicians who are unaware of these disorders will often attempt to treat the patient's physical complaint by directing treatment to the somatic structures associated with the complaint. Since these structures are not the origin of the symptoms, treatment will fail. Other mental disorders that need to be considered are malingering, personality traits or coping style, and maladaptive health behavior. These disorders will be discussed in more detail in later chapters.

References

1. Wall PD, Devor M. Sensory afferent impulses originate from dorsal root ganglia as well as from the periphery in normal and nerve injured rats. Pain 1983;17:321–339.
2. Chapman CR, Turner JA. Psychological control of acute pain in medical settings. J Pain Symptom Manage 1986;1:9–20.
3. Magni G, Marchetti M, Moreschi C, Merskey H, Luchini SR. Chronic musculoskeletal pain and depressive symptoms in the National Health and Nutrition Examination. I. Epidemiologic follow-up study. Pain 1993;53:163–168.
4. Sharp LK, Lipsky MS. Screening for depression across the lifespan: A review of measures for use in primary care settings. Am Fam Physician 2002;66:1001–1008.
5. Fernandez E, Milburn TW. Sensory and affective predictors of overall pain and emotions associated with affective pain. Clin J Pain 1994; 10:3–9.
6. Korszun A. Facial pain, depression and stress: Connections and directions. J Oral Pathol Med 2002;31:615–619.
7. Sternbach RA. Pain and "hassles" in the United States: Findings of the Nuprin Pain Report. Pain 1986;27:69–80.
8. Asmundson GJ, Bonin MF, Frombach IK, Norton GR. Evidence of a disposition toward fearfulness and vulnerability to posttraumatic stress in dysfunctional pain patients. Behav Res Ther 2000;38:801–812.
9. Sherman JJ, Turk DC, Okifuji A. Prevalence and impact of posttraumatic stress disorder–like symptoms on patients with fibromyalgia syndrome. Clin J Pain 2000;16:127–134.
10. Riley JL 3rd, Robinson ME, Kvaal SA, Gremillion HA. Effects of physical and sexual abuse in facial pain: Direct or mediated? Cranio 1998; 16:259–266.
11. Schwartz SM, Gramling SE. Cognitive factors associated with facial pain. Cranio 1997;15: 261–266.
12. Von Korff M, Simon G. The relationship between pain and depression. Br J Psychiatry Suppl 1996 Jun;(30):101–108.
13. Carlson CR, Okeson JP, Falace DA, Nitz AJ, Curran SL, Anderson DT. Comparison of psychologic and physiologic functioning between patients with masticatory muscle pain and matched controls. J Orofac Pain 1993;7:15–22.
14. Curran SL, Carlson CR, Okeson JP. Emotional and physiologic responses to laboratory challenges: Patients with temporomandibular disorders versus matched control subjects. J Orofac Pain 1996;10:141–150.
15. Bonica JJ. The Management of Pain. Philadelphia: Lea & Febiger, 1953.
16. Pilling LF. Psychosomatic aspects of facial pain. In: Alling CC, Mahan PE (eds). Facial Pain. Philadelphia: Lea & Febiger, 1977:213-226.
17. Romano JM, Turner JA, Friedman LS, et al. Sequential analysis of chronic pain behaviors and spouse responses. J Consul and Clin Psych 1992;60:777-782.
18. American Psychiatric Association. Diagnostic and Statistical Manual of Mental Disorders: DSM-IV, vol 4. Washington, DC: American Psychiatric Association, 1994.

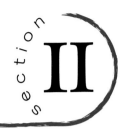

Clinical Considerations of Orofacial Pain

The Various Presentations of Pain

The genesis of pain is poorly understood, if, indeed, it is understood at all. There was a time when it was generally thought that noxious stimulation, meaning tissue-damaging stimulation, was the chief basis for nociception. It was presumed that pain was some kind of gauge of tissue injury: the greater the pain, the greater the injury that had been sustained. Pain occurring without an initiating antecedent was presumed to be generated by psychic phenomena and therefore was not really pain at all.

As the concept of pain modulation evolved, the question of genesis lost much of its significance. It is now recognized that factors other than noxious stimulation are determinants of discomfort. For example, Wall[1] has shown that the degree of pain experienced at the time of injury does not relate to the amount of tissue damage but instead to the attention given the injury. After the initial experience of pain associated with the tissue injury, the amount of continued pain and suffering more closely re-

lates to the consequence of the injury and its treatment. Algogenic substances that accompany inflammation incidental to tissue injury require time to develop and therefore are not immediate determinants in the matter of pain from tissue damage per se. So, structural injury from mechanical, chemical, or thermal trauma, as it relates to the genesis of pain, abounds in uncertainty.

Not All Pains Are Alike

The word *pain* has different meanings to different individuals. Certainly the clinician who attempts to understand and manage pain needs to have a thorough appreciation for the different types of pain that can be encountered. Several types of pains will now be contrasted.

Clinical Versus Experimental Pain

Beecher[2] pointed out that pain as presented by patients—so-called *clinical* or *pathologic pain*—is different from experimental pain induced and studied in the laboratory. The difference is illustrated in the capacity of morphine to give relief. A large dose of morphine does not significantly alter the brief jabs of experimental pain, while a much smaller dose consistently reduces pain that has meaning to the patient. The difference is also borne out in placebo effects. Beecher determined that the average effectiveness of placebos when dealing with clinical pain was about 35%, whereas it was only 3.2% with experimental pain. Nyquist and Eriksson,[3] in commenting on this problem, said, "We interpret our findings to suggest that clinical and experimental pain are explained by different mechanisms and that direct correlations cannot be drawn between them." Bromm[4] believed that experimental pain was actually a measurement of the sensory-discriminative component only, not the aversive-emotional component that is displayed in clinical pain.

It is likely that the emotional significance embodied in clinical pain is the real determinant. Indeed, the purpose of the signal detection (sensory decision) theory for determining the effectiveness of analgesic medications is to minimize this bias factor.[5,6]

gether. Perhaps this increase in pain intensity in the presence of less peripheral nociceptive input may result from a decrease in the effectiveness of the descending inhibitory system (see chapter 4). It follows that a sustained level of discomfort may remain even after the initiating cause has resolved. With chronicity, all pains, regardless of initial type or origin, seem to take on the clinical characteristics of psychologic intensification. As such, some chronic orofacial pain syndromes display features suggestive of depressive illness.[7–9] Treatment measures effective for alleviating acute pain may no longer be applicable. As pain becomes chronic, management options shift from local to systemic modalities. Pain that initially could be managed on a purely dental level may require extensive and coordinated interdisciplinary therapy when it becomes chronic.

It should be noted that there is a definite relationship between intensity and duration of pain. The higher the intensity, the shorter the period that can be tolerated by the sufferer. Low-intensity pain can be sustained for up to 7 hours, whereas maximum-intensity pain can be tolerated for no more than a few seconds. The higher the intensity, the more likely it is that the pain will be intermittent. Only low-intensity pain can be protracted. Intractable pain, regardless of the patient's contention to the contrary, must be either periodic or of extremely low intensity. In fact, intractable pain may be little more than an unpleasant or unwanted sensation.[10,11(pp3–28),12]

Acute Versus Chronic Pain

As the duration of pain input continues, the level of suffering increases even though the intensity of the input remains the same. In fact, protracted input may result in a high level of discomfort, even if the intensity decreases or the input disappears alto-

Primary Versus Secondary Pain

The site where pain is felt may or may not identify the location of the source of pain. If the pain does in fact emanate from the structures that hurt, it constitutes a primary nociceptive input. If, however, the true source of pain is located elsewhere, the area of discomfort represents secondary pain. Secondary pains are called *heterotopic pains* (see chapter 4). The clinical significance of these pains will be described in future chapters.

Stimulus-Evoked Versus Spontaneous Pain

Most primary somatic pains result from stimulation of neural structures that innervate the site. The actual stimulus may be obscure and positive identification difficult, but the clinical characteristics displayed by stimulus-evoked pain relate to the location, timing, and intensity of the stimulus. Some pains, however, occur spontaneously and do not require a stimulating force. Neuropathic pain may be felt spontaneously along the peripheral distribution of the affected nerve, while heterotopic pains may occur spontaneously as far as the site of pain is concerned.

Somatic Versus Neuropathic Pain

Pain emanating from a particular area may result from noxious stimulation of the somatic structures. When this occurs, the nociceptive impulses are being received and transmitted by normal components of the sensory nervous system. Such pain is referred to as *somatic pain*. This type of pain presents with clinical characteristics that relate to the effect of stimulation of normal neural structures. Quite a different type of pain, however, may emanate not from abnormality in the somatic structures but from abnormality in the neural components that innervate the area. Such pain is

termed *neuropathic*. This type of pain presents clinical characteristics that relate to the type and location of the neural abnormality rather than to noxious stimulation as such.

Superficial Versus Deep Somatic Pain

Pains emanating from the cutaneous and mucogingival tissues present clinical characteristics that are similar to other exteroceptive sensations. They are precisely localized by the patient and relate faithfully to provocation in timing, location, and intensity. In contrast, pains resulting from stimulation of deeper musculoskeletal and visceral structures resemble other proprioceptive and interoceptive sensations. As such, they are more diffusely felt, respond less faithfully to provocation, and frequently initiate secondary effects such as referred pain.

Musculoskeletal Versus Visceral Pain

All deep somatic pains are not alike. Deep somatic pains that emanate from muscles, bones, joints, tendons, ligaments, and soft connective tissue bear a close relationship to the demands of biomechanical function. Such pain also yields a graduated response to noxious stimulation. Visceral structures, however, are innervated by high-threshold receptors, so that pain usually is not felt until the threshold level is reached. Such pains therefore do not ordinarily yield a graduated response to noxious stimulation and are less responsive to biomechanical function.

Normal Neural Activities: Central and Peripheral Mechanisms

With the discovery of the normal ongoing barrage of afferent signals generated in the dorsal root ganglia and the countered action of the brainstem descending inhibitory mechanism, a better concept of pain inception and accentuation has developed. It is known that peripheral nerve injury accentuates the normal ongoing barrage of afferent signals.[13] Likewise, it is known that nonpainful sensation conducted by the superficial cutaneous nerves effectively accentuates the inhibitory activity of the descending mechanism, thus shifting the balance away from painful sensation experience. This activity has been more broadly called the *diffuse noxious inhibitory control*[14] (see chapter 4). There is good reason to presume that most, if not all, exteroceptive sensory input, including that of the special senses, has a similar counterbalancing effect on the dorsal ganglion source of sensory impulses.

The important issue here is that central mechanisms may actually be the chief factor in the inception of pain, rather than any peripheral input. Indeed, pain may be felt in the absence of noxious stimulation when the descending inhibitory mechanism is deficient, when the ganglionic barrage is accentuated, or both. Likewise, little or no pain may be sensed from otherwise painful causes when the descending mechanism more effectively acts to arrest the passage of impulses to the higher centers. It is known that both peripheral and central influences affect the action of this inhibitory mechanism.[14-16]

There are many possibilities, both peripheral and central, that may exert an influence on what is felt as pain. We are just beginning to learn the significance of these factors. The antinociceptive action of superficial stimulation (for example, pressure, massage, analgesic balms, vibration, thermal applications, hydrotherapy, counterirritation, transcutaneous electrical nerve stimulation) is quite well known. The inhibitory effect of distraction, physical activity, and calm serenity as contrasted with the excitatory effect of attention, fear, anxiety, and consequences very likely also involves activity of the descending inhibitory mechanism and the diffuse noxious inhibitory control.

With the discovery of the axon transport system and the antidromic passage of neurotransmitters and other neurochemicals peripherally, a better understanding of the importance of the neurogenic component of inflammation is developing (see chapter 4). Since cutaneous effects of wheals (edema) and flare (hyperemia) are now known to result from such antidromic activity,[17] the intimate relationship between neural activities and inflammation makes it difficult to decide what part of an inflammatory process generates pain and what part is actually the result of pain. In other words: Is the muscle painful because of local tissue reasons such as overuse, or is the central nervous system (CNS) responsible for the muscle soreness by way of antidromic neurogenic inflammation? This is an important question that must be appreciated and understood by the clinician, since the treatment of these two conditions is very different.

Inflammatory Pain

The traditional concept of noxious stimulation as the initiating origin of pain stems from an inflammatory process. Tissue injury initiates an inflammatory reaction that characteristically induces pain. The symptoms relate to the conditions that prevail, such as: *(1)* the kind, extent, and location of injury; *(2)* the reactivity of the injured structures; *(3)* the degree of confinement of the inflammatory exudate; and *(4)* the phase of inflammation.

Inflammatory pain is due chiefly to the action of prostaglandins and bradykinin, substances released by the inflammatory process. They act in conjunction with each other to increase local vasodilation and capillary permeability as well as alter the sensitivity and receptivity of receptors in the area[18-23] (see chapter 4). Thus, the pain threshold is lowered so that nociceptors become more sensitive to stimulation, and higher-threshold mechanoreceptors are sensitized to a wider variety of stimuli. As a result, spontaneous primary pain and stimulation-evoked primary hyperalgesia take place. Along with these local effects, there is a prostaglandin-like substance released in the CNS that sensitizes nociceptive interneurons to mechanical and chemical stimuli and renders neural pathways related to inflammatory pain more sensitive to the action of opiates. This has been called *prostaglandin hyperalgesia.*[24]

Pain of inflammatory origin may involve different kinds of tissue innervated by receptors with different reactive responses. For example, superficial pain may be inflammatory, such as that of dermatitis or gingivitis. Examples of musculoskeletal inflammatory pain are those of myositis and cellulitis. Visceral inflammatory pain may be expressed as that of lymphadenitis or arteritis. Inflammatory neuropathic pain may be manifested as neuritis. Many physical ailments are inflammatory, and pain of the inflammatory type is part of the symptom complex.

It should be noted that inflammation due to local tissue injury is a normal immune response that initiates the healing process.[25] The pain generated by inflammation functions to alert the subject to its presence. This type of pain exerts a protective inhibitory influence on biomechanical activity, and it serves to monitor the progress toward recovery of the injured part. Inflammation therefore should be looked upon as a protective and beneficial body function. Failure of the immune system to respond appropriately invites disaster. Artificial suppression of the inflammatory process to minimize pain may be counterproductive therapeutically. The recognition of inflammatory pain should alert the examiner to the need for cause-related therapy.

Noninflammatory Pain

It is likely that noninflammatory pain is a much more common source of suffering than inflammatory pain. This concept, however, is certainly not the traditional approach to explaining pain. Most clinicians have been trained to establish a diagnosis that ends in "itis" (eg, tendonitis, gastritis, otitis). This suggests that the tissue or organ described is inflamed. This is certainly not true of many pain disorders. By this time it is hoped that the reader has an appreciation for the many conditions that exist in the somatic tissues and CNS that may create pain in the absence of inflammation.

It is useful to diagnostically separate inflammatory pains from noninflammatory pains because of their different clinical presentations and courses. As previously stated, true tissue inflammation is a result of an immune response that causes certain changes in local tissues, such as reddening, increased temperature, and edema. Inflammation follows a relatively predictable time course, getting worse and then, with healing (with or without therapy), getting better. Most pains do not show these characteristics, at least not at the clinical level, and are therefore considered to be noninflammatory pains. For example, in this text neurogenic inflammation will not be considered in the category of a true inflammatory disorder, since it does not seem to present with the obvious local clinical symptoms associated with inflammation. It is acknowledged that this separation may not be distinguishable or appropriate; however, it does offer some diagnostic advantages.

Noninflammatory pain may originate from somatic (*soma* is Latin for body) or neurogenous structures. Some of the more common disorders and features of these two categories will be presented here, with a more complete description to follow in future chapters.

Somatic Pain

Somatic pains are pains that originate from body structures and may be divided into two main types: superficial and deep.

Superficial somatic pains

Superficial somatic pains have their origin in cutaneous tissues of the skin or the mucogingival tissues of the mouth. These tissues provide information from the environment.

Deep somatic pains

Deep somatic pains originate from all of the structures that are located deep within the envelope, with the exception of the neural structures. Deep somatic structures are either musculoskeletal structures or visceral structures (the supply system). Within these two categories fall some of the most common pains of human suffering, specifically, muscle pains and vascular pains.

Musculoskeletal pains

Noninflammatory muscle pain is the most common type of somatic pain, and yet it remains very poorly understood. A great deal of mystery continues to shroud myogenous pain in general; this affects clinicians and patients alike. Without a good understanding of this pain one cannot effectively manage the patient's complaints. Muscle pain may frequently occur in relationship to systemic responses. Some pains are a result of a protective response called *co-contraction* (formally called muscle splinting). Co-contraction may result from any alteration in sensory or proprioceptive input. It also may be a response to deep pain or even the threat of injury. If this condition is protracted, *delayed-onset muscle soreness* (or local muscle soreness) may result.

Another painful muscle condition is *myofascial trigger point pain*. This type of pain is characterized by localized areas of hypersensitive bands of muscle fibers called trigger points. These trigger points often produce heterotopic pains that dominate the patient's complaints.

Occasionally muscle pain may originate from a combination of peripheral factors and the CNS. This may induce contraction of the entire muscle, called a *myospasm*. When muscle pain becomes protracted, myositis may dominate in the clinical presentation. True muscle inflammation, however, is rare unless associated with trauma or other injury.

An additional type of muscle pain may originate solely from the CNS. This condition is termed *centrally mediated myalgia* and is dependent on the neurogenic inflammation produced antidromically by the central mechanisms.

Musculoskeletal pains also include the articular surfaces of joints and their associated structures. Various types of arthritides can be a source of deep pain. When discussing orofacial pains, the temporomandibular joint becomes the joint of interest.

Visceral pains

Visceral pains originate from tissues associated with the supply system. Structures that are of concern in the orofacial region are visceral mucosa (sinus), tooth pulps, and glandular, ocular, and auricular structures. Vascular tissues of the orofacial structures may become painful secondary to inflammation. Such conditions are called *vasculitis* and *arteritis*. The greatest source of vascular pain, however, comes from neurogenic inflammation of the vessel walls. Since the origin of the neurogenic inflammation is the afferent nerve that innervates the vessel wall, this type of pain is termed *neurovascular pain*, also called *migraine*. Migraine may likely represent one of the most common pain complaints known to humans.[26] Unfortunately, vascular pain continues to be poorly understood by health professionals. Gross[27] has shown that blood vessels are innervated by afferent neurons of both the somatic and visceral nervous systems. Nociceptive impulses arising from vascular structures therefore may be mediated by either or both of these pathways.

It was originally thought that neurovascular pain was initiated chiefly by dilation of small arteries, which distorted and noxiously stimulated afferent fibers in vascular and perivascular tissues. Vasoconstricting medications such as ergotamine tartrate, which reduce the dilation and amplitude of pulsation of arteries, decrease the pain. Pressure applied to the carotid artery also diminishes the pain.[11(pp3–28)] The presumption, however, that vasodilation is the primary cause of neurovascular pain is no longer tenable, because spontaneous dilation of cranial arteries does not cause pain in normal subjects. Rather, dilating drugs provide relaxation of arteries but do not cause pain. Only algogenic substances such as bradykinin and histamine can evoke vasodilation and pain.[28] It is more likely that a neurogenic inflammation within the trigeminal neurovascular complex is re-

sponsible for this type of neurovascular pain (see chapter 16).

Systemic factors, more than local factors, seem to play the major role in the incidence of neurovascular pain. These pains seem to occur more commonly in certain "pain patients," called *hypernoceptors*, who are thought to have some deficiency in opioid peptides and neurotransmitters of the antinociceptive system.[28] Serotonin deficiency in the CNS has been identified with the incidence of neurovascular pain.[29-32] Administration of histamine to known "migraine patients" consistently precipitates an attack of pain, while nonmigrainous persons do not react in this way.[33] Patients with neurovascular pain frequently display a characteristic emotional overlay with personality features of insecurity with tension.[34] This may be manifested as inflexibility, conscientiousness, meticulousness, perfectionism, and resentment. Frustration, fatigue, and prostration seem to set the stage for an attack.[11(pp3–28)] In the light of serotonin depletion, which also characterizes depressive states,[35,36] the emotional symptoms and the pain may simply represent different facets of a common problem.[37-39]

Early on, Wolff[11(pp3–28)] described four conditions that seemed to contribute to the discomfort of neurovascular pain: *(1)* dilation of blood vessels, *(2)* local edema of the painful site, *(3)* edema of the vessel wall and perivascular tissue, and *(4)* associated muscle pain (especially in the occipital area). It has been shown that attacks of migraine without aura (see chapter 16) display accompanying increased electromyographic activity in pericranial muscles.[40,41]

It appears that tension-type headache (commonly associated with myofascial pain) and neurovascular headache (especially migraine without aura) have much in common.[28,42] The clinical complaint frequently comprises elements of both varieties of pain. It is likely that the systemic factors in these conditions stem from a common cause, and the peripheral symptoms may represent little more than different facets of a common problem. The psychologic implications of both conditions therefore are of great importance.

Since neurovascular pain appears to be originating in the vessel, it is perfectly logical to consider this a type of visceral pain. However, recent information alters our original view of this most common and complex type of pain. It appears that the phenomenon of neurovascular pain begins with a triggering of a trigeminal neurovascular mechanism. Since the initiating factor appears to be associated with neurogenic mechanism, the classification of migraine will be discussed in this text under the category of neurovascular pain disorders (see chapter 16).

Neuropathic Pain

Some clinical pains arise from abnormalities in the neural structures themselves and are therefore called *neuropathic pains.* Neuropathic pains can be confusing to the clinician, since the clinical examination in the area of the reported pain reveals no somatic tissues changes. The clinical examination reveals no reason for the pain condition. The novice clinician is likely to jump to the conclusion that this is a psychogenic pain. An understanding of neuropathic pain is fundamental in the management of orofacial pains since it is common in the head and neck. These pains may be divided into two groups, according to their presentation: paroxysmal neuropathic pains and continuous neuropathic pains.

Paroxysmal neuropathic pains

Some neuropathic pains have a clinical course that reveals very high and sudden levels of pain, followed by periods of total remission of symptoms. These sudden electrical-like volleys of pain are typically felt in the exact distribution of the involved nerve. These shock-like pains are called *paroxysmal pains* and are usually momentary and severe. They are often triggered by relatively mild mechanical stimulation at a site in the peripheral distribution of the same nerve involved in the neuralgia. The pains are often recurrent, with no pain experienced between the episodes. Paroxysmal neuralgias are named for the nerve that is affected, for example, trigeminal neuralgia (originally known as *tic douloureux*).

Paroxysmal trigeminal neuralgia is one of the most painful conditions known to humans, yet it remains an enigma to many health professionals. It is thought that paroxysmal neuralgic pains are closely associated with demyelination of the nerve fiber. Myelination of peripheral neurons helps to isolate the transmission of impulses within the single neuron. Transfer of signals from one neuron to another normally takes place only at synapses. If the myelin sheath is lost, however, neural impulses can be transferred to a neighboring neuron. Kerr[43] observed that demyelination of peripheral neurons can lead to the ephaptic transmission of impulses. (An *ephapse* is a point of lateral contact, other than a synapse, between nerve fibers across which impulses are conducted directly through the nerve membranes from one fiber to the other.) Experimental demyelination leads to antidromically propagated extraction potentials, as well as some post-discharge activity followed by refractory periods.[44] Short-term peripheral nerve compression is usually painless and rarely lasts more than a few seconds.[45,46] Continued compression causes local demyelination without a loss of axonal continuity. Chronic nerve entrapment causes demyelination initially, followed by progressive axonal degeneration. In traumatic neuroma, ephaptic cross-excitation may be a factor in the generation of pain.[47]

Fig 6-1 Transverse section through the posterior rootlet of the human trigeminal nerve that illustrates an area of unusually abundant unmyelinated fibers and several myelinated fibers (original magnification × 10,000). (From Kerr FWL. Fine structure and functional characteristics of the primary trigeminal neuron. In: Hassler R, Walker AE (eds). Trigeminal Neuralgia: Pathogenesis and Pathophysiology. Stuttgart: Thieme, 1970. Used with permission.)

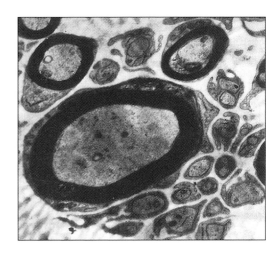

Fig 6-2 Proliferative degenerative changes in a myelinated fiber in trigeminal neuralgia (original magnification × 10,700). (From Kerr FWL. Pathology of trigeminal neuralgia: Light and electron microscopic observations. J Neurosurg 1967;26: 151–156. Used with permission.)

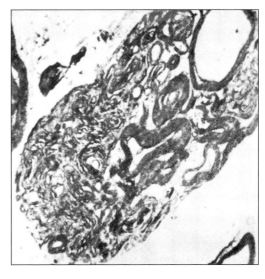

It is therefore widely accepted that trigeminal neuralgia is associated with demyelination of axons in the gasserian ganglion, the dorsal root, or both (Figs 6-1 and 6-2).[48-53] The cause of the demyelination can be associated with constant and chronic pressure from an adjacent structure. It has been suggested that this condition may be related to an aberrant branch of the superior cerebellar artery that lies on the trigeminal nerve root.[54-56] It may also be caused by an aneurysm,[57,58] a posterior fossa tumor,[59-63] a cerebellopontine angle tumor,[64-67] any other expanding lesion, and even brainstem diseases from strokes.[68] When other symptoms are present, the clinician must investigate these potential causes. For example, if an intracranial tumor is responsible there may be a diminished corneal reflex, masseter muscle weakness, facial muscle weakness, or hypoesthesia. Another cause of trigeminal neuralgia that needs to be considered is multiple sclerosis.[69,70]

Continuous neuropathic pains

As this category suggests, continuous neuropathic pains present as an ongoing, unremitting pain condition. The intensity of the pain may increase or decrease but will never completely go away. Continuous neuropathic pains fall into one of the following three categories: metabolic polyneuropathies, neuritis, or deafferentation pains. Some of these conditions may be enhanced by local sympathetic activity and are therefore called *sympathetically maintained pains*.

Metabolic polyneuropathies

Continuous neuropathic pain can arise secondary to a metabolic condition. Since the metabolic condition is systemic, many neurons can be affected in multiple sites. When this occurs, the general term used is *metabolic polyneuropathy*. Much controversy exists regarding the exact mechanisms by which a systemic condition can create nociception, but often demyelination is suspected. The neuropathy is named by the condition that has created it. The literature describes many different metabolic polyneuropathies, but only the more common ones will be discussed in this text. Some of the more common polyneuropathies that the clinician should be aware of are diabetic neuropathies,[71] hypothyroid neuropathies,[72] alcoholic neuropathies,[73] and nutritional neuropathies.[74] Each of these conditions will be presented in more detail in chapter 17.

Neuritis

Neuritis, sometimes referred to as *neuritic neuralgia,* is clinically characterized as an ongoing, unremitting, burning sensation in the peripheral distribution of the affected nerve.[11(pp3–28, 652–655),75,76] The distribution of neuritic pain closely follows dermatomes, which have been previously described (see chapter 4). The symptom picture depends on the fiber population of the nerve as well as on the kind and degree of involvement of each fiber type. Other sensory, motor, and autonomic symptoms may therefore accompany the complaint of pain. Neuritis pains can be of four general types: peripheral neuritis, herpes zoster, postherpetic neuralgia, and entrapment neuropathies.

Like many other clinical pain disorders, the neural mechanism of a peripheral neuritis is poorly understood. It is usually presumed that an inflammatory condition of the nerve is responsible for the production of nociception impulses. The reason for such inflammation may be obscure. Metabolic and toxic disorders as well as neurovascular phenomena and viral infections are possible etiologic agents.

Herpes zoster is one of the more commonly known types of neuritis.[75,76] It is generally agreed that the pain of herpes zoster stems from a viral infection of the ganglion, dorsal root, or medullary tract of the involved nerve. The threshold of C fibers is lowered, thus making them more sensitive to nociceptive stimuli. The reactivity of A-delta fibers, however, appears to be partially or completely abolished.[77]

The exact pathogenesis of herpes zoster is not known,[78] but it is caused by herpesvirus varicella.[11(pp8–23),48,79–82] It is thought that the virus travels to the dorsal root or ganglion during primary varicella infection, where it remains latent within neurons until the immune response of the host falls below a critical level.[83] At that time it becomes activated and fulminates, especially under conditions of local trauma or malignancy or when other therapy utilizes steroids, irradiation, or antimetabolites. Herpes zoster appears to be the unmasking of a latent virus that, when activated, travels along the peripheral nerve to produce active disease. It is thought that chicken pox can be contracted from a patient with herpes zoster, but not vice versa.[84]

Approximately 10% of patients who suffer with herpes zoster seem to progress into a clinical condition known as *postherpetic neuralgia.*[83,85,86] Fifty percent of zoster patients over 60 years of age also seem to progress to the same condition.[78,87] Postherpetic neuralgia is a much more severe and lasting pain condition. The mechanisms and management will be discussed in chapter 17.

Deafferentation pains

Crushing or cutting a peripheral nerve induces anesthesia by interrupting the afferent impulses. This loss of afferent input into the CNS is called *deafferentation*. Although one might assume that terminating afferent input could only result in anesthesia, clinical case reports reveal that a variety of other symptoms may develop. As strange as it might appear, one of these symptoms may be pain. It is possible, therefore, to have a patient report a painful area of the tissue that is numb (called *anesthesia dolorosa*). The understanding of this condition has greatly curtailed the ablative procedures once performed to eliminate pain.

Since it is part of a cell, a damaged peripheral sensory axon causes reactions in other peripheral and central cells that are in functional communication with the damaged neuron.[88] Deafferentation pains seem to arise from both peripheral and central mechanisms.[89-91] Some deafferentation pains seem to have a greater input from the periphery, while others seem more centrally mediated. Although it may be difficult to determine the precise mechanism for any given pain condition, it may be therapeutically important to separate peripheral origins from central origins. Therefore deafferentation pains can be divided into two types: peripheral neuroma pain (eg, traumatic neuralgia, stump pain) and centrally mediated neuropathic pain (eg, phantom limb pain, atypical odontalgia).

The neural changes that take place as the result of peripheral deafferentation affect both the peripheral axons and the central terminals. Cutting the nerve peripheral to the dorsal ganglion arrests the afferent barrage of impulses and halts the movement of transport substances. Only limited anatomic degeneration takes place in the central terminals of the afferent fibers.[92] Some sprouts may find their proper neurilemma tubes, and relatively normal reinnervation may ensue. However, in other cases, the regenerating axons may not find their proper neurilemma tubes. They may bundle into a disorganized, random overgrowth of intertwined extraneural and intraneural tissue and Schwann cells. Such a mass of newly developed neural tissue is called a *neuroma*. The neuropathic pain that results is thought to be largely to the result of ephaptic transfer of neural impulses generated by pressing or stretching the nerve tissue mass.[93,94] Sprouts and axons peripheral to the site of damage become sensitive to norepinephrine,[95,96] which is generated by activity in the sympathetic efferents. They also possibly become sensitive to acetylcholine.[97] Retrograde shrinkage of axons proximal to the site of damage slows conduction velocity. Degenerative changes in the dorsal ganglion cells and central terminals yield an abnormal, unbalanced input. Sprouting produces an increased number of small fibers proximal to the injury. In the dorsal horn, nearby intact afferents appear to have the ability to excite cells formerly dominated by the cut afferents, and spinal cord cells begin to respond to the nearest intact afferents. Thus, the sensory receptive field is enlarged.[88]

The peripheral effects of deafferentation may be chiefly attributed to alien innervation and mismatch and to sensitization of peripheral axons to autonomic activity. The central effects relate primarily to the loss of C-fiber function, which normally maintains organization of the cord with respect to inhibitory mechanisms and the size of receptive fields. Deafferentation therefore markedly reduces normal inhibitory influences and enlarges the receptive fields.[92,98]

The discovery by Wall and Devor[13] that dorsal ganglion cells normally initiate and maintain an ongoing, low-level background barrage of afferent signals may help to elucidate deafferentation phenomena. They observed that this ganglionic source of afferent input increases considerably in response to peripheral nerve injury. Since the clinical symptoms of deafferentation are masked by the normal sensibility of sufficient regenerated neurons, depending on the extent and manner of such regeneration, there may be some regression of deafferentation symptoms when adequate regeneration takes place.

Deafferentation of peripheral nerves may induce various sensory symptoms, which include paresthesia, dysesthesia, hyperesthesia, hyperalgesia, and spontaneous pain. Symptoms may be felt not only in the region of the initial anesthesia but also in a considerably larger area. Anesthesia dolorosa and phantom pain are examples. Deafferentation effects have been identified following the extraction of pulps from teeth,[99] minor oral surgery,[100] and endodontic therapy.[101] Alling[102] reported that, according to a national survey, dysesthesia of the lingual nerve occurred once per 1,756 patients, with 13% persisting longer than 1 year, while dysesthesia of the inferior alveolar nerve occurred once in 241 patients, with 3.5% persisting longer than 1 year. Goldberg et al[103] reported that, in 500 consecutive procedures in private practice, dysesthesia occurred in 1.2% of the cases, but only one persisted longer than 6 months. Wofford and Miller[104] reported dysesthesia of 15 inferior alveolar nerves and 4 lingual nerves following the removal of 576 impacted mandibular third molars. All the dysesthesias except that of one lingual nerve resolved within 6 months. Of 52 inferior alveolar nerves with altered sensation following sagittal ramus osteotomy and mandibular advancement, Upton et al[105] reported that 53.8% returned to normal (meaning that 46.2% did not). Although some phantom pains may originate from peripheral nerve injury,[106] some do not.[107] This finding reveals the complexity of deafferentation pain conditions.

Sympathetically maintained pains

In certain circumstances, continuous neuropathic pains can be influenced by the local efferent activity of the sympathetic nervous system. Evidence of this condition is demonstrated by the clinical observation that a regional blockade of the sympathetic nervous system in certain patients can produce immediate and complete relief of the pain.[108,109] Likewise, electrical stimulation of the sympathetic nervous system in some patients can increase painful conditions.[110] It should be noted that, in normal patients, sympathetic blockade does not reduce pain, nor does stimulation of sympathetic neurons produce pain. With this understanding it is now appreciated that the sympathetic nervous system may actually enhance and/or maintain the continuous neuropathic pain condition. When this occurs the condition, is called a *sympathetically maintained pain.*

Most sympathetically maintained pains begin with some type of peripheral tissue damage.[111,112] This tissue damage excites the C fibers, and nociceptive impulses are carried into the CNS to synapse with a second-order neuron such as a wide dynamic range (WDR) neuron.[112] During healing, the WDR neuron can become sensitized, which reduces its threshold so that even normal activity of the low-threshold, myelinated mechanoreceptors (A-delta and A-beta) can be perceived not as pressure or touch but instead as noxious (ie, hyperalgesia or allodynia). The neuroplasticity seen in the WDR neuron can continue to maintain the hyperalgesic state, even after healing of the tissue is complete (see chapter 17).

Normal efferent sympathetic activity results in the release of norepinephrine at the peripheral receptor sites in the target organ. In the cutaneous tissues, this is predominantly the capillaries. Under normal conditions, this release of norepinephrine does not affect primary sensory neurons. However, if the primary neurons have been sensitized by neuroplastic changes, this release of norepinephrine can excite the A-delta and A-beta receptors, which continue to excite the WDR neurons, thus developing a self-maintaining loop. It is thought that even normal sympathetic activity (sympathetic tone) can be responsible for maintaining the pain. Certainly any increase in sympathetic activity would likely increase the pain condition. One can quickly appreciate that increased levels of emotional stress would likely aggravate this condition.

The most common pain described by patients with this condition is one of a burning quality. This condition was originally called *causalgia*. The term was used to describe pain associated with major nerve injury. Later, the term *reflex sympathetic dystrophy* was adopted to describe a group of clinical presentations associated with minor nerve injury. The most recent attempt to categorize these pain conditions is *chronic regional pain syndromes*. These conditions will be described in detail in chapter 17.

Other Causes of Orofacial Pains

Intracranial Pain

Primary intracranial head pain is rare. The parenchyma of the brain, including the vessels found within it, most of the dura and pia-arachnoid, the ependymal lining of the ventricles, and the choroid plexuses, are not sensitive to pain. The great venous sinuses and their tributaries from the surface of the brain, parts of the dura at the base, the dural arteries, and the cerebral arteries at the base of the brain are sensitive to pain. Stimulation of intracranial pain-sensitive structures on or above the superior surface of the tentorium cerebelli results in pain felt in the trigeminal distribution, whereas stimulation on or below the inferior surface of the tentorium cerebelli results in pain felt in the distribution of the glossopharyngeal and vagus cranial nerves and the upper cervical spinal nerves. Intracranial pain results from the following[12]:

1. Traction on veins that pass from the surface of the brain to the venous sinuses, on the middle meningeal arteries, and on the large arteries at the base of the brain and their main branches
2. Displacement of the great venous sinuses
3. Distension and dilation of intracranial arteries
4. Inflammation of pain-sensitive structures of the head
5. Pressure by such lesions as tumors on nerves containing afferent pain fibers

Brain tumors may cause pain by encroachment on pain-sensitive structures or by reason of pressure or weight. Malignant tumors may involve neural structures directly. Brain tumors involving the trigeminal root and ganglion may be divided into four groups[113]:

1. Cerebellopontine angle tumors usually do not cause typical trigeminal neuralgia. Of 44 cases of meningioma, Nguyen et al[114] reported that nine had ipsilateral intermittent sharp lancinating pain somewhat similar to trigeminal neuralgia. They reported that the common symptoms associated with the pains were ipsilateral trigeminal nerve deficits, hearing loss, and occasional ipsilateral facial muscle weakness. Hypoesthesia is considerably more common than pain.
2. Middle cranial fossa tumors may cause high-intensity paroxysms of 10 to 15 minutes' duration. Usually the pain, if any, is a sustained aching and burning sensation associated with areas of hypoesthesia.
3. Extracranial tumors that invade the ganglion from beneath may cause prolonged

high-intensity paroxysms of burning pain. Anesthesia also may be the result.

4. Tumors arising from the outer layers of the ganglion cause a neuritic type of pain accompanied by other sensory and motor signs. Usually other nerves are simultaneously involved. Such pain is nonparoxysmal.

Neoplasm Pain

Benign tumors may be quite painless unless they encroach on pain-sensitive structures by their mass or weight and, as such, induce somatic-type discomfort. Malignant neoplasms may induce pain by somatic encroachment as well as by neural involvement.[115] Thus, cancer may induce a chronic structural pain syndrome.

The Contribution of Neuroplasticity to Chronic Pain Conditions

In recent years some extremely important insight has been gained that helps us better understand chronic pain. We now know that there can be changes in the manner by which the second-order neurons process neural impulses entering the CNS. As discussed in earlier chapters, the primary afferent neuron carries impulses into the CNS to synapse in the nucleus caudalis with the second-order neuron, which carries the impulses on to higher centers. The second-order neuron may be a WDR neuron or a nociceptive-specific neuron. If there is continued stimulation of the primary afferent neuron (C fiber), there will also be continued production of excitatory

neurotransmitters in the synapse, such as substance P,[116] neurokinin A,[117] somatostatin,[118] and calcitonin gene-related peptide.[119] The continued presence of these neurotransmitters can alter the sensitivity of the second-order neuron. This alteration in the neuron is further increased with the release of certain excitatory amino acids, such as glutamate and aspartate.[120,121] These amino acids activate the N-methyl-D-aspartic acid (NMDA) receptors located on the second-order neurons.[122] The NMDA receptors are involved in the induction and maintenance of the central sensitization of the dorsal horn neurons. In other words, with continued nociceptive input, the second-order neuron becomes increasingly sensitized, allowing the next impulses to depolarize the neuron even more quickly. This change in the processing of second-order neuron is called *central sensitization* or *neuroplasticity.*

As a second-order neuron becomes sensitized, it not only responds more quickly to the next impulse, but it also responds faster to the other converging neurons. Therefore the receptive field from where the impulse originates begins to widen or broaden. When a WDR neuron becomes sensitized, the normally nonnoxious impulses carried by the A-delta and A-beta fibers can be misinterpreted as nociceptive. This phenomenon may be responsible for certain hyperalgesic and allodynic states (for example, light touch to the face producing an extremely high level of pain).

It is now known that electrical stimulation of C fibers located in cutaneous tissues can create an increase in the activity of the dorsal horn neurons that lasts up to 10 minutes longer than the stimulation itself.[123] This is even more dramatic when deep structures are stimulated. When rat muscles are noxiously stimulated, the dorsal horn nociceptive neurons remain activated or sensitized for up to 50 minutes after the stimulus has been terminated.[123] It is now becoming evident that once the

NMDA receptors are activated, the processing of impulses by the neuron can change, and this change may actually result in a permanent sensitization of the neuron. If this neuroplasticity is prolonged or permanent, primary nociceptive input is no longer needed for pain. The clinical findings, therefore, would reveal a patient who continues to report pain and suffering, yet the examination fails to find any somatic tissue damage that might explain the pain. This, in essence, is chronic pain.

The concept of neuroplasticity has certainly changed the way we evaluate and manage pain. Its ramifications are enormous. For example, if any tissue damage produces neuroplasticity that lasts far longer than the stimulus itself, then the potential for permanent neuroplastic changes is always a risk. If this is true, then one could certainly appreciate the benefit of local anesthetic each and every time tissue is to be surgically injured. In the dental office this is generally the normal procedure. This, however, is not the case in the operating room. When a patient is placed under general anesthesia, the nociceptive impulses created at the surgical site are blocked from reaching the cortex at the brainstem level. Therefore the C fibers stimulated at the site of the surgical trauma carry the nociceptive impulses into the dorsal horn (or spinal tract nucleus) and excite the second-order neurons. This nociceptive input is allowed to sensitize these neurons, creating neuroplasticity, even though the anesthetized patient feels no pain. Upon awakening, the patient feels an increased postoperative pain secondary to the sensitized second-order neurons. With this in mind, it seems very logical that postoperative pain and perhaps even chronic pain disorders can be minimized by the use of local anesthetic that blocks nociceptive input at the surgical site in conjunction with general anesthetics.[124]

An understanding that neuroplasticity can contribute to any pain condition is basic to pain management. A protracted toothache risks a chance of becoming an ongoing pain condition even after the tooth has been extracted. We now realize that pain can no longer be thought of as a simple symptom that resolves with proper management of somatic tissues. Pain can actually be the disease itself. With this in mind, the importance of immediate management of acute pain becomes obvious and relevant.

Other Considerations

Pain may result from numerous causes other than specific inflammatory conditions or other myogenous, vascular, or neuropathic phenomena. Pain may occur spontaneously with no identifiable cause of any kind. It may constitute an integral part of pathologic and pathophysiologic conditions of all types. Alterations in the endogenous antinociceptive mechanisms may occur. A degree or so of elevation in body temperature may induce pain in many structures. The general response to abnormal endocrine, metabolic, emotional, allergic, or toxic conditions may include a component of pain. Direct noxious stimulation by various mechanical, thermal, and chemical insults may induce pain. Cutaneous structures are sensitive to all such stimuli. The periosteum is especially reactive to compressive force; ligaments and fascia respond to distortion, strain, and traction; tendons and muscle tissue are particularly sensitive to torque and stretching. Glands react especially to pressure, while hollow viscera are sensitive to distention. Some structures are not pain-sensitive at all, for example, articular surfaces of joints and the parenchyma of the brain.

Headache is perhaps the most frequent of all regional pain complaints. Most intermittent head pains are heterotopic manifestations. Being secondary in type, most such headaches are not as much a diagnostic concern for the pain itself as for the primary sources of deep somatic pain that initiate them.

Psychologic intensification of pain is a normal modulation phenomenon. If pain is intensified until it continues in the absence of significant peripheral input, a state of pain chronicity becomes evident. The psychogenic component of chronic pain syndromes of all types becomes a significant management problem. Pains may be the result of conversion hysteria or the painful hallucinations of schizophrenia.

Some pains result from therapeutic efforts. Although such phenomena may relate to the modulating effects of management, there are instances when dental or masticatory therapy directly initiates a pain problem. Treatment based on an incorrect or incomplete diagnosis may terminate this way. Therapy applied at the site of heterotopic pain rather than at the true source may cause injury. Injudicious occlusal grinding may increase the sensitivity of teeth. Alteration of the occlusal relationship may initiate pain involving muscles and temporomandibular joints, as well as the teeth and periodontal structures. Any procedure (even if it is corrective and otherwise beneficial) that alters the proprioceptive and sensory input may initiate protective co-contraction, and if it is not properly managed, it can develop into delayed-onset muscle soreness or even centrally mediated myalgia. Overzealous therapy, a rapid change in the functional relationship, or an unwise selection of treatment may initiate a condition that has a component of pain. Many dental procedures, especially those that involve surgery, entail therapeutic hazards that can result in pain. Accidents happen, complications arise, and unexpected results may follow therapy. Some procedures, such as the surgical interruption of nociceptive pathways, may generate irreversible sequelae that can offset the possible benefit.

The incidence of iatrogenic pain is sufficient to warrant a high degree of caution on the part of all types of clinicians. The ancient maxim "At least do no harm" should be heeded always.

References

1. Wall PD. On the relation of injury to pain. Pain 1979;6:253–264.
2. Beecher HK. The use of chemical agents in the control of pain. In: Knighton RS, Dumke PR (eds). Pain. Boston: Little, Brown, 1966:221–239.
3. Nyquist JK, Eriksson MBE. Effects of pain treatment procedures on thermal sensibility in chronic pain patients [abstract]. Pain 1981; 11(suppl 1):91.
4. Bromm B. Evoked cerebral potential and pain. In: Fields HL, Dubner R, Cervero F (eds). Proceedings of the Fourth World Congress on Pain: Seattle, vol 9, Advances in Pain Research and Therapy. New York: Raven Press, 1985: 305–329.
5. Chapman CR. An alternative to threshold assessment in the study of human pain. In: Bonica JJ (ed). International Symposium on Pain, vol 4, Advances in Neurology. New York: Raven Press, 1974:115–121.
6. Clark WD. Pain sensitivity and the report of pain: An introduction to sensory decision theory. Anesthesiology 1974;40:272–287.
7. Yap AU, Tan KB, Chua EK, Tan HH. Depression and somatization in patients with temporomandibular disorders. J Prosthet Dent 2002;88:479–484.
8. Sipila K, Veijola J, Jokelainen J, et al. Association between symptoms of temporomandibular disorders and depression: An epidemiological study of the Northern Finland 1966 Birth Cohort. Cranio 2001;19:183–187.
9. Kleinknecht RA, Mahoney ER, Alexander LD. Psychosocial and demographic correlates of temporomandibular disorders and related symptoms: An assessment of community and clinical findings. Pain 1987;29:313–324.

10. Dalessio DJ, Silberstein SD. Wolff's Headache and Other Head Pain, ed 6. New York: Oxford University Press, 1993.

11. Wolff HG. Headache and Other Head Pain, ed 2. New York: Oxford University Press, 1963.

12. Wolff HG, Wolf S. Pain, ed 2. Springfield, IL: Thomas, 1958.

13. Wall PD, Devor M. Sensory afferent impulses originate from dorsal root ganglia as well as from the periphery in normal and nerve injured rats. Pain 1983;17:321–339.

14. Kakigi R. Diffuse noxious inhibitory control. Reappraisal by pain-related somatosensory-evoked potentials following CO_2 laser stimulation. J Neurol Sci 1994;125:198–205.

15. Bradley RM. Basic Oral Physiology. Chicago: Year Book, 1981.

16. Fields HL. Pain. New York: McGraw-Hill, 1987: 59–78.

17. Levine J, Basbaum AI. The peripheral nervous system and the inflammatory process [abstract]. Pain 1987;31(suppl 4):109.

18. Burgess PR, Perl ER. Cutaneous mechano-receptors and nociception. In: Iggo A (ed). Handbook of Sensory Physiology. Heidelberg: Springer, 1973:29–78.

19. Beitel RE, Dubner R. The response of unmyelinated (C) polymodal nociceptors to thermal stimuli applied to monkey's face. J Neurophysiol 1976;35:1160–1175.

20. Lim RJS. Pain. Ann Rev Physiol 1970;32: 269–288.

21. Handwerker HO. Influences of algogenic substances and prostaglandins on the discharges of unmyelinated cutaneous nerve fibers identified as nociceptors. In: Bonica JJ, Liebeskind JC, Albe-Fessard DG (eds). Proceedings of the Second World Congress on Pain, vol 3, Advances in Pain Research and Therapy. New York: Raven Press, 1979:41–45.

22. Ahlquist ML, Franzen OG, Edwall LGA. Quality of pain sensations following local application of algogenic agents on the exposed human tooth pulp: A psychophysical and electrophysiological study. In: Fields HL, Dubner R, Cervero F (eds). Proceedings of the Fourth World Congress on Pain: Seattle, vol 9, Advances in Pain Research and Therapy. New York: Raven Press, 1985:351–359.

23. Hedenberg-Agnusson B, Ernberg M, Alstergren P, Kopp S. Pain mediation by prostaglandin E_2 and leukotriene B_4 in the human masseter muscle. Acta Odontol Scand 2001;59:348–355.

24. Ferreira SH. Prostaglandins: Peripheral and central analgesia. In: Bonica JJ, Lindblom U, Iggo A (eds). Proceedings of the Third World Congress on Pain, vol 5, Advances in Pain Research and Therapy. New York: Raven Press, 1983:627–634.

25. Roitt IM, Brostoff J, Male DK. Immunology. St Louis: Mosby, 1985.

26. Bassoe P. Migraine. JAMA 1933;101:599–612.

27. Gross D. Pain and autonomic nervous system. In: Bonica JJ (ed). International Symposium on Pain, vol 4, Advances in Neurology. New York: Raven Press, 1974:93–103.

28. Sicuteri F. Headache as the most common disease of the antinociceptive system: Analogies with morphine abstinence. In: Bonica JJ, Liebeskind JC, Albe-Fessard DG (eds). Proceedings of the Second World Congress on Pain, vol 3, Advances in Pain Research and Therapy. New York: Raven Press, 1979:359–365.

29. Appenzeller O. Headache: Clinical and pathogenetic aspects. In: Bonica JJ, Liebeskind JC, Albe-Fessard DG (eds). Proceedings of the Second World Congress on Pain, vol 3, Advances in Pain Research and Therapy. New York: Raven Press, 1979:345–358.

30. Dvilansky A, Rishpon S, Nathan L. Release of platelet 5-hydroxytryptamine by plasma taken from patients during and between migraine attacks. Pain 1976;2:315–318.

31. Anthony M, Hinterberger H, Lance JW. Plasma serotonin in migraine and stress. Arch Neurol 1967;16:544–552.

32. Anthony M, Hinterberger H, Lance JW. The possible relationship of serotonin to the migraine syndrome. Res Clin Stud Headache 1969;2:29–42.

33. Krabbe AA, Olesen J. Headache provocation by continuous intravenous infusion of histamine: Clinical results and receptor mechanisms. Pain 1980;8:253–259.

34. Stronks DL, Tulen JH, Pepplinkhuizen L, et al. Personality traits and psychological reactions to mental stress of female migraine patients. Cephalalgia 1999;19:566–574.

35. Seltzer S, Marcus R, Stoch R. Perspectives in the control of chronic pain by nutritional manipulation. Pain 1981;11:141–148.

36. Braccili T, Montebello D, Verdecchia P, et al. Evaluation of anxiety and depression in childhood migraine. Eur Rev Med Pharmacol Sci 1999;3:37–39.

37. Johansson F, Von Knorring L. A double-blind controlled study of a serotonin uptake inhibitor (zimeldine) versus placebo in chronic pain patients. Pain 1979;7:69–78.

38. Materazzo F, Cathcart S, Pritchard D. Anger, depression, and coping interactions in headache activity and adjustment: A controlled study. J Psychosom Res 2000;49:69–75.

39. Mongini F, Ciccone G, Ibertis F, Negro C. Personality characteristics and accompanying symptoms in temporomandibular joint dysfunction, headache, and facial pain. J Orofac Pain 2000;14:52–58.

40. Clifford T, Lauritsen M, Bakke M. Electromyography of pericranial muscles during treatment of spontaneous common migraine attacks. Pain 1982;14:137–147.

41. Bakke M, Tfelt-Hansen P, Olesen J, Moller E. Action of some pericoronal muscles during provoked attacks of common migraine. Pain 1982;14:121–135.

42. Olesen J. Clinical and pathophysiological observations in migraine and tension-type headache explained by integration of vascular, supraspinal and myofascial inputs. Pain 1991;46: 125–132.

43. Kerr FWL. Correlated light and electron microscopic observations on the normal trigeminal ganglion and sensory root in man. J Neurosurg 1967;26:132–137.

44. Burchiel KJ. Abnormal impulse generation in focally demyelinated trigeminal roots. J Neurosurg 1980;53:674–683.

45. Howe JF, Loeser JD, Calvin WH. Mechanosensitivity of dorsal root ganglia and chronically injured axons: A physiological basis for the radicular pain of nerve root compression. Pain 1977; 3:25–41.

46. Rosomoff HL. Do herniated disks produce pain? In: Fields HL, Dubner R, Cervero F (eds). Proceedings of the Fourth World Congress on Pain: Seattle, vol 9, Advances in Pain Research and Therapy. New York: Raven Press, 1985: 457–461.

47. Ochea J, Noorrdenbes W. Pathology and disordered sensation in local nerve lesions: An attempt at correlation. In: Bonica JJ, Liebeskind JC, Albe-Fessard DG (eds). Proceedings of the Second World Congress on Pain, vol 3, Advances in Pain Research and Therapy. New York: Raven Press, 1979:67–90.

48. Sweet WH. Trigeminal neuralgia. In: Alling CC, Mahan PE (eds). Facial Pain. Philadelphia: Lea & Febiger, 1977:71–93.

49. Kerr FWL. Fine structure and functional characteristics of the primary trigeminal neuron. In: Hassler R, Walker AE (eds). Trigeminal Neuralgia: Pathogenesis and Pathophysiology. Stuttgart: Thieme, 1970:11–21.

50. Kerr FWL, Miller RH. The pathology of trigeminal neuralgia: Electron microscopic studies. Arch Neurol 1966;15:308–309.

51. Rappaport ZH, Devor M. Trigeminal neuralgia: The role of self-sustaining discharge in the trigeminal ganglion. Pain 1994;56:127–138.

52. Devor M, Amir R, Rappaport ZH. Pathophysiology of trigeminal neuralgia: The ignition hypothesis. Clin J Pain 2002;18:4–13.

53. Devor M, Govrin-Lippmann R, Rappaport ZH. Mechanism of trigeminal neuralgia: An ultrastructural analysis of trigeminal root specimens obtained during microvascular decompression surgery. J Neurosurg 2002;96:532–543.

54. Jannetta P. Arterial compression of the trigeminal nerve at the pons in patients with trigeminal neuralgia. J Neurosurg 1967;26:159–162.

55. Linskey ME, Jho HD, Jannetta PJ. Microvascular decompression for trigeminal neuralgia caused by vertebrobasilar compression. J Neurosurg 1994;81:1–9.

56. Jannetta PJ. Microsurgical management of trigeminal neuralgia. Arch Neurol 1985;42:800.

57. Soyka D. Etiology and therapy of trigeminal neuralgia [in German]. Neurochirurgia (Stuttg) 1990;33(suppl 1):11–13.

58. Kikuchi K, Kamisato N, Sasanuma J, Watanabe K, Kowada M. Trigeminal neuralgia associated with posterior fossa arteriovenous malformation and aneurysm fed by the same artery [case report] [in Japanese]. Neurol Med Chir (Tokyo) 1990;30:918–921.

59. Mursch K, Ludwig HC, Behnke-Mursch J, Markakis E. Trigeminal neuralgia as symptom of an infratentorial space-occupying process [in German]. Schmerz 1997;11:263–267.

60. Kuroki A, Kayama T, Song J, Saito S. Removal of petrous apex meningioma and microvascular decompression for trigeminal neuralgia through the anterior petrosal approach. Case report. Neurol Med Chir (Tokyo) 1999;39: 447–451.

61. Mase G, Zorzon M, Capus L, Biasutti E, Vitrani B, Cazzato G. Trigeminal neuralgia due to contralateral meningioma of the posterior cranial fossa. J Neurol Neurosurg Psychiatry 1994;57: 1010.

62. Puca A, Meglio M. Typical trigeminal neuralgia associated with posterior cranial fossa tumors. Ital J Neurol Sci 1993;14:549–552.

63. Tsubaki S, Fukushima T, Tamagawa T, et al. Parapontine trigeminal cryptic angiomas presenting as trigeminal neuralgia. J Neurosurg 1989;71:368-374.

64. Wegrzyn ZM. Trigeminal neuralgia and tumors of the cerebellopontile angle [in Polish]. Neurol Neurochir Pol 1983;17:245-251.

65. Celik SE, Kocaeli H, Cordan T, Bekar A. Trigeminal neuralgia due to cerebellopontine angle lipoma. Case illustration. J Neurosurg 2000;92:889.

66. Matsuka Y, Fort ET, Merrill RL. Trigeminal neuralgia due to an acoustic neuroma in the cerebellopontine angle. J Orofac Pain 2000;14: 147-151.

67. Ren M, Chen X, Xu L. Cholesteatoma of the cerebellopontine angle presented as trigeminal neuralgia [in Chinese]. Zhonghua Er Bi Yan Hou Ke Za Zhi 2000;35:446-448.

68. Kim JS, Kang JH, Lee MC. Trigeminal neuralgia after pontine infarction. Neurology 1998;51: 1511-1512.

69. Zvartau-Hind M, Din MU, Gilani A, Lisak RP, Khan OA. Topiramate relieves refractory trigeminal neuralgia in MS patients. Neurology 2000;55:1587-1588.

70. Leandri M, Lundardi G, Inglese M, et al. Lamotrigine in trigeminal neuralgia secondary to multiple sclerosis. J Neurol 2000;247:556-558.

71. Thomas P. Metabolic neuropathy. J R Coll Physicians Lond 1973;7:154-160.

72. Pollard JD, McLeod JG, Honnibal TG, Verheijden MA. Hypothyroid polyneuropathy. Clinical, electrophysiological and nerve biopsy findings in two cases. J Neurol Sci 1982;53: 461-471.

73. Walsh JC, McLeod JG. Alcoholic neuropathy. An electrophysiological and histological study. J Neurol Sci 1970;10:457-469.

74. Windebank A. Polyneuropathy due to nutritional deficiency and alcoholism. In: Dyck PJ, Thomas P, Griffin J, Low P, Poduslo JF (eds). Peripheral Neuropathy, ed 3. Philadelphia: Saunders, 1993:1310-1321.

75. Dekonenko EP, Leont'eva I, Martynenko IN, et al. Neuritis of the facial nerve and its connection with herpes viruses [in Russian]. Zh Nevrol Psikhiatr Im S S Korsakova 2000;100:58-59.

76. Murakami S, Sugita T, Hirata Y, Yanagihara N, Desaki J. Histopathology of facial nerve neuritis caused by herpes simplex virus infection in mice. Eur Arch Otorhinolaryngol 1994:S487-S488.

77. Bigelow N, Harrison L, Goodell H. Studies on pain: Quantitative measurements of two pain sensations of the skin with reference to the nature of the hyperalgesia of peripheral neuritis. J Clin Investig 1945;23:503-516.

78. Lobato RD, Madrid JL. Clinical and physiopathological mechanisms of postherpetic neuralgia. Clin J Pain 1987;2:253-257.

79. Stookey B, Rausohoft J. Trigeminal Neuralgia. Springfield, IL: Thomas, 1959.

80. Reuler JB, Chang M. Herpes zoster: Epidemiology, clinical features and management. South Med J 1984;77:1149-1156.

81. Furuta Y, Ohtani F, Kawabata H, Fukuda S, Bergstrom T. High prevalence of varicella-zoster virus reactivation in herpes simplex virus-seronegative patients with acute peripheral facial palsy. Clin Infect Dis 2000;30:529-533.

82. Murakami S, Honda N, Mizobuchi M, Nakashiro Y, Hato N, Gyo K. Rapid diagnosis of varicella zoster virus infection in acute facial palsy. Neurology 1998;51:1202-1205.

83. Oxman MN. Varicella and herpes zoster. In: Fitzpatrick TB, Eisen AZ, Wolff KD (eds). Dermatology in General Medicine. New York: McGraw-Hill International, 1979:1600-1616.

84. Loeser JD. Herpes zoster and postherpetic neuralgia. Pain 1986;25:149-164.

85. Reuler JB, Chang M. Herpes zoster: Epidemiology, clinical fractures and management. South Med J 1984;77:1149-1156.

86. Zaal MJ, Volker-Dieben HJ, D'Amaro J. Risk and prognostic factors of postherpetic neuralgia and focal sensory denervation: A prospective evaluation in acute herpes zoster ophthalmicus. Clin J Pain 2000;16:345-351.

87. Watson CP, Evans RJ, Watt VR, Birkett N. Postherpetic neuralgia: 208 cases. Pain 1988;35: 289-297.

88. Wall PD. Changes in damaged nerves and their sensory consequences. In: Bonica JJ, Liebeskind JC, Albe-Fessard DG (eds). Proceedings of the Second World Congress on Pain, vol 3, Advances in Pain Research and Therapy. New York: Raven Press, 1979:39-52.

89. Loeser JD. Definition, etiology, and neurological assessment of pain originating in the nervous system following deafferentation. In: Bonica JJ, Lindblom U, Iggo A (eds). Proceedings of the Third World Congress on Pain, vol 5, Advances in Pain Research and Therapy. New York: Raven Press, 1983:701-711.

90. Nikolajsen L, Ilkjaer S, Kroner K, Christensen JH, Jensen TS. The influence of preamputation pain on postamputation stump and phantom pain. Pain 1997;72:393–405.

91. Nikolajsen L, Jensen TS. Phantom limb pain. Br J Anaesth 2001;87:107–116.

92. Wall PD. Alterations in the central nervous system after deafferentation: Connectivity control. In: Bonica JJ, Lindblom U, Iggo A (eds). Proceedings of the Third World Congress on Pain, vol 5, Advances in Pain Research and Therapy. New York: Raven Press, 1983:677–689.

93. Gregg JM, Walter JR, Driscoll R. Neurosensory studies of trigeminal dysesthesia following peripheral nerve injury. In: Bonica JJ, Liebeskind JC, Albe-Fessard DG (eds). Proceedings of the Second World Congress on Pain, vol 3, Advances in Pain Research and Therapy. New York: Raven Press, 1979:311–315.

94. Inbal R, Rousso M, Ashur H. Collateral sprouting in skin and sensory recovery after nerve injury in man. Pain 1987;28:141–154.

95. Ochoa JL, Torebjork E, Marchettini P. Mechanisms of neuropathic pain: Cumulative observations, new experiments, and further speculation. In: Fields HL, Dubner R, Cervero F (eds). Proceedings of the Fourth World Congress on Pain: Seattle, vol 9, Advances in Pain Research and Therapy. New York: Raven Press, 1985: 431–450.

96. Devor M, Rappaport Z. Pain and the pathophysiology of damaged nerve. In: Fields H (ed). Pain Syndromes in Neurology. London: Butterworths, 1990:47–83.

97. Diamond J. The effect of injecting acetylcholine into normal and regenerating nerves. J Physiol (Lond) 1959;145:611–629.

98. Wall PD. Mechanisms of acute and chronic pain. In: Kruger L, Liebeskind JC (eds). Neural Mechanisms of Pain, vol 6, Advances in Pain Research and Therapy. New York: Raven Press, 1984:95–104.

99. Hu JW, Dostrovsky JO, Lenz YE, Ball GJ, Sessle BJ. Tooth pulp deafferentation is associated with functional alterations in the properties of neurons in the trigeminal spinal tract nucleus. J Neurophysiol 1986;56:1650–1658.

100. Gregg JM. Posttraumatic pain: Experimental trigeminal neuropathy. J Oral Surg 1971;29: 260–267.

101. Gobel S, Binck JM. Degenerative changes in primary trigeminal axons and in neurons in nucleus caudalis following tooth pulp extirpation in the cat. Brain Res 1977;132:347–354.

102. Alling CC. Dysesthesia of the lingual and inferior alveolar nerves following third molar surgery. J Oral Maxillofac Surg 1986;44:454–457.

103. Goldberg MH, Nemarich AN, Marco WP. Complications after mandibular third molar surgery: A statistical analysis of 500 consecutive procedures in private practice. J Am Dent Assoc 1985;111:277–279.

104. Wofford DT, Miller RI. Prospective study of dysesthesia following odontectomy of impacted mandibular third molars. J Oral Maxillofac Surg 1987;45:15–19.

105. Upton LG, Rajvanakarn M, Hayward JR. Evaluation of the regeneration capacity of the inferior alveolar nerve following surgical trauma. J Oral Maxillofac Surg 1987;45:212–216.

106. Howe JF. Phantom limb pain: A re-afferentation syndrome. Pain 1983;15:101–107.

107. Melzack R, Loeser JD. Phantom body pain in paraplegics: Evidence for a central pattern generating mechanism for pain. Pain 1978;4: 195–210.

108. Livingston WK. Pain Mechanisms. New York: Macmillan, 1943.

109. Bonica JJ. Causalgia and other reflex sympathetic dystrophies. In: Bonica JJ, Liebeskind JC, Albe-Fessard DG (eds). Proceedings of the Second World Congress on Pain, vol 3, Advances in Pain Research and Therapy. New York: Raven Press, 1979:141–166.

110. Walker AE, Nulson F. Electrical stimulation of the upper thoracic portion of the sympathetic chain in man. Arch Neurol Psychiatry 1948; 59:559–567.

111. Campbell JN, Raja SN, Meyer RA. Painful sequelae of nerve injury [abstract]. Pain 1987; 31(suppl 4):334.

112. Roberts W. A hypothesis on the physiological basis for causalgia and related pains. Pain 1986; 24:297–311.

113. Cushing H. The major trigeminal neuralgias and their surgical treatment. Am Med Sci 1920; 160:157–168.

114. Nguyen M, Maciewicz R, Bouckoms A. Facial pain symptoms in patients with cerebellopontine angle tumors: A report of 44 cases of cerebellopontine angle meningioma and a review of the literature. Clin J Pain 1986;2:3–9.

115. Foley KM. The treatment of pain in the patient with cancer. Can Assoc Radiol J 1986;36: 194–215.

116. Go VLW, Yaksh TL. Release of substance P from the cat spinal cord. J Physiol (Lond) 1987; 391:141–167.

117. Duggan AW, Hope PJ, Jarrott B, Schaible HG, Fleetwood-Walker SM. Release, spread and persistence of immunoreactive neurokinin A in the dorsal horn of the cat following noxious cutaneous stimulation. Studies with antibody microprobes. Neuroscience 1990;35:195–202.

118. Morton CR, Hutchison WD, Hendry IA. Release of immunoreactive somatostatin in the spinal dorsal horn of the cat. Neuropeptides 1988;12:189–197.

119. Morton CR, Hutchison WD. Release of sensory neutopeptides in the spinal cord: Studies with calcitonin gene-related peptide and galanin. Neuroscience 1990;31:807–815.

120. Skilling SR, Smullin DH, Larson AA. Extracellular amino acid concentrations in the dorsal spinal cord of freely moving rats following veratridine and nociceptive stimulation. J Neurochem 1988;51:127–132.

121. Sorkin LS, Westlund KN, Sluka KA, Dougherty PM, Willis WD. Neural changes in acute arthritis in monkeys. IV. Time course of amino acid release into the lumbar dorsal horn. Brain Res Rev 1992;17:39–50.

122. Woolf CJ, Thompson SWN. The induction and maintenance of central sensitization is dependent on N-methyl-D-aspartic acid receptor activation; implications for the treatment of postinjury pain hypersensitivity states. Pain 1991; 50:293–299.

123. Cook AJ, Woolf CJ, Wall PD, McMahon SB. Dynamic receptive field plasticity in rat spinal cord dorsal horn following C-primary afferent input. Nature 1987;325:151–153.

124. Wall PD. The prevention of postoperative pain. Pain 1988;33:289–290.

Category Classification of Orofacial Pains

This chapter will present a means of assessing the pain complaint and describe a diagnostic "road map" that will lead the examiner toward an accurate classification of pain disorders, which becomes a valuable diagnostic tool. The more sophisticated the classification, however, the greater the requirement for a good understanding of pain mechanisms and examination techniques.

Pain Diagnosis

Diagnosis is by far the most difficult aspect of managing a patient's pain problem. Because of this difficulty, many therapists fail to make the proper diagnosis. In fact, the majority of treatment failures arise directly out of misdiagnosis. It is only through proper diagnosis that effective therapy can be selected and instituted.

The first prerequisite in classifying pain is a common language with which to communicate intelligibly. Considerable improvement has been made in the meaning of terms used to describe pain. Some defini-

tions listed in a standard medical dictionary[1] are not precise enough to prevent ambiguity and misunderstanding. The International Association for the Study of Pain has taken the lead in defining such terms more precisely.[2–5] A list of definitions as used in this text may be found at the back of the book. The reader is encouraged to become familiar with them.

The most elementary classification of pain is that which lists the anatomic locations where pain is felt. An example of such a classification follows:

1. Head and neck pain
2. Thoracic pain
3. Abdominal pain
4. Extremity pain

Subdivisions of head and neck pain would include orofacial pains, headaches, and cervical pains. This text will discuss primarily orofacial pains; however, the clinician must have an appreciation for other pain conditions of the head and neck so that proper diagnosis is possible. Other texts should be reviewed for a more complete understanding of headaches and cervical pain disorders.

Table 7-1 Important Categories of the International Headache Society's Classification of Headache[7]

Part One: Primary headaches
1. Migraine
2. Tension-type headache
3. Cluster headache and other trigeminal autonomic cephalalgias
4. Other primary headaches

Part Two: Secondary headaches
5. Headache attributed to head and/or neck trauma
6. Headache attributed to cranial or cervical vascular disorder
7. Headache attributed to nonvascular intracranial disorder
8. Headache attributed to substances or their withdrawal
9. Headache attributed to infection
10. Headache attributed to disorder of homeostasis
11. Headache or facial pain attributed to disorder of cranium, neck, eyes, ears, nose, sinuses, teeth, mouth, or other facial or cranial structures
12. Headache attributed to psychiatric disorder

Part Three: Cranial neuralgias, central and primary facial pain, and other headaches
13. Cranial neuralgias and central causes of facial pain
14. Other headache, cranial neuralgia, central or primary facial pain

Used with permission.

A simple classification of pain disorders is often used to record the patient's subjective complaint. For example, it might list the complaint as headache, toothache, chest pain, backache, or leg pain. It should be understood, however, that this type of classification identifies only the site where pain is felt and not necessarily the location of its true source. A pain listed as a "toothache" could be of dental origin and require dental therapy. But it could also be a heterotopic manifestation of some myogenous, vascular, or neuropathic condition that would require treatment at quite a different level. Therefore, such a classification has very little diagnostic or therapeutic value.

More refined pain classifications require additional knowledge of pain behavior and a greater diagnostic effort. To classify pain by the location of its source requires an understanding of heterotopic pains and entails the need for diagnostic differentiation between primary pain and its secondary effects. Thus, "toothache" in such a classification might become pulpal pain, periodontal pain, or heterotopic pain when its true site of origin is determined. It should be obvious that this more accurate classification of the patient's complaint implies important therapeutic considerations.

In 1988, the International Headache Society published the first edition of the "Classification and diagnosis criteria for headache disorders, cranial neuralgias and facial pain."[6] In 2004 this classification was revised.[7] This classification attempts to separate all headaches according to etiology and involved structures. Although this classification has been most useful in unifying international groups, it relies heavily on the clinician's preexisting knowledge of each condition. In this classification (Table 7-1), the area of orofacial pain and temporomandibular disorders falls mostly in section 11, which is listed as "Headache or facial pain attributed to disorder of cranium, neck, eyes, ears, nose, sinuses, teeth, mouth, or other facial or cranial structures." Although this section includes many temporomandibular and orofacial pain disorders, it falls short in helping the clinician diagnose and ultimately treat the patient's pain condition. This classification also fails to consider the psychologic aspect of the pain condition.

An understanding of the genesis of pain can help to refine a pain classification. Previous chapters in this text have described in detail how nociceptive input from different tissues of the body can produce pain. An important concept presented was that the clinical characteristics of the pain can be useful in identifying the tissues or structures that are responsible for the pain. A reasonable classification for pain disorders, therefore, would be based on the structures that are responsible for producing the nociceptive input (the true origin of the pain). However, even this type of classification does not consider the psychologic factors that may influence or even cause the pain disorder. For the clinician to fully classify the pain disorder, he or she must consider both the somatosensory input and the psychosocial input. A complete pain classification must assess the pain condition on two levels or axes. One axis represents the physical factors that are responsible for the nociceptive input, and the other axis represents the psychologic factors that influence the pain experience. In this text, Axis I will depict the physical factors and Axis II will depict the psychologic factors. In evaluating any pain disorder, both axes must be considered before a diagnosis can be established and proper therapy selected. Therapy that addresses only one axis will likely fail if the other axis is a major contributor to the pain disorder.

As already discussed, some pain disorders are influenced by one axis more than the other. For example, acute pains are commonly related more to Axis I factors than Axis II factors. Therefore, acute pains often respond well to therapies directed toward the somatosensory input. Chronic pains, however, often have significant Axis II factors, and therefore therapies directed only to somatosensory inputs will likely fail

(see chapter 5). This concept is essential to the successful management of pain.

Axis I (Physical Conditions)

Axis I represents the physical conditions that are responsible for the initiation of nociceptive impulses. These conditions can be classified according to the tissues that produce the nociception. The following is a list of orofacial structures that provide the basis for a classification of orofacial pains:

1. Cutaneous and mucogingival pains
2. Mucosal pains of the pharynx, nose, and paranasal sinuses
3. Pains of dental origin
4. Pains of the musculoskeletal structures of the mouth and face
5. Pains of the visceral structures of the mouth and face
6. Pains of the neural structures of the mouth and face

Axis II (Psychologic Conditions)

Axis II represents the psychologic conditions that can either produce or influence the pain experience. The American Psychiatric Association has developed a comprehensive classification for mental disorders.[8] Only the categories that may be associated with pain will be discussed in this text. For a more complete review of all mental disorders, the clinician should review this document. Mental disorders that need to be considered as Axis II factors are:

1. Anxiety disorders
2. Mood disorders
3. Somatoform disorders
4. Other conditions, such as psychologic factors affecting a medical condition

Categories of Orofacial Pains

For the clinician to begin classifying orofacial pain disorders, he or she must first be able to differentiate the signs and symptoms associated with each category. In this section, physical and psychologic factors will be separated and identified. This begins the process of diagnosis and represents the most important process for the successful management of pain. Without proper diagnosis, appropriate therapy cannot be selected.

A reliable pain classification needs to be based on symptomatology. This requires an understanding of the clinical characteristics displayed by the different categories of pain. It is on the basis of the subjective symptoms and objective signs of the nociceptive condition under examination that proper identification is made. If one fully appreciates the concept of pain modulation, understands and can differentiate primary pain from secondary pain, has some knowledge of pain genesis, can identify the categories of pain by their clinical characteristics, and appreciates psychologic factors, a truly sophisticated and useful classification of orofacial pains is possible. As concepts have evolved in recent years, this pain classification has undergone considerable metamorphosis. It represents a logical classification for orofacial pains that conforms well to current knowledge of nociceptive mechanisms and psychologic factors. Table 7-2 outlines these classification categories.

Axis I Categories (Physical Conditions)

The various tissues of the body contribute to the physical conditions that are responsible for nociceptive input that can eventually produce pain. These tissues can be divided into two broad categories: somatic and neurogenous. As explained in chapter 1, neurogenous tissues are those tissues that comprise the communication system, while somatic tissues comprise all other body tissues. The somatic structures are the envelope, the musculoskeletal system, the supply system, and the special sensory organs. Remember also that the manner by which each system communicates with the neurologic system is perceived differently by the brain and brainstem. Therefore, pain felt from each type of somatic tissue can be differentiated from pain of the other somatic tissues by unique clinical characteristics. An understanding of these characteristics is essential in establishing the proper diagnosis.

Somatic pain

Somatic pains occur in response to the stimulation of normal neural receptors. Local conditions such as inflammation increase the receptivity of the neural structures, so that stimulation becomes more evident. Reduced central inhibitory control of the passage of peripheral impulses to the higher centers also causes less intense peripheral stimulation to become more noxious. The degree of pain therefore does not necessarily relate to the intensity of the stimulus.

The neural structures involved in such pain reception and transmission are presumed to be normal, and the sensation serves to warn, alert, or inform the individual of the noxious stimulation. The conscious sensation of pain under such conditions is an added component to the voluminous sensory input that the brain receives constantly, and it serves the purpose of preparing the patient for the appropriate response. Afferent neurons of both the peripheral (somatic) and autonomic (visceral) nervous systems participate in this mechanism.

Table 7-2 Orofacial Pain Classification

Axis I (Physical conditions)
I. Somatic pain
  A. Superficial somatic pain
    1. Cutaneous pain
    2. Mucogingival pain
  B. Deep somatic pain
    1. Musculoskeletal pain
      a. Muscle pain
        i. Protective co-contraction
        ii. Local muscle soreness
        iii. Myofascial pain
        iv. Myospasm
        v. Centrally mediated myalgia
      b. Temporomandibular joint pain
        i. Ligamentous pain
        ii. Retrodiscal pain
        iii. Capsular pain
        iv. Arthritic pain
      c. Osseous and periosteal pain
      d. Soft connective tissue pain
      e. Periodontal dental pain
    2. Visceral pain
      a. Pulpal dental pain
      b. Vascular pain
        i. Arteritis
        ii. Carotidynia
      c. Neurovascular pain
        i. Migraine
        ii. Tension-type headache
        iii. Cluster headache and other
          trigeminal autonomic cephalalgias
        iv. Other primary headaches
        v. Neurovascular variants
      d. Visceral mucosal pain
      e. Glandular, ocular, and auricular pain

II. Neuropathic pain
  A. Episodic neuropathic pains
    1. Paroxysmal neuralgia pain
      a. Trigeminal neuralgia
      b. Glossopharyngeal neuralgia
      c. Geniculate neuralgia
      d. Superior laryngeal neuralgia
      e. Nervus intermedius
      f. Occipital neuralgia
    2. Neurovascular pain (already listed
      under visceral pain)

  B. Continuous neuropathic pains
    1. Peripherally mediated pain
      a. Entrapment neuropathy
      b. Deafferentation pain
        i. Traumatic neuroma pain
      c. Neuritic pain
        i. Peripheral neuritis
        ii. Herpes zoster
    2. Centrally mediated pain
      a. Burning mouth disorder
      b. Atypical odontalgia (phantom pain)
      c. Postherpetic neuralgia
      d. Complex regional pain syndromes
        (CRPS)
      e. Sympathetically maintained pain
    3. Metabolic polyneuropathies
      a. Diabetic neuropathy
      b. Hypothyroid neuropathy
      c. Alcoholic neuropathy
      d. Nutritional neuropathies

Axis II (Psychologic conditions)
I. Mood disorders
  A. Depressive disorders
  B. Bipolar disorders
  C. Mood disorders resulting from a medical
    condition
II. Anxiety disorders
  A. Generalized anxiety disorders
  B. Posttraumatic stress disorders
  C. Anxiety disorders arising from a medical
    condition
III. Somatoform disorders
  A. Undifferentiated somatoform disorders
  B. Conversion disorders
  C. Pain disorders
  D. Hypochondriasis
IV. Other conditions
  A. Malingering
  B. Psychological factors affecting a medical
    condition
    1. Personality traits or coping style
    2. Maladaptive health behavior
    3. Stress-related physiologic response
  C. Any other mental disorders not men-
    tioned in this classification

The clinical characteristics of pain that originates in superficial structures are distinctly different from those of pain of deep origin. It is by these differences that the two types of somatic pain are distinguished.

Superficial somatic pain

The external surface of the body is richly innervated with receptors and sensory fibers of different types. These constantly feed information concerning the organism's environment to the somatosensory cortex. Not only does such sensation establish full conscious contact between the organism and its surroundings; it also furnishes the impetus for involuntary reflex activity. Superficial sensation serves a protective function so the organism may react appropriately to the constant and varied environmental threat to its well-being, comfort, and survival.

The sensory system provides input at conscious levels to allow precise definition of the physical characteristics of the stimulus, including its modality, location, duration, and intensity. Pain emanating from these superficial structures presents characteristics at a conscious level of the definition of the physical properties of the noxious stimulus. These qualities are inherent in superficial somatic pain and furnish the examiner with a means of identifying it.

Superficial pains have a bright, stimulating quality.[9-11] This probably results from the alarm reaction that such discomfort tends to create. As part of the environmental threat, superficial pain causes the patient to react in such a way as to escape the threat (fight-or-flight reaction). The more severe the superficial pain, the more pronounced this stimulating quality becomes.

Superficial pains can be correctly located by the patient, ie, the patient is aware precisely of where he or she hurts and is able to describe the location of the pain with anatomic accuracy.

Since the source of superficial pain is noxious stimulation of the very structures that hurt, the location of the pain clearly identifies where to look for its cause: the site of pain and the origin of the pain are identical. In fact, if the cause of the pain is not immediately evident or reasonably explicable, the diagnosis of superficial pain should be questioned.

Since superficial somatic pain is the result of a lowered pain threshold and since the site of pain and the location of its true source are the same, the discomfort that results from provocation at the site of pain relates faithfully to the stimulus. This means that the reaction is immediate, it is proportional to the intensity of the stimulus, it lasts as long as the stimulus, and there is no reference of pain to other normal structures. Superficial pain responds faithfully to provocation. Effects of central sensitization, such as referred pain, secondary hyperalgesia, local autonomic effects, and secondary muscle co-contraction, are not observed.

Since superficial pain emanates from the surface tissue, application of a topical anesthetic interrupts the pain. It should be noted that neither neuropathic pain felt in superficial tissues nor pain referred from deeper structures to the surface is arrested by the application of topical local anesthesia.

Two types of superficial orofacial pain are recognized, namely, *cutaneous pain* and *mucogingival pain*.

To summarize, the following clinical characteristics are displayed by superficial somatic pain:

1. The pain has a bright, stimulating quality.
2. Subjective localization of the pain is excellent and anatomically accurate.
3. The site of pain identifies the correct location of its source.
4. Response to provocation at the site of pain is faithful in incidence, intensity, and location.
5. The application of a topical anesthetic at the site of pain temporarily arrests it.

Deep somatic pain

Sensory innervation of the deeper structures of the body supplies the somatosensory cortex with a constant inflow of information monitoring all the internal functioning of the body. No doubt the information has a certain precision of definition as to the physical characteristics of the stimulus, including its modality, location, duration, and intensity, but this information is normally below conscious levels unless volition brings it to the attention of the subject. Functions that require precise definition of the physical characteristics of the stimulus, such as the action of skeletal muscles, are attended by some conscious sensation that is fairly precise for location. Most functions that operate at an involuntary level, such as the action of smooth muscle, are attended by sensations that remain below conscious levels unless unusual conditions prevail, such as distension, pressure, sustained hyperemia, or inflammation.[12,13] In such cases the conscious sensation usually is that of diffusely located and poorly defined discomfort or pain.

Deep pain has a dull, depressing quality[9,11,14] and sometimes causes a sickening sensation of nausea. The background sensation may be punctuated by momentary lancinating pains that the patient describes as stimulating and exciting. Such lancinating pain is usually initiated by sudden traction, distension, or distortion of deep tissues.

The depressing effect of pain arising in deeper body structures and mediated by either deep somatic or visceral afferent fibers is likely to be a manifestation of withdrawal reaction. In contrast to the alarm effect from an environmental threat that is witnessed in superficial pain, the usual reaction to discomfort emanating from deeper structures is to prepare the subject for conservation and recovery. Therefore a decrease in somatic skeletal activity occurs in favor of increased visceral function. The characteristic quality of deep pain is that the discomfort induces a depressing effect leading to inactivity and withdrawal, sometimes accompanied by weariness, depression, weakness, or lowered blood pressure.[15]

Deep pain is less accurately localizable by the patient. Some pains of deep origin, such as those from skeletal muscle or from the periodontal ligament, are fairly localizable. However, such localizing sensation is considerably less accurate, and the ability of the patient to describe the painful site anatomically is less certain than with the superficial pain. The area where pain is sensed is usually larger than the site from which it arises. Many deep pains, such as those emanating from the dental pulp or from blood vessels, are hardly localizable, and the patient's anatomic description of where he or she feels the pain may be diffuse indeed. Some deep pains produce central sensitization, so that the pain may be referred to otherwise normal structures and the descriptive location of the pain is nonanatomic.

Because of the variable and inconsistent localizability of deep pain, the site of pain may not indicate the true origin. This applies especially to pains that occur spontaneously or in response to normal function. Pain provoked by manual palpation and manipulation more accurately identifies its true location, and this diagnostic maneuver often can be useful to isolate otherwise vague and diffusely located pain sites. Muscle and organ pains especially show this trait. It is true that the site of some deep pains may clearly identify the origin, but even then it is considerably less precise and dependable than with superficial pain. Although some deep pains are felt in sites that are much larger than the true source of pain, others may be felt in entirely normal structures. Since these variables are characteristic of deep pain, it behooves the examiner to take measures that prove the location of the pain source, rather than depending on the site of pain for this information.

Deep pain may not be proportional to the stimulus. Although some deep pains (usually those with better localization behavior) respond rather faithfully to a stimulus, the response is not as faithful as with superficial pain. In contrast, some deep pains manifest little relationship between stimulus and response, and others cannot be provoked by manual palpation or the demands of function. Although the lack of faithful response to provocation is characteristic of deep pain (sometimes greater, sometimes less than the intensity of provocation would suggest), true summation effects are not seen. Therefore, triggering of intense pain by light touch or superficial movement is not characteristic of deep pain disorders.

One of the most important identifying clinical characteristics of deep pain is its tendency to display effects caused by central sensitization or hyperexcitability.[9,14] Deep pain input tends to provoke referred pains, secondary hyperalgesia, localized autonomic effects, and secondary muscle co-contraction. This tendency relates to the continuity, severity, and duration of the deep pain input. When diagnostic evidence of such central excitatory effects is observed, a deep pain disorder must be suspected and a serious diagnostic search made for the primary pain source. Great care must be exercised not to confuse secondary pain effects, which may actually be the patient's clinical complaint, with the primary pain source, which may be relatively silent and therefore asymptomatic to the patient. It is the manifestation of such secondary effects that creates much of the diffuse variability and spreading effect of some deep pains. Certainly, these effects are largely responsible for the confusion that surrounds many deep pain disorders and the therapeutic failure that sometimes occurs.

Usually, deep pain is not arrested by the application of a topical anesthetic, except when it arises from visceral mucosa such as the nasal mucosa in so-called "sinus head-ache." Analgesic blocking of the nerve that mediates the primary painful impulses usually arrests deep pain, and this technique is useful diagnostically in localizing the source of such pains (see chapter 8). Vascular pains, however, may not respond well to ordinary analgesic blocking.

To summarize, the following clinical characteristics are displayed by deep somatic pain:

1. The pain has a dull, depressing quality.
2. Subjective localization of the pain is variable and somewhat diffuse.
3. The site of pain may or may not identify the correct location of its true source.
4. Response to provocation at the site of pain is fairly faithful in incidence and intensity but not in location.
5. Secondary central excitatory effects frequently accompany the deep pain.

There are two distinct types of deep somatic pain, namely, *musculoskeletal pain* and *visceral pain*. Musculoskeletal pain involves the action of receptors that respond to varying degrees of stimulation. Such pain therefore yields a graduated response to stimulation. Musculoskeletal pain relates intimately to biomechanical function. It can be localized to the degree that such a sense of localization is required in the course of normal functioning. Musculoskeletal pain is further subdivided into *(1)* muscle pain, *(2)* temporomandibular joint pain, *(3)* osseous and periosteal pain, *(4)* soft connective tissue pain, and *(5)* dental pain of periodontal origin. Muscle pains include protective co-contraction, local muscle soreness, myofascial pain, myospasm, myositis, and centrally mediated myalgia. Temporomandibular joint pain includes ligamentous pain, retrodiscal pain, capsular pain, and arthritic pain.

Visceral pain involves the action of high-threshold receptors of the interoceptive type. Such pain is not usually felt until the threshold is reached. Unless inflammatory, it does not present a graduated response to stimulation. It has little or no relationship to biomechanical function and is poorly localizable by the subject. Visceral pain is further subdivided into *(1)* neurovascular pain; *(2)* vascular pain; *(3)* dental pain of pulpal origin; *(4)* visceral mucosal pain; and *(5)* glandular, ocular, and auricular pain. Neurovascular pains are common and can be subdivided into *(1)* migraine, *(2)* tension-type headache, *(3)* cluster headache and other trigeminal autonomic cephalalgias, *(4)* other primary headaches, and *(5)* neurovascular variants.

Neuropathic pain

Neuropathic pains are those that are generated within the nervous system itself.[16] Stimulation of receptors and nerve fibers is therefore unnecessary. Stimulation may cause summation effects, so that the evoked response may be wholly disproportionate to the stimulus. A common clinical characteristic of neuropathic pain is the lack of any obvious source of the nociception. Since the pain originates in the neural structures, the somatic structures appear normal. This clinical presentation is a real challenge for the clinician because neuropathic and psychogenic pains both present with no obvious clinical findings. In earlier years, before neuropathic pains were appreciated, most of these patients were assumed to have a psychologic problem that was causing the pain. This was a very unfortunate assumption and very frustrating for patients. In fact, even today many patients are given a primary psychiatric diagnosis by the naïve, uninformed clinician. Most informed pain clinicians agree that true psychogenic pain is rare. This does not mean that a psychologic disorder does not exist (Axis II). In fact, as already mentioned, the longer one suffers with pain, the greater the likelihood of a coexisting condition such as depression, anxiety, hostility, or frustration. But these conditions may be second-ary to the pain and not the primary diagnosis. Informing a neuropathic pain patient that his pain condition is "all in his head" can be a devastating blow.

Neuropathic pains are commonly associated with other neurologic symptoms such as burning, hyperalgesia, dysesthesia, and even sometimes anesthesia. Heterotopic pain is also common. Neuropathic pain can present as either *episodic* or *continuous*. Since this characteristic is useful for classifying neuropathic pains, it will be discussed further in this text.

Episodic neuropathic pains

Episodic neuropathic pains are characterized by periods of very intense pains followed by total remission. These pains may last from seconds to hours, depending on the type. Usually, the individual is able to localize the site of pain quite well. The site, however, does not identify the correct source, since many of these pains are projected heterotopic pains. Response to provocation at the site of pain is unfaithful. Since these pains will demonstrate periods of total remission, secondary symptoms associated with central excitatory effects are not usually seen. Episodic neuropathic pains are classified into two categories: *paroxysmal neuralgic pains* and *neurovascular pains*.

Paroxysmal neuralgic pains are characterized by a bright, stimulating, burning quality that simulates superficial somatic pain, from which it must be differentiated. These pains are said to be *paroxysmal;* hence the name *paroxysmal neuralgia*. The pain is extremely intense but rarely lasts more than 20 to 30 seconds. Between episodes the individual will be normal, without pain. Neuralgic pains are categorized according to the affected nerve, for example, trigeminal neuralgia. Other neuralgias are glossopharyngeal neuralgia, geniculate neuralgia, superior laryngeal neuralgia, and nervus intermedius neuralgia.

Neurovascular pains are characterized by periods of intense, debilitating, pulsating pain that typically lasts from 6 to 8 hours. These pains have already been classified within the visceral pain category. They are mentioned here because of studies that have demonstrated that their etiology is likely to begin with a neuromechanism. Neurovascular pains will be discussed under the category of visceral pains, since their clinical characteristics are more typical of visceral pains.

Continuous neuropathic pains
Continuous neuropathic pains result from interference with the normal transmission of afferent impulses by primary sensory neurons. Many of these pains are felt as a persistent, ongoing, unremitting, burning sensation. These pains may have some fluctuation in intensity but no periods of total remission. These will often show an enlargement of the receptive field and diminished central inhibitory activity. They occur from a variety of conditions, but trauma or some other form of damage to the neuron is common. Continuous neuropathic pains are classified into three categories: (1) peripherally mediated pain, (2) centrally mediated pain, and (3) metabolic polyneuropathies. The peripherally mediated neuropathic pains are subdivided into three subcategories: entrapment neuropathies, deafferentation pains, and neuritic pains. Centrally mediated neuropathic pains are subdivided into two subcategories: burning mouth disorders and atypical odontalgia (phantom pain).

In some instances, a continuous neuropathic pain can be influenced by activity of the sympathetic nervous system in the area of the problem. When this occurs, the neuropathic condition is referred to as a *sympathetically maintained pain*. In other conditions the sympathetic nervous system has no obvious influence on the pain condition, and this is referred to as *sympathetically independent pain*.

When neuropathic pain conditions become more chronic, they can present with additional clinical signs and symptoms such as extreme allodynia, tissue redness, and swelling. In an attempt to better study and understand these conditions, researchers have developed clinical criteria and termed these conditions *complex regional pain syndromes* (CRPS). The precise description of CRPS will be discussed in chapter 17.

Axis II Categories (Psychologic Conditions)

As already stated, psychologic conditions influence all pains. These conditions have their greatest effects on chronic pains. The longer a patient suffers, the greater the influence of these factors. All clinicians treating pain disorders must be familiar with certain important psychologic factors so that, when indicated, these conditions can be properly addressed.

Psychologic intensification of pain may proceed until the suffering is wholly disproportionate to the peripheral nociceptive input. Although the original pain complaint may have displayed the usual clinical characteristics of somatic or neuropathic pain, as psychologic intensification converts it into a chronic pain disorder, the clinical symptoms take on identifying features. Such pain lacks an adequate source of input that is anatomically related to the site of pain. It may be felt in multiple and sometimes changeable locations. Pain bilaterally may become evident in the absence of bilateral sources of noxious input. The complaint may display unusual or unexpected responses to therapy. It may respond too quickly or too slowly. It may respond in an exaggerated way or with unusual side effects or complications. The response may be followed by a relapse without organic justification, or the condition may remain refractory in spite of otherwise effective therapy. Pains that are greatly influenced by psychologic factors may display changeability in location, intensity, or temporal behavior without a reasonable, identifiable organic cause.

To summarize, the following clinical characteristics are common to pain conditions that are greatly influenced by psychologic factors:

1. The site of pain lacks an adequate, anatomically related source of nociceptive input.
2. The clinical behavior and responsiveness of the pain to reasonable therapy are unusual, unexpected, and nonphysiologic.

The psychologic influence of orofacial pains can be categorized into certain identifiable mental disorders.[8] Although there are numerous disorders, the clinician needs to be familiar with the following common mental disorders, since these can greatly influence the individual's pain experience: *(1)* mood disorders, *(2)* anxiety disorders, *(3)* somatoform disorders, and *(4)* another category that includes many other mental conditions or psychologic factors that affect the outcome of a medical condition.

Each of these major categories can be separated into subcategories. Mood disorders are divided into the depressive disorders, bipolar disorders, and a general category in which the mood disorder is the result of a medical condition.

Anxiety disorders are subdivided into generalized anxiety disorders, posttraumatic stress disorders, and anxiety disorders that are the result of a medical condition.

Somatoform disorders are a group of disorders that are characterized by physical symptoms suggesting a physical disorder for which there are no demonstrable organic findings of known physiologic mechanisms. Strong positive evidence that the symptoms are linked to psychologic factors or conflicts is important. The somatoform disorders are subdivided into undifferentiated somatoform disorders, conversion disorders, pain disorders, and hypochondriasis.

The last category is a broad group of mental disorders that may be related to pain conditions. This category includes malingering and psychologic factors affecting a medical condition, such as certain personality traits or coping styles, maladaptive health behavior, and stress-related physiologic responses.

Each category in Axis I and Axis II conditions will be presented in detail in later chapters, along with treatment strategies.

References

1. Dorland WAN. Dorland's Illustrated Medical Dictionary, ed 27. Philadelphia: Saunders, 1981.
2. Merskey H. Pain terms: A list with definitions and notes on usage. Pain 1979;6:249–252.
3. Merskey H. Pain terms: A supplementary note. Pain 1982;14:205–206.
4. Merskey H, Bogduk N, IASP Task Force on Taxonomy. Classification of Chronic Pain, ed 2. Seattle: IASP Press, 1994:209–214.
5. Merskey H. Pain specialists and pain terms. Pain 1996;64:205.
6. Classification and diagnosis criteria for headache disorders, cranial neuralgias, and facial pain. Headache Classification Committee of the International Headache Society. Cephalalgia 1988;8(suppl 7):1–96.
7. Headache Classification Committee of the International Headache Society. The international classification of headache disorders: 2nd edition. Cephalalgia 2004;24(supp 1):9–160.
8. American Psychiatric Association. Diagnostic and Statistical Manual of Mental Disorders: DSM-IV, ed 4. Washington, DC: American Psychiatric Association, 1994.
9. Bonica JJ. The Management of Pain. Philadelphia: Lea & Febiger, 1990:161–169.
10. Wolff HG, Wolf S. Pain, ed 2. Springfield, IL: Thomas, 1958.

11. Procacci P, Zoppi M, Maresea M. Experimental pain in man. Pain 1979;6:123–140.

12. Cutrer FM. Pain-sensitive cranial structures. In: Silberstein SD, Lipton RB, Dalessio DJ (eds). Wolff's Headache and Other Head Pain, ed 7. New York: Oxford University Press, 2001:50–56.

13. Dalessio DJ. The major neuralgias, postinfectious neuritis, and atypical facial pain. In: Dalessio DJ, Silberstein SD. Wolff's Headache and Other Head Pain, ed 6. New York: Oxford University Press, 1993:345–364.

14. Coffey RJ, Rhoton AL. Pain-sensitive cranial structures. In: Dalessio DJ. Wolff's Headache and Other Head Pain, ed 5. New York: Oxford University Press, 1987:34–50.

15. Dellow PG, Morgan NJ. Trigeminal nerve inputs and central blood pressure change in the rat. Arch Oral Biol 1969;14:295–300.

16. Bowsher D. A camel is a horse designed by a committee. J Pain Symptom Manage 1987;2:237–239.

Principles of
Pain Diagnosis

Every day, patients seek care for the reduction or elimination of pain. Nothing is more satisfying to the clinician than the successful elimination of the patient's pain. This elimination is usually the result of some form of therapeutic intervention. Both the patient and clinician therefore tend to focus on the importance of the therapy. The most important part of managing pain, however, is in understanding the problem and establishing a proper diagnosis. It is only through proper diagnosis that the appropriate therapy can be selected. Diagnosis is not easy. Too often it is overlooked or de-emphasized; yet success cannot be achieved without it. This chapter will describe the necessary components for making the proper diagnosis.

The objective of diagnosis is to accurately identify the what, where, how, and why of the patient's complaint. Pain diagnosis is complicated by some very difficult problems. Pain is a dynamic, changing experience that embraces sensation, emotion, and reaction. Nociception is predominantly subjective in nature, while objective pain behavior reflects consequences as much as cause. A complex pain modulation phenomenon individualizes every painful experi-

ence. These characteristics of pain make the diagnosis and management of obscure pains a sobering and sometimes humbling experience for even the most astute clinician.

One difficulty that many clinicians face is his or her mechanistic approach to disease. We are often very "cause" oriented. The "why" in diagnosis, important as it is, may become a stumbling block when dealing with obscure pain, for there may be no cause at all. An understanding that not all pains are somatic is basic to diagnosis. Neuropathic pains and psychologic factors are not always obvious upon examination. The clinician must be cognitive of the biopsychosocial model of disease. On the other hand, if the condition seems related to an actual stimulus of somatic structures, then identification of the cause is essential for proper management.

Another difficulty of which we must be aware is the temptation to assume that the symptoms of which the patient complains represent the real problem that needs to be investigated and managed. Pain behavior consists of audible and visible signals exhibited by the patient that indicate his or her suffering. These signals have filtered down through a chain of modulating influences, not the least of which are the consequences that attend the whole experience. Thus, the complaint as manifested by suffering may bear little relevance to the real underlying problem. Yet it is the suffering itself that the patient presents for treatment.

Diagnosis of a pain complaint consists essentially of three major steps:

1. Accurate identification of the location of the structure from which the pain emanates.
2. Establishment of the correct pain category that is represented in the condition under investigation. This is a matter of recognizing the clinical characteristics that are displayed. Establishment of the proper pain category is dependent upon a good understanding of the genesis and mechanisms of pain.
3. Choice of the particular pain disorder that correctly accounts for the incidence and behavior of the patient's pain problem. This requires familiarity with the clinical symptoms displayed by pain disorders that occur in the orofacial region.

Evaluation of the Pain Condition

When a patient reports with pain, information must be gathered so that the clinician can determine the proper pain diagnosis. This information is gathered in two forms: the history and the clinical examination. The data collected from the history and examination must be thorough enough to determine not only the physical factors that contribute to the pain disorders, but also the psychologic factors. The main objective of the history and the examination is to locate the true source of the pain that relates to the patient's chief complaint.

All pain complaints merit an interview with the patient to determine the significance of the complaint. Some pains are easy to identify and require little diagnostic effort. In these instances, an elaborate evaluation may not be needed. Other pains require significant evaluation by the clinician. These pains require a very detailed orofacial pain history and examination. The need for a thorough history and examination is determined by the preliminary interview.

Preliminary Interview

The initial contact with the patient and discussion of his or her problem are extremely important. Unless satisfactory professional rapport can be initially established, it may be wise to refer the patient before becoming further involved. The rapport on which proper communication must rest requires sincere effort by both patient and clinician. The patient must be willing to honestly and accurately divulge the information that the clinician needs. He or she must do so cooperatively and with a sincere desire to obtain relief from the complaint. If the patient's intentions and objectives are anything less than this, not only will valuable time and effort be wasted, but chances are, more harm than good will result.

The clinician must feel confident of his or her own competence in the identification and management of pain problems. Any lack of confidence will quickly be sensed by the patient and can destroy the chances of a satisfactory patient-clinician relationship. Moreover, it would be professionally dishonest for a therapist to pursue any course of action for which he felt unprepared. Competence, honesty, patience, and an earnest desire by the therapist to serve the patient are the minimal prerequisites for establishing a satisfactory professional rapport.

At the preliminary interview, sufficient data should be collected to help determine the future course of the examining procedure. Some overall idea of the location, inception, duration, and clinical behavior of the complaint should be obtained. Plans should then be made to either continue the examination, refer the patient to another practitioner, or plan for needed consultations as indicated. Very simple pain problems, such as mucogingival pain of local origin, localized pain due to obvious dental cause, and some cases of typical trigeminal neuralgia, may be solved without extensive examination. More obscure pain complaints justify a carefully planned diagnostic procedure.

It is important to evaluate the patient's pain in terms of what it means to him or her. This is accomplished by obtaining specific and meaningful descriptors from the patient that accurately describe the complaint. Many patients may not have at their disposal an adequate means of communicating such exact information. In his McGill Pain Questionnaire, Melzack[1-4] arranged descriptive adjectives in several groups. Each series of words is arranged in order of increasing intensity. The patient can be instructed to select one word in each series that best describes the complaint. The first group is composed of sensory descriptors that help describe what the discomfort feels like to the patient.

1. Temporal: flicking, quivering, pulsing, throbbing, beating, pounding
2. Spatial: jumping, flashing, shooting
3. Punctate pressure: pricking, boring, drilling, stabbing, lancinating
4. Incisive pressure: sharp, cutting, lacerating
5. Constrictive pressure: pinching, pressing, gnawing, cramping, crushing
6. Traction pressure: tugging, pulling, wrenching

7. Thermal: hot, burning, scalding, searing
8. Brightness: tingling, itchy, smarting, stinging
9. Dullness: dull, sore, hurting, aching, heavy
10. Miscellaneous: tender, taut, rasping, splitting

The second group consists of affective descriptors that yield information about how the patient is reacting to the pain.

1. Tension: tiring, exhausting
2. Autonomic: sickening, suffocating
3. Fear: fearful, frightful, terrifying
4. Punishment: punishing, grueling, cruel, vicious, killing
5. Miscellaneous: wretched, blinding

The third group is a series of evaluative descriptors that tend to classify the intensity of pain.

1. Annoying, troublesome, miserable, intense, unbearable

A fourth group of general descriptors has been added to the questionnaire.

1. Spreading, radiating, penetrating, piercing
2. Tight, numb, drawing, squeezing, tearing
3. Cool, cold, freezing
4. Nagging, nauseating, agonizing, dreadful, torturing

Patients who cannot verbalize the description of their complaint may find these descriptors useful.

When the clinician identifies a complex pain complaint, a more thorough evaluation should be accomplished. This evaluation is composed of two major components: the history and the clinical examination. Information gained during the history and examination should allow the clinician to place the pain complaint into the proper pain category so that effective therapy may be selected. Establishment of the proper diagnosis is the most important task accomplished by the clinician and should never be underemphasized, since it is the basis for successful pain management.

The history needs to investigate all aspects of the pain complaint. It should assess the present location of the pain complaint, the time it began, and a detailed description of the pain as initially felt. An evaluation of the early characteristics of the complaint may give valuable clues to its identification prior to modification. Information concerning the duration and clinical course of the complaint with special reference to efforts at treatment is valuable. The general physical and emotional background for the complaint should be noted, as well as the influence of prior trauma, infection, or systemic illness. All medications currently in use should be listed.

The examination should gather information from clinical, radiographic, and laboratory procedures relative to the oral cavity, masticatory system, and regional musculature. Special information derived from diagnostic analgesic blocking, the effect of diagnostic drugs, and trial therapy may also be helpful.

History for Orofacial Pain

An accurate history is the most important aspect in diagnosing obscure pain. It is far more important than the examination. If the clinician will carefully listen, the patient will report the precise pain problem that exists. The patient may use nonmedical terms; nevertheless, the information should allow the clinician to establish a differential diagnosis. The examination can then be used to further clarify the proper pain category or disorder. Much thought should therefore be given to the skillful interviewing of the patient.

History taking can be accomplished in one of two forms: oral or written. An oral history provides some advantages over the written history in that it allows the clinician to meet the patient and establish important rapport. It also allows the patient to express feelings and experiences in his or her own words. The clinician can often gain insight regarding the patient's feelings concerning past experiences, anger, fear, hostility, and disability. Oral history taking allows the clinician to gain information in a logical sequence, asking appropriate questions as needed. The major disadvantage of the oral history is that it relies heavily on the clinician's ability to remember all aspects of the history so that no important information is missed. A written history form can eliminate this concern. With a written history form, all important aspects can be included and the patient can fill the form out leisurely in advance of the appointment. Although this type of history is certainly more reliably complete, it may be frustrating to the patient when the questions do not adequately allow him or her to depict the problem.

In many offices both types of histories are used. The written form is completed in advance of the appointment. This is reviewed by the clinician before actually meeting the patient. Then, when the patient is seated, the clinician allows the patient to verbalize the pain complaint while establishing the important doctor/patient rapport. Any confusing items observed in the written history can then be clarified.

Table 8-1 lists important features that should be included in a thorough orofacial pain history. Each item will be discussed in more detail.

The Chief Complaint

A good starting point in history taking is to obtain an accurate description of the patient's chief complaint. This should first be taken in the patient's own words and then restated in technical language as indicated. If the patient has more than one pain complaint, each complaint should be noted and when possible placed in a list according to its significance to the patient. Each complaint needs to be evaluated according to each factor listed in the history outline. Once this has been accomplished, each pain complaint should be assessed with respect to its relationship to any of the other complaints. Some complaints may be secondary to another complaint, while others may be independent. An understanding of these relationships is basic to management.

Location of the pain

The patient's ability to locate the pain with accuracy is diagnostic. However, the examiner should always guard against assuming that the site of pain necessarily identifies the true source of pain, ie, the structure from which the pain actually emanates. The patient's description of the location of the complaint identifies only the site of pain. It is the examiner's responsibility to determine whether it is also the true source of the pain. Sometimes, what appears to be adequate cause at the site of pain may mislead both the patient and the doctor, such as visible superficial herpetic lesions or deep tenderness to manual palpation.

It is very helpful to provide the patient with a drawing of the head and neck and ask him or her to outline the location of the pain (Figs 8-1a to 8-1c). This allows the patient to reflect in his or her own way any and all of the pain sites. The patient can also draw arrows revealing any patterns of pain referral. These drawings can give the clinician significant insight regarding the

location and even the type of pain the patient is experiencing.

Onset of the pain

It is important to assess any circumstances associated with the initial onset of the pain complaint. These circumstances can give great insight as to etiology. For example, in some instances, the pain complaint began immediately following a motor vehicle accident. Trauma can frequently cause a pain

---

Table 8-1 Features to Include in an Orofacial Pain History

A. The chief complaint (perhaps more than one)
1. Location of the pain
2. Onset of the pain
   a. Association with other factors
   b. Progression
3. Characteristics of the pain
   a. Quality of the pain
   b. Behavior of the pain
      i. Temporal nature
      ii. Frequency
      iii. Duration
   c. Intensity
   d. Concomitant symptoms
   e. Flow of the pain
4. Aggravating and alleviating factors
   a. Physical modalities
   b. Function and parafunction
   c. Sleep disturbances
   d. Medications
   e. Emotional stress
5. Past consultation and/or treatments
6. Relationship to other complaints

B. Past medical history

C. Review of systems

D. Psychologic assessment

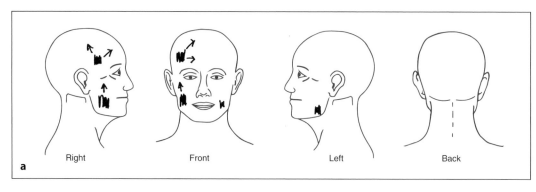

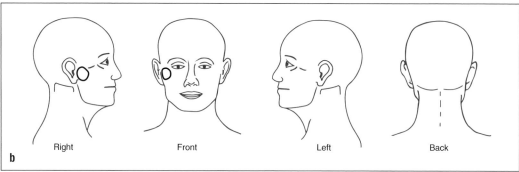

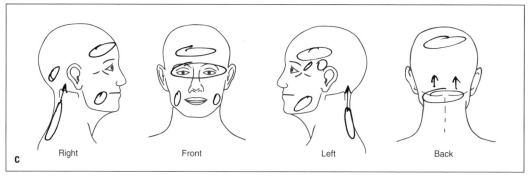

Fig 8-1 Asking the patient to draw the location of the pain and any patterns of referral on a drawing of the head and neck can be very helpful. *(a)* Example of how a patient with masticatory muscle pain described her pain. Note the broad areas of pain and the radiating patterns of referral. *(b)* Example of how a patient experiencing temporomandibular joint (TMJ) pain described the location of her pain. *(c)* Locations of the pain felt by a patient suffering with myofascial pain in the cervical region with referral to the head, initially described as "headache."

condition, and knowing this not only gives insight as to etiology but also enlightens the examiner to other considerations such as other injuries, related emotional trauma, and possible litigation. The onset of some pain conditions is associated with systemic illnesses or jaw function, or may even be wholly spontaneous. It is important that the patient presents the circumstances associated with the initial onset in chronologic order so that proper relationships can be evaluated.

It is equally important to ask the patient what he or she believes caused the pain condition. This may provide great insight into the patient's view of the pain. In many instances the patient knows precisely what caused the condition. Even if the patient is confused as to cause, the examiner may gain valuable information that is useful in management. For example, this question may reveal anger associated with blame for the pain condition. It is important to know whether the patient believes the pain has been caused by mistreatment or another practitioner. This type of anger may greatly influence future treatment outcome.

Characteristics of the pain

The characteristics of the pain need to be precisely described by the patient, ie, the quality, behavior, intensity, concomitant symptoms, and manner of flow of the pain.

Quality of the pain

The quality of pain should be classified according to how it makes the patient feel. This classification is usually termed *bright* or *dull*. When pain has a stimulating or exciting effect on the patient, it is classified as bright. When the pain has a depressing effect that causes the patient to withdraw to some extent, it is classified as dull. It is important that such judgment be wholly independent of pain intensity, variability, temporal characteristics, or any accompanying

lancinating exacerbations that may punctuate the basic underlying painful sensation.

Further evaluation of the quality of pain should be made to classify it as pricking, itching, stinging, burning, aching, or pulsating. Many pains, of course, require more than a single designation. Bright, tingling pain is classified as a pricking sensation, especially when mild and stimulating. Superficial discomfort that does not reach pain threshold intensity may be described as itching. As the intensity increases, the pain may take on a pricking, stinging, aching, or burning quality. Deep discomfort that does not reach pain threshold intensity may be described as a vague, diffuse sensation of pressure, warmth, or tenderness. As the intensity increases, the pain may take on a sore, aching, throbbing, or burning quality. When the discomfort has an irritating, hot, raw, caustic quality, it is usually described as burning. Most pains have an aching quality. Some increase noticeably with each heartbeat and are described as pulsating or throbbing.

Behavior of the pain

The behavior of the pain should be evaluated according to frequency or temporal behavior, as well as its duration and localizability.

Temporal behavior reflects the frequency of the pain as well as the periods between episodes of the pain. If the suffering distinctly comes and goes, leaving pain-free intervals of noticeable duration, it is classified as *intermittent* or *episodic*. If such pain-free intervals do not occur, it is classified as *continuous*. Intermittency should not be confused with variability, in which there may be alternate periods of high-level and low-level discomfort. Intermittent pain implies the occurrence of true intermissions or pain-free periods during which comfort is complete. This temporal behavior should not be confused with the effect of medications that induce periods of comfort by analgesic action. When episodes of pain, whether continuous or intermittent, are separated by an extended period of freedom from discomfort, only to be followed by another similar episode of pain, the syndrome is said to be *recurrent*.

The *duration* of individual pains during an episode is an important descriptive feature that aids in pain identification. A pain is said to be *momentary* if its duration can be expressed in seconds. Longer-lasting pains are classified in minutes, hours, or a day. A pain that continues from one day to the next is said to be *protracted*.

The *localization behavior* of the pain should be included in its description. If the patient is able to define the pain to an exact anatomic location, it is classified as *localized pain*. If such description is less well defined and somewhat vague and variable anatomically, it is termed *diffuse pain*. Rapidly changing pain is classified as *radiating*. A momentary cutting exacerbation is usually described as *lancinating*. More gradually changing pain is described as *spreading*, and if it progressively involves adjacent anatomic areas, the pain is called *enlarging*. If it changes from one location to another, the complaint is described as *migrating*. Referred pain and secondary hyperalgesia are clinical expressions of secondary pain.

Intensity of the pain

The intensity of the pain should be established by distinguishing between mild and severe pain. This can be based on how the patient appears to react to the suffering. Mild pain is associated with pain that is described by the patient but without a display of visible physical reactions. Severe pain is associated with significant reactions of the patient to provocation of the painful area. One of the best methods of assessing the intensity of the pain is with a visual analogue scale. The patient is given a piece of paper with a line that has "no pain" written on one end and "the worst possible pain

experienced ever" written on the other end. The patient is then asked to place a mark on the location of the line that best describes the pain at that time. A scale of 0 to 5 or 0 to 10 can be used to assess the intensity of the pain, with 0 indicating no pain and 10 indicating the most pain possible. This scale is not only helpful for the initial assessment of pain, but is also useful at follow-up appointments to evaluate the success or failure of therapies.[5]

Concomitant symptoms

All concomitant symptoms, such as sensory, motor, or autonomic effects that accompany the pain, should be included. Sensations such as hyperesthesia, hypoesthesia, anesthesia, paresthesia, or dysesthesia should be mentioned. Any concomitant change in the special senses affecting vision, hearing, smell, or taste should be noted. Motor changes expressed as muscular weakness, muscular contractions, or actual spasm should be recognized. Various localized autonomic symptoms should be observed and described. Ocular symptoms may include lacrimation, injection of the conjunctivae, pupillary changes, and edema of the lids. Nasal symptoms include nasal secretion and congestion. Cutaneous symptoms may include changes in skin temperature or color, sweating, and piloerection. Gastric symptoms include nausea and indigestion.

Manner of flow of the pain

The *manner of flow* informs the clinician whether the individual pains are steady or paroxysmal. A flowing type of pain, although it may vary in intensity or be distinctly intermittent, is described as *steady*. Such pain is to be distinguished from *paroxysmal pain*, which characteristically consists of sudden volleys or jabs. The volleys may vary considerably in both intensity and duration. When they occur frequently, the pain may become nearly continuous.

Aggravating and alleviating factors

Effect of functional activities

The effect of functional activities should be observed and described. Common biomechanical functions include such activities as movement of the face, jaw, or tongue and the effects of swallowing, head position, and body position. The effect of such activities as talking, chewing, yawning, brushing the teeth, shaving, washing the face, turning the head, stooping over, or lying down should be noted. In addition, the effect of emotional stress, fatigue, and time of day should be recorded.

The pain may be triggered by minor superficial stimulation, such as touch or movement of the skin, lips, face, tongue, or throat. When triggered by such activities, it is well to distinguish between merely incidental stimulation of overlying tissues and stimulation that is the result of functioning of the joints and muscles themselves. The former is true triggering, while the latter is pain induction. This distinction can usually be made by stabilizing the joints and muscles with a bite block to prevent their movement while the other structures are stimulated or moved. If uncertainty exists, the distinction can be made more positively by utilizing local anesthesia. Topical anesthesia of the throat effectively arrests triggering in the glossopharyngeal nerve distribution. Mandibular block anesthesia stops triggering from the lower lip and tongue. Infraorbital anesthesia arrests triggering from the upper lip and maxillary skin. None of these procedures prevents the induction of true masticatory pain.

Parafunctional activities should also be assessed. The patient should be questioned regarding bruxism, clenching, or any other oral habit. One should remember that often these activities occur at subconscious levels and therefore the patient may not report them accurately.

Effect of physical modalities

The patient should be questioned regarding the effectiveness of hot or cold on the pain condition. The patient should be asked whether other modalities, such as massage or transcutaneous electrical nerve stimulation therapy, have been tried, and if so, what the results were. The results of such therapies may shed light on the type of pain condition and its therapeutic responsiveness.

Medications

The patient should report all past and present medications taken for the pain condition. Dosages should be acquired, along with the frequency taken and effectiveness in altering the chief complaint. It is also helpful to know who prescribed these medications, since their input may also shed light on the pain condition.

Emotional stress

As has already been discussed, emotional stress can be a major contributing factor to the pain condition. In some instances, however, emotional stress may not be a major factor but instead an aggravating factor. When this is present, patients will report that although their pain is present at all times it seems to be accentuated during times of increased stress. It is important for both the clinician and the patient to recognize this relationship.

Sleep quality

There appears to be a relationship between some pain conditions and the quality of the patient's sleep.[6-13] It is important, therefore, that quality of sleep be reviewed. Patients who report poor-quality sleep should be questioned regarding the relationship of this finding with the pain condition. Particular notice should be taken when the patient reports waking during the night in pain or when the pain actually wakens the patient.

Litigation

During the interview it is important to inquire whether the patient is involved in any form of litigation related to the pain complaint. This information may help the clinician better appreciate all conditions surrounding the pain. The presence of litigation does not directly imply secondary gains, but this condition may be present.

Past consultations and treatments

During the interview, all previous consultations and treatments should be thoroughly discussed and reviewed. This information is extremely important in avoiding repetition of tests and therapies. If information is incomplete or unclear, the previous treating clinician should be contacted and appropriate information requested. Clinical notes from previous treating clinicians can be extremely helpful in deciding future treatments.

When a patient reports previous treatment with an occlusal appliance, the patient should be asked to bring the appliance to the evaluation appointment. The previous success of this treatment should be reported and the appliance evaluated. This evaluation may shed light on future treatment considerations.

Relationship to other pain complaints

As previously discussed, some patients may report more than one pain complaint. When more than one complaint is reported, the clinician needs to evaluate each aspect of each complaint separately. Once each complaint is evaluated according to all the above-mentioned criteria, the relationship of one complaint to the others should be ascertained. Sometimes a pain complaint may actually be secondary to another complaint. In these instances, effective management of the primary pain complaint will likely also resolve the secondary pain complaint. In other instances, one complaint may be totally independent of another complaint. When this exists, individual therapy may need to be directed to each complaint. Identification of the relationship between these complaints is essential and best determined by the history.

Medical History

Since pain can be a symptom related to many physical illnesses and disorders, it is essential that the past and present medical condition be carefully evaluated. Any past serious illnesses, hospitalizations, operations, medications, or other significant treatments should be discussed in light of the present pain complaint. When indicated, treating physicians should be contacted for additional information. It may also be appropriate to discuss your proposed treatment with the patient's primary practitioner when significant health problems are present.

Review of Systems

A complete history should also include appropriate questions concerning the present status of the patient's general body systems. Questions should investigate the present health status of the following systems: cardiovascular (including lungs), digestive, renal, and liver, as well as the peripheral and central nervous systems. Any abnormalities should be noted and any relationship with the pain complaint should be determined.

Psychologic Assessment

As pain becomes more chronic, psychologic factors relating to the pain complaint become more common. Routine psychologic evaluation may not be necessary with acute pain; however, with chronic pain it becomes essential. It may be difficult for the general practitioner to confidently evaluate psychologic factors. For this reason, chronic pain patients are best evaluated and managed by a multidisciplinary approach.

There are a variety of measuring tools that can be used to assess the psychologic status of the patient. Turk and Rudy[14] have developed the Multidimensional Pain Inventory (MPI). This scale evaluates three pain profiles: adaptive coping, interpersonal distress, and dysfunctional chronic pain. Dysfunctional chronic pain is a profile of severe pain, functional disability, psychologic impairment, and low perceived life control.

Another useful tool is the Symptom Check List 90 (SCL-90).[15] This evaluation provides both a depression scale and a scale measuring the severity of nonspecific physical symptoms (the somatization subscale). Assessment of these factors for a chronic pain patient is essential.

Often the general practitioner may not have immediate access to psychologic evaluation support. In this instance, the practitioner may elect to use IMPATH[16] or the TMJ Scale.[17,18] These two scales have been developed for use in the private dental practice to assist in evaluating clinical and certain psychologic factors associated with orofacial pains. Although these scales are helpful, they are not as complete as the above psychologic tests and certainly do not replace the personal evaluation of a clinical psychologist.

As discussed in chapters 6 and 7, there are a number of psychologic conditions that can contribute to or actually be responsible for pain disorders. One category of psychologic conditions is the *somatoform disorders*. These disorders are characterized by complaints of physical symptoms for which there are no demonstrable organic findings or known physical mechanisms.

When pain is the chief complaint, this disorder is called a *somatoform pain disorder*.[19] Another type of somatoform disorder is a *conversion disorder*. The essential feature of this disorder is an alteration or loss of physical functioning that suggests a physical disorder, but instead of the presence of an actual physical disorder, the symptoms are an apparent expression of a psychologic conflict or need. The symptoms are not intentionally produced, yet they cannot be explained by any physical disorder or known pathophysiologic mechanism. A third type of somatoform disorder is *hypochondriasis*. The essential feature of this disorder is preoccupation with the fear of having—or the belief that one has—a serious disease, based on the patient's interpretation of physical signs or symptoms as evidence of physical illness.

Psychologic assessment is also important in identifying other mental disorders such as mood disorders (ie, depression) and anxiety disorders (ie, posttraumatic stress disorder). There is also a broad category that includes psychologic factors that are affecting a physical condition. In this category, the psychologic factor may not be significant enough to warrant its own disorder but in fact it does affect an existing condition. This category may likely be the most common psychologic condition associated with chronic orofacial pain disorders.

Psychologic assessment is an essential part of the orofacial pain history. The manner by which it is performed will vary according to the expertise of the clinician. As pain disorders become more chronic, it is best for the clinician to rely on a trained clinical psychologist or psychiatrist for this evaluation.

Summary of History

Once the history has been taken, the clinician should be able to accurately and completely describe the pain condition. For example, a typical narrative description of trigeminal neuralgia involving the right mandibular division of the trigeminal nerve would be as follows:

Patient presents with a 1-year history of severe pain in the mandibular right dental and alveolar process area spontaneously triggered by light touch and movement of the lower lip. The complaint is described as recurrent episodes of bright, burning pain that occur intermittently in repeated paroxysms, lasting a few seconds each time and felt in the same precise anatomic location with little or no variation from time to time. No secondary pains are noticed. The paroxysms are excited by all functional activities that cause minor stimulation of the lower lip. The pains are accompanied by contraction of facial muscles, but no other concomitant neurologic effects are seen. The pain is not relieved or prevented by any medications. The patient does not present with any significant psychologic conditions, although he does admit that the pain has increased his general anxiety level secondary to not knowing when the next pain will strike.

Clinical Examination for Orofacial Pain

An effective examination form helps the practitioner obtain essential data with the least expenditure of time and effort. Ensuring that such data are complete is important in the identification of pain. An examination form should be as simple and flexible as possible so as to be readily adaptable to the many different pain problems that present themselves.

The purpose of the clinical examination is to identify any variations from the normal health and function of the orofacial structures. The examination should include an assessment of nonmasticatory structures, such as the neurologic status, as well

as evaluation of the eyes, ears, and neck. If abnormal findings are identified, an immediate referral to the appropriate specialty is indicated. The examination should also include an assessment of the masticatory structures.

Locating the Source of Pain

Although the history is important in identifying the site of pain, it is the examination that is most helpful in locating the true source of the pain. The clinician should always be suspicious of heterotopic pains, since they are so common in the orofacial structures. Remember, for therapy to be effective, it must be directed toward the source of pain, not the site. Of course, this is no problem if the pain is primary pain, since both the site and source are in the same location. If, however, the pain is referred, this presents an interesting twist. When referred pains are present, the clinician may often have a tendency to direct therapy to the site of pain as directed by the patient. Of course this type of therapy will fail, since it will not affect the cause of the pain. The astute pain clinician will always be suspicious of referred pain and will always clinically confirm the source of the pain.

Primary pains can be differentiated from referred pains by their characteristics during local provocation (Fig 8-2a). Remember, referred pains are wholly dependent upon the original source of the pain. Therefore, when a source of pain is located during an examination, palpation of the source will not only increase the pain at the source but will also likely increase the pain at the referred site (Fig 8-2b). If palpation of the site of pain does not increase the pain, one should be suspicious of a referred site of pain. If the information gained during the examination is not complete enough to identify the pain, then selective local anesthetic blocking of selected tissues may be needed. Local anesthetic blocking of the site of pain will not decrease the pain, since it does not interrupt the true source of the pain (Fig 8-2c). On the other hand, when the source of pain is anesthetically blocked (Fig 8-2d), the pain will be reduced not only at the source, but also at the site. When the clinician is confused regarding the true source of the pain, local anesthetic blocking should be used. In some instances it may be the only way to locate the true source of pain. Pain therapists need to be familiar with the various local anesthetic blocks used in the head and neck. These will be discussed later in this chapter.

The following four rules summarize the examination techniques used to differentiate primary pain from referred pain:

1. Local provocation of the site of pain does not increase the pain.
2. Local provocation of the source of pain increases the pain, not only at the source but also at the site.
3. Local anesthetic blocking of the site of pain does not decrease the pain.
4. Local anesthetic blocking of the source of pain decreases the pain at the source as well as the site.

An orofacial pain examination should thoroughly evaluate all structures of the orofacial region. Table 8-2 provides a summary of a comprehensive examination.

General Examination

Vital signs

For the clinician to become well acquainted with the patient, vital signs should be taken. Although this information may not always be helpful in making a diagnosis, in some instances it may prove to be a major contributor to the pain. Certain headaches may be associated with hypertension. Systemic infections are often associated with elevated body temperature. Increased breathing rates are often associated with an up-regulation of the sympathetic nervous system. Therefore, blood pressure, pulse rate, respiration rate, and body temperature should be assessed, especially when the pain condition is obscure and unexplained.

Cranial nerve evaluation

The 12 cranial nerves supply sensory information to and motor impulses from the brain. Any gross problem relating to their functions must be identified so that abnormal conditions can be immediately and appropriately addressed. The orofacial pain therapist does not need to be trained as a neurologist. In fact, a cranial nerve examination need not be a complex evaluation. Any clinician who regularly evaluates pain problems can test the gross function of the cranial nerves to evaluate for any neuropathic disorders. Each nerve can be assessed with the following simple evaluation procedures.

Olfactory nerve

The first cranial nerve has sensory fibers originating in the mucous membrane of the nasal cavity and provides the sensation of smell. It is tested by asking the patient to detect differences between the odors of peppermint, vanilla, and chocolate. (It is helpful to have these available in the office for testing.) It must also be determined whether or not the patient's nose is obstructed. This can be done by asking the patient to exhale nasally onto a mirror. Fogging of the mirror from both nostrils indicates adequate air flow.

Optic nerve

The second cranial nerve, also sensory, with fibers originating in the retina, provides for sight. It is tested by having the patient cover one eye and read a few sentences. The other

Figs 8-2a to 8-2d Proper examination procedures are necessary to identify the true source of the pain. When one is unsure of the source of pain the following sequence should be followed.

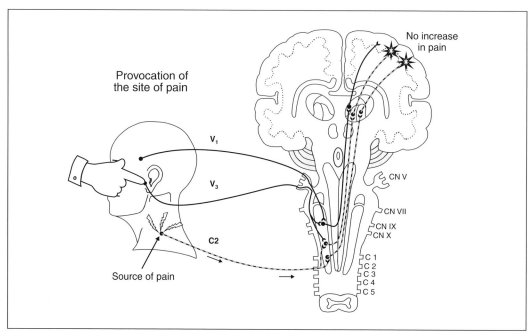

Fig 8-2a Provocation of the site of pain does not increase the pain.

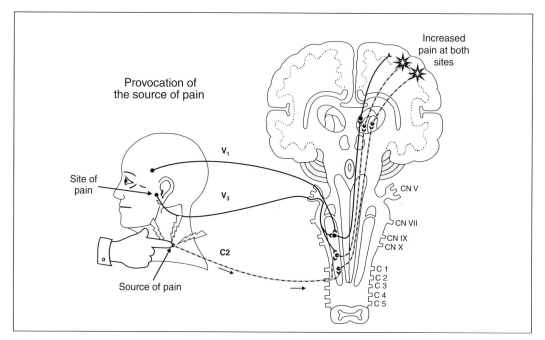

Fig 8-2b Provocation of the source of pain increases the pain, not only at the source but also at the site.

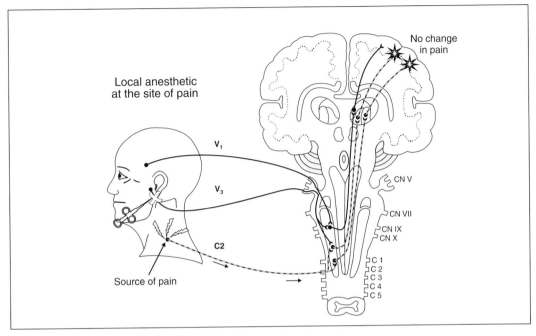

Fig 8-2c Local anesthesia at the site of pain fails to reduce the pain.

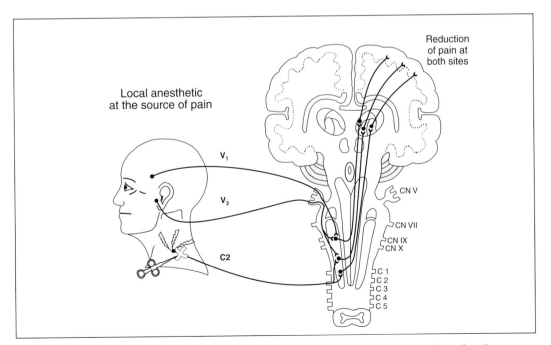

Fig 8-2d Local anesthesia at the source of pain reduces the pain at the source as well as the site.

Table 8-2 Summary of a Comprehensive Clinical Examination

A. General examination
1. Vital signs
   a. Blood pressure
   b. Pulse rate
   c. Respiration rate
   d. Temperature
2. Cranial nerve evaluation
3. Eye evaluation
4. Ear evaluation
5. Cervical evaluation
6. Balance and coordination

B. Muscle examination
1. Palpation
   a. Pain and tenderness
   b. Trigger points and pain referral

C. Masticatory evaluation
1. Range of mandibular movement
   a. Measurements
   b. Pain
2. Temporomandibular joint evaluation
   a. Pain
   b. Dysfunction
3. Oral structures
   a. The mucogingival tissues
   b. The teeth
   c. The periodontia
   d. The occlusion

D. Other diagnostic tests
1. Imaging
2. Laboratory tests
3. Psychologic assessment and/or psychologic provocation tests

---

eye is checked in the same manner. The clinician assesses the visual field by standing behind the patient and slowly bringing the fingers from behind around into view (Fig 8-3). The patient should report when the fingers first appear. There normally will be no variation between when they are seen on the right and on the left.

Oculomotor, trochlear, and abducent nerves
The third, fourth, and sixth cranial nerves, which supply motor fibers to the extraocular muscles, are tested by having the patient follow the clinician's finger as the clinician makes an X (Fig 8-4). Both eyes should move smoothly and similarly as they follow the finger. The pupils should be of equal size and rounded and should react to light by constricting. The accommodation reflex is tested by having the patient change focus from a distant to a nearby object. The pupils should constrict as the object (the finger) approaches the patient's face. Not only should they both constrict to direct light, but each should also constrict to light

directed in the other eye (consensual light reflex) (Fig 8-5).

Trigeminal nerve
The fifth cranial nerve is both sensory (from the face, scalp, nose, and mouth) and motor (to the muscles of mastication). Sensory input is tested by lightly stroking the face with a cotton tip bilaterally in three regions: forehead, cheek, and mandible (Fig 8-6). This will give a rough idea of the function of the ophthalmic, maxillary, and mandibular branches of the trigeminal nerve. The patient should describe similar sensations on each side. The trigeminal nerve also contains sensory fibers from the cornea. The corneal reflexes can be tested by observing the patient's blink in response to light touch on the cornea with a sterile cotton pledget or tissue. Gross motor input is tested by having the patient clench while the clinician feels both masseter and temporal muscles (Fig 8-7). The muscles should contract equally bilaterally.

Fig 8-3 Checking the patient's visual field (optic nerve): With the patient looking forward, the examiner's fingers are brought around to the front from behind. The initial position at which the fingers are seen marks the extent of the visual field. Right and left fields should be very similar.

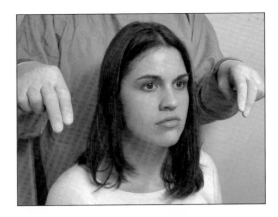

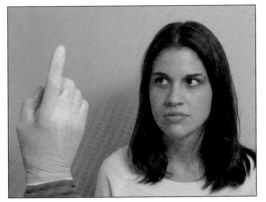

Fig 8-4 Checking the patient's extraocular muscles: Without moving the patient's head, the examiner asks the patient to follow the finger as it makes an X in front of the patient. Any variation in right or left eye movement is noted.

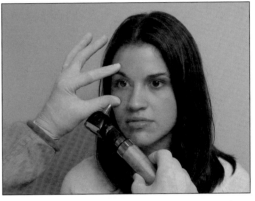

Fig 8-5 Constriction of the pupil can be seen when light is directed toward the eye. The opposite pupil should also constrict, demonstrating the consensual light reflex.

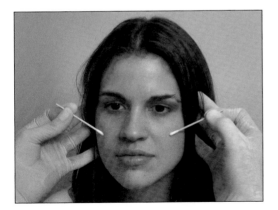

Fig 8-6 Cotton tip applicators can be used to compare discrimination of light touch between the right and left maxillary branches of the trigeminal nerve. The ophthalmic and mandibular branches are also tested.

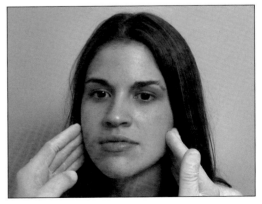

Fig 8-7 Motor function of the trigeminal nerve to the masseter muscles is tested by asking the patient to clench the teeth together while the examiner feels for bilateral contraction.

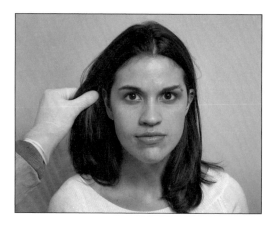

Fig 8-8 Gross hearing can be evaluated by asking the patient if she can hear the sound of rubbing a strand of hair between the finger and thumb. Any difference in hearing between the right and left ear is noted.

Facial nerve

The seventh cranial nerve also is sensory and motor. The sensory component, which supplies taste sensations from the anterior portion of the tongue, is tested by asking the patient to distinguish between sugar and salt using just the tip of the tongue. The motor component, which innervates the muscles of facial expression, is tested by asking the patient to raise both eyebrows, smile, and show the lower teeth. During these movements, any bilateral differences should be recorded.

Acoustic nerve

Also called the vestibulocochlear nerve, the eighth cranial nerve supplies the senses of balance and hearing. The patient should be questioned regarding any recent changes in upright posture or in hearing, especially if they were associated with the problem that initiated the office visit. If there is a question regarding balance, the patient should be asked to walk heel-to-toe along a straight line. Gross hearing can be evaluated by rubbing a strand of hair between the first finger and thumb near the patient's ear and noting any difference between right and left sensitivities (Fig 8-8).

Glossopharyngeal and vagus nerves

The 9th and 10th cranial nerves are tested together because they both supply fibers to the back of the throat. The patient is asked to say "ah,'" and the soft palate is observed for symmetric elevations. The gag reflex is tested by touching each side of the pharynx.

Accessory nerve

The spinal accessory nerve supplies fibers to the trapezius and sternocleidomastoid muscles. The trapezius is tested by asking the patient to shrug the shoulders against resistance. The patient is then asked to tilt the head to one side while the clinician resists the movement (Fig 8-9). The sternocleidomastoid is tested by having the patient look first to the right and then to the left against resistance. Any differences in muscle strength between sides should be noted.

Hypoglossal nerve

The 12th cranial nerve supplies motor fibers to the tongue. To test it, the patient is asked to protrude the tongue and note any uncontrolled or consistent lateral deviation is noted. The strength of the tongue can also be evaluated by having the patient push laterally against a tongue blade.

Fig 8-9 The spinal accessory nerve is tested by asking the patient to move the head laterally to one side against resistance. The examiner assesses for equal muscle strength between the right and left sides.

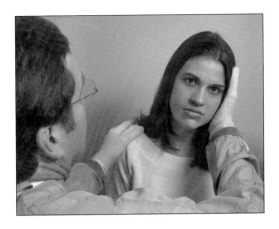

Autonomic function

The parasympathetic functioning of the oculomotor (third cranial) nerve has already been checked by testing pupillary accommodation to light. That of the facial (seventh cranial) and glossopharyngeal (ninth cranial) nerves can be checked by lacrimation and salivation. The parasympathetic functioning of the vagus (10th cranial) nerve can be checked by testing the carotid sinus reflex by which the heart rate is reduced in response to pressure on the internal carotid artery at the level of the cricoid cartilage. A deficit in cranial sympathetic functioning is recognized by the presence of Horner syndrome, which presents with narrowing of the palpebral fissure, ptosis of the upper lid, elevation of the lower lid, constriction of the pupil, and facial anhidrosis.

Superficial reflexes

The corneal reflex has already been tested by closure of the eyelids in response to irritation of the cornea by touching with a sterile cotton applicator. It involves afferent impulses transmitted by the trigeminal (fifth cranial) nerve and efferent motor impulses via the facial (seventh cranial) nerve. The palatal reflex is involuntary swallowing in response to stimulation of the soft palate. It involves afferent impulses trans-

mitted by the trigeminal (5th cranial) and glossopharyngeal (9th cranial) nerves and efferent motor impulses via the glossopharyngeal (9th cranial) and vagus (10th cranial) nerves. The pharyngeal or gag reflex is contraction of the constrictor muscle of the pharynx, which is elicited by touching the posterior wall of the pharynx. It involves afferent impulses transmitted by the glossopharyngeal (9th cranial) nerve and efferent motor impulses via the glossopharyngeal (9th cranial) and vagus (10th cranial) nerves.

As previously stated, any abnormalities found during the cranial nerve examination should be viewed as important and should be assessed with respect to their relationship to the pain condition. The purpose of this evaluation is to determine with certainty whether referral to a neurologist is essential and justified. When one or more of the following conditions are observed, immediate neurologic consultation is indicated:

1. Unexplained areas of significant facial hypoesthesia
2. Loss of normal corneal reflex
3. Persistent muscular weakness
4. Simultaneous involvement of otherwise unrelated nerve trunks

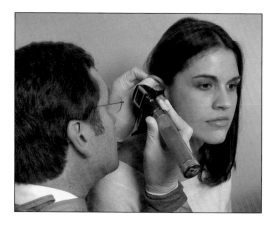

Fig 8-10 An otoscope is used to visualize the tympanic membrane.

Eye evaluation

The patient is questioned regarding his or her vision and any recent changes, especially any associated with the reason for seeking treatment. As in the cranial nerve examination, simple techniques will be sufficient in testing gross vision. The patient's left eye is covered and he or she is asked to read a few sentences from a paper. The other eye is then similarly examined. Any diplopia or blurriness of vision is noted, as well as whether this relates to the pain problem. Pain felt in or around the eyes is noted, along with whether reading affects the pain. Reddening of the conjunctivae should be recorded, along with any tearing or swelling of the eyelids.

Ear evaluation

Ear pain is a common source of facial pain and needs to identified so that proper therapy can be instituted. The proximity of the ear to the TMJ and muscles of mastication, as well as their common trigeminal innervation, frequently creates pain referral between these structures. Any clinician who treats orofacial pains should become proficient at examining the ear for gross pathology. Hearing should be checked as in the eighth cranial nerve examination. Infection

of the external auditory meatus (otitis externa) can be identified by simply pushing inward on the tragus. If this causes pain, there could be an external ear infection and the patient should be immediately referred to an otolaryngologist. An otoscope is necessary to visualize the tympanic membrane for inflammation, perforations, or fluid (Fig 8-10).

Remember that the clinician's role is to identify the source of pain. When ear disease is suspected, the patient should be referred to an otolaryngologist for a more thorough evaluation and appropriate treatment. On the other hand, normal findings from an otologic examination may be taken as encouragement to continue to search for the true source of pain or dysfunction.

Cervical evaluation

As described in chapter 4, cervicospinal pain and dysfunction can be referred to the orofacial structures. Since this is a frequent occurrence, it is important to evaluate the neck for pain or movement difficulties. A simple screening examination for craniocervical disorders is easily accomplished. The mobility of the neck is examined for range and symptoms. The patient is asked to look first to the right and then to the left (Fig 8-11a). There should be at least 70 de-

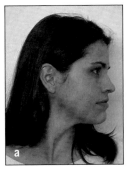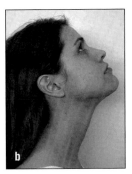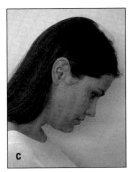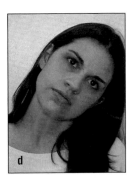

Fig 8-11 Examination for craniocervical disorders. The patient is asked to *(a)* look to the extreme left and then the extreme right, *(b)* look upward fully, *(c)* look downward fully, and *(d)* bend the neck to the right and left. Normal ranges are listed in the text. Pain associated with any movement is noted, as is any restriction in normal range of movement.

grees of rotation in each direction.[20] Next, the patient is asked to look upward as far as possible (extension) (Fig 8-11b) and then downward as far as possible (flexion) (Fig 8-11c). Normally, the head should extend upward some 60 degrees and flex downward 45 degrees.[20] Finally, the patient is asked to bend the neck to the right and left (Fig 8-11d). This should be possible to approximately 40 degrees each way.[20]

Any pain is recorded and any limitation of movement carefully investigated to determine whether its source is a muscular or a vertebral problem. When patients with limited range of movement can be passively stretched to a greater range, the source is usually muscular (known as a soft end feel). Patients with vertebral problems cannot normally be stretched to a greater range (known as a hard end feel). If the clinician suspects that the patient has a craniocervical disorder, proper referral for a more complete cervicospinal evaluation may be indicated. This is very important, since craniocervical disorders can be closely associated with some orofacial pain disorder symptoms.[21]

Balance and coordination

Each patient should be asked whether he or she is experiencing any problems with balance or coordination. If there is a positive response, a few simple tests can help determine the significance of these complaints. The patient is asked to close the eyes and attempt to touch a finger to the nose. This is repeated with both hands to give the clinician some appreciation of the patient's proprioceptive abilities. The patient can also be asked to walk along a straight line on the floor with the toe of one shoe touching the heel of the other. Significant balancing problems can be quickly identified. The presence of a balance or coordination problem should be assessed with respect to its relationship with the pain disorder. Proper referral may be indicated.

Muscle Examination

No pain is associated with the normal function or palpation of a healthy muscle. By contrast, a frequent clinical sign of compromised muscle tissue is pain. The condition that brings about compromised or unhealthy muscle tissue may be physical abuse or trauma, such as overstretching or receiving a blow to the muscle tissue itself. Often muscles become compromised through increased activity. As the number and duration of contractions increase, so also do the physiologic needs of the muscle tissues. Increased muscle tonicity or hyperactivity, however, may decrease blood flow to the muscle tissues, lowering the inflow of nutrient substances needed for normal cell function while accumulating metabolic waste products. This accumulation of metabolic wastes and other algogenic substances can cause muscle pain.[22,23]

The degree and location of muscle pain and tenderness are identified during direct palpation of the muscle.

Palpation

A widely accepted method of determining muscle tenderness and pain is digital palpation.[24-26] A healthy muscle does not elicit sensations of tenderness or pain when palpated. Deformation of compromised muscle tissue by palpation can elicit pain.[27] Therefore, if a patient reports discomfort during palpation of a specific muscle, it can be deduced that the muscle tissue is a source of pain.

Pressure algometry has become a useful adjunct in evaluating muscle tenderness and myofascial trigger point sensitivity.[28-33] The pressure algometer provides a means of objective quantitative documentation of myalgia.[34]

Palpation of the muscle is accomplished mainly with the palmar surface of the middle finger, with the index finger and forefinger testing the adjacent areas. Soft but firm pressure is applied to the designated muscles, with the fingers compressing the adjacent tissues in a small circular motion. A single firm thrust of 1 or 2 seconds' duration is usually better than several light thrusts. During palpation the patient is asked whether it hurts or is merely uncomfortable.

For the muscle palpation examination to be most helpful, the degree of discomfort is ascertained and recorded. This is often a difficult task. Pain is subjective and is perceived and expressed quite differently from patient to patient. Yet the degree of discomfort in the structure can be important in recognizing the patient's pain problem and is also an excellent method for evaluating treatment effects. An attempt is made, therefore, not only to identify the affected muscles but also to classify the degree of pain in each. When a muscle is palpated, the patient's response is placed in one of four categories.[25,35-36] A zero (0) is recorded when the muscle is palpated and there is no pain or tenderness reported by the patient. A 1 is recorded if the patient responds that the palpation is uncomfortable (tenderness or soreness). A 2 is recorded if the patient experiences definite discomfort or pain. A 3 is recorded if the patient shows evasive action or eye tearing or verbalizes a desire not to have the area palpated again. The pain or tenderness of each muscle is recorded on an examination form, which will assist with diagnosis and later be used in the evaluation and assessment of treatment progress.

A routine orofacial muscle examination includes palpation of the following muscles or muscle groups: temporalis, masseter, sternocleidomastoid, and posterior cervical (eg, the splenius capitis and trapezius). For increased efficiency of the examination, both right and left muscles are palpated simultaneously. The technique of palpating each muscle will be described.

Temporalis

The temporalis is divided into three functional areas, which must be independently palpated. The anterior region is palpated above the zygomatic arch and anterior to the TMJ (Fig 8-12a). Fibers of this region run essentially in a vertical direction. The middle region is palpated directly above the TMJ and superior to the zygomatic arch (Fig 8-12b). Fibers in this region run in an oblique direction across the lateral aspect of the skull. The posterior region is palpated above and behind the ear (Fig 8-12c). These fibers run in an essentially horizontal

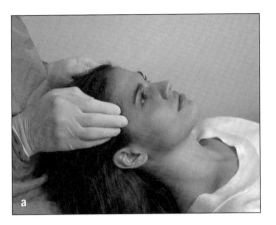
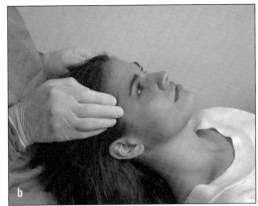
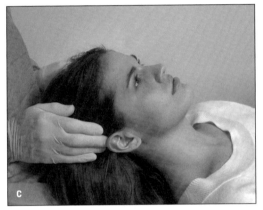
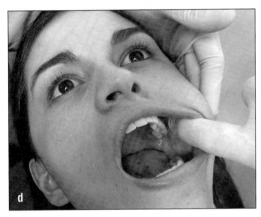

Fig 8-12 Palpation of *(a)* the anterior, *(b)* the middle, and *(c)* the posterior regions of the temporal muscles. *(d)* Palpation of the tendon of the temporalis. The fingers of both hands (one intraorally, the other extraorally) move simultaneously up the anterior border of the ramus until the coronoid process and the attachment of the tendon of the temporalis are felt.

direction. If uncertainty arises regarding the proper placement of the fingers, the patient is asked to clench the teeth together. The temporalis will contract and the fibers should be felt beneath the fingertips. It is helpful to be positioned behind the patient and to use the right and left hands to palpate respective muscle areas simultaneously. During palpation of each area, the patient is asked whether it hurts or is only uncomfortable, and the response is classified as 0, 1, 2, or 3, according to the previously described criteria.

When evaluating the temporalis muscle, it is important to also palpate its tendon.

The fibers of the temporalis muscle extend inferiorly to converge into a distinct tendon that attaches to the coronoid process of the mandible. It is common for some temporomandibular disorders to produce temporalis tendonitis, which can create pain in the body of the muscle as well as referred pain behind the adjacent eye (retroorbital pain). The tendon of the temporalis is palpated by placing the finger of one hand intraorally on the anterior border of the ramus and the finger of the other hand extraorally on the same area (Fig 8-12d). The intraoral finger is moved up the anterior border of the ramus until the coronoid pro-

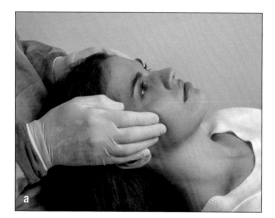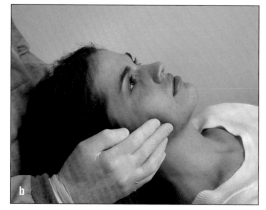

Fig 8-13 *(a)* Palpation of the deep masseters at their superior attachment to the zygomatic arches. *(b)* Palpation of the superficial masseters near the lower border of the mandible.

cess and the tendon are palpated. The patient is asked to report any discomfort or pain.

Masseter

The masseter is palpated bilaterally at its superior and inferior attachments. First, the fingers are placed on each zygomatic arch (just anterior to the TMJ). They are then dropped down slightly to the portion of the masseter attached to the zygomatic arch, just anterior to the joint (Fig 8-13a). Once this portion (the deep masseter) has been palpated, the fingers drop to the inferior attachment on the inferior border of the ramus. The area of palpation is directly above the attachment of the body of the masseter (ie, the superficial masseter) (Fig 8-13b). The patient's response is recorded.

Sternocleidomastoid

Although the sternocleidomastoid (SCM) does not function directly in moving the mandible, it is specifically mentioned because it often becomes symptomatic with temporomandibular disorders and can be a source of pain felt in the face. The palpation is done bilaterally near its insertion on the outer surface of the mastoid fossa, be-

hind the ear (Fig 8-14a). The entire length of the muscle is palpated, down to its origin near the clavicle (Fig 8-14b). The patient is asked to report any discomfort during the procedure. Also, any trigger points found in this muscle are noted, since they are frequent sources of referred pain to the temporal, joint, and ear area.

Posterior cervical muscles

The posterior cervical muscles (trapezius, longissimus [both capitis and cervicis], splenius [both capitis and cervicis], and levator scapulae) are the major muscles responsible for cervical function. They originate at the posterior occipital area and extend inferiorly along the cervicospinal region. Because they are layered over each other, they are sometimes difficult to identify individually.

In palpating these muscles, the examiner's fingers slip behind the patient's head. Those of the right hand palpate the right occipital area, and those of the left hand the left occipital area, at the origins of the muscles. The patient is questioned regarding any discomfort. The fingers move down the length of the neck muscles through the cervical area, and any patient discomfort is

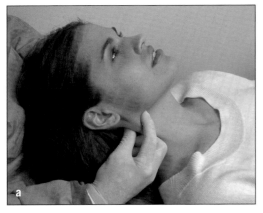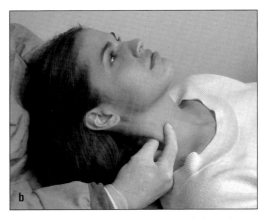

Fig 8-14 Palpation of the SCM muscles. The full length of this muscle should be palpated, from its attachment to the mastoid process down to the clavicle.

recorded (Fig 8-15). It is important to be aware of trigger points in these muscles, since they are a common source of frontal headache.

The *splenius capitis* is palpated for general pain or tenderness as well as for trigger points. Its attachment to the skull is a small depression just posterior to the attachment of the SCM (Fig 8-16). Palpation is begun at this point and moves inferiorly as the muscle blends into the other neck muscles. Any pain, tenderness, or trigger points are recorded.

The *trapezius* is an extremely large muscle of the back, shoulder, and neck that (like the SCM and the splenius) does not directly affect jaw function but is a common source of headache pain and is easily palpated. The major purpose of its palpation is not to evaluate shoulder function but to search for active trigger points that may be producing referred pain. The trapezius commonly has trigger points that refer pain to the face. In fact, when facial pain is the patient's chief complaint, this muscle should be one of the first sources investigated. The upper part is palpated from behind the SCM, inferolaterally to the shoulder (Fig 8-17), and any trigger points are recorded.

There are three muscles that are basic to jaw movement but impossible to palpate. These muscles are the *inferior lateral pterygoid,* the *superior lateral pterygoid,* and the *medial pterygoid.* The inferior and superior lateral pterygoids reside deep within the skull, originating on the lateral wing of the sphenoid bone and the maxillary tuberosity and inserting on the neck of the mandibular condyle and the TMJ capsule. The medial pterygoid has a similar origin, but it extends downward and laterally to insert on the medial surface of the angle of the mandible. All three muscles receive their innervation from the mandibular branch of the trigeminal nerve.

Since these muscles cannot be palpated, they are best evaluated by functional manipulation. Functional manipulation utilizes the concept that a painful muscle will not only be tender to palpation but will also be painful to contraction and/or stretching of the muscle. For example, a painful inferior lateral pterygoid muscle will produce increased pain when the patient is asked to push the mandible forward against resistance. If pain is increased during resisted protrusion of the mandible, the inferior lateral pterygoid should be sus-

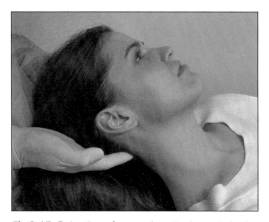

Fig 8-15 Palpation of muscular attachments in the occipital region of the neck. The fingers should then be brought inferiorly down the cervical spine area to examine these muscles for pain or tenderness.

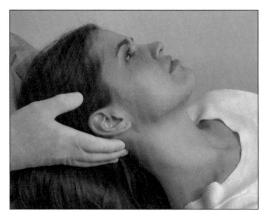

Fig 8-16 The splenius capitis is palpated at its attachment to the skull just posterior to the SCM.

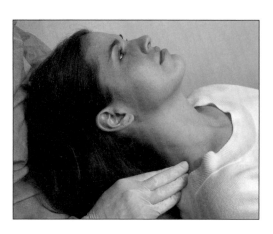

Fig 8-17 The trapezius is palpated as it ascends into the neck structures.

pected as a source of pain. A more detailed description of functional manipulation can be found in other texts.[25]

Trigger points and pain referral

A thorough muscle palpation examination should identify not only generalized muscle tenderness and pain, but also the small, hypersensitive trigger points associated with myofascial pain. As stated in chapter 4, trigger points act as sources of deep pain input that can produce central excitatory effects. It is important that these areas be identified and recorded. To locate trigger points, the examiner palpates the entire body of each muscle. Generalized muscle pain may not exist in a muscle with trigger points. In recording examination findings, it is important to differentiate between generalized muscle pain and trigger point pain, since the diagnosis and treatment are often different.

Trigger points are clinically identified as specific hypersensitive areas within the muscle tissue. Often a small, firm, tight band of muscle tissue can be felt. Active trigger points represent a source of deep pain and can therefore produce referred pain.[37] When referred (heterotopic) pain is detected, one should remember that it is wholly dependent on the conditions of the trigger points (the source of the pain). This means that if active referring trigger points are provoked, the referred pain will usually be increased; this becomes a significant diagnostic observation in relating pain complaints to their source. For example, when a patient's chief complaint is headache, careful palpation of the aforementioned neck muscles for trigger points will demonstrate its source. When a trigger point is located, application of pressure to it will usually increase the headache (referred) pain.

The specific pattern of referred pain from various trigger point locations has been outlined by Simons et al.[38] An understanding of these common referral sites may help the clinician who is attempting to diagnose an orofacial pain problem. Anesthetic blocking of the trigger point often eliminates the referred headache pain and thus becomes an important diagnostic tool.

Masticatory Evaluation

Since the masticatory structures can be a significant source of orofacial pain, the examination must include a thorough evaluation of these structures for pain and dysfunction. The following criteria have been found useful and dependable for accurate identification and localization of masticatory pain sources.[39]

1. The pain should relate directly and logically to the movements and functioning of the mandible incidental to mastication.
2. Tenderness in the masticatory muscles or the TMJs should be discernible by manual palpation or functional manipulation.
3. Analgesic blocking of a tender muscle or joint should confirm the presence and precise location of such pain.

An examination of masticatory structures should include evaluation of range of mandibular movement, the TMJs, and the oral structures.

Range of mandibular movement

The normal range of mouth opening when measured interincisally is between 53 and 58 mm.[40-42] Even a 6-year-old child can normally open a maximum of 40 mm or more.[43,44] Since muscle symptoms are often accentuated during function, it is common for patients to present with a restricted pattern of movement. The patient is asked to open slowly until pain is first felt. At that point, the distance between the incisal edges of the maxillary and mandibular anterior teeth is measured (Fig 8-18a). This is the maximum comfortable opening. The patient is next asked to open maximally (Fig 8-18b). This is recorded as the maximum opening. In the absence of pain, the maximum comfortable opening and maximum opening are the same. If a person has a 5-mm vertical overlap of the anterior teeth, and the maximum interincisal distance is 57 mm, the mandible has actually moved 62 mm in opening. With people who have extreme deep bites, these measurements must be considered when determining the normal range of movement.

A restricted mandibular opening is considered to be any distance less than 40 mm. Only 1.2% of young adults open less than 40 mm.[43] One must remember however, that 15% of the healthy elderly population open less than 40 mm.[42] Less than 40 mm of mouth opening therefore seems to represent a reasonable point to designate restriction, but one should always consider the patient's age and body size.

The path taken by the midline of the mandible during maximum opening should also be observed. In the healthy masticatory system, there is no alteration in the straight opening pathway. Any alterations in opening are recorded. Two types of alteration

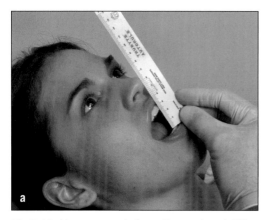 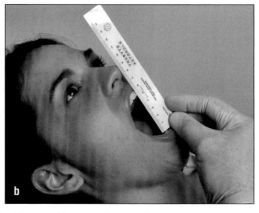

Fig 8-18 Measurement of mouth opening. *(a)* The patient is asked to open the mouth and stop when pain is first felt. A millimeter ruler is used to measure the distance from the incisal edge of the mandibular incisor to the maxillary incisor. This measurement is the comfortable mouth opening. *(b)* The patient is then asked to open as wide as possible, even in the presence of pain. This is considered the maximum mouth opening.

can occur: deviations and deflections. A *deviation* is any shift of the jaw midline during opening that disappears with continued opening (a return to midline) (Fig 8-19a). It is usually due to a disc derangement in one or both joints and is a result of the condylar movement necessary to get past the disc during translation. Once the condyle has overcome this interference, the straight midline path is resumed. A *deflection* is any shift of the midline to one side that becomes greater with opening and does not disappear at maximum opening (does not return to midline) (Fig 8-19b). It is a result of restricted movement in one joint. The source of the restriction varies and must be investigated.

Restricted movements of the mandible are caused by either extracapsular or intracapsular sources. The former are generally the muscles and therefore relate to a muscle disorder. The latter are generally associated with disc/condyle function and the surrounding ligaments and thus are usually related to a disc derangement disorder. Extracapsular and intracapsular restrictions present different characteristics.

Extracapsular restrictions typically occur with elevator muscle spasms and pain. These muscles tend to restrict translation and thus limit opening. Pain in the elevator muscles, however, does not restrict lateral and protrusive movements. Therefore, with this type of restriction, normal eccentric movements are present but opening movement is restricted, primarily because of pain. The point of restriction can range anywhere from 0 to 40 mm interincisally. It is common with this type of restriction for the patient to be able to increase opening slowly, but the pain is intensified (soft end feel).

Extracapsular restrictions often create a deflection of the incisal path during opening. The direction of the deflection depends on the location of the muscle that causes the restriction. If the restricting muscle is lateral to the joint (as with the masseter), the deflection during opening will be to the ipsilateral side. If the muscle is medial (as with the medial pterygoid), the deflection will be to the contralateral side.

Intracapsular restrictions typically present a different pattern. A disc derangement dis-

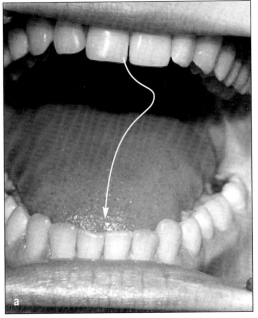
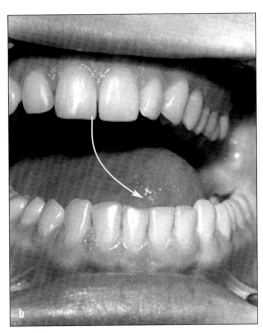

Fig 8-19 Alterations in the opening pathway. *(a)* Deviation. The opening pathway is altered but returns to a normal midline relationship at maximum opening. *(b)* Deflection. The opening pathway is shifted to one side and becomes greater with opening. At maximum opening the midline is deflected to its greatest distance. (From Okeson JP. Management of Temporomandibular Disorders and Occlusion, ed 5. St Louis: Mosby-Year Book, 2003:271. Used with permission.)

order, such as a disc dislocation (see chapter 13), very decisively restricts translation of that joint. Typically, the restriction is in only one joint and limits mandibular opening in that joint primarily to rotation (25 to 30 mm interincisally). At this point, further movement is restricted not because of pain but because of structural resistance in the joint. When intracapsular restrictions are present, deflection of the incisal path during opening is always to the ipsilateral (affected) side.

Pain produced during mouth opening commonly occurs from either a muscle disorder or a joint disorder. When limited mouth opening is present the clinician needs to pursue the reason for the restriction. Testing the "end feel" can be helpful. The end feel describes the characteristics of the joint when an attempt is made to increase mouth opening passively[45] by gently placing downward force on the mandibular incisors with the fingers to increase the interincisal distance (Fig 8-20). This force should be light but steady. If the end feel is "soft," increased opening can be achieved, but it must be done slowly. A soft end feel suggests muscle-induced restriction.[46] If no increase in opening can be achieved, the end feel is said to be "hard." Hard end feels are likely associated with intracapsular sources, such as a disc dislocation.[25]

TMJ evaluation

The TMJs should be examined for any signs or symptoms associated with pain and dysfunction. Radiography and other imaging techniques can also be useful and will be discussed.

Pain or tenderness of the TMJs is determined by digital palpation of the joints,

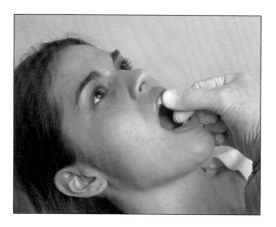

Fig 8-20 Checking the "end feel." Gentle but steady pressure is placed on the incisors for approximately 5 to 6 seconds. A gradual increase in mouth opening indicates a soft end feel (usually associated with a masticatory muscle disorder).

both when the mandible is stationary and during dynamic movement. The fingertips are placed over the lateral aspects of both joint areas simultaneously. If uncertainty exists regarding the proper position of the fingers, the patient is asked to open and close a few times. The fingertips should feel the lateral poles of the condyles passing downward and forward across the articular eminences. Once the position of the fingers over the joints has been verified, the patient relaxes and medial force is applied to the joint areas (Fig 8-21a). The patient is asked to report any symptoms, and they are recorded with the same numeric code that was used for the muscles. After the symptoms are recorded in a static position, the patient opens and closes and any symptoms associated with this movement are recorded (Fig 8-21b). As the patient opens maximally, the fingers should be rotated slightly posteriorly to apply force to the posterior aspect of the condyle (Fig 8-21c). Posterior capsulitis and retrodiscitis are clinically evaluated in this manner.

To evaluate the TMJ effectively, one must have a sound understanding of the anatomy in the region. When the fingers are placed properly over the lateral poles of the condyles and the patient is asked to clench, very little to no movement is felt. However, if the fingers are misplaced only 1 cm anterior to the lateral pole and the pa-

tient is asked to clench, the deep portion of the masseter can be felt contracting. This very slight difference in positioning of the fingers may influence the examiner's interpretation regarding the origin of the pain. Also, it is important to be aware that a portion of the parotid gland extends to the region of the joint and parotid symptoms can arise from this area. The examiner must be astute in identifying whether the symptoms are originating from joint, muscle, or gland, since the basis of treatment will be determined by this evaluation.

Dysfunction of the TMJs can be separated into two types: joint sounds and joint restrictions. Joint sounds can be generally divided into either clicks or crepitation. A click is a single sound of short duration. If it is relatively loud, it is sometimes referred to as a pop. Crepitation is a multiple gravel-like sound described as grating and complicated.[47] Crepitation is most commonly associated with osteoarthritic changes of the articular surfaces of the joint.[48]

Joint sounds can be perceived by placing the fingertips over the lateral surfaces of the joint and having the patient open and close. Often they may be felt by the fingertips. A more careful examination can be performed by placing a stethoscope over the joint area. Not only will the character of any joint sounds be recorded (clicking versus crepitation), but also the degree of

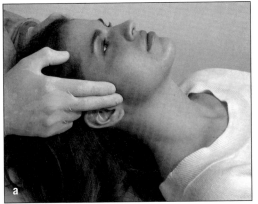

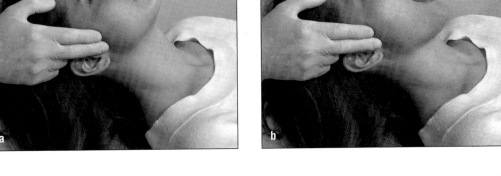

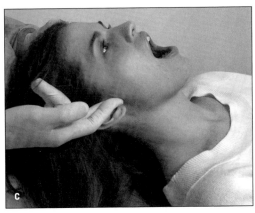

Fig 8-21 Palpation of the TMJ. *(a)* Lateral aspect of the joint with the mouth closed. *(b)* Lateral aspect of the joint during opening and closing. *(c)* With the mouth fully open, the finger is moved behind the condyle to palpate the posterior aspect of the joint.

mandibular opening associated with the sound. In addition, it is equally important to note whether the sound occurs during opening or closing or can be heard during both these movements (ie, a reciprocal click; see chapter 13).

The presence or absence of joint sounds gives insight regarding disc position. One should be aware, however, that the absence of sounds does not always mean normal disc position. In one study[49] 15% of silent, asymptomatic joints showed disc displacements on arthrograms. Information received during examination of the joints needs to be evaluated with respect to all other examination findings.

The dynamic movements of the mandible are observed for any irregularities or restric-

tions. The characteristics of intracapsular restrictions have already been described in connection with the muscle examination. Any mandibular movements that either are restricted or have unusual pathway characteristics are recorded. Their relationship to pain should also be noted.

Oral structures

The gingiva and entire oral mucosa should be tested by touch, pinprick, and manual palpation to identify areas of abnormal sensibility. Visual inspection of the superficial mucogingival tissues of the mouth and throat is done to identify hyperemia, inflammation, abrasion, ulceration, neoplasm, or other abnormality.

There is no doubt that pains about the mouth and face stem most frequently from local dental causes, and a thorough examination of the teeth is an indispensable part of the orofacial examination. Odontogenous pains have the propensity to simulate many other pain disorders, and a very careful examination is needed to arrive at a correct differential diagnosis.

The teeth, especially on the side in question, should be examined individually to yield the following data:

1. Sensitivity or tenderness without provocation
2. Sensitivity or tenderness due to occlusal function
3. Sensitivity to touch, percussion, or probing with a dental explorer
4. Tenderness from pressure directed down the long axis of the tooth
5. Tenderness from pressure exerted laterally on the tooth
6. Response to thermal shock (warmth may be applied via a heated instrument, while chilling may be done by applying ethyl chloride on a cotton applicator. The tooth should be isolated with celluloid strips, especially when adjacent metallic fillings are present or when it is covered with an artificial dental crown.)
7. Response to electric pulp tester (each tooth should be isolated with celluloid strips, especially when adjacent metallic fillings are present, and care should be taken to differentiate between pulpal and gingival responses.[50])
8. Radiographic evidence of pathologic change
9. Evidence of occlusal trauma
10. Evidence to justify direct exploration of the tooth

The periodontal condition, especially in the region of the pain, should be evaluated carefully. Gingival tissue color and surface texture should be noted. A periodontal probe should be used to identify any loss of gingival attachment or pocketing that might be associated with the pain. The tooth should be percussed apically and laterally to determine any relationship to the pain. Radiographs should be obtained to help identify any changes in the alveolar bone support for the teeth.

For many years, the dental profession placed significant emphasis on the occlusal contact pattern of the teeth and pain in the orofacial structures. In more recent years, this significance of this relationship has been questioned. A review of the literature can be found in other texts.[51,52] Although the controversy continues, the relationship is likely to be associated with occlusal conditions that create significant orthopedic instability between the mandible and the cranium.

It is important for the clinician to assess the occlusal relationship between the mandible and the maxilla when masticatory pains are present. This can be accomplished by placing the mandible in its most orthopedically stable relationship with the cranium and observing the occlusion of the teeth. A simple method of finding the stable joint position utilizes a bilateral manual manipulation technique.[25] It begins with the patient lying back and the chin pointed upward (Fig 8-22a). Lifting the chin upward places the head in an easier position to locate the condyles near the superior anterior position, which is the most stable relationship of the condyle in the fossa. The four fingers of each hand are placed on the lower border of the mandible (Figs 8-22b and 8-22c). It is important that the fingers be located on the bone and not in the soft tissues of the neck. Next, both thumbs are placed over the symphysis of the chin so they touch each other (Figs 8-22d and 8-22e). When the hands are in this position, the mandible is guided by upward force placed on its lower border and angle with the fingers, while at the same time the thumbs press downward and backward on

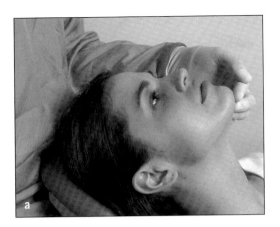

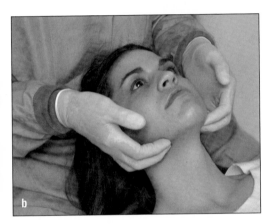

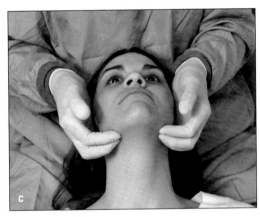

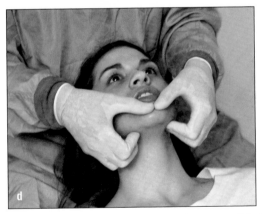

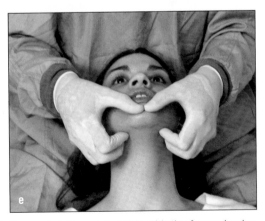

Fig 8-22 *(a)* Successful guidance of the mandible into its most stable relationship with the fossae begins with having the patient recline and directing the chin upward. *(b and c)* The four fingers of each hand are placed along the lower border of the mandible with the small fingers behind the mandibular angles. They should be positioned on the bone and not in the soft tissues of the neck. *(d and e)* The thumbs meet over the symphysis of the chin. Once the hands are properly positioned, gentle force is placed downward on the chin, with upward and forward force applied to the angle of the mandible. This allows the condyles to be seated into a superior anterior position in the fossae.

the chin. The overall force on the mandible is directed so the condyles will be seated in their most superoanterior position, braced against the posterior slopes of the eminences. Firm but gentle force is needed to guide the mandible so as not to elicit any protective reflexes.

The mandible is positioned with a gentle arcing until it freely rotates around the stable joint position. This arcing consists of short movements of 2 to 4 mm. Once the mandible can be slightly rotated in an opening and closing position, force is firmly applied by the fingers to seat the condyles in their most superoanterior position. The mouth is slowly closed with the condyles in this position, and the occlusal contacts of the teeth are observed. If orthopedic stability is present, the teeth should occlude in their maximum intercuspation with no slide. If orthopedic stability is not present, a significant shift will occur as the teeth are brought into intercuspal position. Only shifts of 2 mm or more should be considered a significant finding, since smaller shifts seem to be within most patients' tolerances. The clinician should remember that the presence of a significant shift does not in itself represent an etiology for orofacial pain. Many patients with significant shifts have no pain symptoms. The clinician must evaluate this information together with all of the other information gained from the history and examination to make a diagnosis.

Other Diagnostic Tests

Imaging

Various types of imaging techniques can be used to gain additional insight regarding the health and function of the masticatory structures. When painful symptoms arise from the orofacial structures, radiographs of the teeth, sinuses, and TMJs can be help-

ful. Radiographs of the TMJs will provide information regarding the morphologic characteristics of the bony components of the joint and about certain functional relationships between the condyle and the fossa.

Common films of the TMJs are the transcranial view, the transpharyngeal view, and the panoramic view (Figs 8-23a to 8-23c). When additional information is needed, tomography can be helpful (Fig 8-23d). When soft tissue imaging is needed, magnetic resonance imaging (MRI) may be useful. Periapical and bitewing films are appropriate to assess dental and periodontal conditions, while a Waters' projection is helpful for evaluating sinus disease.

Unfortunately, neither the articular disc nor the actual articular surfaces can be seen radiographically. Only the subarticular bone and the intervening "space" are seen on the film. Also, usually the central articulating relationship of these subarticular osseous structures is not recorded (except by the tomographic method). Rather, what is seen on the film is the lateral contour of the joint. This interarticular space may not accurately represent the true thickness of the articular disc. If actual osseous disease is observed on the flat plate, tomographic visualization is the best technique for accurate evaluation. The usual open and closed views of the joint can give some information about joint structure and the extent of condylar movement. The reason for joint restriction should be determined by a combination of radiographic findings and clinical and history findings.

Laboratory tests

When the clinician is suspicious of significant medical problems, medical laboratory testing may be needed to confirm a diagnosis. This is especially true for arthritides such as rheumatoid arthritis, psoriatic arthritis, and hyperuricemia. Blood studies may also be helpful in ruling out systemic

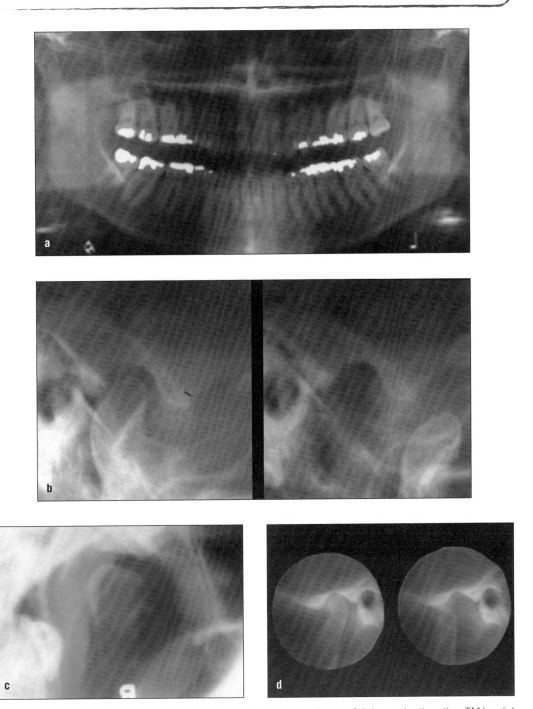

Fig 8-23 Examples of several types of radiographs that can be useful in evaluating the TMJs. (a) Panoramic view, an excellent method to screen the orofacial structures. (b) Transcranial view, closed and open views. (c) Transpharyngeal view; note the osteophyte. (d) Tomographic view, closed and open views.

infections or other systemic conditions, such as diabetes.

The following are indications for a medical consultation:

1. Obvious illness, as indicated by the patient's appearance and behavior and by the medical history questionnaire
2. The presence of obscure illness, as indicated by the medical history questionnaire
3. Evidence obtained during the history interview that the pain complaint may primarily relate to physical or emotional illness
4. Evidence obtained during the clinical examination that systemic factors may be present and need investigating
5. Determination that the pain disorder does not stem from orofacial structures
6. Indication that the pain disorder coexists with or is aggravated by some systemic condition that should be approached at a medical level

Psychologic assessment

As mentioned earlier, as pain becomes more chronic, psychologic factors relating to the pain complaint become more common. For acute pain patients, psychologic evaluation is usually unnecessary; however, with chronic pain patients, it becomes essential. Since confident evaluation of psychologic factors may be difficult for the general practitioner, chronic pain patients are best evaluated and managed by a multidisciplinary approach.

There are a variety of measuring tools that can be used to assess the psychologic status of the patient. These include the MPI,[14] which evaluates how the pain experience is affecting the patient, and the SCL-90,[15] which provides an assessment of the following nine psychologic states: somatization, obsessive-compulsive behavior, interpersonal sensitivity, depression, anxiety, hostility, phobic anxiety, paranoid ideation, and psychoticism. Assessing these factors is essential when evaluating the chronic pain patient.

A general practitioner without immediate access to psychologic evaluation support may elect to use IMPATH[16] or the TMJ Scale,[17,53] two scales developed for use by dental practitioners to assist in evaluating clinical and certain psychologic factors associated with orofacial pains. These scales can assist the dental clinician in identifying whether psychologic issues are an important aspect of a patient's pain condition. Although these scales are helpful, they are not as complete as the MPI or SCL-90 and certainly do not replace the personal evaluation of a clinical psychologist.

If during the examination the clinician becomes suspicious of significant psychologic factors, certain provocation tests may be helpful. One such test is to evaluate how the patient responds to an attempt to induce pain purely by suggestion. This may be done by pressing firmly on the painful site and strongly suggesting to the patient that he will feel the pain simultaneously in the corresponding site on the opposite normal side. If he does in fact complain of similar pain on the opposite side, the emotional overlay is probably great. Or the reverse may be tried: the clinician may attempt to relieve the pain purely by suggestion. The examiner presses firmly at the corresponding site on the opposite, normal side and strongly suggests that by doing so the patient will sense relief of pain at the site in question. If the pain is thus substantially relieved by this maneuver, significant psychologic factors are likely to be present.

Another testing device is trial placebo therapy, although this method has not been looked upon with favor by some investigators.[54] It should be remembered that a normal placebo effect may account for up to 40% of the effectiveness of any form of treatment, especially in emotionally tense individuals.[55-57] Therefore, to evaluate placebo therapy, the results up to this percentage must be discounted. Testing can be done by prescribing a definite plan of treatment utilizing only placebo medications and suggesting to the patient that definite benefit will occur at a specified time. If such benefit occurs according to the specified time schedule and the benefit is substantially greater than 40%, it may be presumed that the purely psychologic element is important.

Establishing the Pain Category

Once the history and examination have been completed, the clinician should have a significant understanding of the patient's pain complaint. The next step in diagnosis is to place the pain complaint into the proper pain category. This can only be accomplished if the clinician has a complete understanding of all the possibilities. When one appreciates that different pain categories are characterized by different symptoms, diagnosis becomes more simplified. The pain classification in Fig 8-24 can be used as a "road map" to direct the clinician to an accurate diagnosis. Remember, it is only through proper diagnosis that appropriate therapy can be selected. Therefore, establishment of the proper diagnosis is the most critical and often the most difficult task for the clinician.

The proper category may be established by answering the following six questions:

Is the Pain Chronic or Acute?

As described earlier, pain may be considered chronic if it continues after a normal healing time has elapsed. The classic definition of chronic pain is pain that has lasted longer than 6 months. The important diagnostic consideration is that the longer pain is present, the greater the possibility of significant psychologic factors. As stated earlier, all pains have to some degree a psychologic component (Axis II). It is important to identify early those patients who may have a significant Axis II diagnosis, since these conditions are managed differently than the Axis I disorders. If the patient is experiencing chronic pain, some Axis II disorders are almost always present, even if only within the category of psychologic factors affecting a medical condition.

The following clinical evidence should provide the clinician with suspicion that significant psychologic factors may be associated with the chronic pain condition:

1. Progressive inadequacy of local cause
2. Progressive nonphysiologic behavior of the pain
3. Withdrawal from normal daily activities
4. Progressive emotional and/or physical deterioration
5. Mood changes (depression)
6. Evidence of significant anxiety
7. Significant alterations in sleep patterns
8. Preoccupation or obsession with the pain condition

Is the Pain Somatic or Neuropathic?

Assuming that Axis II factors are not a dominant feature of the patient's complaint, the next diagnostic issue is whether the pain stems from somatic structures supplied by normal neural elements (somatic pain) or from abnormal neural structures (neuropathic pain). Recognition of evidence of neuropathic pain therefore is of prime importance.

Neuropathic pains include the following clinical characteristics:

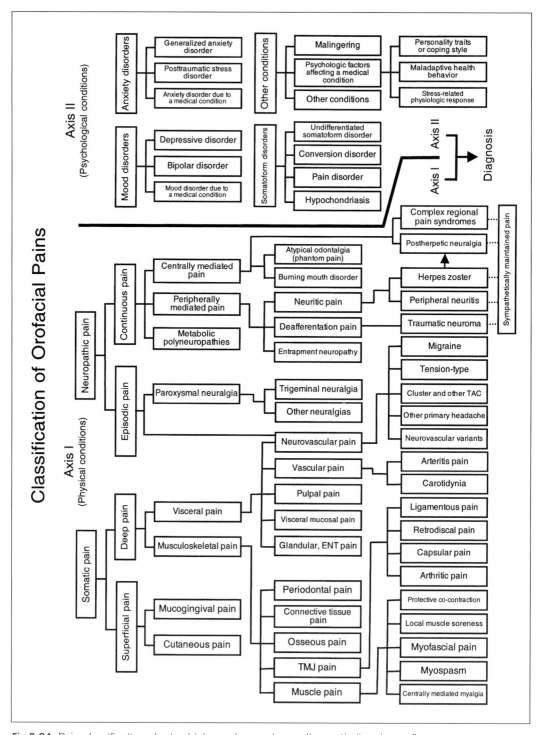

Fig 8-24 Pain classification chart, which can be used as a diagnostic "road map."

Fig 8-25 The major categories of neuropathic pain disorders.

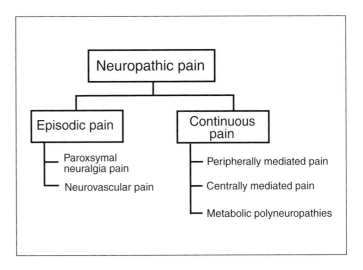

1. Burning-type pains that are spontaneous, triggered, or ongoing and unremitting
2. Pains that occur disproportionately to the stimulus
3. Pains that are accompanied by other neurologic symptoms
4. Pains that are initiated or accentuated by efferent sympathetic activity in the area

Neuropathic orofacial pains are classified as either episodic or continuous. Episodic pains are pains that will appear for a time and then completely resolve. There are two categories of episodic pains: paroxysmal neuralgic pains or neurovascular pains. Continuous neuropathic pains are present constantly, although they may fluctuate between mild and severe. There are three categories of continuous neuropathic pains according to the origin of the dysfunction: peripherally mediated pain, centrally mediated pain, and metabolic polyneuropathies (Fig 8-25). In some instances, the sympathetic nervous system may promote or maintain these pains; when this condition is present the pain is said to be sympathetically maintained.

Is the Pain Primary or Secondary?

Assuming that evidence of neuropathic pain is absent from the patient's complaint, the next diagnostic issue is whether the problem is a true primary pain or a secondary manifestation, such as referred pain or secondary hyperalgesia. Since there is no definitive treatment for secondary pains other than identifying and managing the primary source, it is of extremely importance that secondary pains be clearly recognized and primary pain sources be identified.

Differentiation of secondary pain from primary pain is accomplished by the rules described earlier in this chapter. Secondary pains are not increased by local provocation, unless it is a site of secondary hyperalgesia. Secondary pains are not arrested by anesthesia at the site of pain. Secondary pain that is felt superficially as a touchy or sensitive area (secondary hyperalgesia) is not arrested by a topical anesthetic applied to the site of pain. Secondary pain that is felt more deeply as an area of palpable ten-

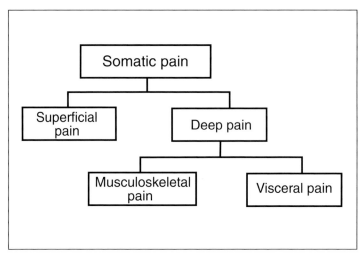

Fig 8-26 The major categories of somatic pain disorders.

derness is not arrested by analgesic blocking of that area.

Primary pain is present when local provocation of the site of pain increases the pain. Primary pains are arrested by local anesthesia at the site of pain. Primary somatic pain emanating from superficial skin or the mucogingival tissue is arrested by application of topical anesthetic at the site of pain. Primary somatic pain emanating from musculoskeletal or visceral structures is felt as tenderness to manual palpation or functional manipulation. This type of primary pain is arrested by analgesic blocking of that area.

Is the Pain Superficial or Deep?

Assuming that the patient's complaint is positively identified as a primary somatic pain and is not a result of reference or secondary hyperalgesia, the next diagnostic issue is whether it stems from superficial or deep somatic structures (Fig 8-26).

Superficial somatic pain displays the following clinical characteristics, by which it can be recognized:

1. The pain is a bright, stimulating sensation that is precisely localizable by the patient.
2. Response to local provocation is faithful in location, duration, and intensity.
3. The pain remains "clean-cut," without secondary manifestations such as reference, secondary hyperalgesia, autonomic symptoms, and/or muscle effects.
4. The pain is arrested by topical anesthesia at the site of pain.

Deep somatic pain displays the following clinical characteristics, by which it can be recognized:

1. The pain is a duller, more depressing sensation that is less precisely localizable by the patient.
2. Response to local provocation is less faithful, especially with regard to location and size.

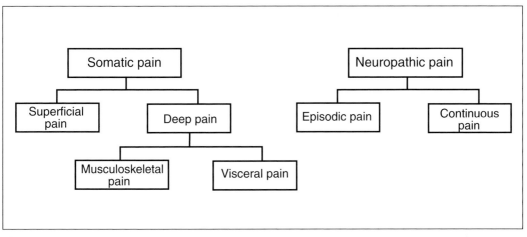

Fig 8-27 The major pain chart used to help identify the proper category represented by the patient's pain complaint.

3. The pain frequently exhibits secondary manifestations such as referred pain, secondary hyperalgesia, autonomic symptoms, and/or muscle effects.
4. The pain is arrested by analgesic blocking of the site of pain.

Is the Pain Musculoskeletal or Visceral?

If the primary pain that represents the patient's complaint originates from deep somatic structures, the next diagnostic issue is whether it is of musculoskeletal or visceral origin (Fig 8-27).

Musculoskeletal structures are primarily engaged in biomechanical function, and pain from such structures as muscles, bone, joints, ligaments (including periodontal ligaments), and soft connective tissue exhibits two characteristic clinical features: it is related intimately to biomechanical function, and the response to provocation is a gradient reaction that is proportional to the stimulus.

Visceral structures are primarily engaged in metabolic rather than biomechanical functions, and pain from such structures as blood vessels, glands, viscera, and tooth pulps exhibits two characteristic clinical features: it occurs irrelevant to biomechanical function, and it is relatively nonresponsive to local provocation until a threshold level is reached.

The answers to this series of questions should clearly establish the category of the patient's pain complaint and place the examiner in an excellent position to make a final diagnosis.

Is the Pain Inflammatory?

One more question may be useful therapeutically as well as diagnostically. This question relates to whether or not the pain disorder is associated with an inflammatory condition. Inflammatory pain may have its source in superficial somatic, deep somatic, or neuropathic structures. When this type of pain is suspected, the cause of the inflammatory process must be identified and eliminated to resolve the pain.

Inflammatory pain can usually be recognized by the following clinical features:

1. Concomitant signs of inflammation are present, such as swelling, redness, heat, and dysfunction.
2. The pain reflects the type, intensity, location, and phase of inflammatory reaction.
3. The pain follows an inflammatory time frame, meaning that it requires time to develop, plateau, and resolve.

Choosing the Correct Pain Disorder

Once the patient's pain complaint has been placed into the proper category, the clinician needs to select the precise diagnosis from within that category. This requires accurate knowledge of the clinical symptoms and behavior of all such pain disorders. The clinician's knowledge of the many possible orofacial pain disorders is of great importance. Remember, a clinician can never diagnosis a condition that he has never heard about. The most important pain disorders in each category will be discussed in the third section of this book.

Confirmation of the Clinical Diagnosis

Before undertaking definitive therapy, confirmation of the clinical diagnosis is advisable. There are four methods that can help confirm the diagnosis: diagnostic analgesic blocking, utilization of diagnostic drugs, consultations, and trial therapy.

Diagnostic Analgesic Blocking

Indications

The value of local anesthetic injections, as well as the application of topical anesthetics to identify and localize pain, cannot be overemphasized. This method is essential when differentiating primary pains from secondary pains. It is equally useful to identify the pathways that mediate peripheral pain and to localize pain sources. Very often, when the source of pain is difficult to identify, local anesthetic blocking of related tissues is the key to making the proper diagnosis. The examiner should therefore become skilled in the use of this valuable diagnostic tool. Muscle injections can also be useful for diagnostic purposes as well as for therapy. Local anesthetic blocking not only provides valuable diagnostic information, but in some pain disorders it can also provide therapeutic value. This is especially true for myofascial pain and myospasms.

Another indication for analgesic blocking is to help educate the patient to the source of his or her pain problem. Often patients do not appreciate the concept of pain referral, and it can be quite convincing to the patient when blocking a remote site reduces or even eliminates the chief complaint. This can be a very valuable educational tool.

The armamentarium

The armamentarium needed to provided anesthetic blocks is already present in almost every dental office. It begins with an aspirating syringe and both short and long 27-gauge needles. The length needed depends on the structure that is targeted. Alcohol and/or povidone-iodine swipes are also need to clean the site to be injected. Sterile 2 × 2 gauze pads should be available to apply to the injection site to control bleeding. Clean, disposable gloves are also needed.

The type of local anesthetic used may vary according to the type and purpose of the particular injection. When only diagnostic information is needed, the use of short-acting drugs is most desirable. Usually a solution without a vasoconstricting agent is best. Good anesthesia for skeletal muscle requires a nonvasoconstricting solution due to the vasodilating effect of epinephrine-like substances on such tissue. This reverse effect on muscle tissue is sometimes forgotten and may account for the transient anesthesia of poor quality sometimes obtained when muscles are injected for diagnostic purposes.

It has been demonstrated that local anesthetics have a measure of myotoxicity. Procaine appears to be the least myotoxic of the local anesthetics in common use.[38] Mild inflammatory reactions follow the injection of 1% and 2% procaine hydrochloride as well as isotonic sodium chloride.[58] Single injections of either procaine or isotonic saline cause no muscle necrosis.[59] The longer-acting and stronger anesthetics induce more severe inflammation and occasionally coagulation necrosis of muscle tissue.[60] Regeneration takes place in about 7 days. Solutions containing epinephrine cause greater muscle damage.[61] To minimize the danger of muscle damage in analgesic blocking for both diagnostic and therapeutic purposes, low concentrations of procaine are advisable, and such injections should be spaced at least 7 days apart. Since procaine is not available in dental Carpules, the dentist may select 2% lidocaine or 3% mepivacaine[62] without a vasoconstrictor. When a longer-acting anesthetic is indicated, 0.5% bupivacaine may be used.[63] Although bupivacaine is sometimes indicated for joint pain (auriculotemporal nerve block), it should not be routinely used with muscle injections because of its myotoxicity.[64]

The diagnostic use of local anesthetics in muscles should be curtailed to actual need. It should be noted that, despite some myotoxicity, the diagnostic and therapeutic use of local anesthesia in the management of myogenous pain disorders is clinically justified. Many diagnostic procedures and therapeutic modalities are attended by some risk. Note, for example, the destructive effects of radiation in radiography. All anesthetics and most medications are toxic to some degree. The inherent risks therefore must be weighed against the benefits derived. Reasonable judgment should be exercised in the application of all procedures that entail a measure of risk to the patient.

General rules

When any injection is to be performed, the following fundamental rules for local anesthesia should always be observed.

1. The clinician should have a sound knowledge of the anatomy of all structures in the region that is to be injected. The purpose of an injection is to isolate the particular structure that is to be blocked. Therefore, the clinician must know the precise location and appropriate technique used to get the needle tip to the desired structure. The clinician also needs a sound understanding of all the important structures in the area that should be avoided during the injection.
2. The clinician should have a sound knowledge of the pharmacology of all solutions that will be used.
3. Any injection into inflamed or diseased tissues must be avoided.
4. Strict asepsis should be maintained at all times.
5. The clinician should always aspirate before injecting the solution to ensure the needle is not in a blood vessel.

Types of injections

Diagnostic and therapeutic anesthetic blocks are divided into three types according to the structures that are targeted: muscle injections, nerve block injections, and intracapsular injections. Each of these will be discussed separately, since the indications and techniques vary.

Muscle injections

Injection of a muscle can be very valuable in determining the source of a pain disorder. In some instances, muscle injections can provide therapeutic value. For example, the injection of local anesthetic into a myofascial trigger point can result in significant pain reduction long after the anesthetic has been metabolized.[38,65,66] In myofascial pain, the patient presents with a firm, taut band of muscle tissue that is quite painful to palpate. This is known as a trigger point and is often responsible for producing a pattern of pain referral.[38] When this is suspected, the trigger point can be injected with local anesthetic and the resulting pattern of pain referral is shut down. The precise mechanisms of trigger point pain and the indications for treatment will be reviewed in chapter 12. When it has been determined that injection of the trigger point is indicated, the following sequence should be followed:

1. The trigger point is located by placing the finger over the muscle, and firm pressure is applied to locate the tight band. The finger is moved across the band so that it can be felt to "snap" under the pressure of the finger. Once the band is identified, the finger is moved up and down the band until the most painful area is located (Fig 8-28a).
2. Once the trigger point is located, the tissue over the trigger point is cleaned with alcohol. The trigger point is then trapped between two fingers so that when the needle is placed into the area the tight band will not slip away (Fig 8-28b).
3. The needle tip is then inserted into the tissue superficial to the trigger point and it is penetrated to the depth of the tight band (Fig 8-28c). It is often helpful to

receive feedback from the patient regarding the accuracy of your needle placement. Usually the patient can tell immediately when you have entered the trigger point. Once the needle tip is at the proper depth, the syringe is aspirated to ensure it is not located in a vessel. Then a small amount of anesthetic is deposited in the area (1/4 of a Carpule).

4. Once the initial anesthetic is deposited, it is useful to "fan" the needle tip slightly. This is done by withdrawing the needle halfway, changing the needle direction slightly, and re-entering into the firm band to the same depth (Fig 8-28d). The needle tip should not be completely removed from the tissue. This manipulation of the needle tip should be repeated several times, especially if the patient has not confirmed that the needle tip was in the area of exquisite tenderness. At each site the syringe is aspirated and a small amount of anesthetic can be deposited. In some instances the muscle will be felt to quickly contract. This is known as the "twitch response" and usually helps confirm that the needle is properly placed. Although the presence of a twitch response is favorable, not all muscles demonstrate this, and successful pain reduction can often be achieved without it.
5. Once the injection is completed, the needle is withdrawn completely and sterile gauze is held over the injection site with slight pressure for 20 to 30 seconds to assure good hemostasis (Fig 8-28e).

This general technique is used for most muscle injections; however, the unique anatomy of each muscle may demand slight variations. It is extremely important that the clinician be familiar with the anatomy of the muscle to be injected so as to avoid disturbing any neighboring structures. This text cannot review the anatomy of all the muscles that may need to be injected; therefore it is recommended that appropriate gross anatomy texts be reviewed before the

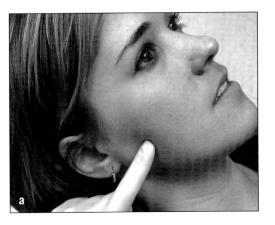

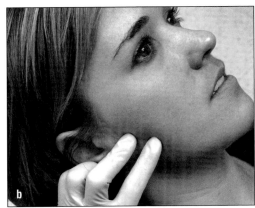

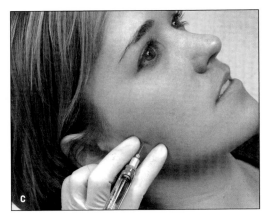

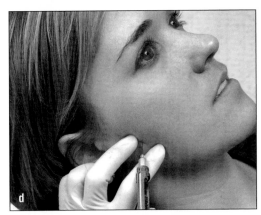

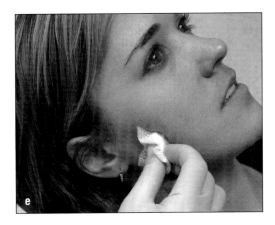

Fig 8-28 The technique used for trigger point injections. *(a)* The trigger point is located by placing the finger over the muscle and applying firm pressure to locate the tight band. *(b)* The trigger point is then trapped between two fingers, so that when the needle is placed into the area the tight band will not slip away. *(c)* The needle tip is inserted into the tissue superficial to the trigger point and is penetrated to the depth of the tight band. *(d)* Once the initial anesthetic is deposited, it is useful to "fan" the needle tip slightly. This is done by withdrawing the needle halfway, changing the needle direction slightly, and re-entering into the firm band, again halfway. *(e)* Once the injection is completed, the needle is withdrawn and a sterile gauze is held over the injection site with slight pressure for 20 to 30 seconds to assure good hemostasis.

clinician proceeds with an injection. Some of the muscles that can be easily injected are the masseter (Fig 8-28), temporalis (Fig 8-29), SCM (Fig 8-30), splenius capitis (Fig 8-31), posterior occipital muscles (Fig 8-32), and the trapezius (Fig 8-33). The orofacial pain specialist should become familiar with the anatomic features of these muscles and surrounding structures so that safe and predictable injections can be performed routinely.

Nerve block injections

Diagnostic nerve blocks can be very useful in identifying whether a painful structure is a site or source of pain. When diagnosis is the primary purpose for the injection, a short-acting local anesthetic should be used without a vasoconstrictor. In some instances, long-term pain relief may be therapeutically indicated. This may be appropriate for certain chronic pain conditions when prolonged relief of pain can be used to interrupt pain cycling and hopefully reduce central sensitization. When long-term anesthesia is indicated, a long-term local anesthetic, such as bupivacaine with a vasoconstrictor, may be a better choice.

Some of the important nerve blocks that should be considered are *dental blocks,* the *auriculotemporal nerve block,* the *infraorbital nerve block,* and the *stellate ganglion nerve block.*

The practicing dental clinician uses dental blocks routinely in dental treatments. It should be remembered that these same injections can provide valuable diagnostic information. The common nerve blocks used are the *inferior alveolar nerve block,* the *posterior superior nerve block,* the *mental nerve block,* and *infiltration blocks,* often administered in various areas of the maxillary arch. The techniques used for these blocks will not be reviewed here, since they are routinely used in the dental office. Although these blocks are mostly used for anesthesia during dental procedures, their diagnostic value should not be overlooked. For exam-

ple, an inferior alveolar nerve block will completely eliminate any source of pain coming from the mandibular teeth on the side of the injection. This block is useful in distinguishing dental pain from muscle or joint pain, since it blocks only the dental structures. This is very important diagnostic information, especially when a patient's chief complaint is toothache. If a mandibular toothache is truly of dental origin, an inferior alveolar nerve block will eliminate the pain. If, however, the toothache is actually a referred pain to the tooth, the block will not change the pain.

When identifying pain sources, it is vital that the clinician ask the patient the proper questions. If the patient has a nonodontogenic toothache and an inferior alveolar nerve block is administered, the pain will not be resolved, even though the tissues become anesthetized. If the doctor asks whether the area is numb, the patient will respond positively. This may lead the clinician to assume that the pain has resolved when this is not the case. The clinician needs to carefully phrase the question after giving the patient local anesthesia. The clinician should ask the question in this manner: "Now I realize that your jaw is numb, but does it still hurt?" The patient will certainly feel numb, but the important question is "Does it still hurt?" This is a critical concept to appreciate when differentiating the odontogenic toothache from the nonodontogenic toothache (as will be discussed in chapter 11).

A very important nerve block that all orofacial pain clinicians should become very familiar with is the *auriculotemporal nerve block.* This nerve block has very significant diagnostic value. The auriculotemporal nerve innervates approximately 90% of the TMJ.[67] Therefore, if the TMJ is a source of pain, this nerve block will quickly eliminate the pain. Since the TMJ area is a frequent site of pain referral, this block is very valuable and indicated to help identify when the joint is actually a source of pain. In fact,

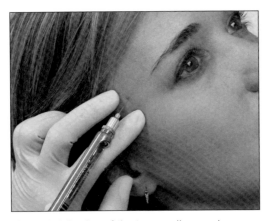

Fig 8-29 Injection of the temporalis muscle.

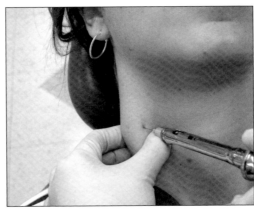

Fig 8-30 Injection of the SCM muscle from an anterior approach, which will help avoid vital deep structures.

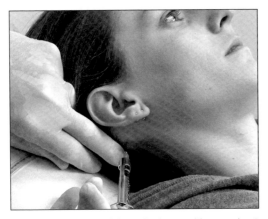

Fig 8-31 Injection of the splenius capitis muscle at its attachment to the skull slightly distal to the mastoid process.

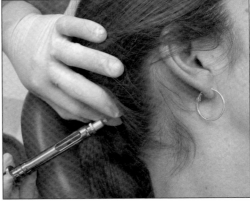

Fig 8-32 Injection of the posterior occipital muscles at their attachments to the skull.

Fig 8-33 Injection of a common site for a trigger point in the trapezius muscle.

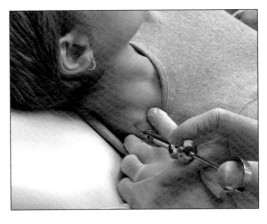

any time there is irreversible treatment planned for the TMJ, such as surgery, this block can help confirm the need for such treatment. If an auriculotemporal nerve block does not resolve the pain, aggressive therapies should not be considered until the true source of the pain is identified.

Some clinicians anesthetize the TMJ by injecting directly into the joint or into the retrodiscal structures. Although this may be effective, it also can traumatize delicate joint structures. A less traumatic method is to anesthetize the joint structures by blocking the auriculotemporal nerve before its fibers reach the joint (Fig 8-34a). The auriculotemporal nerve can be blocked by first cleaning the tissue and then passing a 27-gauge needle through the skin just anterior and slightly above the junction of the tragus and the earlobe (Figs 8-34b and 8-34c). The needle is then advanced until it touches the posterior neck of the condyle. The needle is then repositioned in a more posterior direction until the tip of the needle is able to pass behind the posterior neck of the condyle (Fig 8-34d). Once the neck of the condyle is felt, the tip of the needle is carefully moved slightly behind the posterior aspect of the condyle in an anteromedial direction to a depth of 1 cm (Fig 8-34e). The syringe is then aspirated, and if no blood is seen, the solution is deposited.[68] If the true source of pain is the joint, the pain should be eliminated or certainly significantly decreased within 4 to 5 minutes.

In cases of trauma to the face, the infraorbital nerve can be injured, resulting in continuous neuropathic pain (see chapter 17), and performance of an *infraorbital nerve block* may have some therapeutic value. This nerve transverses below the eye to exit from the infraorbital foramen, located in the inferior border of the orbit. This nerve goes on to innervate the facial structures below the eye and some of the lateral aspects of the nose. It can be blocked by either an extraoral or an intraoral approach. When the

extraoral approach is used, the foramen is identified by palpation of the inferior border of the orbit, feeling for a slight notch. The notch represents the exit of the infraorbital nerve. Once the notch is located, the tissue is cleaned and the needle is placed to the depth of the notch and into the foramen when possible (Fig 8-35a). When the intraoral approach is used, the notch is found in the same manner as previously described. The middle finger is used to maintain the position of the notch, while the index finger and thumb are used to retract the lip. The needle is placed into the mouth, and the tip is inserted into the vestibule and directed upward to the notch (Fig 8-35b). In some instances, a long 27-gauge needle may be needed to reach the foramen with this technique.

In certain instances, sympathetic activity may contribute to the pain condition. Such pains are called *sympathetically maintained pains* (see chapter 17). A *stellate ganglion block* is indicated when there is suspicion that the orofacial pain complaint is mediated by the afferent sympathetic pathways or is dependent on sympathetic efferent activity.[69–73] The sympathetic fibers descend from the hypothalamus to the dorsal horn in the region of T2 and T3, where they exit the spinal column to enter the sympathetic chain. From there they ascend to the stellate ganglion and exit to innervate the facial structures. When sympathetic activity is suspected of contributing to a patient's pain, it can be diagnostically confirmed by blocking the stellate ganglion with local anesthetic. This injection will block most of the sympathetic innervation to the face. This injection is performed in the anterior region of the neck, just lateral to the larynx. Because of the close proximity of other significant structures in the region of the stellate ganglion, this injection is not performed in a routine dental setting. Some of the structures of concern are the vagus and phrenic nerves. If these nerves are affected by the local anesthetic during the proce-

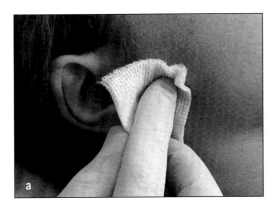

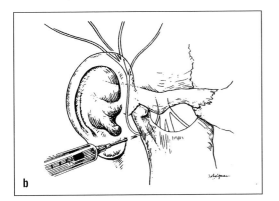

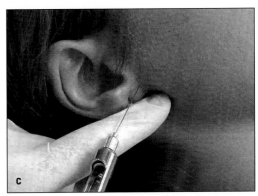

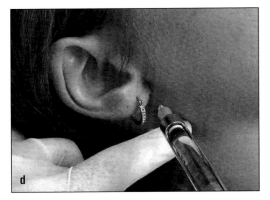

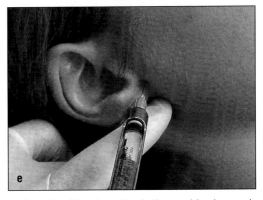

Fig 8-34 Auriculotemporal nerve block. *(a)* The tissue at the site of the injection is thoroughly cleansed. *(b)* Drawing showing the proper needle placement for an auriculotemporal nerve block as well as the position of the auriculotemporal nerve as it traverses the posterior aspect of the condyle. (From Donlon et al.[72p544] Used with permission.) *(c)* The needle is placed slightly anterior to the junction of the tragus and earlobe and is penetrated until the posterior neck of the condyle is felt. *(d)* The needle is then repositioned in a more posterior direction until the tip of the needle is able to pass behind the posterior neck of the condyle. *(e)* Once the needle tip passes beyond the neck of the condyle, the syringe is again positioned in a more anterior direction and the tip is inserted behind the neck of the condyle. The total depth of the needle is approximately 1 cm. The syringe is then aspirated, and if there is no blood drawn back into the syringe, the anesthetic solution is deposited. Placement of the needle in this manner will minimize anesthetization of the facial nerve.

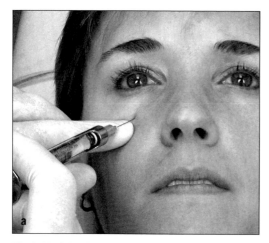 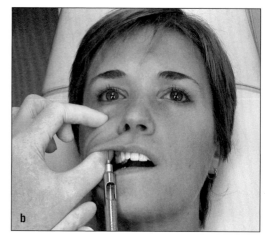

Fig 8-35 Injection of the infraorbital nerve. *(a)* During an extraoral approach, the infraorbital foramen is palpated (notch) and the needle tip is placed directly into the opening of the foramen. *(b)* During the intraoral approach, the foramen is first located extraorally and the position is maintained by a finger. The needle is placed into the vestibule and moved superiorly until the tip is located at the foramen. For this injection, a long-gauge needle is used.

dure, the patient may have difficulty breathing or possible cardiac complications. The clinician must be prepared to manage any medical complication that arises, such as maintaining the patient on ventilation during the period of anesthesia. It is important that the orofacial clinician be familiar with the indications for analgesic blocking of the stellate ganglion, but not necessarily the precise technique, since this is a very specialized procedure. An anesthesiologist with proper training and facilities should be called upon to make this injection.

Intracapsular injections

On occasion an injection directly into the TMJ is indicated. This type of injection would be indicated for therapeutic reasons, not diagnosis. Diagnostic information is derived from performing the auriculotemporal nerve block, but a therapeutic injection would be indicated when it is appropriate to introduce some medication to the joint structures.

Injection of an anti-inflammatory medication such as hydrocortisone into the joint has been advocated[74-79] for the relief of pain and restricted movements. A single intra-articular injection seems to be most helpful in older patients; however, less success has been observed[76] in patients under age 25. Although a single injection is occasionally helpful, an earlier study[80] reported that multiple injections may be harmful to the structures of the joint and should be avoided. Another long-term follow-up study of intra-articular corticosteroid injections for TMJ osteoarthritis, however, was more encouraging.[78] Injection of corticosteroids has also been reported to improve acute TMJ symptoms resulting from rheumatoid arthritis, without long-term adverse sequelae.[78]

Another injectable solution that is used for intracapsular injections is sodium hyaluronate. Although not a local anesthetic, sodium hyaluronate has been suggested for the treatment of TMJ articular disease.[77,81] Studies of sodium hyaluronate for the treatment of disc displacements and disc

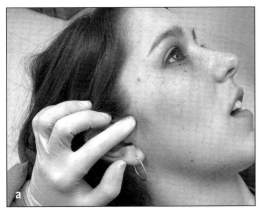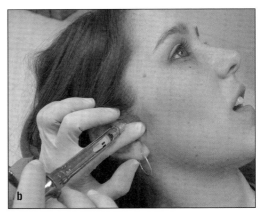

Fig 8-36 The intracapsular TMJ injection. *(a)* The lateral pole of the condyle is located. *(b)* The patient is asked to open the mouth slightly, and the tip of the needle is placed just below the zygomatic arch and slightly posterior and superior to the condylar pole. The needle is angulated slightly anterior to avoid the retrodiscal tissues.

dislocations without reduction are promising.[82-84] Some studies[85-87] have found that the use of sodium hyaluronate following arthrocentesis of the TMJ can be helpful in reducing pain (see chapter 13). The use of sodium hyaluronate in the TMJ is limited at this time, since it has not yet received approval for this use in the United States.

Normally, the superior joint space is the target for an intracapsular (intra-articular) injection, because it is the largest joint space and it is the simplest to consistently locate. The joint can be entered by first locating the lateral pole of the condyle. This can be assisted by asking the patient to open and close the mouth (Fig 8-36a). Once the pole is located, the clinician asks the patient to open slightly and palpates directly above to locate the zygomatic arch. The tissue is cleaned and the tip of the needle is placed just below the zygomatic arch and slightly posterior and superior to the condylar pole. The needle is angulated slightly

toward the anterior to avoid the retrodiscal tissues (Fig 8-36b). Once the capsule is penetrated, the tip of the needle will be in the superior joint space. The solution is then deposited and the needle removed. A sterile gauze is held over the injection site for a few seconds to assure hemostasis. The patient is then asked to open and close the mouth a few times to distribute the solution throughout the joint space.

Often a successful intra-articular injection will leave the patient with an immediate acute malocclusion on the ipsilateral side. Since there is very little area in the superior joint space, the introduction of additional fluid will temporarily cause an increase in the joint space, which leads to the separation of the posterior teeth on the same side of the injection. This will resolve in a few hours. The patient should be made aware of this condition so that it does not lead to any unnecessary concern or emotional stress.

Diagnostic Drugs

There are some drugs that have very specific effects on certain pain disorders. For example, the triptans can often quickly abort neurovascular pains. Therefore, if a patient's pain condition has neurovascular quality, a single dose of a product such as sumatriptan succinate may completely abort the headache. When this occurs, the medication can be used to confirm the diagnosis of migraine. Another example of a medication that has diagnostic value is the use of indomethacin for paroxysmal hemicrania. This medication is often used to confirm the diagnosis of paroxysmal hemicrania.

In the medical literature, confirmation of pain due to myocardial ischemia is usually accomplished by use of a test dose of nitroglycerin beneath the tongue. The drug relaxes smooth muscle, principally in the smaller blood vessels, and therefore dilates the arterioles, especially in the coronary circulation. Treatment with this drug is contraindicated in early myocardial infarction, severe anemia, glaucoma, increased intracranial pressure, and idiosyncrasy, and therefore this trial should be left in the hands of the physician.

Consultations

On occasion, pain problems require medical, otolaryngologic, orthopedic, neurologic, rheumatologic, or psychologic consultation for proper identification of the pain disorder. Judgment on the part of the examiner is required to guide the patient through the examination procedure to arrive at a firm diagnosis in the most direct, time-saving, and economic manner. Elaborate diagnostic and consultative procedures should not be routine. However, if the problem justifies it, every avenue of exploration should be used to arrive at a confirmed working diagnosis.

Trial Therapy

A short period of trial therapy is often a good means of confirming a diagnosis, provided that the examiner is familiar with the effectiveness of placebo therapy. This is particularly true with patients who have significant Axis II diagnoses. These factors must be taken into account when evaluating the results of trial therapy. One form of trial therapy is the use of oxcarbazepine to help confirm a doubtful diagnosis of paroxysmal neuralgia. This medication has no analgesic action for musculoskeletal pains; therefore, if it reduces the pain it confirms a neuropathic diagnosis. If the relief is well beyond the 40% maximum pain reduction that can be attributed to placebo, this suggests the diagnosis of paroxysmal neuralgia. One should guard against assuming that absence of effect from this drug excludes neuralgia. This would be a serious error, since not all neuralgias respond to this medication.

Trial therapy for muscular pains is useful to help confirm the diagnosis. This includes the use of vapocoolant sprays, analgesic blocking of the painful muscles, controlled physiotherapy, and the use of muscle relaxants. If definite benefit accrues from such therapy, a firm diagnosis of muscle pain becomes justified.

If an acute attack of temporomandibular arthralgia is suspected to be the result of hyperuricemia, a period of trial therapy consisting of colchicine can be useful. If the condition is chronic, colchicine combined with a uricosuric agent such as probenecid is helpful. Such medications should be given under medical supervision. If the arthralgia responds favorably to such therapy, the diagnosis should stand confirmed, and further medical care would be appropriate.

Multiple Categories of Pain

In managing pain problems about the mouth and face, one should avoid assuming that the complaint necessarily involves only a single category of pain. On many occasions, two or more types of pain may coexist, which may make establishing the proper diagnoses even more difficult. An early indication of this complication may come with the series of questions that constitute the second step of making the diagnosis. Difficulty in obtaining clear answers to these questions should alert the examiner to this possibility. Management difficulties are also likely to follow. When more than one diagnosis is suspected, the clinician needs to carefully evaluate the history and examination findings and separate the conditions. Once the conditions are separated and properly diagnosed, it is often therapeutically helpful to list all the diagnoses in order of their severity and/or patient concerns. Accomplishing this will help develop a treatment plan that will affect the patient's symptoms in the most positive and immediate manner. Understanding this concept leads to more effective patient management.

References

1. Melzack R. The McGill Pain Questionnaire: Major properties and scoring methods. Pain 1975;1:277–299.
2. Grushka M, Sessle BJ. Applicability of the McGill Pain Questionnaire to the differentiation of "toothache" pain. Pain 1984;19:49–57.
3. Corson JA, Schneider MJ. The Dartmouth Pain Questonnaire: An adjunct to the McGill Pain Questonnaire. Pain 1984;19:59–69.
4. Melzack R. The short-form McGill Pain Questionnaire. Pain 1987;30:191–197.
5. Breivik EK, Bjornsson GA, Skovlund E. A comparison of pain rating scales by sampling from clinical trial data. Clin J Pain 2000;16:22–28.
6. Moldofsky H, Scarisbrick P. Induction of neurasthenic musculoskeletal pain syndrome by selective sleep deprivation. Psychomatic Med 1976;38:35–44.
7. Moldofsky H, Scarisbrick P, England R, Smythe H. Musculoskeletal symptoms and non-REM sleep disturbance in patients with "fibrositis" and healthy subjects. Psychosom Med 1986;37:341–351.
8. Moldofsky H, Tullis C, Lue F. Sleep related myoclonus in rheumatic pain modulation disorder (fibrosis syndrome). J Rheumatol 1986;13:614–617.
9. Molony RR, MacPeek DM, Schiffman PL, et al. Sleep, sleep apnea, and the fibromyalgia syndrome. J Rheumatol 1986;13:797–800.
10. Yatani H, Studts J, Cordova M, Carlson CR, Okeson JP. Comparison of sleep quality and clinical and psychologic characteristics in patients with temporomandibular disorders. J Orofac Pain 2002;16:221–228.
11. Rollman GB, Gillespie JM. The role of psychosocial factors in temporomandibular disorders. Curr Rev Pain 2000;4:71–81.
12. Sayar K, Arikan M, Yontem T. Sleep quality in chronic pain patients. Can J Psychiatry 2002;47:844–888.
13. McCracken LM, Iverson GL. Disrupted sleep patterns and daily functioning in patients with chronic pain. Pain Res Manage 2002;7:75–79.
14. Turk DC, Rudy TE. Toward a comprehensive assessment of chronic pain patients: A multiaxial approach. Behav Res Ther 1987;25:237–249.
15. Derogatis LR. SCL-90-R: Administration, Scoring and Procedures Manual-II for the Revised Version. Towson, MD: Clinical Psychometric Research, 1977.
16. Fricton J, Nelson A, Monsein M. IMPATH: Microcomputer assessment of behavioral and psychosocial factors in craniomandibular disorders. Cranio 1987;5:372–381.
17. Levitt SR, McKinney MW, Lundeen TF. The TMJ scale: Cross-validation and reliability studies. Cranio 1988;6:17–25.
18. Levitt SR. Predictive value of the TMJ Scale in detecting clinically significant symptoms of temporomandibular disorders. J Craniomandib Disord Facial Oral Pain 1990;4:177–185.
19. American Psychiatric Association. Diagnostic and Statistical Manual of Mental Disorders: DSM-IV, ed 4. Washington, DC: American Psychiatric Association, 1994.

20. Clark GT. Examining temporomandibular disorder patients for craniocervical dysfunction. J Craniomandib Pract 1984;2:55–63.
21. Clark GT, Green EM, Dornan MR, Flack VF. Craniocervical dysfunction levels in a patient sample from a temporomandibular joint clinic. J Am Dent Assoc 1987;115:251–256.
22. Keele KD. A physician looks at pain. In: Weisenberg M (ed). Pain: Clinical and Experimental Perspectives. St Louis: Mosby, 1975:45–52.
23. Delcanho RE. Masticatory muscle pain: A review of clinical features, research findings and possible mechanisms. Aust Prosthodont J 1995;9:49–59.
24. Mahan PE, Alling CC. Facial Pain. Malvern, PA: Lea & Febiger, 1991:145–151.
25. Okeson JP. History and examination for temporomandibular disorders. In: Management of Temporomandibular Disorders and Occlusion, ed 5. St Louis: Mosby-Year Book, 1993:245–320.
26. McNeill C. Temporomandibular Disorders: Guidelines for Classification, Assessment, and Management. Chicago: Quintessence, 1993: 64–65.
27. Frost HM. Musculoskeletal pains. In: Alling CC, Mahan PE (eds). Facial Pain. Philadelphia: Lea & Febiger, 1977:140–157.
28. Reeves JL, Jaeger B, Graff-Radford SB. Reliability of the pressure algometer as a measure of myofascial trigger point sensitivity. Pain 1986; 24:313–321.
29. Jensen K, Andersen HO, Olesen J, Lindblom U. Pressure-pain threshold in human temporal region. Evaluation of a new pressure algometer. Pain 1986;25:313–323.
30. Fischer AA. Instruments for pain diagnosis in clinical practice: Pressure algometers for measurement of pain sensitivity and documentation for tender spots; tissue compliance meter for objective quantitative recording of muscle spasm [abstract]. Pain 1987;31(suppl 4):292.
31. Schiffman E, Fricton J, Haley D, et al. A pressure algometer for MPS: Reliability and validity [abstract]. Pain 1987;31(suppl 4):291.
32. Fischer AA. Pressure algometry over normal muscles: Standard values, validity, and reproducibility of pressure threshold. Pain 1987;30: 115–126.
33. Fischer AA. Pressure threshold measurement for diagnosis of myofascial pain and evaluation of treatment results. Clin J Pain 1987;2: 207–214.
34. Jaeger B, Reeves JL. Quantification of changes in myofascial trigger point sensitivity with the pressure algometer following passive stretch. Pain 1986;27:203–210.
35. Moody PM, Calhoun TC, Okeson JP, Kemper JT. Stress-pain relationships in MPD syndrome patients and non-MPD syndrome patients. J Prosthet Dent 1981;45:84–88.
36. Okeson JP, Kemper JT, Moody PM. A study of the use of occlusion splints in the treatment of acute and chronic patients with craniomandibular disorders. J Prosthet Dent 1982;48: 708–712.
37. Travell J, Rinzler SH. The myofascial genesis of pain. Postgrad Med J 1952;11:425.
38. Simons DG, Travell JG, Simons LS. Apropos of all muscles. In: Travell & Simons' Myofascial Pain and Dysfunction: The Trigger Point Manual, ed 2. Baltimore: Williams & Wilkins, 1999: 94–177.
39. Bell WE. Management of temporomandibular joint problems. In: Goldman HM (ed). Current Therapy in Dentistry. St Louis: Mosby, 1970: 398–415.
40. Agerberg G. Maximal mandibular movement in young men and women. Swed Dent J 1974; 67:81–100.
41. Solberg W. Occlusion-related pathosis and its clinical evaluation. In: Clarke JW (ed). Clinical Dentistry. Hagerstown, MD: Harper & Row, 1976:1–29.
42. Bitlar G. Range of jaw opening in an elderly non-patient population [abstract 1225]. J Dent Res 1991;70(special issue):419.
43. Agerberg G. Maximal mandibular movements in children. Acta Odontol Scand 1974;32: 147–159.
44. Vanderas AP. Mandibular movements and their relationship to age and body weight in children with or without clinical signs of craniomandibular dysfunction. Part IV. J Dent Child 1992;59:338–341.
45. McCarroll RS, Hesse JR Naeije M, Yoon CK, Hansson TL. Mandibular border positions and their relationship with peripheral joint mobility. J Oral Rehabil 1987;14:125–131.
46. Hesse J, Naeije M, Hansson TL. Craniomandibular stiffness toward maximum mouth opening in healthy subjects: A clinical and experimental investigation. J Craniomandib Disord Facial Oral Pain 1990;4:257–266.

47. Burch JG. History and clinical examination. In: Laskin DM, American Dental Association (eds). The President's Conference on the Examination, Diagnosis, and Management of Temporomandibular Disorders. Chicago: American Dental Association, 1983:54–59.

48. Bezuur JN, Habets LLH, Jimenez Lopez V, Naeije M, Hansson TL. The recognition of craniomandibular disorders: A comparison between clinical and radiographic findings in eighty-nine subjects. J Oral Rehabil 1988;15:215–222.

49. Westesson PL, Eriksson L, Kurita K. Reliability of a negative clinical temporomandibular joint examination: Prevalence of disk displacement in asymptomatic temporomandibular joints. Oral Surg Oral Med Oral Pathol Oral Radiol Endod 1989;68:551–554.

50. Mumford JM. Toothache and Related Pain. Edinburgh: Churchill Livingstone, 1973.

51. Okeson JP. Causes of functional disturbances in the masticatory system. In: Management of Temporomandibular Disorders and Occlusion, ed 5. St Louis: Mosby-Year Book, 2003, 149–189.

52. McNamara JA Jr, Seligman DA, Okeson JP. Occlusion, orthodontic treatment, and temporomandibular disorders: A review. J Orofac Pain 1995;9:73–90.

53. Levitt SR, McKinney MW. Validating the TMJ scale in a national sample of 10,000 patients: demographic and epidemiologic characteristics. J Orofac Pain 1994;8:25–35.

54. Keats AS. Use of analgesics at bedside. In: Way EL (ed). New Concepts in Pain. Philadelphia: Davis, 1967:143–154.

55. Beecher HK. The use of chemical agents in the control of pain. In: Knighton RS, Dumke PR (eds). Pain. Boston: Little, Brown, 1966:221–239.

56. Stockstill JW. The placebo effect. The placebo effect in the management of chronic myofascial pain: A review. J Am Coll Dent 1989;56:14–18.

57. Amanzio M, Benedetti F. Neuropharmacological dissection of placebo analgesia: expectation-activated opioid systems versus conditioning-activated specific subsystems. J Neurosci 1999;19:484–494.

58. Pizzolato P, Mannheimer W. Histopathologic Effects of Local Anesthetic Drugs and Related Substances. Springfield, IL: Thomas, 1961.

59. Burke GWJ, Fedison JR, Jones CR. Muscle degeneration produced by local anesthesia. Va Dent J 1972;49:33–37.

60. Travell JG, Simons DG. Head and neck pain and muscle guide to introduce the masticatory muscles. In: Myofascial Pain and Dysfunction. A Trigger Point Manual. Baltimore: Williams & Wilkins, 1983:165–332.

61. Yagiela JA, Benoit PW, Buoncristiani RD, Peters MP, Fort NF. Comparison of myotoxic effects of lidocaine with epinephrine in rats and humans. Anesth Analg 1981;60:471–480.

62. Ernest EA. Temporomandibular Joint and Craniofacial Pain. Montgomery, AL: Ernest Publications, 1983:105–113.

63. Laskin JL, Wallace WR, DeLeo B. Use of bupivacaine hydrochloride in oral surgery: A clinical study. J Oral Surg 1977;35:25–29.

64. Guttu RL, Page DG, Laskin DM. Delayed healing of muscle after injection of bupivicaine and steroid. Ann Dent 1990;49:5–8.

65. Fine PG, Milano R, Hare BD. The effects of myofascial trigger point injections are naloxone reversible. Pain 1988;32:15–20.

66. Hameroff SR, Crago BR, Blitt CD, Womble J, Kanel J. Comparison of bupivacaine, etidocaine, and saline for trigger-point therapy. Anesth Analg 1981;60:752–755.

67. Schmidt BL, Pogrel MA, Necoechea M, Kearns G. The distribution of the auriculotemporal nerve around the temporomandibular joint. Oral Surg Oral Med Oral Pathol Oral Radiol Endod 1998;86:165–168.

68. Donlon WC, Truta MP, Eversole LR. A modified auriculotemporal nerve block for regional anesthesia of the temporomandibular joint. J Oral Maxillofac Surg 1984;42:544–545.

69. Moore DC. Stellate Ganglion Block. Springfield, IL: Thomas, 1954.

70. Bonica JJ. The Management of Pain. Philadelphia: Lea & Febiger, 1990:1931–1944.

71. Wang JK, Johnson KA, Ilstrup DM. Sympathetic blocks for reflex sympathetic dystrophy. Pain 1985;23:13–17.

72. Verre M, De Santis F, Glyronakis S, et al. Pharmacological sympathetic block in complex regional pain syndrome [in Italian]. Clin Ther 2002;153:367–372.

73. Hanamatsu N, Yamashiro M, Sumitomo M, Furuya H. Effectiveness of cervical sympathetic ganglia block on regeneration of the trigeminal nerve following transection in rats. Reg Anesth Pain Med 2002;27:268–276.

74. Henny FA. Intra-articular injection of hydrocortisone into the temporomandibular joint. J Oral Surg 1954;12:314–319.

75. Toller PA. Osteoarthrosis of the mandibular condyle. Br Dent J 1973;134:223–231.

76. Toller P. Non-surgical treatment of dysfunctions of the temporo-mandibular joint. Oral Sci Rev 1976;7:70–85.

77. Kopp S, Carlsson GE, Haraldson T, Wenneberg B. Long-term effect of intra-articular injections of sodium hyaluronate and corticosteroid on temporomandibular joint arthritis. J Oral Maxillofac Surg 1987;45:929–935.

78. Wenneberg B, Kopp S, Grondahl HG. Long-term effect of intra-articular injections of a glucocorticosteroid into the TMJ: A clinical and radiographic 8-year follow-up. J Craniomandib Disord 1991;5:11–18.

79. Wenneberg B. Other disorders. In: Zarb GA, Carlsson GE, Sessle BJ, Mohl ND. Temporomandibular Joint and Masticatory Muscle Disorders. St. Louis: Mosby, 1995:367–372.

80. Poswillo D. Experimental investigation of the effects of intra-articular hydrocortisone and high condylectomy on the mandibular condyle. Oral Surg Oral Med Oral Pathol 1970;30:161–173.

81. Kopp S, Wenneberg B, Haraldson T, Carlsson GE. The short-term effect of intra-articular injections of sodium hyaluronate and corticosteroid on temporomandibular joint pain and dysfunction. J Oral Maxillofac Surg 1985;43:429–435.

82. Bertolami CN, Gay T, Clark GT, et al. Use of sodium hyaluronate in treating temporomandibular joint disorders: A randomized, double-blind, placebo-controlled clinical trial. J Oral Maxillofac Surg 1993;51:232–242.

83. Alpaslan C, Bilgihan A, Alpaslan GH, Guner B, Ozgur Yis M, Erbas D. Effect of arthrocentesis and sodium hyaluronate injection on nitrite, nitrate, and thiobarbituric acid-reactive substance levels in the synovial fluid. Oral Surg Oral Med Oral Pathol Oral Radiol Endod 2000;89:686–690.

84. Hirota W. Intra-articular injection of hyaluronic acid reduces total amounts of leukotriene C4, 6-keto-prostaglandin F1alpha, prostaglandin F2alpha and interleukin-1beta in synovial fluid of patients with internal derangement in disorders of the temporomandibular joint. Br J Oral Maxillofac Surg 1998;36:35–38.

85. Sato S, Ohta M, Ohki H, Kawamura H, Motegi K. Effect of lavage with injection of sodium hyaluronate for patients with nonreducing disk displacement of the temporomandibular joint. Oral Surg Oral Med Oral Pathol Oral Radiol Endod 1997;84:241–244.

86. Sato S, Sakamoto M, Kawamura H, Motegi K. Disc position and morphology in patients with nonreducing disc displacement treated by injection of sodium hyaluronate. Int J Oral Maxillofac Surg 1999;28:253–257.

87. Alpaslan GH, Alpaslan C. Efficacy of temporomandibular joint arthrocentesis with and without injection of sodium hyaluronate in treatment of internal derangements. J Oral Maxillofac Surg 2001;59:613–618.

General Considerations in Managing Orofacial Pains

The conditions that generate pain are susceptible to modification. The treatment of people who suffer pain entails the manipulation of those factors that initiate and accentuate pain and/or the institution of means and methods by which patients can better cope with their complaint. The conditions that we may set out to manipulate, therefore, comprise on the one hand such factors as the elimination of etiologic noxious stimuli, the interruption of nociceptive circuits, and the enhancement of the natural mechanisms of pain inhibition. On the other hand, we may elect to direct the main attention toward the patient rather than his or her problem in an effort to help the patient contend more successfully with the "disease." Sternbach[1] has shown that whereas "pain" in acute pain is a symptom of disease, "pain" in chronic pain is the disease itself. Instantly, it should be obvious that pain management is a complex undertaking. Unfortunately, we are just beginning to learn the rules of the game. This much we do know: it is the patient's body that does the healing, not the doctor. The

most that we can do is provide favorable conditions for healing. Our patients must understand that it is they, not we, who determine the final outcome of therapy. Healing is an activity that only the patients can do. We cannot do it for them.

The first step in the treatment of any condition is accurate and complete diagnostic evaluation of what the problem is, what structures are involved, and what conditions account for it. The diagnosis of pain is not a "naming process." It is an understanding of pain genesis, modulating conditions, inhibitory and excitatory mechanisms, secondary effects, accompanying symptoms, and physical and emotional reactions that occur in human beings as distinct individuals. Every patient who presents a pain complaint has a problem that is peculiar to him or her. Yet we as dental practitioners are trained as therapists more than as diagnosticians. We are conditioned to treat, and our patients are conditioned to expect decisive and effective treatment from us. We are more mouth-oriented than patient-oriented. We do well as long as everything is obvious; when we face obscure problems, our conditioning may fail us. Therefore, when we meet an obscure pain complaint, we need to call forth all our best diagnostic capabilities.

It is essential at the very outset to decide whether we are dealing with an acute pain or a chronic pain. We must decide whether the behavioral characteristics suggest somatic or neuropathic pain, whether the pain emanates from superficial or deep structures, and whether the pain is primary or secondary. To skip these basic steps is to invite failure. Very early we need to decide whether the complaint appears to be stimulus-evoked. Will our therapy be directed toward the elimination of a source of noxious stimulation? Will it use techniques that manipulate modulating influences? Will it entail the management of neuropathic pain sources? Will it employ the use of systemic medications? Will psychotherapy likely be utilized? A decision is needed: "Is this a problem that I can handle alone, or do I need help? What kind of help, and from whom?" Ultimate success or failure may well rest upon such early decisions. They should form the overall guidelines for managing the problem at hand. Each case should be individualized. We are not dealing so much with different kinds of problems as with different kinds of people. Genuine caring on the part of the clinician is the one indispensable attribute in good pain management.[2]

Cause-Related Therapy

Many patients who experience orofacial pain have an organic structural cause that is responsible. The main thrust of therapy for such complaints is to identify the cause and eliminate it. The extent to which one

achieves this will determine his or her success in the management of the pain problem. The cause of pain emanating from somatic structures is thought to be due chiefly to the action of algogenic substances, such as bradykinin, histamine, serotonin (5-hydroxytriptamine [5HT]), potassium, and phosphates.[3] The etiology of neuropathic pain is less well understood.

Somatic Pain

Much somatic pain results from trauma, intrinsic injury, infections, and diseases that induce inflammatory reactions. The variety of traumatic conditions, with respect to the type of agent as well as the extent and location of injury, is nearly endless. Inflammatory conditions reactive to abusive use; intrinsic strains; microtraumas; bacterial, fungal, or viral infections; pathologic lesions; and biomechanical dysfunctions are almost without number. At a dental level, inflammatory conditions of the teeth, the supporting structures, and the mucogingival tissues as well as dysfunctional and inflammatory conditions of the temporomandibular joints (TMJs) and masticatory musculature are commonplace. It is known that ischemia liberates bradykinin,[4-6] that hemolyzed red blood cells in muscle tissue liberate potassium ions, and that phosphates, histamine, and 5HT are liberated from blood platelets.[7-9] Some of the visceral somatic structures elicit pain without such evident cause. Vascular pain involves more than simple vasodilation; it is likely that algogenic substances are involved.[10-12]

There are occasions when the somatic condition that generates pain is refractory to therapy, and the complaint persists as chronic structural pain. Cancer presents this problem. Some masticatory pains, such as inflammatory arthritis, may also fall into this category.

Neuropathic Pain

The matter of eliminating the cause of neuropathic pain presents problems. Some benefit may come from anti-inflammatory therapy for inflammatory neuritis pain, and symptomatic neuralgia may respond to neurosurgical elimination of the neuropathy. A traumatic neuroma in accessible scar tissue can be excised, but in some instances the neuroma may return. Generally, however, many neuropathic pains, such as idiopathic neuralgia and deafferentation, cannot be managed by cause-related therapies. These therapies will be discussed in chapter 17.

Pain Related to Psychologic Disorders

When Axis II diagnoses predominate the pain complaint, an entirely different treatment strategy is often indicated. Any therapies that alter somatic or neurogenous structures should be avoided. Therapy should be directed toward the factors or conditions that relate to the specific psychologic disorder. Sometimes pharmacologic agents or physical therapy modalities may be helpful, but they should not be used as a substitute for proper psychotherapy. Psychotherapies are best provided by trained personnel, and referral may be indicated if these professionals are not immediately available (see chapter 18).

Therapeutic Modalities

Table 9-1 lists the many different approaches that should be considered when managing orofacial pain disorders. The appropriateness of each modality is determined by the specific diagnosis. Each modality will be reviewed in this chapter. The specific use of these modalities will be discussed in the chapters that review each orofacial pain disorder.

Pharmacologic Therapy

Although analgesics are the drugs used most frequently in the management of patients in pain, several other classes of pharmaceuticals are useful for palliative and cause-related therapy. Some drugs bind to known receptors, which are cellular components with which the natural body chemicals (ligands) interact to produce physiologic responses. Some drugs (agonists) mimic rather closely the action of the natural substances. Other drugs (antagonists or blocking agents) prevent those actions. For example, morphine (agonist) binds to certain receptors (mu and kappa) in the central nervous system (CNS) that normally interact with the natural endorphins (ligands); this interaction is prevented by naloxone (antagonist or blocking agent).

Some drugs act by neutralizing the effect of certain enzymes, thus producing a physiologic effect indirectly. The class of antidepressant drugs known as monoamine oxidase (MAO) inhibitors act to increase the concentration of 5HT, dopamine, and norepinephrine in the cerebrospinal fluid (CSF) by reducing their natural breakdown through an inhibitory action on the enzyme MAO. Aspirin produces an anti-inflammatory effect by inhibiting the action of the enzyme cyclooxygenase (COX), which normally metabolizes arachidonic acid into prostaglandins as the result of local tissue injury. Other drugs act in still different ways, and the action of many is not known.

Since drugs induce both intentional (primary) and unintentional (secondary) effects, the selection of the best drug in a given situation requires careful considera-

---

Table 9-1 Therapeutic Modalities for the Management of Orofacial Pain Disorders

A. Pharmacologic therapy
1. Analgesic agents
   a. Nonnarcotic agents
   b. Narcotic agents
   c. Adjuvant analgesics
2. Anesthetic agents
   a. Topical anesthetics
   b. Injectable local anesthetics
3. Anti-inflammatory agents
4. Muscle relaxants
5. Antidepressants
6. Antianxiety agents
7. Vasoactive agents
8. Norepinephrine blockers
9. Antimicrobial agents
10. Antiviral agents
11. Antihistamine agents
12. Anticonvulsive agents
13. Neurolytic agents
14. Uricosuric agents
15. Dietary considerations

B. Physical therapy
1. Modalities
   a. Sensory stimulation
   b. Ultrasound
   c. Electrogalvanic stimulation (EGS)
   d. Deep heat
2. Manual techniques
   a. Massage
   b. Spray and stretch techniques
   c. Exercise
   d. Physical activity

C. Psychologic therapy
1. Counseling
2. Behavioral modification training
   a. Stress-reduction training
   b. Relaxation training
   c. Physical self-regulation

---

tion of the various effects that may occur. When two or more drugs are ingested, their possible interactions should be understood. Some combinations are clearly incompatible; some drugs potentiate the action of others; some act synergistically. To properly gauge dosage, one should be familiar with the estimated half-life of the medication being used, especially if a sustained effect is desired. A drug's half-life is the time necessary for the plasma concentration to decrease by 50%. A relatively steady blood level can usually be achieved after five doses are administered at periods that correspond to the drug's half-life.[13]

Medications of different kinds play an important role in the management of patients with pain. Their proper use is a major concern. It is the clinician's responsibility to be adequately familiar with the drug being administered and with the patient who is receiving it, so that safety and effectiveness are ensured. Individualization is necessary.

Many things need to be known about a medication: indications and contraindications for its use, drug incompatibilities, mode of administration, mode of breakdown or metabolism, safe and toxic dosages, side effects, and possible complications. The clinician should be prepared to recognize and effectively deal with such things as sensitivity to the drug, undesirable side effects, toxicity, idiosyncrasy, anaphylaxis, and other untoward reactions to its use. He or she should know about the possibility of potentiation of other medications being used, synergisms, dependence, and the probability of addiction.

Adequate medical supervision and emergency care should always be available if needed. All these responsibilities rest firmly upon the prescribing doctor, and they cannot be abrogated. If the clinician is not prepared to accept these responsibilities, he or she should place pharmacologic management of the patient in the hands of someone who is.

Analgesic agents

Medications that reduce pain are an important class of drugs useful in pain control. As a general rule, the objective of analgesics should not be to eliminate pain altogether; instead, they should make the pain tolerable, since pain has some value in monitoring progress in the patient's condition. It helps guide the patient as to when his or her actions are excessive or abusive. The American Pain Society[13] has classified analgesic drugs into three groups: nonnarcotic analgesics, narcotic analgesics, and adjuvant analgesics.

Nonnarcotic analgesics

The nonnarcotic analgesics, which include aspirin and the nonsteroidal anti-inflammatory drugs (NSAIDs), have four major actions: analgesic, antipyretic, antiplatelet, and anti-inflammatory. They differ from narcotic analgesics in three ways: *(1)* they presumably prevent the formation of prostaglandin E by inhibitory action on the enzyme COX; *(2)* they do not produce tolerance, physical dependence, or addiction; and *(3)* they have a ceiling effect, whereby increasing the dosage beyond peak limits does not increase the analgesic effect, although it may affect its duration. Representative of such analgesics are aspirin, ibuprofen (Motrin), and ketoprofen (Orudis), which have relatively short half-lives, and nabumetone (Relafen) and naproxen (Naprosyn), which have relatively longer half-lives and therefore are longer-acting.

Also included in the nonnarcotic group are acetaminophen, which has no antiplatelet or anti-inflammatory action, and choline magnesium trisalicylate, which lacks antiplatelet action.[13] The nonnarcotic analgesics are general-purpose medications indicated for use in the treatment of mild to moderate pain and chronic cancer pain. Aspirin and the NSAIDs prolong bleeding time and therefore are contraindicated with anticoagulant therapy and other coagulation deficiency conditions. It is thought that the antiplatelet action is beneficial to those at risk for cardiac attacks. Gastric irritation is a common side effect of these drugs. Acetaminophen is approximately equipotent to aspirin but has no antiplatelet or anti-inflammatory action.

Prostaglandin E_2 is metabolized from arachidonic acid through action of the enzyme COX. There are two identified isomers of COX: COX_1 and COX_2. The action of COX_1 produces prostaglandins that play a physiologic "housekeeping" role in renal parenchyma, gastric mucosa, platelets, and other tissues. It aids in maintaining normal function. Inhibition of COX_1 is responsible for gastrointestinal toxicity. COX_2 is present in most tissues in small amounts. It is expressed primarily in sites of inflammation and produces prostaglandins that are involved in inflammation and mitogenesis. Therefore, if COX_2 is inhibited, the inflammatory response is reduced, which results in less nociception and pain.[14-16] In recent years there has been a strong interest in the "COX_2 inhibitor" drugs, which may reduce pain without the adverse side effects of gastrointestinal irritation. An interesting finding is that COX_2 may also play a role in pain inhibition in the CNS.[17,18] Examples of COX_2 inhibitor drugs available are celecoxib (Celebrex), rofecoxib (Vioxx), and valdecoxib (Bextra).

Narcotic analgesics

Morphine-like drugs act through CNS receptors to induce a peripheral analgesic effect.[19,20] They depress nociceptive neurons while stimulating nonnociceptive cells.[21] Both aspirin and morphine inhibit the release of bradykinin, but aspirin inhibits its release regardless of the type of noxious stimulus, while morphine inhibits its release when mediated by neural mechanisms.[22] There is evidence that part of morphine-induced analgesia is contributed indirectly by the release of endogenous opioid peptides.[23] There is also some evidence that opiates exert an inhibitory influence on the release of substance P.[24] There is no hard evidence that the addition of codeine to NSAIDs yields any measurable increase in analgesic effect.[25] As with all drug therapy, it is the responsibility of the prescribing practitioner to know the proper dosage, indications, contraindications, incompatibilities, and signs of toxicity and/or side effects of prescribed medications. The prescribing clinician should be prepared to cope with any ill effects induced by narcotic therapy.

Narcotic analgesics comprise three classes of drugs: morphine-like agonists, mixed agonists-antagonists, and partial agonists. Included among the morphine-like agonists are codeine, hydrocodone, oxycodone, meperidine, propoxyphene, morphine, hydromorphone, methadone, levorphanol, oxymorphone, and heroin. Representative of the mixed agonist-antagonist drugs are pentazocine, nalbuphine, and butorphanol. Buprenorphine is a partial agonist.

Narcotic medications cause constipation, and therefore stool softeners and laxatives may need to be provided. The clinician should carefully individualize the selection of drug, the mode of administration, and the dosage. Narcotics are best administered on a regular time schedule, rather than as needed, to minimize unnecessary pain periods that may require increased dosage attendant with overmedication and increased toxicity. Side effects should be recognized and treated appropriately. The clinician should be watchful for tolerance, physical dependence, and/or addiction (psychologic dependence). *Tolerance* means that larger doses are required to obtain a satisfactory analgesic effect. *Physical dependence* means that withdrawal symptoms accompany abstinence. *Addiction* means compulsive craving for the drug and the need to use it for effects other than the relief of pain.

Narcotics are useful in managing severe acute pain and chronic cancer pain but are not generally indicated for the management of most chronic orofacial pain disorders. However, there are a few orofacial pain conditions that are so poorly controlled that narcotic medications may be considered. Typically these conditions are continuous neuropathic pain disorders, where we now better understand the pain mechanisms but often still lack the ability to eliminate the pain. When narcotics are considered for long-term management of benign pain conditions, both the patient and the therapist need to be aware of all the risks and complications. Long-term narcotic use should not be taken lightly. Narcotics should be considered only when other medications, both analgesic and nonanalgesic, have failed to control the pain, and the quality of the patient's life is so diminished that the therapist must step in and provide relief. When this occurs, a contract should be established between the patient and the therapist, clarifying the responsibilities of each. The therapist needs to commit to evaluating the patient on a regular basis (eg, monthly) to determine the appropriateness of the pain relief and evaluate any adverse side effects as well as the psychologic state of the patient. Depression is a common occurrence in chronic pain patients, and this condition needs to be regularly evaluated, and when indicated, managed. The patient needs to agree to take the medication only as directed and not change any dosage without the consent of the therapists. The patient must agree to receive pain medication from the therapist only and keep the therapist informed of any change in his or her medical condition. The patient must agree in advance that he or she will submit to a drug screening test at any time the therapist feels it is in order. Any lost medication will not be replaced unless a full explanation is accepted by the therapist. Having the patient sign a formal narcotic contract before beginning long-term narcotic management helps emphasize to the patient the seriousness of the agreement. Any violation of the contract results in discontinuation of the use of narcotic medications. If the patient has been taking the medication for a long time, a treatment-withdrawal program is developed or the patient is sent to a formal drug rehabilitation center, whichever is deemed more appropriate.

Adjuvant analgesics

The drugs listed as adjuvant analgesics are those that enhance the analgesic effect of other medications or have independent analgesic activity in certain situations. They are not primarily used as an analgesic, but in certain conditions with certain disorders they may reduce the pain experience. These include tricyclic antidepressants,[26] antihistamines, caffeine, dextroamphetamine, steroids, phenothiazines, and anticonvulsants. Many of these will be discussed in the following pages.

Anesthetic agents

Local anesthetics have an essential role in pain management, both diagnostically and therapeutically. Anesthetic agents can be used either topically or within the tissues by injection.

Topical anesthetics

Topical anesthetics may be used as solutions, sprays, ointments, or lozenges. Water-soluble ointments containing a topical anesthetic and a germicide are useful for managing dental alveolitis.

Analgesic balms are agents that give soothing, palliative relief of inflammatory pain of both superficial and deep somatic categories when applied topically to exposed or ulcerated tissue. Aloe vera juice is an ancient remedy for superficially generated inflammatory pain. It is an ingredient of compound benzoin tincture. Balsam of Peru, eugenol, and guaiacol are other well-known balms. Applied in various forms as liquid, ointment, or cement-like or adhesive dressings, analgesic balms are extremely useful in the palliative control of pain emanating from exposed or ulcerated cutaneous and mucogingival tissues, exposed dentin, and acute alveolitis.

Sometimes topical anesthetics such as lidocaine or benzocaine can be mixed with other medications to enhance the pain-relieving effect. For example, in some peripheral neuropathies a combination of lidocaine, amitriptyline, and carbamazepine (Tegretol) can provide pain relief. When this is found to be helpful and the painful area is intraoral, a dental stent can be fabricated to place over the painful area so that the medication will be maintained in the correct area for a longer period of time (Figs 9-1a and 9-1b).

Injectable local anesthetics

A variety of injectable local anesthetics are available in different concentrations, both with and without a vasoconstricting agent. Long-acting local anesthetics such as bupivacaine hydrochloride (Marcaine) are useful, although they entail a higher risk of toxicity. Proper dosage, correct technique, adequate precautions, and readiness for emergencies are essential to the safety and effectiveness of all local anesthetics. Resuscitative equipment, oxygen, and other resuscitative drugs should be instantly available, and adequate training in their proper use is necessary. Since most untoward reactions with local anesthetics follow accidental intravascular injection, aspiration prior to injection of any medication is a standard must.

The use of local anesthesia to control surgical pain and diagnostically to identify nociceptive pathways and primary sources of pain is commonplace (Fig 9-2). The ther-

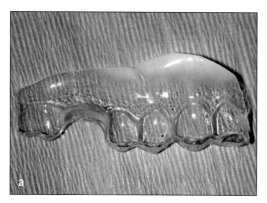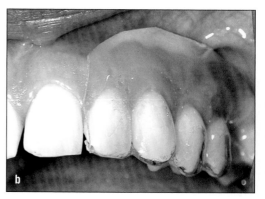

Fig 9-1 *(a)* When topical medications are used in the mouth, a stent can be fabricated that can be used to shield the medication from the tongue and saliva. *(b)* The medication is placed onto the involved tissue and the stent is placed over the teeth to keep the medications in place longer.

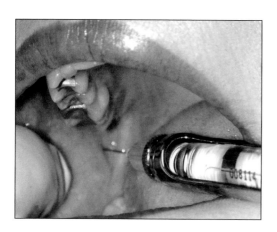

Fig 9-2 An inferior alveolar nerve block can be a very important tool to differentiate primary pain from heterotopic pain. It is especially helpful in identifying toothache, since this block does not anesthetize other common sources of pain such as the muscles or joints.

apeutic use of analgesic blocking is less well known. Four facets of this modality of pain control are useful at a clinical level, namely: *(1)* to arrest primary pain input, *(2)* to interrupt pain cycling, *(3)* to resolve myofascial trigger point activity, and *(4)* to induce a sympathetic blockade.

Arresting primary pain input. Primary deep pain input is an important factor, not only in initiating heterotopic pains and secondary muscle effects, but also in perpetuating them. For example, the pain of local

muscle soreness by its own central excitation tends to perpetuate cyclic muscle pain (see chapter 12). The arrest of cyclic muscle pain by analgesic blocking has marked therapeutic value; it shuts off this perpetuating influence. This can be done by anesthetizing the muscle itself (Fig 9-3). Since myotoxicity of local anesthetics may restrict the choice of agent to short-acting anesthetics of low potency, it is preferable to block the nociceptive pathway rather than the muscle proper. Long-acting, potent anesthetics can then be used with rela-

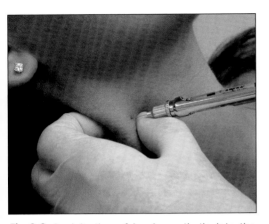

Fig 9-3 An injection of local anesthetic into the sternocleidomastoid muscle can be useful to help differentiate primary pain from heterotopic pain. When heterotopic pain is present, this injection will reduce the pain even in a remote site, such as the TMJ.

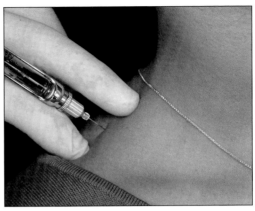

Fig 9-4 When myofascial pain is present, a trigger point in the trapezius muscle can produce pain referral in the ipsilateral face and temple area. An injection of local anesthetic in the trapezius trigger point can reduce the pain in this area as well as reduce the heterotopic face pain.

tive impunity, and thus the benefits of arresting the deep pain input can be extended.

Interruption of pain cycling. On the basis of clinical evidence, a cycling mechanism appears to complicate several pain disorders that occur in the orofacial region. When such cycling is effectively interrupted by local anesthetic blockage of nociceptive impulses at the primary source or somewhere along its mediating pathway, remission of pain may significantly outlast the period of anesthesia. It is thought that this prolonged relief may be the result of a decrease in the sensitization of the second-order neuron after the nociceptive input is terminated. Such remission indicates that a therapeutic effect has been achieved. When such an effect can be obtained with a short-acting anesthetic, a greater therapeutic effect usually results from the use of a longer-acting drug.

Repeated analgesic blocking of the pathway that subserves the peripheral receptors

that trigger trigeminal neuralgia may induce an extended period of remission. Analgesic blocking of the primary source of pain input may effectively arrest some myofascial trigger point pains in the facial region. Myospasm of masticatory muscles can be influenced favorably, if not resolved completely, by one or more analgesic blocks of the nociceptive pathway that serves the muscle.

Trigger point therapy. It is well known that the injection of a short-acting, aqueous local anesthetic of low myotoxicity at a myofascial trigger point located in muscle tissue effectively resolves the referred pain phenomena that characterize myofascial pain syndromes[27,28] (Fig 9-4). Several authors[29-31] believe that such therapy is required when the trigger point is located in a muscle tendon. The technique used for trigger point injections has been described in chapter 8.

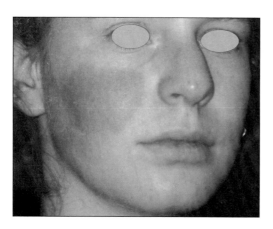

Fig 9-5 This patient reveals a very specific area of the check that is red and warm. This area has been affected by unusual sympathetic activity. When this is present, the clinician needs to evaluate the contribution of the sympathetic nervous system in the pain condition. A stellate ganglion block may be helpful to determine the role of the sympathetic nervous system in the pain condition (sympathetically maintained pain).

Sympathetic blockade. The diagnostic analgesic blocking of afferent sympathetic pathways to identify pain mediated by such neurons is well known (Fig 9-5). The stellate ganglion block is the one usually used for afferent sympathetic routes from the head.[32-35] Analgesic blocking at the same site also arrests the efferent sympathetic impulses and constitutes an ipsilateral sympathetic blockade as far as the orofacial region is concerned. It is reported that daily stellate ganglion analgesic blocking is as effective as guanethidine for the treatment of reflex sympathetic dystrophy.[33,36] Thompson[37] reported that half of his 120 cases of causalgia were relieved by repeated sympathetic analgesic blocks. Procacci et al[38] reported that, in 11 of their 30 subjects with reflex sympathetic dystrophy of the limbs, a significant increase in cutaneous pain threshold developed after analgesic blocking of the sympathetic ganglia on the affected side. Wetchler and Wyman[39] reported that all 23 of their patients with acute herpes zoster of the ophthalmic nerve had excellent pain relief and freedom from cutaneous scarring by treatment with daily analgesic blocks of the stellate ganglion. Three of this group, however, complained of postherpetic neuralgia at the 6-month follow-up.

The three pain disorders for which analgesic blocking of the stellate ganglion appears to be specifically indicated are *(1)* sympathetically maintained deafferentation pains, such as reflex sympathetic dystrophy[40-44]; *(2)* herpes zoster[45-47]; and *(3)* postherpetic neuralgia.[48] With both reflex sympathetic dystrophy and acute herpes zoster, early treatment appears to be the key to success. For postherpetic neuralgia, Milligan and Nash[48] reported that 75% of their patients were helped if sympathetic blockade was performed within the first year.

Anti-inflammatory agents

In addition to the anti-inflammatory analgesics, several similar nonsteroidal medications are used chiefly for their anti-inflammatory effect. They are mildly analgesic and antipyretic. The specific action of all such medications is not known. The therapeutic effect appears to relate to the inhibition of prostaglandin biosynthesis. All such drugs should be used with caution, especially when protracted therapy is needed. Good medical supervision is appropriate. These agents do not alter the course of disease; they only suppress the symptoms of inflammation—hence their usefulness in the management of inflammatory pain.

Corticosteroids exert a potent anti-inflammatory effect, presumably by acting to inhibit prostaglandin biosynthesis. However, they also cause profound and varied metabolic effects and modify the body's immune responses to diverse stimuli. They are eminently useful medications but require considerable care in administration. Extended use should be done only under close medical supervision. Their suppressive effect on inflammation may mask infection. They are contraindicated for systemic fungal and herpes simplex infections. Corticosteroid ointments are available in different strengths and with different bases. They are useful for topical application of the drug.

Devor et al[49,50] reported that locally applied corticosteroid rapidly and effectively arrested the pain from damaged nerve fibers in experimental neuromas. They suggested that it acts directly on the membrane rather than as an anti-inflammatory.

Muscle relaxants

Medications that tend to relax skeletal muscle have some value, especially in the management of myogenous pains. If prescribed in sufficient dosage to induce real muscle relaxation, however, the patient cannot remain ambulatory or safely continue his or her usual activities. Use of potent relaxants, such as succinylcholine chloride, should be restricted to hospitalized patients and administered under expert supervision. The intravenous (IV) use of methocarbamol also requires special care. Some muscle relaxants are anticholinergic and therefore display physical symptoms incidental to that action. There are also some incompatibilities with which the prescribing clinician should be familiar. Although the use of muscle relaxants with fully ambulatory patients has some value, if no more than placebo effect, the actual amount of relaxation achieved is equivocal.

Antidepressants

Some patients with neurovascular pain and patients with chronic pain who verbalize reactive depression may respond to the judicious use of antidepressant medications. The tricyclic antidepressants increase the availability of 5HT and norepinephrine in the CSF. The demethylated tricyclics make 5HT proportionately more available and induce some sedative effect. They are useful in treating agitated depression. The monomethylated tricyclics make norepinephrine proportionately more available and induce some CNS stimulation. They are used more for retardant depression.[51]

Tricyclic antidepressants have been used with some success for a variety of chronic pain conditions.[52-55] It has been demonstrated that a low dose of amitriptyline (10 mg) just before sleep can have an analgesic effect on chronic pain after several weeks of use.[56-59] This clinical effect is not related to any antidepressive action, since antidepressive dosages are from 10 to 20 times higher. Although tricyclic antidepressants increase the available 5HT in the CSF, they may not have inherent analgesic properties. In normal subjects, they have no greater effect on pain than does placebo.[60] Ward et al[61] reported that all moderately to severely depressed individuals in this study complained also of pain, with headache being the most frequent complaint. Patients who obtained minimal antidepressant effect from tricyclics also obtained minimal analgesic effect.

The MAO inhibitors increase the available 5HT, norepinephrine, and dopamine in the CSF by inhibiting their breakdown. They potentiate the action of sympathomimetic substances and may induce a hypertensive crisis. The use of all antidepressant agents should be under adequate medical supervision.

Serotoninergic antidepressant medications are useful in the management of some chronic pain disorders.[62-64] Antidepressant therapy, however, is not effective for deafferentation dysesthesia.[65] Amitriptyline has a pain-relieving action in postherpetic neuralgia that is not primarily linked with its serotoninergic and antidepressant effect.[64,66] Although amitriptyline has a beneficial effect on some chronic pains, it does not appear to have the same positive effect on acute pain.[67] It has been reported that subanalgesic doses of antidepressant drugs potentiate the action of morphine.[68,69]

Although the tricyclics have been helpful for some neuropathic pains, their side effect profile can be formidable. Common side effects are drowsiness and anticholinergic effects (ie, dry mouth, constipation). In the 1980s a new class of antidepressants was introduced: the selective serotonin reuptake inhibitors (SSRIs). These new antidepressants have better efficacy on mood disorders, with significantly fewer side effects. Some of the commonly used SSRIs are fluoxetine (Prozac), venlafaxine (Effexor), paroxetine (Paxil), sertraline (Zoloft), nefazodone (Serzone), fluvoxamine (Luvox), citalopram (Celexa), and escitalopram (Lexapro). As we study these drugs more completely, we appreciate that noradrenaline can also be affected and therefore subcategories are arising. For example, venlafaxine is a serotonin and noradrenergic reuptake inhibitor (SNaRI). Mirtazapine (Remeron) is considered a noradrenergic and specific serotoninergic antidepressant (NaSSA). Reboxetine (Edronax), a newer medication available in Europe, has its primary effect on the reuptake of noradrenaline and therefore is considered a noradrenaline reuptake inhibitor (NaRI). Venlafaxine, an SNaRI, has received the most investigation and has been shown to be effective in the treatment of different kinds of pain, with a side-effect profile that is significantly better than that of the tricyclic antidepressants.[70] The other new antidepressants have been studied less extensively; thus, only anecdotal therapeutic results and experimental works have been found and reported. Further evidence-based research in the safety and efficacy of these promising agents for pain relief is warranted.

Caution should be exercised in the administration of tricyclic antidepressants, especially in patients with a history of cardiac disease. A potentially serious outcome may accompany overdosing as well as combinations with other drugs such as antihistamines, beta-blockers, calcium-channel blockers, SSRIs, and anticonvulsants.[71] It is well that such medications be administered with medical supervision and consent.

Antianxiety agents

Numerous sedative and tranquilizing medications are available, some of which also have muscle relaxant action. The major tranquilizers, such as the phenothiazines, are very useful in pain control by reducing the modulating effects of anxiety and apprehension. They are not addictive. They may display some objectionable side effects, however, and therefore require careful monitoring. Extrapyramidal effects are not uncommon. Protracted use has caused tardive dyskinesia.

The minor tranquilizers, such as meprobamate and diazepam, have the advantage of fewer side effects. Their muscle relaxant action is also useful. But they present a serious potential for drug tolerance and for dependence, and abuse of such drugs is commonplace. When utilized for pain control, they are best prescribed for limited periods only. When protracted use is needed, different drugs should be used periodically so that neither dependence nor tolerance is permitted to occur. Tranquilizers appear to exert some potentiating effect on narcotic analgesics.[72]

Clonazepam is a benzodiazepine that may have some pain-reducing effects in certain neuropathic pain disorders.[73,74] This medication has specifically been use with some success in burning mouth disorders.[75,76]

Vasoactive agents

Neurovascular pain disorders may be favorably influenced by the alpha-adrenergic blocking action of ergotamine tartrate, which causes a stimulating effect on the smooth muscle of peripheral and cranial blood vessels. It is available in several different preparations, both with and without the addition of caffeine. The caffeine enhances this vasoconstricting effect without increasing the dosage. Its effect appears to be greatest on the pulsatile component of neurovascular pain. The drug has several contraindications, including peripheral vascular and coronary heart disease, hypertension, and pregnancy.

Beta-adrenergic blocking agents that decrease vasodilator responses to beta-adrenergic receptor stimulants may have value in neurovascular pain disorders, even though the mechanism for the antimigraine effect has not been established.[77] The successful use of beta-blockers in the treatment of phantom limb pain has also been reported.[78] Somatostatin has been reported to inhibit the effect of the release of substance P from peripheral sensory nerve terminals. Since substance P induces effects that resemble some of the symptoms of neurovascular pain disorders, such as cluster headache, the use of somatostatin has been investigated as a possible treatment modality. It is reported to be as effective as ergotamine tartrate in the treatment of cluster headache.[79]

5HT receptors have been strongly implicated in the mechanism of migraine headache. Many of the drugs that are effective in migraine are believed to affect one or more of the various 5HT receptors. Methysergide, cyproheptadine, and dihydroergotamine (DHE) interact with the $5HT_2$ receptor. Sumatriptan and DHE interact at the $5HT_{1A}$ and $5HT_{1D}$ receptors.[80,81]

Norepinephrine blockers

In lieu of analgesic blocking of the stellate ganglion for the control of sympathetically maintained pains about the orofacial region, the norepinephrine blocking agent guanethidine has been used.[82] It appears to block the uptake of norepinephrine by sensitized deafferentated axons. The clinical benefit outlasts the pharmacologic actions.[83,84] Bonelli et al[36] reported that IV administration of guanethidine once every 4 days for a total of four blocks was equal in effectiveness to daily stellate ganglion analgesic blocks for 8 days. In a controlled, randomized, double-blind, crossover study of 12 reflex sympathetic dystrophy patients, Lief et al[85] reported that weekly IV injections of guanethidine or reserpine achieved equally significant short-term pain relief. Levine and Basbaum[86] reported that both guanethidine- and reserpine-induced sympathectomy decreased the severity of joint inflammation and pain, especially in rheumatoid arthritis.

Antimicrobial agents

A variety of antibiotic and other antimicrobial drugs is available for both topical and systemic administration. The choice depends on the type of organism represented in the infection. Culturing and susceptibility testing to identify the best-suited drug are good practice. The antinociceptive benefit of such agents relates to the resolution of the infection that causes pain.

It is very interesting to note that some antibiotics may actually have analgesic qualities.[87,88] This can be very confusing to the patient and the clinician. For example, when a patient is treated with an antibiotic for a toothache and the pain resolves, it is immediately assumed that the antibiotic has eliminated the organism responsible for the infection and ultimately the pain. Although this is logical, it may not be true. The fact that an antibiotic reduces pain does not mean there is an infection present. Too often a patient is repeatedly placed on an antibiotic because it reduces the pain, and the clinician assumes the bacterial infection is produced by a resistant strain of organisms. Long-term antibiotic therapy creates significant risk factors for the patient, and such therapy should not be continued when pain relief is the only therapeutic effect. The clinician needs good evidence of an actual infection if antibiotic therapy is to be continued.

Antiviral agents

Acyclovir and famciclovir are effective drugs for treating infections caused by such viruses as herpes simplex (HSV-1, HSV-2) and herpes zoster.[89-93] They may be administered topically,[94] orally, or by IV. They appear to be more effective in the treatment of primary infections than recurrent episodes.[95] Johnson reported that an experimental herpes vaccine proved effective in animal studies for both HSV-1 and HSV-2.[96] Famciclovir (Famvir) is an orally administered prodrug of the antiviral agent penciclovir.[93] Its unique pharmacokinetic profile makes it an efficacious, convenient, and well-tolerated alternative to the more traditionally prescribed acyclovir. Famciclovir is used for the acute treatment and suppressive therapy of recurrent genital herpes as well as for herpes zoster and its debilitating comorbidities. Famciclovir allows patients to manage or prevent symptoms, thereby significantly improving their quality of life. Its favorable safety profile makes it a good treatment choice for the elderly as well as for immunocompromised patients, including those infected with human immunodeficiency virus.

Antihistamine agents

Antihistamines counteract the vasodilator action of histamine by blocking certain histamine receptors. Many antihistamine preparations are available. They may be useful in allergic responses and some neurovascular pain disorders. A direct analgesic effect has been reported for several antihistamines (diphenhydramine, hydroxyzine, orphenadrine, pyrilamine).[97-101] Combination of an antihistamine with acetaminophen has a greater analgesic effect than acetaminophen alone.[101]

Anticonvulsive agents

It is generally considered that anticonvulsive medications are useful in certain pain conditions, specifically neuropathic pains. An extensive review of the literature, however, fails to significantly support this assumption.[102] Nevertheless, the clinical judgment of many clinicians is that this class of medications helps neuropathic pain patients.

One of the oldest and still commonly used anticonvulsives is carbamazepine (Tegretol). Carbamazepine has been the mainstay medication for trigeminal neuralgia for many years. In fact, some neurologists suggest that if the pain associated with trigeminal neuralgia is not controlled with carbamazepine, then it is not trigeminal neuralgia. This is not a documented statement. Unfortunately, carbamazepine is associated with considerable side effects related to bone marrow suppression and blood dyscrasia. Pretreatment blood studies are necessary, and careful monitoring at regular intervals during treatment is essential for patient safety. Active medical supervision is a prerequisite during its use. There are a number of contraindications and drug incompatibilities with which one must be familiar before prescribing. When tolerated, however, this medication can provides significant benefits for trigeminal and glossopharyngeal neuralgias.[103-105]

Today there are several other anticonvulsive drugs that can be useful in neuropathic pain disorders and that have far fewer side effects. Gabapentin (Neurontin), oxcarbazepine (Trileptal), and topiramate (Topamax) are a few of these drugs. Sometimes a combination of anticonvulsive drugs can be used,[106] but this is only recommended if a single drug is not adequate to satisfy the patient's needs.

Neurolytic agents

A neurolytic medication is one that actually destroys a nerve. Neurolytic medications were thought to be very useful in pain management, until the profession began to better understand deafferentation pain. Now we appreciate that destruction of a nerve can actually lead to a pain condition. For this reason, neurolytic agents are rarely used today. The most common neurolytic drug used to destroy peripheral nerves is 95% ethyl alcohol.[107] Sometimes phenol is added. Although it is an effective neurolytic, its denervating effect does not preclude regeneration of the peripheral axons and therefore gives only temporary relief.[108] The hazards of neuritis, extensive local fibrosis, and deafferentation effects restrict its use in modern practice.

Glycerol has also been used as a neurolytic agent.[109,110] The successful use of glycerol (0.30 mL) injected into the retrogasserian space for the treatment of trigeminal neuralgia has been reported.[111] About 90% of the patients remained pain-free after one or two injections. About 60% noticed slight numbness, but otherwise there were no significant sensory effects. No dysesthesia or anesthesia dolorosa was observed. It is thought that glycerol acts upon demyelinated axons assumed to be involved in the triggering mechanism of neuralgia.

Uricosuric agents

Antihyperuricemic agents are needed in the treatment of hyperuricemia involving the TMJs. Although its specific action is unknown, colchicine suppresses acute attacks of gout and relieves the pain generated by such attacks. For the treatment of chronic gouty arthritis, probenecid is useful. It is a uricosuric and renal tubule blocking agent that inhibits the reabsorption of urates in the tubules of the kidney. By thus increasing the excretion of uric acid, the serum urate level is lowered. However, probenecid may induce exacerbations of acute gout, however, and should not be used until the acute symptoms are controlled with colchicine. A combination of the two medications is useful in treating chronic gouty arthritis that is complicated by occasional recurrent attacks of acute gout. Gout can involve the TMJ.[112-114]

Dietary considerations

The possibility of dietary manipulation to influence a number of physical complaints, including pain, has come under serious investigation in recent years. Although it is logical that diet would have a significant effect on the patient's ability to recover from injury or adapt, the data are not impressive. One of the chief relationships between diet and pain that has been investigated is L-tryptophan, which converts into 5HT. Brain and spinal cord serotoninergic neurons are actively involved in nociceptive responses as well as in the analgesic effects of opiates. On the basis of pharmacologic, surgical, electrophysiologic, and dietary manipulative data, it is evident that increased activity of 5HT interneurons is associated with analgesia and enhanced drug potency.[115] Hosobuchi et al[116] and Schwarz et al[117] reported that when patients with chronic pain who were unable to obtain pain relief from 30 mg of IV morphine in divided doses due to drug tolerance were placed on diets supplemented with 4 g of L-tryptophan a day for several weeks, they were able to achieve significant pain relief from opiates. They were also able to lead more active lives, even while reducing their daily opiate intake. Seltzer et al[118,119] reported significant elevation of pain tolerance by the dietary supplementation of L-tryptophan. Cheng and Pomeranz[120] reported that naloxone-reversible analgesia induced by electroacupuncture was significantly increased when dietary D-phenylalanine and D-leucine were added.

The synthesis of brain 5HT is dependent on the availability of plasma tryptophan, 90% of which is bound to albumin and must compete with other amino acids at the blood-brain barrier.[121] It is estimated that only about 2% of plasma tryptophan is hydroxylated by tryptophan hydroxylase to form the precursor to 5HT.[122] This conversion requires the presence of adequate vitamin B$_6$.[123] Brady et al[124] reported that, in a double-blind study, the 10 chronic pain patients included in their study obtained a measure of relief by taking 4 g of L-tryptophan per day and consuming a low-protein, low-fat, high-carbohydrate diet for 8 weeks. Seltzer et al[125] reported a reduction in clinical pain and elevated pain tolerance for randomly selected chronic maxillofacial pain patients as the result of 4 weeks of tryptophan supplement therapy.

The dietary considerations in pain therapy, especially for neurovascular pain and fibromyalgia,[117,126–130] are becoming more popular. As more is learned about the role of neurotransmitters and protein fractions such as glutamic acid, substance P, glycine, gamma-aminobutyric acid, cholecystokinin, and somatostatin, a variety of dietary manipulations and additional medicinal forms of therapy likely will become available.[131] The dietary approach would not be expected to influence the management of acute pain complaints, however, because of the time factor. Like other nutritional approaches to disease, several weeks are usually required for the effects of dietary therapy to become apparent clinically.

Physical Therapy

Modalities

Physical therapy modalities refer to those treatments that utilize an instrument, device, or agent to accomplish the desired effect. These are sensory stimulation, ultra-sound, electrogalvanic stimulation (EGS), and deep heat.

Sensory stimulation

Sensory stimulation can be divided into several categories according to the tissue and mode of stimulation: cutaneous, transcutaneous, and percutaneous.

Cutaneous stimulation. Although the stimulation of skin has been used to obtain relief from pain since ancient times, it has only been during the last few decades that some understanding of the mechanism involved has come to light, along with a revival of many old remedies. The effect occurs through stimulation of thick myelinated cutaneous afferents, A-beta neurons chiefly.[132,133] Whether other inhibitory mechanisms are involved remains to be determined.

There are many forms of cutaneous stimulation that effectively attenuate pain. Perhaps the oldest and most natural is pressing or rubbing the skin over the site of injury. Superficial massage is an important means of reducing pain (Fig 9-6). It is enhanced by adding a stimulating substance such as alcohol or menthol ointment.

Counterirritation is an age-old pain remedy.[134] Mustard plasters can still be remembered by many. It is well known that mild stimulation of nociceptors also increases pain-inhibitory mechanisms. A mixture of aconite and iodine has been used for this purpose by dental clinicians. Currently, vapocoolant therapy is important in relieving myofascial trigger point pain (Fig 9-7). Initially thought to be effective through its local anesthetic action, it is now recognized that the vapocoolant mildly stimulates the cutaneous nociceptors as well as the thicker A-beta fibers. Thus, the body's pain inhibitory system is activated. As long ago as 1902, ethyl chloride was strayed on the eardrum to alleviate the pain of otitis media.[135] Kraus[136] introduced the use of ethyl chloride spray for the treatment of

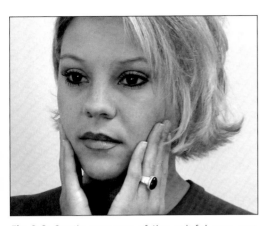

Fig 9-6 Gentle massage of the painful area can often reduce pain. The reduction of pain may be due to gate-control mechanisms. Deep massage can be used for musculoskeletal pains and may provide pain relief by altering the local tissue status.

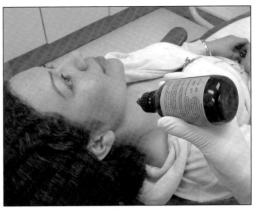

Fig 9-7 A vapocoolant spray can be applied to the symptomatic muscles to reduce the pain. The reduction of pain is likely due to gate-control mechanisms. Vapocoolant spray can also be used during a spray and stretch technique, which is used to treat the trigger points associated with myofascial pain.

painful motion in 1941. Travell advocated its use in 1949 for the treatment of somatic trigger areas[137] and in 1952 for treating skeletal myospasms.[138] Schwartz[139] applied it to the treatment of painful mandibular movement in 1954.

Intermittency is an essential element in vapocoolant therapy and probably is the reason why it is more effective than are other forms of thermal therapy. Thick afferents adapt quickly to stimulation and therefore are more reactive to gradient changes. The application of heat and cold to obtund pain is very old. It has long been known to be more effective when the heat and cold are applied alternately for brief periods (Fig 9-8). Infrared heat is another form of cutaneous stimulation.

The use of mechanical vibration to relieve pain is an old pain remedy. It has been reported that at least one third of patients obtain complete relief from dental pain by this method, and the period of relief outlasts the stimulation by several hours.[140-143] Mechanical vibration also enhances the effect of transcutaneous electrical stimula-

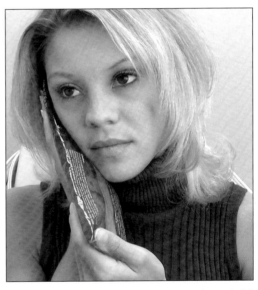

Fig 9-8 Application of moist heat to the painful area may help reduce the pain. When heat is not helpful, ice can be tried.

tion in about half the subjects.[144] Lundeberg[145] reported that in a study of 267 patients with chronic neuropathic or musculoskeletal pain treated with vibratory stimulation, 59% achieved more than 50% relief.

Hydrotherapy is another form of cutaneous stimulation, especially for neck and back pains of muscle origin. Agitated circulating bath water has a therapeutic effect, and a brisk stream of shower water directed against the neck and back gives considerable relief. On the whole, cutaneous stimulation as a therapeutic tool for the management of pain has not been fully utilized.

Transcutaneous stimulation. It is said that in ancient times, electric fish were used to relieve pain.[146] During the last century there have been several attempts to utilize electrical stimulation for this purpose. The method was resurrected by Wall and Sweet[147] in 1967 as the result of the gate-control theory verbalized by Melzack and Wall[132] 2 years earlier. Soon, transcutaneous electrical nerve stimulation (TENS) became a popular form of pain control (Figs 9-9a and 9-9b). The units employed a low-intensity faradic current at high frequency (50 to 100 Hz) applied to the skin through electrodes attached by conduction paste. No discomfort was felt. It was remarkably effective in relieving pains of various types and was innocuous except for an occasional rash from the conduction paste. Being portable, the mechanism could be worn and used by subjects at will.

In 1972 the American public became aware of traditional Chinese acupuncture methods through media coverage. This initiated a wave of nociceptive research to explain this "miracle from the Orient." It was not until the discovery of the endogenous antinociceptive system in 1975 that a plausible explanation for acupuncture became available. Research into electroacupuncture (EA) on a worldwide scale established a relationship between it and the newly discovered endorphins. Although some confusion still exists and conflicting reports appear, the following summarizes the present understanding of transcutaneous stimulation methods.[148,149]

TENS utilizes a high-frequency (50 to 100 Hz) but very low-intensity electric current. It is used to stimulate the nonnociceptive A-beta cutaneous afferents that activate the descending pain-inhibitory mechanism without involving the opioid peptides.[150,151] It may be felt as a tingling or vibratory sensation with no phasic muscle contraction; some minor tonic contraction may occur in nearby muscles. Its action is immediate and generally restricted to the segment that is stimulated, and it induces few or no aftereffects. Therapeutic benefit is negligible. It does not depend on skin location where impedance is low, but if applied at such sites (acupoints), an EA effect may result. The analgesic effect ranges from 50% to 70%.[152,153]

EA utilizes a low-frequency (2 Hz) but high-intensity electric current. It is applied at specific cutaneous sites, the so-called acupoints. It is used to stimulate the muscle nociceptors (group III and group IV afferents), which in turn activate the endogenous antinociceptive system. Phasic muscle contraction and pulsing muscle pain are required. The antinociceptive effect is not immediate but requires an induction period of 15 to 20 minutes. Some therapeutic effect may result.[154] The analgesia may be either segmental or general. The segmental relief of pain is thought to involve the CSF enkephalin level, while the general effects appear to involve the action of beta-endorphin secreted by the pituitary gland into the bloodstream.[155,156]

Antinociception of the teeth and mouth occurs segmentally by application of EA at the intraorbital acupoint; more general effects come from the HoKu acupoint, located between the thumb and index finger. The best results are obtained by simultaneous and bilateral use of both acupoints.

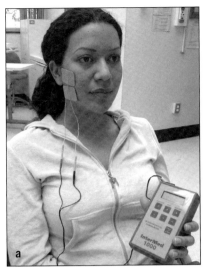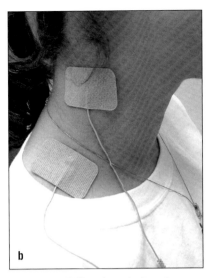

Fig 9-9 *(a)* Surface electrode pads are attached to a TENS unit and placed over a painful masseter muscle. Mild electrical stimulation can be used to reduce pain. *(b)* TENS being used to reduce trapezius muscle pain.

A comparison of the two methods of transcutaneous sensory stimulation on a clinical level indicates that both are effective if properly applied and yield satisfactory relief from pain in 50% to 70% of subjects. The antinociceptive mechanism that is involved in either case is of more academic than clinical value. The two techniques have much in common and often overlap. It seems to matter little whether they are used separately or conjointly.[157-161] Cold laser (helium-neon) stimulation at acupoints is as effective as EA and has the advantage of being practically painless.[162-164]

Although Sweet[165] did not find transcutaneous sensory stimulation useful in the management of tic douloureux, Melzack[166] reported significant relief from peripheral nerve injury pain, phantom limb pain, shoulder/arm pain, and low back pain. Sodipo[167] reported that acupuncture was beneficial in 60% of patients with chronic pain. It has been reported useful in the management of tension headache.[168,169] It

can also effect mood changes that resemble those of opioids.[170]

Percutaneous stimulation. Percutaneous stimulation is done by electrodes that penetrate the skin. Such methods have been used by neurosurgeons for many years. Subcutaneous nerve stimulation by an electric current produces prolonged analgesia that is not reversible by naloxone, which indicates that it does not recruit the opioid peptides. Tolerance is not developed, and it can be administered with other analgesic medications, including narcotics.[171,172]

Lawrence[173] introduced a form of percutaneous stimulation. It is electric stimulation of the periosteum by insulated needles. He used 9 to 12 V at 100 to 300 Hz for 45 minutes. He kept the stimulation intensity at a level just perceived by the subject. He reported results that were subjectively superior to EA and TENS for the relief of chronic pain.

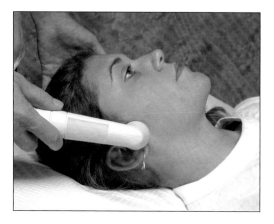

Fig 9-10 Ultrasound can be helpful for the symptomatic relief of pain that has its origin in the musculoskeletal structures.

Ultrasound

Ultrasound is a method of producing an increase in the temperature at the interface of the tissues and therefore affects deeper tissues than does surface heat.[174] Not only does ultrasound increase the blood flow in deep tissues, it also seems to separate collagen fibers. This improves the flexibility and extensibility of connective tissues.[175] It has been suggested[176,177] that surface heat and ultrasound be used together, especially in the treatment of posttrauma patients (Fig 9-10).

Ultrasound has also been used[178-180] to administer drugs through the skin, by a process known as *phonophoresis*. For example, 10% hydrocortisone cream is applied to an inflamed joint and the ultrasound transducer is then directed at the joint. The effects of salicylates and other topical anesthetics can also be enhanced in this manner.

EGS

EGS[181,182] utilizes the principle that electrical stimulation of a muscle causes it to contract. A rhythmic electrical impulse is applied to the muscle, creating repeated involuntary contractions and relaxations. The intensity and frequency of these can be varied according to the desired effect, and they will help to break up myospasms as well as increase blood flow to the muscles. Both effects lead to a reduction of pain in compromised muscle tissues. Muscle pulsing has been reported to yield favorable results with the myofascial pain-dysfunction syndrome.[183]

Deep heat therapy

Physiotherapy in the form of penetrating heat has value in treating patients with pain. Diathermy and ultrasound are used for this purpose. The judicious use of deep heat is beneficial in treating inflammatory pain. Although it has been employed to help relieve myospasm activity, its effects are equivocal. It is reported to be a useful adjunct in the treatment of myofascial trigger point pain.[28]

Manual techniques

Massage

As just stated, mild stimulation of cutaneous sensory nerves exerts an inhibitory influence on pain.[134] Thus, gentle massage of the tissues overlying a painful area can often reduce pain perception. The patient can be taught gentle self-massage techniques and is encouraged to do this as needed for the reduction of pain. The technique is often helpful.

Deep massage can be even more helpful than gentle massage in reducing pain and re-establishing normal muscle function. Deep massage, however, must be provided by another individual, such as a physical therapist. Deep massage can assist in mobilizing tissues, increasing blood flow to the area, and eliminating trigger points.[184] It is often most effective when it follows 10 to 15 minutes of preparation of the tissues with deep, moist heat. The deep heat tends to relax the muscle tissues, decreasing pain and enhancing the effectiveness of the deep massage.

Spray and stretch techniques

The primary physiotherapeutic technique for the treatment of myofascial trigger points is so-called spray and stretch.[184] A mixture of fluorocarbons is used as the vapocoolant (Fluori-Methane, Gebauer Chemical). A spring-capped bottle with a calibrated nozzle that delivers a fine stream is needed. While the muscle is moderately stretched just short of pain, the vapocoolant is applied by using parallel sweeps in one direction, traveling toward the reference area. The nozzle is held 15 to 18 inches away from the skin, and the stream is directed at an acute angle of about 30 degrees. The sweeps are made at the rate of about 4 in/s. After two or three sweeps, the muscle should be rewarmed. At the end of the treatment, moist heat should be applied and range-of-motion exercises instituted. The best results are obtained by first spraying, then stretching, using care not to stretch to the point of pain, and then spraying again. It is thought that the vapocoolant modulates the pain so that more manipulation is possible without discomfort. It should be noted that painfully stretching a muscle with myofascial triggers may induce a muscle spasm. Other forms of physiotherapy applicable to the treatment

of myofascial trigger points include ischemic compression, deep massage and kneading, and ultrasound. Ischemic compression is done by applying 20 to 30 pounds of pressure at the trigger site for 1 minute while the muscle is stretched just short of pain.[184]

Exercise

Forceful contraction of antagonist muscles causes reflex relaxation of an agonist muscle. This principle of reciprocal inhibition is useful in the treatment of masticatory myospasms.[185] For example, a spastic elevator muscle is relaxed by exercises that open the mouth against resistance. Retrusion of the protruded mandible against resistance tends to relax a spastic inferior lateral pterygoid muscle.

It has been reported that stimulation of muscle proprioceptors tends to normalize excessive electromyographic (EMG) activity in painful spastic skeletal muscles.[186] When using this principle, resumption and maintenance of normal muscular activity in masticatory muscles is beneficial as long as pain is not generated by the activity.

For a muscle to maintain its normal resting length, occasional stimulation of the inverse stretch reflex is necessary. This is accomplished by occasionally stretching the muscle. An immobilized muscle not only loses its strength by disuse atrophy, it also shortens due to myostatic contracture.[187] Exercises that stimulate both the muscle spindles (contraction) and the Golgi tendon organs (stretching) are therefore needed to maintain normality of muscles. So-called functional manipulation is useful physiotherapy. Exercise elevates the pain threshold.[188,189]

Physical activity

In patients with chronic pain, the maintenance of physical activity is an important part of therapy, since patients tend to withdraw and take to their beds. Fordyce et al[190] found that, during periods when the pain is increased, extending exercises to the limit of patient tolerance was significantly beneficial: the more exercises performed, the fewer the pain behaviors displayed. The maintenance of physical activity kept the body in better condition and reduced time in bed. Individuals who maintain levels of aerobic fitness seem to feel better, sleep better, and concentrate better.

Psychologic Therapy

Psychologic therapies are oriented toward minimizing the Axis II factors that either influence or create the pain disorder. These therapies can be generally categorized into two types: counseling and behavioral modification training.

Counseling

As already discussed, all pain disorders are influenced to some degree by psychologic factors. The therapist should always keep this in mind when first managing a pain condition. The first therapy that should be offered to the patient is education. Educating the patient about his or her pain condition can have marked therapeutic value. Many patients experiencing pain have increased levels of anxiety, emotional stress, and depression secondary to the pain itself. Often, much of this distress can be reduced by proper education. The following five factors should be included when initially discussing the pain condition with the patient:

Provide a definitive diagnosis
Most patients would like to know exactly what is causing their pain. Understanding the source of pain is often the beginning of the healing process. The clinician should inform the patient, as precisely as possible, of the exact etiology of the pain. Since pain complaints are often complex, this may be a difficult task. When a specific diagnosis is

impossible on the first visit, the patient should at least be informed as to the general type and category of pain he or she is experiencing. Several probable diagnoses should be explained, with a more specific diagnosis to come with additional tests. The circumstance that should be avoided is the clinician leaving the patient with the idea that he or she does not know the reason for the pain. If this occurs, the patient will likely think the worst, and anxiety and emotional stress levels will increase the pain experience. Remember, attention and consequence are two major factors in pain and suffering. Both attention and consequence increase when the source of pain is unknown.

If the clinician has no clue as to the source of the pain, it is his or her obligation to immediately refer the patient to the proper medical or dental personnel who can help with the diagnosis. Time is of essence in addressing pain and suffering.

Provide assurance
Life-threatening disorders that present as orofacial pains are rare but certainly can exist. It is important to immediately identify and refer patients with these disorders (ie, neoplasia) to proper specialists. Most orofacial pains, however, are not life-threatening. This is especially true of the musculoskeletal disorders of the masticatory system known collectively as temporomandibular disorders (TMD). Once the clinician has properly ruled out significant life-threatening disorders, he or she should provide assurance to the patient that the disorder is benign and in many cases quite common. It is important that the patient knows the significance of the condition so that proper attention can be placed. Often when a patient learns that the pain is not coming from cancer but instead a muscle cramp, the pain experience may be greatly reduced.

The excitatory influence of attention directed toward the complaint can be countered by distraction, by directing the mind toward more positive thinking, and by a good measure of physical activity. Pleasurable sensations derived from suggested diversionary activities can be employed to counter the painful experience.

Explain the problem in appropriate terms

Most patients want to know exactly where their pain comes from, how it started, and how it can be treated. This information will usually reduce anxiety and emotional stress associated with the pain, as well as provide the patient with realistic consequences for the pain. In general, therefore, this explanation can reduce suffering. The clinician should be careful to use terminology to which the patient can relate and understand. When appropriate, drawings or models can be helpful.

Apprehension concerning the consequential damage and the expectancy of future threat to the patient's well-being cause psychologic intensification of the painful experience. This can be reversed by an open discussion of the realistic consequences that exist and the true expectations that the particular problem holds for the patient. The patient should be made to understand that there may be little relationship between the level of discomfort and the true significance of its cause.

Do not deny the patient's pain

As mentioned in chapter 1, pain is a very individual experience. A condition that may be quite painful to one individual may not be very painful to another. The clinician should always keep this in mind when talking with patients. There is absolutely no benefit to denying the patient's pain. In fact, this behavior can be quite devastating to the patient. The clinician should always be supportive of the patient and provide proper explanation for the pain. In those conditions when psychologic factors are predominant (Axis II), the psychologic factors should be properly introduced so that

it does not appear that the clinician is suggesting that the patient is "crazy." In some instances this is may be difficult, but it is essential for proper management. It may be helpful to emphasize the physical conditions first and then discuss how the psychologic factors can greatly enhance these conditions. A warm, caring attitude by the clinician is imperative.

Provide realistic expectations

Most patients who seek treatment for a pain condition want, and expect, complete relief from their pain along with return to normal function. These expectations may not be realistic, and the patient needs to be aware of this fact when beginning treatment. Once the pain disorder has been explained to the patient, realistic expectations for the treatment should be presented. It is often helpful to explain the natural course of the disorder to the patient. It is necessary, therefore, that the clinician knows the natural course of the disorder, which may not always be apparent. For example, in the past, many TMD were thought to be progressive, yet recent studies have not supported this concept.[191-193] As always, the clinician's knowledge of the disorder is basic to treatment and proper expectations.

The patient should be aware that the symptoms of a pain condition often follow a cyclic course. It is common, therefore, to experience both decreases and increases in the pain during treatment. When the patient is told this before treatment begins, reccurrence of pain is better tolerated and accepted.

These five factors should be considered with all patients who present with pain, regardless of the specific conditions. When significant psychologic factors have been identified, however, specific counseling may be indicated. Some formal psychotherapy is needed in many Axis II disorders such as significant depression, anxiety, or emotional stress. Many somatoform disorders require psychiatric consultation. A small percentage of TMD that are refractory to nonsurgical therapy may need psychotherapy, rather than more aggressive surgical treatment.[194] In most Axis II disorders, local peripheral therapy, including surgery, should be restricted to a secondary role in management. The chief therapeutic effort should be systemic, psychologic, or both.

Fordyce[195] considered that some pains are behavioral and for the most part learned. To a considerable degree, pain is controlled by consequences in the environment. The modification of such consequences may be needed for pain management to be effective. Pain behavior may be unlearned by manipulation of consequences, such as withdrawing positive reinforcements and rewarding better behavior. Such contingency management usually requires full knowledge and cooperation, not only from the patient but also from all those in close personal contact with him or her. This includes family members, doctors, nurses, therapists, and aides.[196]

Since pain behavior is learned, it can be unlearned. Illness behavior should simply be ignored, while wellness behavior should be rewarded by attention and loving care. Severe pain can be made tolerable by replacing the suffering with something better to do, like doing something that benefits others. The patient should be encouraged to engage in activities that direct one's attention away from oneself. Coping with pain is a matter of attitude: "After all, it is only pain. I not only can live peaceably with it, I can overcome it!"[190]

Melzack[197] pointed out the importance of coping strategies in chronic pain, because some pains may last a lifetime. The objective in such cases is not to abolish the pain but to make it bearable. Melzack trained his subjects to reach a meditational state, thus gaining the benefits of distraction, response to suggestion, relaxation, and the development of voluntary control over the pain. Strong suggestion is essential to psychologic approaches for pain management.

Sternbach[198] assumed that pain behavior was acquired and therefore modifiable. Subjective improvement followed behavioral improvement. He utilized social modeling, conditioning, and cognitive forms of therapy.

Roberts[199] focused therapy not on nociceptive sources or the alteration of an emotional state, but directly on patient behavior. His objective was to rehabilitate the patient rather than to alleviate the pain. He avoided all strategies that focused on pain per se, eg, analgesics, electrical stimulation, analgesic blocking, and biofeedback training.

A more detailed description of therapies for each Axis II disorder will be presented in chapter 18.

Behavioral modification training

Often, patients can significantly alter their pain experiences by modifying certain aspects of their routine daily activities. These modifications should be encouraged, since they provide the patient an active role in treatment. Patients who can influence their own symptoms gain a great psychologic edge over those who cannot. These activities reduce the feelings of helplessness and hopelessness that too often accompany chronic pain conditions. Two types of behavioral modification are stress-reduction training and relaxation training.

Stress-reduction training

Many patients who have orofacial pain and/or functional disturbance of the masticatory system are not aware of the possible relationship between their problem and emotional stress. It would be surprising to think any differently, since their symptoms arise from structures in the masticatory system. Therefore, when a patient comes to the clinician with pain symptoms, the first treatment is to educate the person regarding the relationship of emotional stress and anxiety to the problem. An awareness of this relationship must be created before any treatment begins. It is common for the patients to deny the presence of high levels of emotional stress in their life. One must be sure, therefore, that the patient is aware that stress is a common everyday experience and not a neurotic or psychotic disorder.

Emotional stress can also be controlled to some extent voluntarily. Once the stressors are identified, the patient is encouraged, when possible, to avoid them. For example, if stress is increased by driving through heavy traffic, alternate routes should be developed that will avoid major traffic areas. When stress is caused by specific encounters at work, these should be avoided.

Obviously, though, all stressors cannot and should not be avoided. Some stressors are positive and help motivate the individual toward particular goals. As Hans Selye[200] once wrote, "Complete freedom from stress is death." When negative stressors cannot be completely avoided, the frequency and duration of exposure to them should be reduced.

Patients should be encouraged when possible to remove themselves from stressors and substitute other activities that they enjoy—such as allowing more time for sports, hobbies, or recreational activities. For some patients, this may include some quiet time alone. It should be an enjoyable time and an opportunity to forget their stressors. Such activities are considered to be external stress-releasing mechanisms and to lead to an overall reduction of emotional stress experienced by the patient.

Regular exercise may also be an active external stress-releasing mechanism. It is encouraged for patients who find it enjoyable. Obviously it will not be suitable for all patients, and general body condition and health must always be considered before patients are advised to initiate an active exercise program.

Relaxation training

Training the patient in the art of relaxation can be a great benefit in several ways. First, it requires regular quiet periods of time away from stressors. The training sessions are in themselves a type of relaxation therapy. Second, it aids in reducing the level of activity of the autonomic nervous system, which is often up-regulated in the pain patient.[201] This training should be oriented toward reducing muscle activity, slowing breathing rate, lowering blood pressure, and decreasing skin temperature. These techniques are called *physical self-regulation* and will be discussed in detail in the next section of this chapter.

A patient can be trained to relax effectively via several techniques. One that has been well researched is *progressive relaxation*. Most of these techniques used in dentistry are modifications of Jacobson's method,[202] developed in 1968. Jacobson suggested that the patient tense the muscles and then relax them until the relaxed state can be felt and maintained. The patient is instructed to concentrate on relaxing the peripheral areas (hands and feet) and to move progressively centrally to the abdomen, chest, and face. Results can be enhanced by having the patient relax, preferably by lying down in a quiet, comfortable environment with the eyes closed.[203] The relaxation procedures are slowly explained in a calm and soothing voice. An audiotape of the procedures can be developed to aid in the technique. The patient listens to the tape at the training session in the office, and then, after understanding what is to be accomplished, takes the tape home with instructions to listen at least once a day to become proficient at relaxing the muscles. As proficiency increases, the muscle symptoms will decrease.

Relaxation techniques have been demonstrated to be effective in several studies.[204-213] It would appear to be best accomplished by well-trained therapists during frequent visits to help and encourage proper relaxation habits. Although it is not harmful to send the patient home to learn the technique alone, it is less likely that good results will be achieved by mere simple explanations of the relaxation procedures.[214] Also, the best results are achieved over months of training and not just a week or two.

Another form of progressive relaxation utilizes a reverse approach. Instead of asking the patient to contract the muscle and then relax, the muscles are passively stretched and then relaxed.[215-217] It appears that this technique is also effective in teaching progressive relaxation and has one major inherent advantage over the Jacobson technique. Patients with muscle pain disorders often produce pain when asked to contract their muscles. This increase in pain makes relaxation more difficult. In contrast, gentle stretching of the muscles seems to assist in relaxation. Many pain patients find this technique more suitable than the Jacobson technique.

Progressive relaxation techniques are the most common method of promoting relaxation. Other training methods also encourage relaxation but are used to a lesser degree. Self-hypnosis,[218-220] meditation,[221,222] yoga,[222,223] and even music[224-227] can all promote relaxation and may help reduce levels of emotional stress. They likewise are best learned and applied with help from a trained therapist.

Hypnotherapy can be a useful antinociceptive method, provided the pain is not a result of psychoneurosis. Some suffering is too "valuable" to the patient to be given up, due to secondary gains. It has even been suggested that personality disintegration may follow the sudden withdrawal of pain.[228] Therefore, some form of psychiatric screening should precede the use of hypnosis in the management of a pain problem.

The effectiveness of hypnosis depends largely on the susceptibility of the subject to suggestion. A direct-induction technique may be quite satisfactory in highly susceptible subjects. Indirect induction, however, is equally effective and is superior in less-susceptible individuals.[229] Hypnosis is clinically effective for a large number of patients presenting with symptoms of severe

pain of organic origin.[230] Almost all patients derive some benefit through the placebo effect and relaxation. Some well-hypnotized individuals can block high-intensity pain of organic origin. Chronic pain usually requires behavioral modification as well.[231] Hypnotherapy is especially useful in the management of pain associated with burns.[232] Although the issue is still unsettled, there is some evidence that long-term reduction of pain by hypnotherapy involves the endorphins.[233-235]

Although the relaxation of muscles would appear to be a simple procedure, often it is not. Patients, especially those experiencing pain, frequently find it difficult to learn to relax their muscles effectively. They can sometimes benefit from immediate feedback regarding the success or failure of their efforts.

One method of achieving this is with biofeedback, a technique that assists the patient in regulating bodily functions that are generally controlled unconsciously. It has been used to help patients alter such functions as blood pressure, blood flow, and brain wave activity and can assist in muscle relaxation. It is accomplished by electromyographically monitoring the state of contraction or relaxation of the muscles through placement of surface electrodes over the muscles to be monitored.[236] Among facial muscles, the masseter is often selected. When full-body relaxation is the goal, the frontalis muscle is commonly monitored. The electrodes are connected to a monitoring system that lets the patient see the spontaneous electrical activity in the muscles being assessed. The monitor provides feedback by way of a scale or a digital readout or sometimes even a light-bar mechanism. Most biofeedback units also give auditory feedback, which is beneficial for patients who relax best with their eyes closed. When a patient tenses the muscles, high readings appear on the scale or an elevated tone is heard. When the muscles are relaxed, these signals are lowered. The patient attempts to lower the readings or the tone. This can be achieved by any relaxation technique, but progressive relaxation is encouraged, since it is easily accomplished at a later date when the biofeedback instrument is not available. Once the patient can achieve low levels of activity in the muscles, the next instruction is to become familiar with the sense or feeling of relaxation. When this has been accomplished and low levels of muscle activity have been adequately sensed, the patient can be more adept in regaining this state at a later time, even without the aid of the biofeedback instrument, and is encouraged to work toward achieving this goal. A progressive relaxation tape can aid in the training.[237]

Several studies report the usefulness of relaxation training in the management of headaches.[238-243] Sternbach[244] stated that biofeedback could not be expected to help unless the clinical condition presented symptoms of peripheral vasomotor origin. In other words, he questioned the use of biofeedback in management of certain neurovascular pains, such as migraine. Turner and Chapman[245] reported that, although biofeedback may be helpful with some headaches and some TMJ pain, it was not helpful in chronic pain. Sherman et al[246] reported substantial benefit from muscle relaxation training in the treatment of phantom limb pain. Half of their patients obtained virtually complete relief from pain. Large and Lamb[247] reported that a significant correlation existed between subjective pain levels and surface EMG activity and that EMG feedback was superior to other methods of relaxation, but not in reducing the subjective pain level. Nouwen[248] reduced significantly the EMG activity in paraspinal muscles by EMG feedback training, but it did not reduce the pain. Brooke and Stenn[249] reported on 174 patients with myofascial pain who were randomly treated by physiotherapy, occlusal splinting, biofeedback, or relaxation training without biofeedback. The biofeedback-assisted relax-

ation was reported to be as effective as either physiotherapy or occlusal splinting, but it was no more effective than relaxation training without the feedback assistance.

Relaxation training with or without the aid of biofeedback training appears to have merit in the overall management of masticatory problems in that it does reduce EMG activity. Its actual value in reduction of pain, however, is rather variable. Relaxation of muscles seems to be accomplished more readily by the use of biofeedback techniques.

For many years it has been clinically obvious that occlusal disengagement induces a substantial benefit for the discomfort of TMD. This constituted the treatment used by Costen[250] when he inserted thin cork wedges between the teeth. Disengaging the teeth seems to put the masticatory muscle at rest; however, the precise manner by which pain is reduced is very controversial.[251]

Occlusal disengagement can be accomplished voluntarily by training the individual to keep the teeth from contacting during nonfunctional times. The individual is instructed to not allow the teeth to contact unless he is eating, speaking, or swallowing. Most individuals are unaware of putting their teeth together at nonfunctional times, and so they must first become cognitively aware of this occurrence. Once they appreciate that tooth contacts do occur during nonfunctional times (eg, driving the car, working on the computer) the patient actively attempts to keep the teeth apart. The patient is instructed to lightly buff air between the lips and then gently seal the lips. The patient should note that the teeth are not in contact, and the mandible is resting in the muscle sling provided by the elevator muscles. The patient is asked to repeat this every time he or she finds the teeth together. This altered behavior can be very powerful in allowing muscles to relax and reduce pain.

The teeth can also be disengaged with interocclusal appliances (Fig 9-11). Although interocclusal appliances seem to have a pos-

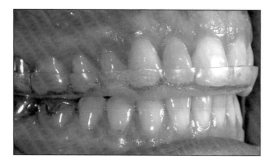

Fig 9-11 An occlusal appliance can be used to help manage certain TMD.

itive effect on TMD symptoms, the exact mechanism is not easily explained and likely to vary in different patients and different disorders.[251] Occlusal appliances may be classified according to their intended function, either as stabilization or muscle relaxation appliances or as mandibular repositioning appliances. Stabilization appliances are particularly useful in the management of masticatory muscle pain. These appliances tend to normalize sensory and proprioceptive impulses generated by the occlusal condition, thereby shutting off the afferent input that initiates muscle co-contraction and aggravates muscle pain conditions. Mandibular repositioning appliances are used to improve the condyle-disc relationship associated with some painful intracapsular disorders.

The concept of physical self-regulation
When an orofacial pain disorder is acute, immediate therapy directed to an obvious etiology is normally sufficient to reduce and often eliminate symptoms. However, when symptoms are prolonged, management becomes far more difficult. Chronic orofacial pain disorders are often not resolved by simple dental or medical procedures (eg, an occlusal appliance). This is likely the result of the presence of other significant factors that are not strongly linked to the dental condition. Some of these factors may be psychosocial issues that are associated with characteristic changes in brain-controlled physiology. In an interesting study by Phillips et al,[252] patients with acute TMD symptoms were evaluated psychosocially but not offered any formal treatment. These individuals were then recalled in 6 months to determine the status of their TMD symptoms. Philips reported that individuals who continued to experience TMD symptoms were different in several psychosocial considerations from those who no longer experienced symptoms. Chronic TMD individuals had more anxiety disorders and depressive disorders than those who had recovered. Differences were also reported between men and women. Men who developed chronic TMD were more likely to demonstrate a personality disorder, while women were more likely to demonstrate a significant degree of a major psychopathology. The important thought here is that some individuals may have certain psychosocial issues and altered physiologic responses to innocuous stimuli that make them more prone to becoming chronic pain sufferers. Prior emotional traumas experienced by an individual can chronically up-regulate the autonomic nervous system. This up-regulation and disturbed physiology may make it more difficult for an individual to recover from a recent injury or onset of symptoms, thus leading to a chronic condition. This is why, as orofacial pain becomes chronic, a team approach should be considered. The minimal team for chronic TMD includes a

dentist, a psychologist, and a physical therapist, or practitioners who have a combination of skills from each of these disciplines.

A reasonable treatment approach in managing chronic TMD and orofacial pain is to develop interventions that address the specific characteristics commonly found in chronic orofacial patients. In our research laboratory at the University of Kentucky, we have developed a program of research[253,254] that suggests that persons with chronic muscle-related orofacial pains are distinguished by five characteristics. First, these individuals report significant pain intensity in comparison to other pain patients and they are also more sensitive to painful stimuli in the trigeminal region. This sensitivity to painful stimuli is consistent with research findings in other orofacial pain settings.[255,256] Second, pain patients report significant levels of fatigue that impairs normal functioning. This fatigue may be closely related to the third important characteristic, depression, which is common among these patients. Our data, however, further suggest that a significant component of the fatigue is not linked to depression itself. A fourth characteristic of these patients is that breathing patterns are disrupted, so that end-tidal carbon dioxide levels are lower in these patients than in comparable controls. This finding suggests that altered breathing patterns may be contributing to the overall "physical dysregulation" reported by these patients. Finally, pain patients report significant sleep disturbances involving either sleep-onset difficulties or disruptive awakenings. These five characteristics represent a constellation of symptoms indicative of "autonomic dysregulation" and provide direction for the application of specific intervention strategies to address the underlying physiologic disturbances that may be contributing to the maintenance of the pain disorder.

The following is a treatment approach for chronic orofacial pains that is based on the interpretations of our research findings developed by Drs Peter Bertrand and Charles Carlson in 1993. The focus of this treatment is on (1) addressing the pain and fatigue as physiologic disturbances in need of correction, (2) managing autonomic dysregulation, (3) altering dysfunctional breathing patterns, and (4) improving sleep. Since this approach involves entrainment of specific skills to alter physiologic parameters, the approach has been called *physical self-regulation training* (PSR). A training manual for PSR was developed by Drs Carlson and Bertrand in 1995 to codify and standardize the procedures.[257] In 2001, Drs Bertrand and Carlson conducted a randomized, controlled clinical trial of the PSR approach in a clinical sample of orofacial pain patients at the National Naval Dental Center in Bethesda, Maryland.[258] The clinical trial included randomization of 44 patients with an average age of 34.6 years and with pain lasting for 52 months into either a group receiving PSR or a group receiving standard dental care (SDC) that included a stabilization appliance. Both treatments resulted in significant decreases in pain intensity and life interference from the pains 6 weeks after treatment was initiated. At 6 months' follow-up, however, the PSR group reported less pain than the SDC group. Comfortable and maximum mouth opening improved for both groups initially as well. At the 6-month follow-up, the PSR group had greater comfortable and maximum mouth opening than did the SDC group. These results provide support for the use and continued evaluation of the PSR approach for managing orofacial pains.

The PSR approach consists of eight areas of education and training.

1. First, patients are provided with an explanation of their condition and an opportunity to develop personal ownership of the problem.
2. The patients are given instructions regarding the rest positions for structures in the orofacial region[259] and the impor-

tance of diminishing muscle activation by recognizing whether head and neck muscle responses are relevant for specific tasks.

3. Specific skills are provided for improving awareness of postural positioning, especially of the head and neck regions. This is termed *proprioceptive re-education*, and the rationale for this is further elaborated by Carlson et al.[258]

4. A skill for relaxing upper back tension is also imparted to patients through an exercise involving gentle movement of the rhomboid muscle groups.

5. A brief progressive relaxation procedure involving the positioning of body structures is given to patients, along with instructions to take at least two periods during daily activities to deeply relax muscles and reduce tension.

6. This training is followed by specific diaphragmatic breathing entrainment instructions, so that patients regularly take time to breathe with the diaphragm at a slow, relaxed pace when the body's major skeletal muscles are not being employed in response to stimuli.

7. Patients are given instructions for beginning sleep in a relaxed position, along with other sleep hygiene recommendations.

8. Finally, patients are provided with instructions on the role of fluid intake, nutrition, and exercise for the restoration of normal functioning.

The entire PSR program is presented within a framework that focuses on understanding pain as a physiologic disturbance that is best managed by addressing those disturbances through rest, nutrition, tissue repair, behavioral regulation of autonomic functioning, and appropriate activity. The PSR approach focuses on limiting any activity that increases the sense of discomfort or pain to promote the return of pain-free function.

Our clinical experience in working with PSR over the past 12 years suggests it is a valuable treatment for a variety of orofacial pain conditions. Although it was initially designed predominantly for masticatory muscle pain disorders, we have found it helpful in managing many intracapsular disorders as well. PSR assists in the management of intracapsular disorders by enabling recognition of inappropriate muscle activity that can lead to co-contraction and inhibition of efficient synovial fluid diffusion into previously overloaded joints. By reducing muscle loading, PSR helps reestablish normal function with pain-free range of motion. In fact, PSR is helpful in most pain conditions because it enables the patient to gain control of many physiologic functions and reverse "dysregulation" of their physiologic systems. For those interested in adding this approach to their clinical practices, a more detailed description of the PSR approach can be obtained elsewhere.[257,258] While more clinical trials are needed to further evaluate the PSR approach, our current data, both from controlled scientific study and clinical practice, indicate that patients can receive substantial benefit from PSR training.

Considerations Related to Chronic Orofacial Pain

Most of the many orofacial pain disorders seen in the general practice of dentistry represent problems of short duration. With proper therapy, these disorders can be completely resolved. However, when orofacial pain disorders persist, more chronic and often complex pain disorders can develop. With chronicity, orofacial pain disorders become even more influenced by the CNS, resulting in a more regional or occasionally even global pain condition. Often, cyclic muscle pain also becomes an important feature that perpetuates the condition.

As a general rule, chronic pain is considered to be pain that has been present for 6 months or longer. However, the duration of pain may not be the most important factor in determining chronicity. Some pains are experienced for years but never become chronic pain conditions. Likewise, some pain conditions become clinically chronic in a matter of months. The additional factor that must be considered is the continuity of the pain. When a pain experience is constant, with no periods of relief, the clinical manifestations of chronicity develop quickly. On the other hand, if the pain is interrupted with periods of remission (no pain), the condition may never reveal the symptoms and behaviors associated with chronic pain. For example, cluster headache is an extremely painful neurovascular pain condition that may last for years and never become a chronic pain disorder. The reason for this is because significant periods of relief occur between episodes of pain. Conversely, the constant pain associated with centrally mediated myalgia, when left untreated, can develop the clinical manifestations of chronicity within several months.

The clinician must recognize that as pain complaints progress from acute to chronic, the effectiveness of local treatment is greatly reduced. Chronic pain disorders most often need to be managed by a multidisciplinary approach. In many instances, the dental practitioner alone is not equipped to manage these disorders. It is important, therefore, for the dental clinician to recognize chronic pain disorders and consider referring the patient to a team of appropriate therapists who are better able to manage the pain condition.

Perpetuating Factors

There are certain conditions or factors that, when present, may prolong the orofacial pain condition. These factors are known as *perpetuating factors* and can be divided into those of a local source and those of a systemic source.

Local perpetuating factors

The following conditions represent local factors that can be responsible for the progression of a relatively simple acute orofacial pain disorder into a more complex chronic pain condition.

Protracted cause
If the clinician fails to eliminate the cause of an acute orofacial disorder, a more chronic condition is likely to develop.

Recurrent cause
If the patient experiences recurrent episodes of the same etiology that produced an acute orofacial pain disorder, it is likely that the disorder will progress to a more chronic condition (eg, bruxism, repeated trauma).

Therapeutic mismanagement
When a patient is improperly treated for an acute orofacial pain disorder, symptoms do not readily resolve. This can lead to a more chronic condition. This type of perpetuating factor emphasizes the importance of establishing the proper diagnosis and quickly initiating effective therapy.

Systemic perpetuating factors

The following conditions represent systemic factors that can be responsible for the progression of an acute orofacial pain disorder into a chronic orofacial pain condition.

Continued emotional stress

Since increased emotional stress can be an etiologic factor in the development of an orofacial pain muscle disorder, continued experience of significant levels of emotional stress can represent a perpetuating factor that may advance the condition to a more chronic orofacial pain disorder.

Down-regulation of the descending inhibitory system

As mentioned in earlier chapters, the descending inhibitory system represents a group of brainstem structures that regulates ascending neural activity. An effective descending inhibitory system minimizes nociceptive input as it ascends to the cortex. If this system becomes less efficient, increased nociception can reach the cortex, resulting in a greater pain experience. It is unclear what factors lead to a down-regulation of the system, but this concept may help in part to explain the marked differences in individuals' responses to various events or conditions. Perhaps factors such as nutritional deficiency and physical fitness play a role. Although a decrease in the function of the descending inhibitory system seems to fit the clinical presentation of continued pain problems, these factors have yet to be documented adequately.

Sleep disturbances

Sleep disturbances appear to be commonly associated with many chronic orofacial pain disorders.[261-265] It is currently unknown whether the chronic pain condition produces a sleep disturbance or whether a sleep disturbance is a significant factor in the initiation of the chronic pain condition. Regardless of this cause-and-effect question, the relationship between sleep disturbances and chronic pain disorders must be recognized, since it may need to be addressed during therapy.

Learned behavior

Patients who experience prolonged suffering can develop an illness behavior that seems to perpetuate the pain disorder. In other words, people learn to be sick instead of well. Patients who present with illness behavior need to receive therapy to promote wellness behavior before complete recovery can be accomplished.

Secondary gain

Chronic pain disorders can produce certain secondary gains for the suffering patient.[266-268] When a patient learns that chronic pain can be used to manipulate normal life events, the patient may have difficulty giving up the pain and going back to normal responsibilities. For example, if chronic pain becomes an excuse to avoid work, it will be difficult for the clinician to resolve the pain problem unless the patient wishes to return to work. It is important for the therapist to recognize the presence of secondary gains so they can be properly addressed. Failure to eliminate secondary gains will lead to failure in resolving the chronic pain disorder.

Depression

Psychologic depression is a common finding in chronic pain patients.[269-276] It is well documented that patients who suffer for long periods of time will frequently become depressed.[277-280] Since depression can result in an independent psychologic problem, it must be properly addressed to manage the patient completely.[281,282] Elimination of the pain problem alone will not necessarily eliminate depression.

This chapter has presented some general considerations in the management of orofacial pain. The remainder of this text will focus on each of the major pain categories, presenting information on diagnosis and specific treatment suggestions.

References

1. Sternbach RA. Chronic pain as a disease entity. Triangle 1981;20:27–32.
2. Degenaar JJ. Some philosophical considerations in pain. Pain 1979;7:281–304.
3. Keele KD. A physician looks at pain. In: Weisenberg M (ed). Pain: Clinical and Experimental Perspectives. St Louis: Mosby, 1975: 45–52.
4. Foreman R, Blair R, Weber R. Effects on T3 to T5 primate spinothalamic tract cells of injecting bradykinin into the heart [abstract]. Pain 1981;11 (suppl 1):212.
5. Zausinger S, Lumenta DB, Pruneau D, Schmid-Elsaesser R, Plesnila N, Baethmann A. Effects of LF 16-0687 Ms, a bradykinin B(2) receptor antagonist, on brain edema formation and tissue damage in a rat model of temporary focal cerebral ischemia. Brain Res 2002;950:268–278.
6. Lehmberg J, Beck J, Baethmann A, Uhl E. Influence of the bradykinin B1/B2-receptor-antagonist B 9430 on the cerebral microcirculation and outcome of gerbils from global cerebral ischemia. Acta Neurochir Suppl 2000; 76:39–41.
7. Becker D. Scientific principles of drug use in dental practice. Part 1: Clinical pharmacokinetics. Compend Contin Educ Dent 1988;9:46–52.
8. Greenberg BD, Tolliver TJ, Huang SJ, Li Q, Bengel D, Murphy DL. Genetic variation in the serotonin transporter promoter region affects serotonin uptake in human blood platelets. Am J Med Genet 1999;88:83–87.
9. Slotkin TA, McCook EC, Ritchie JC, Carroll BJ, Seidler FJ. Serotonin transporter expression in rat brain regions and blood platelets: Aging and glucocorticoid effects. Biol Psychiatry 1997;41:172–183.
10. Fusco M, D'Andrea G, Micciche F, Stecca A, Bernardini D, Cananzi AL. Neurogenic inflammation in primary headaches. Neurol Sci 2003;24(suppl 2):S61–S64.
11. Yonehara N, Yoshimura M. Influence of painful chronic neuropathy on neurogenic inflammation. Pain 2001;92:259–265.
12. Williamson DJ, Hargreaves RJ. Neurogenic inflammation in the context of migraine. Microsc Res Tech 2001;53:167–178.
13. Payne R, Max M, Inturrisi C, et al. Principles of Analgesic Use in the Treatment of Acute Pain and Chronic Cancer Pain. Washington, DC: American Pain Society, 1987.
14. Crossley HL, Bergman SA, Wynn RL. Nonsteroidal anti-inflammatory agents in relieving dental pain: A review. J Am Dent Assoc 1983; 106:61–64.
15. Sheridan P. Flurbiprofen as an alternative pain suppressor to standard analgesic therapy. J Am Dent Assoc 1986;113:671.
16. Guilbaud G, Iggo A, Tegner R. Sensory changes in joint-capsule receptors of arthritic rats: Effect of aspirin. In: Fields HL, Dubner R, Cervero F (eds). Proceedings of the Fourth World Congress on Pain: Seattle, vol 9, Advances in Pain Research and Therapy. New York: Raven Press, 1985:81–89.
17. Cashman J, McAnulty G. Nonsteroidal anti-inflammatory drugs in perisurgical pain management. Mechanisms of action and rationale for optimum use. Drugs 1995;49:51–70.
18. Seibert K, Masferrer J, Zhang Y, et al. Mediation of inflammation by cyclooxygenase-2. Agents Actions Suppl 1995;46:41–50.
19. Ferreira SH. Prostaglandins: Peripheral and central analgesia. In: Bonica JJ, Lindblom U, Iggo A (eds). Proceedings of the Third World Congress on Pain, vol 5, Advances in Pain Research and Therapy. New York: Raven Press, 1983:627–634.
20. Boas RA, Holford NHG, Villiger JW. Clinical pharmacology of opiate analgesia. In: Fields HL, Dubner R, Cervero F (eds). Proceedings of the Fourth World Congress on Pain: Seattle, vol 9, Advances in Pain Research and Therapy. New York: Raven Press, 1985:695–708.
21. Belcher G, Ryall RW. Differential excitatory and inhibitory effects of opiates on nociceptive and nonnociceptive neurons in the spinal cord of the cat. Brain Res 1978;45:303–314.
22. Inoki R, Hayashi T, Kudo T, et al. Effects of aspirin and morphine on the release of a bradykinin-like substance into the subcutaneous perfusate of the rat paw. Pain 1978;5: 53–63.
23. Schlon H, Bentley GA. The possibility that a component of morphine-induced analgesia is contributed indirectly via the release of endogenous opioids. Pain 1980;9:73–84.
24. Tamsen A, Sakurada T, Wahlstrom A, Terenius L, Hartvig P. Postoperative demand for analgesics in relation to individual levels of endorphins and substance P in cerebrospinal fluid. Pain 1982;13:171–183.
25. McQuay HJ, Carroll D, Watts PG, et al. Does adding small doses of codeine increase pain relief after third molar surgery. Clin J Pain 1987;2:197–201.

26. Sharav Y, Singer E, Schmidt E, Dionne RA, Dubner R. The analgesic effect of amitriptyline on chronic facial pain. Pain 1987;31:199–209.

27. Travell JG, Simons DG. Myofascial Pain and Dysfunction: The Trigger Point Manual. Baltimore: Williams & Wilkins, 1983.

28. Simons DG, Travell JG, Simons LS. Travell & Simons' Myofascial Pain and Dysfunction: The Trigger Point Manual, ed 2. Baltimore: Williams & Wilkins, 1999.

29. Kraus H. Clinical Treatment of Back and Neck Pain. New York: McGraw-Hill International, 1970.

30. Hong CZ, Kuan TS, Chen JT, Chen SM. Referred pain elicited by palpation and by needling of myofascial trigger points: A comparison. Arch Phys Med Rehabil 1997;78:957–960.

31. Hong CZ, Simons DG. Pathophysiologic and electrophysiologic mechanisms of myofascial trigger points. Arch Phys Med Rehabil 1998;79:863–872.

32. Bonica JJ. The Management of Pain. Philadelphia: Lea & Febiger, 1990:1931–1944.

33. Singh B, Moodley J, Shaik AS, Robbs JV. Sympathectomy for complex regional pain syndrome. J Vasc Surg 2003;37:508–511.

34. Kohjitani A, Miyawaki T, Kasuya K, Shimada M. Sympathetic activity-mediated neuropathic facial pain following simple tooth extraction: A case report. Cranio 2002;20:135–138.

35. Chaturvedi A, Dash HH. Sympathetic blockade for the relief of chronic pain. J Indian Med Assoc 2001;99:698–703.

36. Bonelli S, Conoscente F, Movilia PG, Restelli L, Francucci B, Grossi E. Regional intravenous guanethidine vs. stellate ganglion block in reflex sympathetic dystrophies: A randomized trial. Pain 1983;16:297–307.

37. Thompson JE. The diagnosis and management of posttraumatic pain syndromes (causalgia). Aust NZ J Surg 1979;49:299–304.

38. Procacci P, Francini F, Zoppi M, Maresca M. Cutaneous pain threshold changes after sympathetic block in reflex dystrophies. Pain 1975;1:167–175.

39. Wetchler BV, Wyman TM. The role of stellate ganglion block in the treatment of acute herpes zoster ophthalmicus [abstract]. Pain 1981;11(suppl 1):120.

40. Loh L, Nathan PW, Schott GD. Pain due to the lesions of central nervous system removed by sympathetic block. Br Med J 1981;282:1026–1028.

41. Wang JK, Johnson KA, Ilstrup DM. Sympathetic blocks for reflex sympathetic dystrophy. Pain 1985;23:13–17.

42. Payne R. Neuropathic pain syndromes, with special reference to causalgia and reflex sympathetic dystrophy. Clin J Pain 1986;2:59–73.

43. Schurmann M, Gradl G, Wizgal I, et al. Clinical and physiologic evaluation of stellate ganglion blockade for complex regional pain syndrome type I. Clin J Pain 2001;17:94–100.

44. Gellman H. Reflex sympathetic dystrophy: Alternative modalities for pain management. Instr Course Lect 2000;49:549–557.

45. Tenicela R, Lovasik D, Eaglstein W. Treatment of herpes zoster with sympathetic blocks. Clin J Pain 1985;1:63–67.

46. Dan K, Higa K, Noda B. Nerve block for herpetic pain. In: Fields HL, Dubner R, Cervero F (eds). Proceedings of the Fourth World Congress on Pain: Seattle, vol 9, Advances in Pain Research and Therapy. New York: Raven Press, 1985:831–838.

47. Yanagida H, Suwa K, Corssen G. The role of sympathetic blockade in terminating acute herpes zoster and preventing postherpetic neuralgia [abstract]. Pain 1987;31(suppl 4):205.

48. Milligan NS, Nash TP. Treatment of postherpetic neuralgia. A review of 77 consecutive cases. Pain 1985;23:381–386.

49. Devor M, Govrin-Lippman R, Raber P. Corticosteroids suppress ectopic neural discharge originating in experimental neuromas. Pain 1985;22:127–137.

50. Devor M, Govrin-Lippmann R, Raber P. Corticosteroids reduce neuroma hyperexcitability. In: Fields HL, Dubner R, Cervero F (eds). Proceedings of the Fourth World Congress on Pain: Seattle, vol 9, Advances in Pain Research and Therapy. New York: Raven Press, 1985:451–455.

51. Allen GD. Dental Anesthesia and Analgesia. Baltimore: Williams & Wilkins, 1984:9–18.

52. Kreisberg MK. Tricyclic antidepressants: Analgesic effect and indications in orofacial pain. J Crainomandib Disord Facial Oral Pain 1988;2:171–177.

53. Lascelles RG. Atypical facial pain and depression. Br J Psychiatr 1966;112:651–659.

54. Brown RS, Bottomley WK. The utilization and mechanism of action of tricyclic antidepressants in the treatment of chronic facial pain: A review of the literature. Anesth Prog 1990;37:223–239.

55. Strumper D, Durieux ME, Hollmann MW, Troster B, den Bakker CG, Marcus MA. Effects of antidepressants on function and viability of human neutrophils. Anesthesiology 2003;98:1356–1362.

56. Sharav Y, Singer E, Schmidt E, Dionne RA, Dubner R. The analgesic effect of amitriptyline on chronic facial pain. Pain 1987;31:199–209.

57. Fields HL. Pain II: New approaches to management. Ann Neurol 1981;9:101–106.

58. Spiegel K, Kalb R, Pasternak GW. Analgesic activity of tricyclic antidepressants. Ann Neurol 1983;13:462–465.

59. Zitman FG, Linssen AC, Edelbroek PM, Stijnen T. Low dose amitriptyline in chronic pain: The gain is modest. 1990;42:35–42.

60. Chapman CR, Butler SH. Effects of doxepin on perception of laboratory induced pain in man. Pain 1978;5:253–262.

61. Ward NG, Bloom VL, Friedel RO. The effectiveness of tricyclic antidepressants in the treatment of coexisting pain and depression. Pain 1979;7:331–341.

62. Feinmann C. Pain relief by antidepressants: Possible modes of action. Pain 1985;23:1–8.

63. Hameroff SR, Cork RC, Weiss JL, et al. Doxepin effects in chronic pain and depression: A controlled study. In: Fields HL, Dubner R, Cervero F (eds). Proceedings of the Fourth World Congress on Pain: Seattle, vol 9, Advances in Pain Research and Therapy. New York,: Raven Press, 1985:761–771.

64. Bowsher D. Factors influencing the features of postherpetic neuralgia and outcome when treated with tricyclics. Eur J Pain 2003;7:1–7.

65. Davidoff G, Guarracini M, Roth E, Sliwa J, Yarkony G. Trazodone hydrochloride in the treatment of dysesthetic pain in traumatic myelopathy: A randomized, double-blind, placebo-controlled study. Pain 1987;29:151–161.

66. Watson CPN, Evans R. A comparative trial of amitriptyline and zimelidine in postherpetic neuralgia. Pain 1985;23:387–394.

67. Kerrick JM, Fine PG, Lipman AG, Love G. Low-dose amitriptyline as an adjunct to opioids for postoperative orthopedic pain: A placebo-controlled trial. Pain 1993;52:325–330.

68. Taiwo YO, Fabian A, Pazoles CJ, Fields HL. Potentiation of morphine antinociception by monoamine reuptake inhibitors in the rat spinal cord. Pain 1985;21:329–337.

69. Levine JD, Gordon NC, Smith R, McBryde R. Desipramine enhances opiate postoperative analgesia. Pain 1986;27:45–49.

70. Mattia C, Paoletti F, Coluzzi F, Boanelli A. New antidepressants in the treatment of neuropathic pain. A review. Minerva Anesthesiol 2002;68:105–114.

71. Roose SP, Glassman AH, Giardina EGU, Walsh BT, Woodring S, Bigger JT. Tricyclic antidepressants in depressed patients with cardiac conduction disease. Arch Gen Psychiatry 1987;44:273–275.

72. Morichi R, Pepeu G. A study of the influence of hydroxyzine and diazepam on morphine antinociception in the rat. Pain 1979;7:173–180.

73. Sindrup SH, Jensen TS. Pharmacotherapy of trigeminal neuralgia. Clin J Pain 2002;18:22–27.

74. Danhauer SC, Miller CS, Rhodus NL, Carlson CR. Impact of criteria-based diagnosis of burning mouth syndrome on treatment outcome. J Orofac Pain 2002;16:305–11.

75. Grushka M, Epstein J, Mott A. An open-label, dose escalation pilot study of the effect of clonazepam in burning mouth syndrome. Oral Surg Oral Med Oral Pathol Oral Radiol Endod 1998;86:557–561.

76. Woda A, Navez ML, Picard P, Gremeau C, Pichard-Leandri E. A possible therapeutic solution for stomatodynia (burning mouth syndrome). J Orofac Pain 1998;12:272–278.

77. Rahimtoola H, Buurma H, Tijssen CC, Leufkens HG, Egberts AC. Incidence and determinants of migraine prophylactic medication in the Netherlands. Eur J Clin Pharmacol 2002;58:149–155.

78. Marsland AR, Weekes JWN, Atkinson RL, Leong MG. Phantom limb pain: A case for beta blockers? Pain 1982;12:295–297.

79. Sicuteri F, Geppetti P, Marabini S, Lembeck F. Pain relief by somatostatin in attacks of cluster headache. Pain 1984;18:359–365.

80. Buzzi MG, Moskowitz MA. The antimigraine drug sumatriptan (GR43175) selectively blocks neurogenic plasma extravasation from blood vessels in dura mater. Br J Pharmacol 1990;99:202–206.

81. Saper JR, Silberstien S, Gordon CD, Hamel RL. Handbook of Headache Management. Baltimore: Williams & Wilkins, 1993:21–22.

82. Livingstone JA, Atkins RM. Intravenous regional guanethidine blockade in the treatment of post-traumatic complex regional pain syndrome type 1 (algodystrophy) of the hand. J Bone Joint Surg [Br] 2002;84:380–386.

83. Noordenbos W. Sensory findings in painful traumatic nerve lesions. In: Bonica JJ, Liebeskind JC, Albe-Fessard DG (eds). Proceedings of the Second World Congress on Pain, vol 3, Advances in Pain Research and Therapy. New York: Raven Press, 1979:91–101.

84. Hannington-Kiff JG. Hyperadrenergic-effected limb causalgia: Relief by IV pharmacologic norepinephrine blockade. Am Heart J 1982; 103:152–153.

85. Lief PA, Reisman R, Rocca A, et al. Intravenous regional guanethidine vs. reserpine for pain relief in reflex sympathetic dystrophy (RSD): A controlled, randomized, double-blind, crossover study [abstract]. Pain 1987;31(suppl 4): 205.

86. Levine J, Basbaum AI. The peripheral nervous system and the inflammatory process [abstract]. Pain 1987;31(suppl 4):109.

87. Suaudeau C, Chait A, Cimetiere C, de Beaurepaire R. Analgesic effects of antibiotics in rats. Pharmacol Biochem Behav 1993;46:361–364.

88. Ocana M, Baeyens JM. Analgesic effects of centrally administered aminoglycoside antibiotics in mice. Neurosci Lett 1991;126:67–70.

89. Corey L, Spear PG. Infections with herpes simplex viruses. N Engl J Med 1986;314:749–757.

90. Reuler JB, Chang M. Herpes zoster: Epidemiology, clinical features and management. South Med J 1984;77:1149–1156.

91. Sklar SH. Herpes zoster, the treatment and prevention of neuralgia with adenosine monophosphate. JAMA 1985;253:1426–1430.

92. Shepp DH, Dandliker PS, Meyer JD. Treatment of varicella-zoster virus infection in severely immunocompromised patients. N Engl J Med 1986;314:208–212.

93. Tyring S. Famiciclovir therapy (famvir) for herpes simplex and herpes zoster infections. Skin Therapy Lett 2001;6:1–2, 5.

94. Rowe NH, Shipman CJ, Drach JC. Herpes simplex virus disease: Implications for dental personnel. J Am Dent Assoc 1984;108:381–382.

95. Raborn GW, McGaw WT, Grace M, Tyrrell LD, Samuels SM. Oral acyclovir and herpes labialis: A randomized, double-blind, placebo-controlled study. J Am Dent Assoc 1987;115:38–42.

96. Johnson S. Advances in dental research. J Am Dent Assoc 1985;111:796.

97. Rumore MM, Schlichting DA. Clinical efficiency of antihistamines as analgesics. Pain 1986;25:7–22.

98. Galeotti N, Ghelardini C, Bartolini A. Antihistamine antinociception is mediated by Gi-protein activation. Neuroscience 2002;109:811–818.

99. Olsen UB, Eltorp CT, Ingvardsen BK, et al. ReN 1869, a novel tricyclic antihistamine, is active against neurogenic pain and inflammation. Eur J Pharmacol 2002;435:43–57.

100. Galeotti N, Ghelardini C, Bartolini A. The role of potassium channels in antihistamine analgesia. Neuropharmacology 1999;38:1893–1901.

101. Sunshine A, Zighelboim I, De Castro A, et al. Augmentation of acetaminophen analgesia by the antihistamine phenyltoloxamine. J Clin Pharmacol 1989;29:660–664.

102. Wiffen P, McQuay H, Carroll D, Jadad A, Moore A. Anticonvulsant drugs for acute and chronic pain. Cochrane Database Syst Rev 2000;(2):CD001133.

103. Loeser JD. The management of tic douloureux. Pain 1977;3:155–162.

104. Harke H, Gretenkort P, Ladleif HU, Rahman S, Harke O. The response of neuropathic pain and pain in complex regional pain syndrome I to carbamazepine and sustained-release morphine in patients pretreated with spinal cord stimulation: A double-blinded randomized study. Anesth Analg 2001;92:488–495.

105. Cruccu G, Leandri M, Iannetti GD, et al. Small-fiber dysfunction in trigeminal neuralgia: Carbamazepine effect on laser-evoked potentials. Neurology 2001;56:1722–1726.

106. Solaro C, Messmer Uccelli M, Uccelli A, Leandri M, Mancardi GL. Low-dose gabapentin combined with either lamotrigine or carbamazepine can be useful therapies for trigeminal neuralgia in multiple sclerosis. Eur Neurol 2000;44:45–48.

107. Vranken JH, Zuurmond WW, Van Kemenade FJ, Dzoljic M. Neurohistopathologic findings after a neurolytic celiac plexus block with alcohol in patients with pancreatic cancer pain. Acta Anaesthesiol Scand 2002;46:827–830.

108. Varghese BT, Koshy RC, Sebastian P, Joseph E. Combined sphenopalatine ganglion and mandibular nerve, neurolytic block for pain due to advanced head and neck cancer. Palliat Med 2002;16:447–448.

109. Westerlund T, Vuorinen V, Kirvela O, Roytta M. The endoneurial response to neurolytic agents is highly dependent on the mode of application. Reg Anesth Pain Med 1999;24: 294–302.

110. Westerlund T, Vuorinen V, Roytta M. The effect of combined neurolytic blocking agent 5% phenol-glycerol in rat sciatic nerve. Acta Neuropathol (Berl) 2003;106:261–270.

111. Hakanson S. Retrogasserian glycerol injection as a treatment of tic douloureux. In: Bonica JJ, Lindblom U, Iggo A (eds). Proceedings of the Third World Congress on Pain, vol 5, Advances in Pain Research and Therapy. New York: Raven Press, 1983:927–933.

112. Barthelemy I, Karanas Y, Sannajust JP, Emering C, Mondie JM. Gout of the temporomandibular joint: Pitfalls in diagnosis. J Craniomaxillofac Surg 2001;29:307–310.

113. Kurihara K, Mizuseki K, Saiki T, Wakisaka H, Maruyama S, Sonobe J. Tophaceous pseudogout of the temporomandibular joint: Report of a case. Pathol Int 1997;47:578–880.

114. Kamatani Y, Tagawa T, Hirano Y, Nomura J, Murata M. Destructive calcium pyrophosphate dihydrate temporo-mandibular arthropathy (pseudogout). Int J Oral Maxillofac Surg 1987;16:749–752.

115. Messing RB, Lytle LD. Serotonin-containing neurons: Their possible role in pain and analgesia. Pain 1977;4:1–21.

116. Hosobuchi Y, Lamb S, Bascom D. Tryptophan loading may reverse tolerance to opiate analgesics in humans: A preliminary report. Pain 1980;9:161–169.

117. Schwarz MJ, Offenbaecher M, Neumeister A, et al. Evidence for an altered tryptophan metabolism in fibromyalgia. Neurobiol Dis 2002; 11:434–442.

118. Seltzer S, Marcus R, Stoch R. Perspectives in the control of chronic pain by nutritional manipulation. Pain 1981;11:141–148.

119. Seltzer S, Stoch R, Marcus R, Jackson E. Alteration of human pain thresholds by nutritional manipulation and L-tryptophan supplementation. Pain 1982;13:385–393.

120. Cheng RSS, Pomeranz B. A combined treatment with D-amino acids and electroacupuncture produces a greater analgesia than either treatment alone; naloxone reverses these effects. Pain 1980;8:231–236.

121. Fernstrom JD, Wurtman RJ. Brain serotonin content: Physiological regulations of plasma neutral amino acids. Science 1972;178:414–416.

122. Van Woert MV, Rosenbaum D. L-5-hydroxytryptophan therapy in myoclonus. In: Fahn S, Rowland LP, Davis JN (eds). Cerebral Hypoxia and Its Consequences, vol 26, Advances in Neurology. New York: Raven Press, 1979:107–115.

123. Shealy CN. Vitamin B6 and other vitamin levels in chronic pain patients. Clin J Pain 1987; 2:203–204.

124. Brady JP, Cheatle MD, Ball WA. A trial of L-tryptophan in chronic pain syndrome. Clin J Pain 1987;3:39–43.

125. Seltzer S, Dewart D, Pollack RL, Jackson E. The effects of dietary tryptophan on chronic maxillofacial pain and experimental pain tolerance. J Psychiatr Res 1982;17:181–186.

126. Alnigenis MN, Barland P. Fibromyalgia syndrome and serotonin. Clin Exp Rheumatol 2001;19:205–210.

127. Sharma V, Barrett C. Tryptophan for treatment of rapid-cycling bipolar disorder comorbid with fibromyalgia. Can J Psychiatry 2001;46: 452–453.

128. Juhl JH. Fibromyalgia and the serotonin pathway. Altern Med Rev 1998;3:367–375.

129. Birdsall TC. 5-Hydroxytryptophan: A clinically effective serotonin precursor. Altern Med Rev 1998;3:271–280.

130. Caruso I, Sarzi Puttini P, Cazzola M, Azzolini V. Double-blind study of 5-hydroxytryptophan versus placebo in the treatment of primary fibromyalgia syndrome. J Int Med Res 1990; 18:201–209.

131. Yaksh TL, Hammond DL. Peripheral and central substrates involved in the rostral transmission of nociceptive information. Pain 1982;13: 1–85.

132. Melzack R, Wall PD. Pain mechanisms: A new theory. Science. 1965;150:971–979.

133. Wall PD. The gate control theory of pain mechanisms: A reexamination and restatement. Brain 1978;101:1–18.

134. Gammon GD, Starr IJ. Studies on the relief of pain by counterirritation. J Clin Invest 1941; 20:13–20.

135. Politzer A. A Textbook of Diseases of the Ear. Philadelphia: Lea Brothers & Co, 1902.

136. Kraus H. The use of surface anesthesia in the treatment of painful motion. JAMA 1941;116: 2582–2583.

137. Travell J. Basis for the multiple uses of local block of somatic trigger areas. Miss Valley Med J 1949;71:13–25.

138. Travell J. Ethyl chloride spray for painful muscle spasm. Arch Phys Med Rehabil 1952;33: 291–298.

139. Schwartz LL. Ethyl chloride treatment of limited painful mandibular movement. J Am Dent Assoc 1954;48:497–507.

140. Ottoson D, Ekbiom A, Hansson P. Vibratory stimulation for the relief of pain of dental origin. Pain 1981;10:37–45.

141. Lundeberg T, Ottoson D, Hakansson S, et al. Vibratory stimulation for the control of intractable chronic orofacial pain. In: Bonica JJ, Lindblom U, Iggo A (eds). Proceedings of the Third World Congress on Pain, vol 5, Advances in Pain Research and Therapy. New York: Raven Press, 1983:555–561.

142. Pantaleo T, Duranti R, Bellini F. Effects of vibratory stimulation on muscular pain threshold and blink response in human subjects. Pain 1986;24:239–250.

143. Sherer CL, Clelland JA, O'Sullivan P, Doleys DM, Canan B. The effect of two sites of high frequency vibration on cutaneous pain threshold. Pain 1986;25:133–138.

144. Hansson P, Ekblom A. Transcutaneous electrical nerve stimulation (TENS) as compared to placebo TENS for the relief of acute orofacial pain. Pain 1983;15:157–165.

145. Lundeberg T. Long-term results of vibratory stimulation as a pain relieving measure for chronic pain. Pain 1984;20:13–23.

146. Kane K, Taub A. A history of local electrical analgesia. Pain 1975;1:125–138.

147. Wall PD, Sweet WH. Temporary abolition of pain in man. Science 1967;155:108–109.

148. Anderson SA. Pain control by sensory stimulation. In: Bonica JJ, Liebeskind JC, Albe-Fessard DG (eds). Proceedings of the Second World Congress on Pain, vol 3, Advances in Pain Research and Therapy. New York: Raven Press, 1979:569–585.

149. Facchinetti F, Sandrini G, Petraglia F, Alfonsi E, Nappi G, Genazzani AR. Concomitant increase in nociceptive flexion reflex threshold and plasma opioids following transcutaneous nerve stimulation. Pain 1984;19:295–303.

150. Hansson P, Ekblom A, Thomsson M, Fjellner B. Influence of naloxone on relief of acute orofacial pain by transcutaneous electric nerve stimulation (TENS) or vibration. Pain 1986;24:323–329.

151. Honig S, Zeale P, Mason A, et al. High-frequency transcutaneous electrical nerve stimulation: Lack of correlation with serum beta-endorphin levels and failure of analgesic reversal with naloxone. Clin J Pain 1987;2:215–217.

152. Augustinsson L, Bohlin P, Bundsen P, et al. Pain relief during delivery by transcutaneous electrical nerve stimulation. Pain 1977;4:59-65.

153. Mannheimer C, Carlsson C. The analgesic effect of transcutaneous electrical nerve stimulation (TNS) in patients with rheumatoid arthritis: A comparative study of different pulse patterns. Pain 1979;6:329–334.

154. Rabinstein AA, Shulman LM. Acupuncture in clinical neurology. Neurology 2003;9:137–148.

155. Peets JM, Pomeranz B. Acupuncture-like transcutaneous electrical nerve stimulation analgesia is influenced by spinal cord endorphins but not serotonin: An intrathecal pharmacological study. In: Fields HL, Dubner R, Cervero F (eds). Proceedings of the Fourth World Congress on Pain: Seattle, vol 9, Advances in Pain Research and Therapy. New York: Raven Press, 1985: 519–525.

156. Hwang BG, Min BI, Kim JH, Na HS, Park DS. Effects of electroacupuncture on the mechanical allodynia in the rat model of neuropathic pain. Neurosci Lett 2002;320:49–52.

157. Fox EJ, Melzack R. Transcutaneous electrical stimulation and acupuncture: Comparison of treatment for low-back pain. Pain 1976;2: 141–148.

158. Eriksson MBE, Sjolund BH, Nielzen S. Long-term results of peripheral conditioning stimulation as an analgesic measure in chronic pain. Pain 1979;6:335–347.

159. Willer JC, Boureau F, Luu M. Differential effects of electroacupuncture (EA) and transcutaneous nerve stimulation (TNS) on nociceptive component (R2) of the blink reflex in man [abstract]. Pain 1981;11(suppl 1):280.

160. Sodipo OA. Transcutaneous electrical nerve stimulation (TENS) and acupuncture: Comparison of therapy for low-back pain [abstract]. Pain 1981;11(suppl 1):277.

161. Chapman CR, Colpitts YM, Benedetti C, Kitaeff R, Gehrig JD. Evoked potential assessment of acupunctural analgesia: Attempted reversal with naloxone. Pain 1980;9:183–197.

162. Bischko JJ. Use of laser beam in acupuncture. Int J Acupuncture Electro Therapeut Res 1980;5:29–36.

163. Barnes JF. Electronic acupuncture and cold laser therapy as adjunct to pain treatment. J Craniomandib Pract 1984;2:148–152.

164. Waker J, Akharrjec LK, Cooney MM. Laser therapy for pain of trigeminal neuralgia [abstract]. Pain 1987;31(suppl 4):85.

165. Sweet WH. Some current problems in pain research and therapy. Pain 1981;10:297–309.

166. Melzack R. Prolonged relief of pain by brief, intense transcutaneous somatic stimulation. Pain 1975;1:357–373.

167. Sodipo JOA. Therapeutic acupuncture for chronic pain. Pain 1979;7:359–365.

168. Ahonen E, Hakumaki M, Mahlanaki S, et al. Acupuncture and physiotherapy in the treatment of myogenic headache patients: Pain relief and EMG activity. In: Bonica JJ, Lindblom U, Iggo A (eds). Proceedings of the Third World Congress on Pain, vol 5, Advances in Pain Research and Therapy. New York: Raven Press, 1983:571–576.

169. Kaptchuk TJ. Acupuncture: Theory, efficacy, and practice. Ann Intern Med 2002;136:374–383.

170. Toyama PM, Heyder C. Acupuncture-induced mood changes reversed by narcotic antagonist naloxone [abstract]. Pain 1981;11(suppl 1):279.

171. Walker JB, Katz RL. Nonopioid pathways suppress pain in humans. Pain 1981;11:347–354.

172. Cottingham B, Phillips PD, Davies GK, Getty CJ. The effect of subcutaneous nerve stimulation (SCNS) on pain associated with osteoarthritis of the hip. Pain 1985;22:243–248.

173. Lawrence RM. Stimulation of the periosteum of the bone for chronic pain reduction [abstract]. Pain 1981;11(suppl 1):112.

174. Esposito CJ, Veal SJ, Farman AG. Alleviation of myofascial pain with ultrasound therapy. J Prosthet Dent 1984;51:106–110.

175. Griffin JE, Karselis TC. Physical Agents for Physical Therapists. Springfield, IL: Thomas, 1982:279–312.

176. Minor MA, Sanford MK. The role of physical therapy and physical modalities in pain management. Rheum Dis Clin North Am 1999;25:233–248, vii.

177. Kahn J. Iontophoresis and ultrasound for postsurgical temporomandibular tissues and paresthesis. Phys Ther 1980;60:307–308.

178. Kleinkort JA, Wood F. Phonopheresis with one percent versus ten percent hydrocortisone [abstract]. Phys Ther 1985;55:1320.

179. Klaiman MD, Shrader JA, Danoff JV, Hicks JE, Pesce WJ, Ferland J. Phonophoresis versus ultrasound in the treatment of common musculoskeletal conditions. Med Sci Sports Exerc 1998;30:1349–55.

180. Shin SM, Choi JK. Effect of indomethacin phonophoresis on the relief of temporomandibular joint pain. Cranio 1997;15:345–348.

181. Jankelson B, Swain CW. Physiological aspect of masticatory muscle stimulation: The Myomonitor. Quintessence Int 1972;3:57–62.

182. Murphy GJ. Electrical physical therapy in treating TMJ patients. J Craniomandib Pract 1983;1:67–73.

183. Wessberg GA, Carroll WL, Dinham R, Wolford LM. Transcutaneous electrical stimulation as an adjunct in the management of myofascial pain-dysfunction syndrome. J Prosthet Dent 1981;45:307–314.

184. Simons DG, Travell JG, Simons LS. Apropos of all muscles. In: Travell & Simons' Myofascial Pain and Dysfunction: The Trigger Point Manual, ed 2. Baltimore: Williams & Wilkins, 1999:94–177.

185. Schwartz L. Disorders of the Temporomandibular Joint. Philadelphia: Saunders, 1959.

186. De Steno CV. The pathophysiology of TMJ dysfunction and related pain. In: Gelb H (ed). Clinical Management of Head, Neck and TMJ Pain and Dysfunction. Philadelphia: Saunders, 1977:1–31.

187. Bechtol CO. Muscle physiology. In: American Academy of Orthopedic Surgeons (eds). International Course Lectures. St Louis: Mosby, 1948.

188. Kemppainen P, Pertovaara A, Huopaniemi T, Johansson G, Karonen SL. Modification of dental pain and cutaneous thermal sensitivity by physical exercise in man. Brain Res 1985;360:33–40.

189. Kemppainen P, Pertovaara A. The contribution of experimental stress to the modulation of dental pain threshold in man [abstract]. Pain 1987;31(suppl 4):414.

190. Fordyce WE, McMahon R, Rainwater G, et al. Pain complaint–exercise performance relationship in chronic pain. Pain 1981;10:311–321.

191. Magnusson T, Egermark I, Carlsson GE. A longitudinal epidemiologic study of signs and symptoms of temporomandibular disorders from 15 to 35 years of age. J Orofac Pain 2000;14:310–319.

192. Tervonen T, Knuuttila M. Prevalence of signs and symptoms of mandibular dysfunction among adults aged 25, 35, 50 and 65 years in Ostrobothnia, Finland. J Oral Rehabil 1988;15:455–463.

193. Egermark I, Carlsson GE, Magnusson T. A 20-year longitudinal study of subjective symptoms of temporomandibular disorders from childhood to adulthood. Acta Odontol Scand 2001;59:40–48.

194. Speculand B, Goss AN, Hughes A, Spence ND, Pilowsky I. Temporomandibular joint dysfunction: Pain and illness behavior. Pain 1983;17:139–150.

195. Fordyce WE. Pain viewed as learned behavior. In: Bonica JJ (ed). International Symposium on Pain, vol 4, Advances in Neurology. New York: Raven Press, 1974:415–422.

196. Fordyce WE. Treating chronic pain by contingency management. In: Bonica JJ (ed). International Symposium on Pain, vol 4, Advances in Neurology. New York: Raven Press, 1974: 583–589.

197. Melzack R. Psychological concepts and methods for the control of pain. In: Bonica JJ (ed). International Symposium on Pain, vol 4, Advances in Neurology. New York: Raven Press, 1974:275–280.

198. Sternbach RA. Fundamentals of psychological methods in chronic pain. In: Bonica JJ, Lindblom U, Iggo A (eds). Proceedings of the Third World Congress on Pain, vol 5, Advances in Pain Research and Therapy. New York: Raven Press, 1983:777–780.

199. Roberts AA. Contingency management methods in the treatment of chronic pain. In: Bonica JJ, Iggo A, Lindblom U (eds). Proceedings of the Third World Congress on Pain, vol 5, Advances in Pain Research and Therapy. New York: Raven Press, 1983:789–794.

200. Selye H. Stress Without Distress. Philadelphia: Lippincott, 1974:32.

201. Carlson CR, Okeson JP, Falace DA, Nitz AJ, Curran SL, Anderson DT. Comparison of psychologic and physiologic functioning between patients with masticatory muscle pain and matched controls. J Orofacial Pain 1993;7: 15–22.

202. Jacobson E. Progressive Relaxation. Chicago: Univ of Chicago Press, 1968.

203. Moller E, Sheik-Ol-Eslam A, Lous I. Deliberate relaxation of the temporal and masseter muscles in subjects with functional disorders of the chewing apparatus. Scand J Dent Res 1971;79: 478–482.

204. Gessel AH, Alderman MM. Management of myofascial pain dysfunction syndrome of the temporomandibular joint by tension control training. Psychosomatics 1971;12:302–330.

205. Goldberg G. The psychological, physiological, and hypnotic approach to bruxism in the treatment of periodontal disease. J Am Soc Psychosom Dent Med 1973;20:75–91.

206. Reading A, Raw M. The treatment of mandibular dysfunction pain. Possible application of psychological methods. Br Dent J 1976;140: 201-205.

207. Blanchard EB, Andrasik F, Evans D, Hillhouse J. Biofeedback and relaxation treatments for headache in the elderly: A caution and a challenge. Biofeedback Self Regul 1985;10:69–73.

208. Larsson B, Melin L. Chronic headaches in adolescents: Treatment in a school setting with relaxation training as compared with information contact and self-registration. Pain 1986; 25:325–336.

209. Dahlstrom L, Carlsson SG. Treatment of mandibular dysfunction: The clinical usefulness of biofeedback in relation to splint therapy. J Oral Rehabil 1984;11:277–284.

210. Lacroix J, Clarke MA, Bock JC, Doxey NC. Muscle-contraction headaches in multiple-pain patients. Treatment under worsening baseline conditions, Arch Phys Med Rehabil 1986;67: 14–18.

211. Hijzen TH, Slangen JL, van Houweligen HC. Subjective, clinical and EMG effect of biofeedback and splint treatment. J Oral Rehabil 1986;13:529–539.

212. Raft D, Toomey T, Gregg JM. Behavior modification and haloperidol in chronic facial pain. South Med J 1979;72:155–159.

213. Erlandson PM, Poppen R. Electromyographic biofeedback and rest position training of masticatory muscles in myofascial pain-dysfunction patients. J Prosthet Dent 1989;62: 335–338.

214. Okeson JP, Moody PM, Kemper JT, Haley JV. Evaluation of occlusal splint therapy and relaxation procedures in patients with temporomandibular disorders. J Am Dent Assoc 1983; 107:420–424.

215. Carlson CR, Ventrella MA, Sturgis ET. Relaxation training through muscle stretching procedures: A pilot case. J Behav Ther Exp Psychiatry 1987;18:121–126.

216. Carlson CR, Collins FL, Nitz AJ, Sturgis ET, Rogers JL. Muscle stretching as an alternative relaxation training procedure. J Behav Ther Exp Psychiatry 1990;21:29–38.

217. Carlson CR, Okeson JP, Falace DA, Nitz AJ, Anderson D. Stretch-based relaxation and the reduction of EMG activity among masticatory muscle pain patients. J Craniomandib Disord Facial Oral Pain 1991;5:205–212.

218. Manns A, Zuazola RV, Sirhan RM, Quiroz M, Rocabado M. Relationship between the tonic elevator mandibular activity and the vertical dimension during the states of vigilance and hypnosis. J Craniomandib Pract 1990;8:163–170.

219. Liossi C, Hatira P. Clinical hypnosis in the alleviation of procedure-related pain in pediatric oncology patients. Int J Clin Exp Hypn 2003; 51:4–28.

220. Spinhoven P, ter Kuile MM. Treatment outcome expectancies and hypnotic susceptibility as moderators of pain reduction in patients with chronic tension-type headache. Int J Clin Exp Hypn 2000;48:290–305.

221. Yocum DE, Castro WL, Cornett M. Exercise, education, and behavioral modification as alternative therapy for pain and stress in rheumatic disease. Rheum Dis Clin North Am 2000;26:145–159, x–xi.

222. Astin JA, Shapiro SL, Eisenberg DM, Forys KL. Mind-body medicine: State of the science, implications for practice. J Am Board Fam Pract 2003;16:131–147.

223. Kabat-Zinn J, Lipworth L, Burney R, et al. Four-year follow-up of a meditation based program for the self-regulation of chronic pain: Treatment outcomes and compliance. Clin J Pain 1987;2:159–173.

224. Bailey LM. Music therapy in pain management. J Pain Sympt Manag 1986;1:25–28.

225. Nilsson U, Rawal N, Enqvist B, Unosson M. Analgesia following music and therapeutic suggestions in the PACU in ambulatory surgery; a randomized controlled trial. Acta Anaesthesiol Scand 2003;47:278–283.

226. Bally K, Campbell D, Chesnick K, Tranmer JE. Effects of patient-controlled music therapy during coronary angiography on procedural pain and anxiety distress syndrome. Crit Care Nurse 2003;23:50–58.

227. Patterson DR, Jensen MP. Hypnosis and clinical pain. Psychol Bull 2003;129:495–521.

228. Pilling LF. Psychosomatic aspects of facial pain. In: Alling CC, Mahan PE (eds). Facial Pain, ed 2. Philadelphia: Lea & Febiger, 1977:213–226.

229. Fricton JR. The effects of direct and indirect hypnotic suggestion for analgesia in high and low susceptible subjects [abstract]. Pain 1981;11(suppl 1):175.

230. Hilgard ER. The alleviation of pain by hypnosis. Pain 1975;1:213–231.

231. Orne MT. Hypnotic methods for managing pain. In: Bonica JJ, Lindblom U, Iggo A (eds). Proceedings of the Third World Congress on Pain, vol 5, Advances in Pain Research and Therapy. New York: Raven Press, 1983:847–856.

232. Toomey TC, Larkin D. Trance as a pain control strategy for the nurse in the burn unit setting [abstract]. Pain 1981;11(suppl 1):113.

233. Stephenson JB. Reversal of hypnosis-induced analgesia by naloxone. Lancet 1978;2:991–992.

234. Finer B, Terenius L. Endorphin involvements during hypnotic analgesia in chronic pain patients [abstract]. Pain 1981;11(suppl 1):27.

235. Moret V, Forster A, Laverriere MC, et al. Mechanism of analgesia induced by hypnosis and acupuncture: is there a difference? Pain 1991; 45:135–140.

236. Neblett R, Gatchel RJ, Mayer TG. A clinical guide to surface-EMG-assisted stretching as an adjunct to chronic musculoskeletal pain rehabilitation. Appl Psychophysiol Biofeedback 2003;28:147–160.

237. Gale EN. Behavioral management of MPD. In: Laskin D, American Dental Association (eds). The President's Conference on the Examination, Diagnosis, and Management of Temporomandibular Disorders. Chicago: American Dental Association, 1983:161–173.

238. Chapman CR, Turner JA. Psychological control of acute pain in medical settings. J Pain Sympt Manag 1986;1:9–20.

239. Egan KJ, Betrus P. Psychological functioning in five pain syndromes: Tension headache, backache, migraine, and temporomandibular and gastrointestinal pain syndromes. Clin J Pain 1987;2:233–238.

240. Chapman SL. A review and clinical perspective on the use of EMG and thermal biofeedback for chronic headaches. Pain 1986;27:1–43.

241. Schwartz MS. Biofeedback and stress management in the treatment of headache. J Craniomandib Disord Facial Oral Pain 1987;1:41–45.

242. Jessup BA, Neufeld RWJ, Merskey H. Biofeedback therapy for headache and other pain: An evaluative review. Pain 1979;7:225–270.

243. Andrasik F. Behavioral treatment approaches to chronic headache. Neurol Sci 2003;24(suppl 2):S80–S85.

244. Sternbach RA. Letter to the editor. Pain 1980; 9:111.

245. Turner JA, Chapman CR. Psychological intervention for chronic pain: A critical review. 1. Relaxation training and biofeedback. Pain 1982;12:1–21.

246. Sherman RA, Gall N, Gormly J. Treatment of phantom limb pain with muscular relaxation training to disrupt the pain-anxiety-tension cycle. Pain 1979;6:47–55.

247. Large RG, Lamb AM. Electromyographic (EMG) feedback in chronic musculoskeletal pain: A controlled trial. Pain 1983;17:167–177.

248. Nouwen A. EMG biofeedback used to reduce standing levels of paraspinal muscle tension in chronic low back pain. Pain 1983;17:353–360.

249. Brooke RI, Stenn PG. Myofascial pain-dysfunction syndrome: How effective is biofeedback-assisted relaxation training? In: Bonica JJ, Lindblom U, Iggo A (eds). Proceedings of the Third World Congress on Pain, vol 5, Advances in Pain Research and Therapy. New York: Raven Press, 1983:809–812.

250. Costen JB. Syndrome of ear and sinus symptoms dependent upon functions of the temporomandibular joint. Ann Otol Rhinol Laryngol 1934;3:1–4.

251. Okeson JP. Occlusal appliance therapy. In: Management of Temporomandibular Disorders and Occlusion. St Louis: Mosby–Year Book, 2003:507–536.

252. Phillips JM, Gatchel RJ, Wesley AL, Ellis E III. Clinical implications of sex in acute temporomandibular disorders. J Am Dent Assoc 2001; 132:49–57.

253. Curran SL, Carlson CR, Okeson JP. Emotional and physiologic responses to laboratory challenges: Patients with temporomandibular disorders versus matched control subjects. J Orofac Pain 1996;10:141–150.

254. Carlson CR, Reid KI, Curran SL, et al. Psychological and physiological parameters of masticatory muscle pain. Pain 1998;76:297–307.

255. Maixner W, Fillingim R, Booker D, Sigurdsson A. Sensitivity of patients with painful temporomandibular disorders to experimentally evoked pain. Pain 1995;63:341–351.

256. Svensson P, Arendt-Nielsen L, Nielsen H, Larsen JK. Effect of chronic and experimental jaw muscle pain on pain-pressure thresholds and stimulus-response curves. J Orofac Pain 1995;9:347–356.

257. Carlson CR, Bertrand P. Self-Regulation Training Manual. Lexington, KY: Univ of Kentucky Press, 1995.

258. Carlson C, Bertrand P, Ehrlich A, Maxwell A, Burton RG. Physical self-regulation training for the management of temporomandibular disorders. J Orofac Pain 2001;15:47–55.

259. Carlson CR, Sherman JJ, Studts JL, Bertrand PM. The effects of tongue position on mandibular muscle activity. J Orofac Pain 1997;11: 291–297.

260. Aigner M, Graf A, Freidl M, et al. Sleep disturbance in somatoform pain disorder. Psychopathology 2003;36:324–328.

261. Moldofsky H, Scarisbrick P. Induction of neurasthenic musculoskeletal pain syndrome by selective sleep stage deprivation. Psychosom Med 1976;38:35–44.

262. Moldofsky H, Scarisbrick P, England R, Smythe H. Musculoskeletal symptoms and non-REM sleep disturbance in patients with "fibrositis" and healthy subjects. Psychosom Med 1986;37:341–351.

263. Moldofsky H, Tullis C, Lue FA. Sleep related myoclonus in rheumatic pain modulation disorder (fibrositis syndrome). J Rheumatol 1986; 13:614–617.

264. Molony RR, MacPeek DM, Schiffman PL, et al. Sleep, sleep apnea and the fibromyalgia syndrome. J Rheumatol 1986;13:797–800.

265. Yatani H, Studts J, Cordova M, Carlson CR, Okeson JP. Comparison of sleep quality and clinical and psychologic characteristics in patients with temporomandibular disorders. J Orofac Pain 2002;16:221–8.

266. Marbach JJ, Lennon MC, Dohrenwend BP. Candidate risk factors for temporomandibular pain and dysfunction syndrome: Psychosocial, health behavior, physical illness and injury. Pain 1988;34:139–151.

267. Burgess JA, Dworkin SF. Litigation and post-traumatic TMD: How patients report treatment outcome. J Am Dent Assoc 1993;124: 105–110.

268. Hopwood MB, Abram SE. Factors associated with failure of trigger point injections. Clin J Pain 1994;10:227–234.

269. Tauschke E, Merskey H, Helmes E. Psychological defence mechanisms in patients with pain. Pain 1990;40:161–170.

270. Marbach JJ, Lund P. Depression, anhedonia and anxiety in temporomandibular joint and other facial pain syndromes. Pain 1981;11: 73–84.

271. Magni G, Marchetti M, Moreschi C, Merskey H, Luchini SR. Chronic musculoskeletal pain and depressive symptoms in the National Health and Nutrition Examination I. Epidemiologic follow-up study. Pain 1993;53:163–168.

272. Auerbach SM, Laskin DM, Frantsve LM, Orr T. Depression, pain, exposure to stressful life events, and long-term outcomes in temporomandibular disorder patients. J Oral Maxillofac Surg 2001;59:628–633.

273. Dworkin SF. Perspectives on the interaction of biological, psychological and social factors in TMD. J Am Dent Assoc 1994;125:856–863.

274. Gallagher RM, Marbach JJ, Raphael KG, Dohrenwend BP, Cloitre M. Is major depression comorbid with temporomandibular pain and dysfunction syndrome? A pilot study. Clin J Pain 1991;7:219–225.

275. Glaros AG. Emotional factors in temporomandibular joint disorders. J Indiana Dent Assoc 2000;79:20–23.

276. Parker MW, Holmes EK, Terezhalmy GT. Personality characteristics of patients with temporomandibular disorders: Diagnostic and therapeutic implications. J Orofac Pain 1993;7:337–344.

277. Fine EW. Psychological factors associated with non-organic temporomandibular joint pain dysfunction syndrome. Br Dent J 1971;131:402–404.

278. Haley WE, Turner JA, Romano JM. Depression in chronic pain patients: Relation to pain, activity, and sex differences. Pain 1985;23:337–343.

279. Hendler N. Depression caused by chronic pain. J Clin Psychiatry 1984;45:30–38.

280. Faucett JA. Depression in painful chronic disorders: The role of pain and conflict about pain. J Pain Symptom Manage 1994;9:520–526.

281. Dworkin RH, Richlin DM, Handlin DS, Brand L. Predicting treatment response in depressed and non-depressed chronic pain patients. Pain 1986;24:343–353.

282. Fricton JR, Olsen T. Predictors of outcome for treatment of temporomandibular disorders. J Orofac Pain 1996;10:54–65.

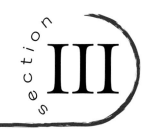

Clinical Pain Syndromes

Cutaneous and Mucogingival Pains

In the orofacial region, primary somatic pain of the superficial type emanates from the skin of the lips, face, outer nares, and outer external auditory canal and from the mucogingival tissues of the oral cavity proper (Fig 10-1). Pains from these structures display clinical features that distinguish them from primary deep somatic pains and from secondary heterotopic manifestations of somatic and neuropathic pain disorders.

Behavior of Cutaneous and Mucogingival Pains

The following are clinical characteristics of superficial somatic pain:

1. The pain has a bright, stimulating quality.
2. Subjective localization of the pain is excellent and anatomically accurate.
3. The site of pain identifies the correct location of its source.
4. Response to provocation at the site of pain is faithful in incidence, intensity, and location.
5. The application of a topical anesthetic at the site of pain temporarily arrests the pain.

Types of Cutaneous and Mucogingival Pain

There are a variety of pains that originate from the cutaneous and mucogingival tissues of the face and oral structures. Many of these conditions are specifically identified by the tissues that are affected. In this chapter, these pains will be simply divided into two categories according to the tissues affected: cutaneous pains and mucogingival pains.

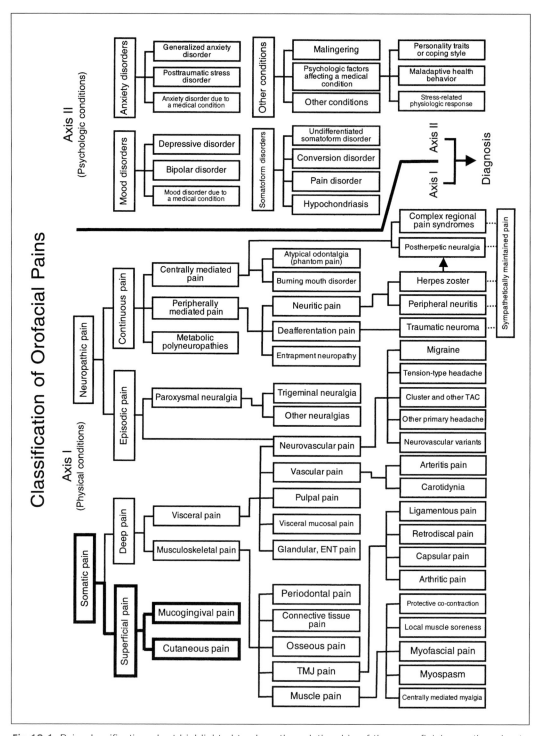

Fig 10-1 Pain classification chart highlighted to show the relationship of the superficial somatic pains to the other orofacial pain disorders.

Cutaneous Pains of the Face

Cutaneous pain is usually described as an itching, pricking, raw, stinging, or burning sensation, depending chiefly on the intensity of the complaint. Stimulation-evoked pain is initially felt as a fast, sharp, pricking pain. Since this is prevented by blocking of A fibers, it is presumed that the initial sensation is mediated by A-delta nociceptive neurons.[1] The initial pricking sensation is followed by a slightly delayed, less sharp, less precisely localized, burning pain that quite assuredly is mediated by C-fiber nociceptive units.

Since the pain is felt precisely at the location of the initiating cause, little diagnostic effort is needed to determine its origin. When the cause of the cutaneous pain is not immediately evident, the examiner should question whether the complaint might be heterotopic, such as referred pain from other deep pain input or projected pain of neuropathic etiology.[2-6] Application of a topical anesthetic at the site of pain temporarily arrests superficial somatic pain. It should be noted, however, that the irritating effect of the medication, when first applied, may initially increase the discomfort.

Caution should be exercised in assuming that a visible lesion at or near the site of pain necessarily represents the primary initiating cause. It may or may not be so. For example, the lesions of herpes zoster stem from a neural disorder and are not the cause of the peripheral pain. Again, one should not assume that the complaint does not emanate from cutaneous structures simply because the etiology is obscure. Subtle forms of noxious stimulation that cause itching and stinging may be encountered. When such confusing situations arise, the use of topical anesthesia to confirm the diagnosis is indicated.

Mucogingival Pains of the Mouth

There may be some question about classifying mucogingival pains in the same category with pains of cutaneous origin, since they are not identical in behavior. For example, mucogingival discrimination of painful sensation does not include the familiar pricking-burning pattern of cutaneous pain. Also, the number of thick fibers innervating the oral mucosa is negligible compared with that of the skin. However, palatal mucosa can sense both itch and tickle, and all oral tissues feel stinging and burning sensations. Mucogingival pains have a bright, stimulating quality, are easily localized, and identify an adequate local cause. These pains respond faithfully to provocation at the site of pain, do not present central excitatory effects, and are arrested by the application of a topical anesthetic at the site of pain. They therefore present the characteristics of superficial somatic pain, by which identification can be made. The true site of origin of such pain is less evident than for cutaneous pain only because of the added difficulty of intraoral examination and failure on the part of the examiner to fully appreciate the implications of oral functioning.

The oral tissues are fragile and easily injured by rubbing against the teeth, tongue, cheeks, and each other during normal use. They are subjected to countless insults from foods, beverages, burns, tobacco, alcohol, toothpastes, mouthwashes, medications, dental defects, dental restorations, dental appliances, objects held in the mouth, habits of clenching the teeth, unusual functional demands, and many more. The oral tissues are reactive to systemic disorders and diseases. The saliva, which normally acts as the oral lubricant, is especially responsive to the effects of emotional stress, physical disorders, diseases, and many medications now in common use. The identification of the cause of pain from these tissues is obviously more difficult than for cutaneous pains, but it should be within the capability of the knowledgeable dental examiner. As with cutaneous pain, when the cause of pain felt in the mucogingival tissues is not immediately evident, the examiner must differentiate between primary pain of mucogingival origin and projected or referred pain that stems from neurogenous or deep somatic sources.

Mucogingival pains are usually described as distinct raw, stinging, or burning sensations. Pains arising from the lining tissues of the oral cavity can be precisely located by the patient. Such pain may be generalized throughout the mouth when the cause widely affects the mucogingival tissues, or it may be isolated if the hyperalgesic area is small. In either case the patient can precisely locate the discomfort. The location changes only as the underlying cause varies. This precision of localization may become less accurate in the deeper recesses of the oral cavity.

The location of pain accurately identifies its source. The pain arises from primary hyperalgesia due to local cause, such as the irritating effect of foods, liquids, mouthwashes, dentifrices, and medications. It may be a result of the abrasive effect of excessive rubbing of the tongue and cheeks, and this effect may be compounded when the quality and quantity of saliva do not afford adequate lubricative protection to the moving tissues. When the salivary deficit is great, normal functioning may become traumatic to the oral tissues. Localized hyperalgesia may occur from numerous causes such as trauma; infection by bacterial, fungal, or viral agents; allergy; and neoplasia. Frequently, one may identify objective signs of hyperemia, inflammation, vesiculation, ulceration, or some other pathosis at the site of pain.

Primary hyperalgesia of the oral lining tissues may show no objective signs, and mucogingival tissues may appear entirely normal. Hyperalgesia may occur with no clinical signs of other tissue change. It is in such instances that the examiner should carefully consider a salivary deficit as the possible etiologic factor.

There is a precise, accurate, and proportional relationship between any noxious stimulation and the resulting discomfort. When no stimulus is applied, little or no discomfort occurs. When the stimulus is increased, the discomfort increases accordingly without summation effects. The pain faithfully reflects the degree of hyperalgesia and the intensity of the stimulus.

Ordinarily, central excitatory effects are not seen as a result of mucogingival pain, even when the pains are severe and continuous. Referred pains, secondary hyperalgesias, and the development of secondary painful muscle co-contraction do not occur. This gives the pain a constancy and sameness that is characteristic.

Since pain of mucogingival origin is an expression of primary hyperalgesia of the tissues that hurt, application of a topical anesthetic to those tissues arrests the pain due to action of the medication on the receptors and pain fibers in the mucogingival tissues. This is an important point of differentiation from referred pain of the superficial type and neuritic pain, neither of which is arrested by the application of topical anesthesia.

Mucogingival pains may result from trauma, allergic responses, local infections, or systemic conditions, or they may present as burning mouth syndromes. Each of these categories will be discussed.

Trauma

Generalized surface injuries cause mucogingival pains, but the etiology is usually so evident that no diagnostic problem is presented. Other signs are present or promptly become apparent, such as hyperemia, inflammation, vesiculation, or ulceration. Such traumatic effects may have mechanical, thermal, or chemical causes, such as scalding with hot foods or liquids (Fig 10-2), excessive smoking or other use of tobacco, abrasions from toothbrushes and other objects, chemical burns (Fig 10-3), accidents as a result of dental treatment, or the use of harmful medications by the patient. Examples of the latter are aspirin burns and injuries produced by toothache remedies.

Traumatic abrasions and decubital ulcerations are common, secondary to poorly fitting dental appliances (Fig 10-4). Exostoses and bony prominences are especially vulnerable to injury, and when severely traumatized, full-thickness mucogingival ulcers may develop and cause exposure and surface devitalization of the underlying cortical bone. Such lesions are slow to heal and cause pain of the superficial somatic variety accompanied by pain characteristics associated with deep pain input. Whenever the periosteal and osseous structures become involved, pains of mixed quality should be expected. This is true not only of the full-thickness ulcers but also of gingival lesions that involve the deeper periodontal structures. Examples of such lesions are acutely inflamed periodontal pockets and superficial infections that spread as cellulitis. Pains of mixed quality are less likely to be arrested by application of a topical anesthetic. They frequently present secondary symptoms of central sensitization.

Allergic responses

Various allergic responses, including stomatitis medicamentosa and stomatitis venenata, may produce rather generalized mucogingival pain, the cause of which may at times be obscure. These conditions are usually accompanied by objective signs of tissue change, and the cause may be established by careful history taking. Stomatitis venenata presents with lesions of the oral mucosa that result from contact with ordinarily innocuous substances, such as denture materials, dentifrices, mouthwashes, lozenges, lipsticks, topical medications, foods, and flavoring materials (Figs 10-5 and 10-6). Sometimes desquamation of the protective surface layers of epithelium occurs and reveals the deeper vascular bed. When the shedding is extensive, the term *desquamative stomatitis* may be applicable.

Stomatitis medicamentosa is an allergic reaction to systemic medications such as antibiotics, sulfonamides, aminopyrine, quinine, arsphenamine, phenolphthalein, barbiturates, mercurials, salicylates, or hormonal birth control. Some cases of erythema multiforme (Fig 10-7), as well as variants described as ectodermosis erosiva pluriorificialis (Stevens-Johnson syndrome) and Behcet syndrome, may represent allergic responses of this type.

Other allergens may cause oral manifestations accompanied by superficial mucogingival pain. At times, such manifestations may require consultation with an allergist. From the standpoint of pain diagnosis, such conditions should be distinguished from localized autonomic effects that result from central excitation. The key to diagnosis relates to one's knowledge of the neuroanatomy of the visceral nervous system. Systemic allergic responses do not follow neuroanatomic patterns and therefore are observed bilaterally and diffusely, whereas localized autonomic effects relate to the anatomic distribution of the neurons involved and are predominantly unilateral.

Local infections

Widespread local infections of the mucogingival tissues cause generalized superficial somatic pain. Usually the accompanying local signs of inflammation and ulceration make the cause of pain obvious. Examples of this are fulminating acute necrotizing ulcerative gingivitis[7-9] (Vincent infection) and fungal infections[10-12] (Figs 10-8 and 10-9).

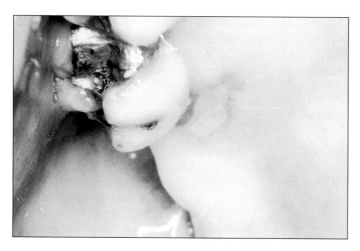

Fig 10-2 Ulcer on palatal tissues secondary to a pizza burn. (Courtesy of Dr John F. Johnson, United States Navy.)

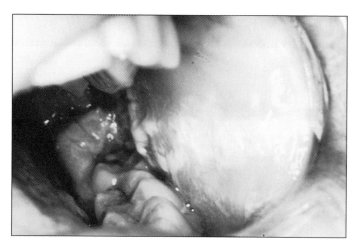

Fig 10-3 Aspirin burn secondary to the placement of an aspirin tablet in the buccal mucosa. (Courtesy of Dr John F. Johnson, United States Navy.)

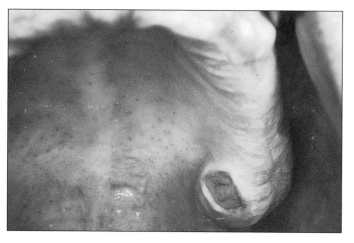

Fig 10-4 Decubital ulcer caused by pressure from a denture.

Fig 10-5 Stomatitis venenata caused by contact with denture base material. Note that the tissue reaction conforms to the shape of the denture base.

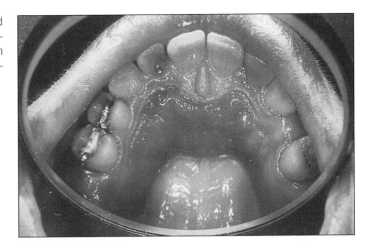

Fig 10-6 Stomatitis venenata resulting from contact with a dentifrice to which the patient was sensitive.

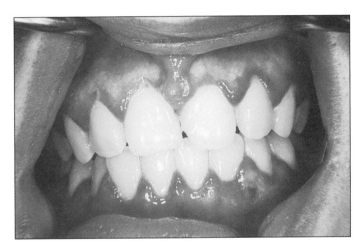

Fig 10-7 Stomatitis medicamentosa expressed clinically as erythema multiforme due to ingestion of a laxative medicine that contained phenolphthalein.

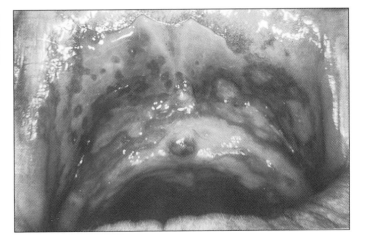

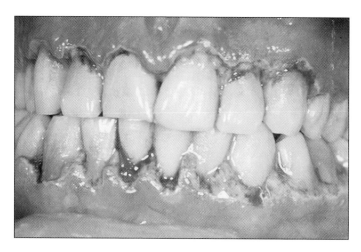

Fig 10-8 Acute necrotizing ulcerative gingivitis (Vincent infection).

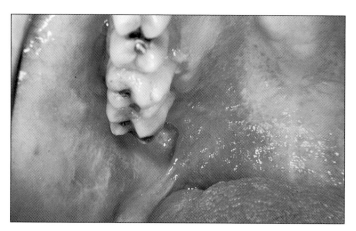

Fig 10-9 Fungal infection of the oral mucosa.

Systemic conditions

Systemic disease may cause oral manifestations that affect the mucogingival tissues and induce generalized superficial somatic pain. Included are nutritional deficiencies, intoxications, exanthematous diseases, anemia and other blood dyscrasias, pellagra, diabetes, pemphigus, and infections. Even pregnancy and general debilitation can affect mucogingival tissues (Fig 10-10). These conditions exhibit objective signs of congestion, so that discoloration and swelling are evident. Such effects frequently occur at sites where other local irritation is present,

such as soft tissue trauma, traumatic occlusion, gingivitis, and periodontal involvement.

Most isolated pains emanating from the oral mucogingival tissues present no diagnostic problem because they are usually associated with local lesions that are clinically evident subjectively and objectively. Two such common disorders are recurrent aphthous stomatitis and herpes simplex infection. Both of these conditions are characterized by recurrent, painful, superficial oral ulcers that persist for 8 to 14 days. They are both associated with a tender regional lymphadenopathy and heal spontaneously, usually without sequelae. There

Fig 10-10 Gingivitis that became acute during the third month of pregnancy and persisted for 5 weeks postpartum.

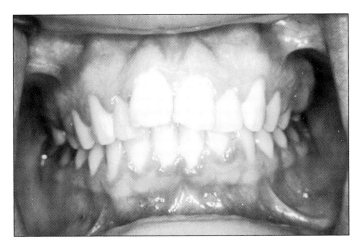

are differences between these conditions, and therefore each will be briefly discussed.

Recurrent aphthous stomatitis

Recurrent aphthous stomatitis is the most common ulcerative disease of the oral cavity, accounting for 90% of all ulcers seen in dental practice and affecting nearly 20% of the general population.[13-15] Aphthous stomatitis appears as an erythematous macula or papilla that undergoes central blanching followed by necrosis and ulceration (Fig 10-11). The ulcers most commonly occur on nonkeratinized, freely movable mucosa, such as the lips, buccal mucosa, tongue, mucobuccal fold, floor of the mouth, or soft palate. They usually occur singly, but on occasion several occur simultaneously. As already mentioned, the ulcers will occur, resolve, and then reoccur at a later date.

The etiology of recurrent aphthous stomatitis is still unknown.[16] Studies suggest that the disorder is an immunopathic process that involves cell-mediated cytolytic activity that leads to decreased tissue integrity.[17,18] Precipitating factors include certain foods (eg, gluten-containing foods, acidic foods, and juices), trauma, stress, hormones, nutritional deficiencies, and chemicals in oral hygiene products[19-22] (Fig 10-12).

Since the etiology is unknown, there is no known cure for recurrent aphthous ulcers; however, in most cases the disease can be controlled to the patient's satisfaction. The patient should be educated about the natural course of the disease and its self-limiting nature. The patient should be told of the noncommunicability of the disease and the benefits of avoiding any precipitating factors, if they are known. During the pain episode, topical anesthetic may be helpful.[23] Topical steroid preparations may also be useful.[24]

Herpes simplex infection

Herpes simplex infects nearly half a million people each year in the United States.[25,26] The initial or primary infection usually occurs early in life, between the ages of 1 and 10 years. Young adults ages 15 to 25 years comprise the second most commonly infected group, with 45% of college students being infected.[27] Herpes simplex infection presents as a cluster of small discrete gray or white vesicles without a red erythematous halo. The vesicles quickly rupture, forming small punctuate ulcers 1 mm or less in diameter. Unlike recurrent aphthous ulcers, herpes simplex usually presents as several small ulcers clustered in a localized area. The lesions are usually found on fixed ker-

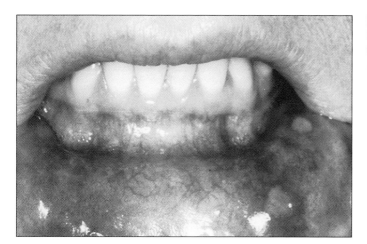

Fig 10-11 Several aphthous ulcers located on the buccal mucosa of the lower lip. (Courtesy of Dr John F. Johnson, United States Navy.)

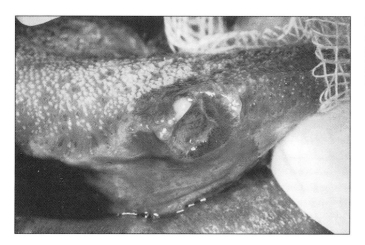

Fig 10-12 A very larger aphthous ulcer that developed following trauma to the tongue. (Courtesy of Dr John F. Johnson, United States Navy.)

atinized mucosa, such as tightly bound periosteum, hard palate, gingiva, and the alveolar ridge.

The etiology of herpes simplex infection is the herpesvirus. There are seven known herpesviruses, two of which are known to occur only in humans: HSV-1 and HSV-2. Both of these viruses produce epithelial disease, enter a latent state, and reactivate at a later date to produce recurrent disease. HSV-1 classically is associated with infection of the orofacial complex, whereas HSV-2 predominantly causes genital infections. Both are natural infections occurring in humans with equal involvement of both

sexes and all races. HSV-1 has affinity for cells of neuroectodermal origin.

Transmission occurs by direct personal contact with infected secretions at mucosal surfaces or abraded skin. The most common portal of entry for HSV-1 is the oral mucosa. The virus binds to the epithelial cell membrane and then penetrates the cell by fusion with the plasma membrane.[28] The virus then affects cellular DNA synthesis, producing balloon degeneration, chromatin condensation, multinucleated giant cell formation, and eventually the lesions.[29,30]

The initial herpes simplex infection may be asymptomatic. It may occur in children and young adults as a pharyngitis or gingivostomatitis. The lesions may be accompanied by fever, malaise, irritability, inability to eat, regional lymphadenopathy, and myalgia. Infection in infants and small children may go undiagnosed.

After the initial episode, the virus can travel to the sensory nerve ganglia and persist within the nucleus in a nonreplicating, dormant (latent) state. The trigeminal ganglia is the most common site of the latent HSV-1 virus. Recurrent herpes simplex is the result of a reactivitation of the virus in the same site of the originally infected nerve. An estimated 98 million cases of recurrent herpes simplex occur in the United States each year.[31] It has been estimated that 35% to 40% of the people who harbor HSV-1 will have recurrent episodes.[32]

The first symptoms of recurrent herpes simplex may be felt as the prodromal symptoms of tingling, throbbing, itching, and burning at the infected site beginning 12 to 24 hours before eruption of the lesion(s). Once the lesions form and erupt, diagnosis becomes obvious. In immunosuppressed patients, recurrent HSV-1 infections may penetrate deeply and disseminate widely.[33]

Treatment of herpes simplex is often determined by the severity of the symptoms. The initial case of herpes simplex can be very painful and widespread, thus demanding treatment. Supportive and palliative care and anti-infective treatments are the basis of managing the primary HSV-1 infection. Rest and isolation are important for limiting transmission and to speed healing. Adequate hydration and nutrition are essential, particularly in small children. Symptoms may be helped with topical anesthetic agents, including diphenhydramine. Antiviral medications such as acyclovir and famciclovir are effective for treating herpes simplex virus (HSV-1, HSV-2).[12,34–38] They may be administered topically,[39] orally, or intravenously (IV). They appear to be more effective in the treatment of primary infections than recurrent episodes.[40]

The *Journal of the American Dental Association* reported an experimental herpes vaccine that proved effective in animal studies for both HSV-1 and HSV-2.[41] Famciclovir (Famvir) is an orally administered prodrug of the antiviral agent penciclovir.[37] Its unique pharmacokinetic profile makes it an efficacious, convenient, and well-tolerated alternative to the more traditionally prescribed acyclovir. Famciclovir allows patients to manage or prevent symptoms, thereby significantly improving their quality of life. Its favorable safety profile makes it a good treatment choice for the elderly and for immunocompromised patients, including those infected with human immunodeficiency virus.

Salicylates, nonsteroidal anti-inflammatory drugs, and acetaminophen may be useful in reducing pain and/or fever. Note that salicylates should be avoided in children to minimize the risk of Reye syndrome.[42]

Recurrent herpes simplex may be precipitated by harsh outdoor elements, stress, menses, trauma, and possibly diet. Therefore, prophylactic measures are the best method of managing the recurrence. Once the recurrence has occurred, topical measures, similar to the primary treatments, may be helpful.

Burning mouth disorders

The complaint of burning mouth, burning tongue, or glossodynia (glossalgia) is common and usually described as a steady, continuous though variable, typical superficial somatic pain.[43] Very frequently, the oral examination reveals a clean, hygienic mouth with little objective evidence of pathosis of any kind. A distinguishing characteristic of this condition is the fact that the location of the pain corresponds to areas of greatest movement, thus revealing the cause as the abrasive effect of the tissues rubbing against themselves and the teeth.

Pain location depends on which tissues are being rubbed and where. At times, hyperemia may be observed, as well as inflammation and ulceration. Secondary infection of the irritated tissues may complicate the symptom picture. There is a tendency for the complaint to improve and worsen in a cyclic pattern, presumably because of the inhibitory effect of pain on functional movements; this permits some regression of the complaint, only to be followed by an exacerbation from increased rubbing when the discomfort eases.

All oral irritants increase the patient's discomfort, especially highly spiced foods, hot liquids, carbonated drinks, strong coffee and tea, certain juices, dentifrices, mouthwashes, and medications. Sometimes mastication becomes so painful that nutritional difficulties arise.

Glossodynia and burning mouth can be caused by a variety of conditions. Often the etiology is located in the actual tissues that are expressing the pain. When local factors are present, this pain condition is truly a superficial somatic pain. Some types of local factors are bacterial or yeast infections (thrush). These conditions can lead to burning symptoms, and when present need to be appropriately managed by antibiotic or antifungal medications.

Xerostomia, or so-called dry mouth syndrome, often accompanies burning mouth and is thought to be etiologically important.[44] Many types of medications can induce xerostomia.[45,46] These include certain antispasmodics, antidepressants, antipsychotics, skeletal muscle relaxants, parkinsonism medications, antiarrhythmic drugs, antihistamines, appetite suppressants, anticonvulsants, anxiolytics, diuretics, and antihypertensives. This has been found to be especially common in the elderly.[47,48] Fox et al[49] found that, although xerostomia was most commonly associated with salivary gland dysfunction, it may be an early symptom of several morbid systemic conditions, including dry gland disease, polyglandular failure syndrome, systemic lupus erythematosus, primary biliary cirrhosis, and autoimmune hemolytic anemia. Autoimmune exocrinopathy (eg, Sjögren syndrome), is still another disorder associated with xerostomia.[50]

The presence of a dry mouth is further compromised by wearing a denture. Dentures normally require more lubrication from saliva than do natural teeth, and therefore a decreased salivary flow can lead to more tissue abrasion and a burning sensation. When this is present, an artificial salivary substitute may be indicated and should help reduce the burning complaint.[51,52]

In a review of 98 cases of burning mouth disorder, Gorsky et al[53] reported that 75% were female, that dentures and medications predominated etiologically, and that glossitis was the only mucosal lesion of significance. It is thought that diminished salivary function due to aging, radiation therapy, mouth breathing from nasal obstruction and other causes, and sustained periods of anxiety, resentment, and/or apprehension may contribute to the condition. Diabetes and anemia appear to have etiologic importance.[54] Quinn[55] reported that tongue-thrusting was common in patients with glossodynia.

When local factors or conditions are found to explain the burning complaint, the condition is a mucogingival pain disorder. However, when no local conditions are found to explain the burning complaint, the clinician needs to think more centrally. In this instance the burning mouth disorder may be more representative of the centrally mediated continuous neuropathic pain conditions. This will be explained more thoroughly in chapter 17.

A diagnostic key to this problem is the application of topical anesthetic to the painful site. Its penetration is too limited to appreciably affect pain sources situated more deeply in the tissues. Heterotopic pains are not affected. Therefore, if application of a topical anesthetic promptly and effectively arrests the pain and induces numbness, the condition truly represents primary hyperalgesia. The diagnosis is confirmed by analgesic lozenges. Regular application of topical anesthesia may be a useful therapy.

Differential Diagnosis

The clinician should always remember that pain felt in the cutaneous or mucogingival tissues may be heterotopic. The decisive diagnostic evidence that the complaint is heterotopic is the failure of an effective topical anesthetic to arrest the pain, even though surface anesthesia is attained. Therapeutic considerations require that the type and source of such heterotopic pain be identified.

Referred pain and/or secondary hyperalgesia induced as a central excitatory effect of deep somatic pain may involve the skin or the oral mucogingival structures. Spontaneous referred pain usually is readily recognized. Stimulus-evoked secondary hyperalgesia, however, can be difficult to identify. The key to diagnosis in either case is to be suspicious that the problem could be a secondary effect of deep pain input located elsewhere.

The diagnostic criteria of this phenomenon relate to identifying the primary pain source. Analgesic blocking or the application of a topical anesthetic at the site where heterotopic pain is felt does not arrest the pain, although some altered sensation may be felt due to the local anesthesia.

Referred pains and areas of hypersensitivity in the mucogingival tissues may occur as a direct result of other deep pain sources such as toothache, earache, sinusitis, temporomandibular arthralgia, myogenous pains, and neurovascular pains. Frequently, other central excitatory effects, such as local autonomic signs and secondary painful muscle effects, may be identified as well.

The following are a few differential diagnoses that should be considered when superficial somatic cutaneous or mucogingival pains are suspected:

- *Heterotopic neuropathic pains* may be projected superficially and present with clinical features that simulate superficial somatic pain. Although these neuropathic pains have not yet been discussed (see chapter 17), differentiation between the two categories of pain is necessary.
- *Paroxysmal neuralgia* may be triggered by stimulation of cutaneous or mucogingival receptors in the peripheral distribution of the same nerve that mediates the pain. In trigeminal neuralgia, the sites of such triggering are predominantly cutaneous, being located especially in the lips. Mucogingival triggering, however, sometimes occurs, with the tongue being a frequent site. Glossopharyngeal trigger sites are located in the pharyngeal mucosa, and pain is induced by swallowing, talking, and chewing. The clinical criterion for identifying mucosal triggering of paroxysmal neuralgia has to do with the summation effects displayed: the triggering provokes pain that is wholly disproportional to the stimulus. Analgesic blocking of the peripheral receptors of the affected nerve prevents the triggering effect of superficial stimulation. Topical anesthesia of mucosal trigger sites, such as those of glossopharyngeal neuralgia, also prevents the paroxysms of pain.
- *Deafferentation pain* may become a complication sequential to trauma, surgery, tooth extraction, or tooth pulp extirpation. The best differential criterion is a history of prior injury. The pain complaint may be accompanied by paresthesia, dysesthesia, anesthesia, hyperesthesia, or hyperalgesia in an area larger than that innervated by the injured nerve. The symptoms may be accentuated by efferent sympathetic activity involving vaso-

motor and glandular function. The pain may be arrested temporarily by analgesic blocking of the stellate ganglion.

- *Traumatic neuralgia* or a *neuroma* is characterized by its location relative to prior injury or surgery and by the specific induction of pain due to compressing or stretching the tissue involved. Topical anesthesia does nothing. However, injection of a drop or so of local anesthetic into the site of pain completely arrests it.

- *Neuritis* that involves cutaneous and mucogingival structures may be difficult to recognize because of its similarity to superficial somatic pain. One clinical criterion for identifying this neuropathic pain is its ongoing, persistent, unremitting character. It is not dependent on superficial stimulation, although such stimulation accentuates the discomfort. A more important criterion, however, is the presence of other neural effects (such as paresthesia, hypoesthesia, anesthesia, and paralysis) that may accompany the neuritic pain. Neuritis of the facial nerve is characterized by paralysis of facial muscles. Analgesic blocking central to the site of neuropathy arrests the pain.

- *Herpes zoster* can be particularly difficult to distinguish from superficial somatic pain unless the typical lesions are present. Cutaneous herpetic lesions are usually recognized because they occur in the neuroanatomic peripheral distribution of the affected nerve, exactly where the pain is felt. The intraoral mucosal lesions of trigeminal and geniculate herpes zoster, however, may be confused with aphthous ulcers. As such, the lesions may be thought to cause the pain. When herpetic lesions are absent, go unnoticed, or are misdiagnosed, leaving only the persistent neuritic pain, diagnosis may be extremely difficult. Perhaps the best criterion is that analgesic blocking does not arrest the pain. If the condition persists for more than a few weeks,

a diagnosis of postherpetic neuralgia is indicated.

The primary superficial somatic pains felt in the cutaneous and mucogingival tissues of the orofacial area need to be distinguished from the following:

1. Heterotopic referred pains, projected pains, secondary hyperalgesias, and autonomic effects that occur secondary to deep somatic pain and neuropathic pains
2. Systemic illness
3. Heterotopic pains of central origin
4. Pains related to psychologic conditions

Therapeutic Options

For the management of primary superficial somatic pains arising from the cutaneous and mucogingival tissues of the orofacial area, the following are therapeutic options (see chapter 9):

1. Analgesics for palliative relief and counseling
2. Cause-related therapy
   a. Identification and treatment of etiologic factors and contributing conditions present
   b. Elimination of all oral irritants
   c. Restriction of oral function within reasonable limits
   d. Antibiotics and antimicrobials, topical and systemic
   e. Antiviral agents, especially for initial episodes[12,34]
   f. For xerostomia[56]: Elimination or reduction of saliva-depressing drugs, chewing paraffin or gum to stimulate salivary flow, use of saliva substitutes,[57,58] and/or electric stimulation of saliva[59]

3. Pharmacologic therapy
   a. Topical anesthetics (liquid, ointment, lozenge)
   b. Analgesic balms
   c. Anti-inflammatory agents
4. Medical consultation

References

1. Ochoa JL, Torebjork HE. Pain from skin and muscle [abstract]. Pain 1981;11(suppl 1):87.
2. Bonica JJ. The Management of Pain. Philadelphia: Lea & Febiger, 1990:169–174.
3. Wolff HG. Headache and Other Head Pain. New York: Oxford University Press, 1963:3–28.
4. Dalessio DJ. The major neuralgias, postinfectious neuritis, and atypical facial pain. In: Dalessio DJ, Silberstein SD. Wolff's Headache and Other Head Pain, ed 6. New York: Oxford University Press, 1993:345–364.
5. Fields HL. Pain. New York: McGraw-Hill, 1987: 79–97.
6. Abraham PJ, Capobianco DJ, Cheshire WP. Facial pain as the presenting symptom of lung carcinoma with normal chest radiograph. Headache 2003;43:499–504.
7. Enwonwu CO, Phillips RS, Falkler WA Jr. Nutrition and oral infectious diseases: State of the science. Compend Contin Educ Dent 2002;23: 431–434, 436, 438 passim; quiz 448.
8. Parameter on acute periodontal diseases. American Academy of Periodontology. J Periodontol 2000;71:863–866.
9. Trieger N. Surgical treatment of periodontal infections. Atlas Oral Maxillofac Surg Clin North Am 2000;8:27–34.
10. Sherman RG, Prusinski L, Ravenel MC, Joralmon RA. Oral candidosis. Quintessence Int 2002;33:521–532.
11. Polak A. Antifungal therapy—State of the art at the beginning of the 21st century. Prog Drug Res 2003;Spec No:59–190.
12. Pallasch TJ. Antifungal and antiviral chemotherapy. Periodontol 2000 2002;28:240–255.
13. Savage NW. Oral ulceration: Assessment and treatment of commonly encountered oral ulcerative disease. Aust Fam Physician 1988;17: 247–250.
14. Casiglia JM. Recurrent aphthous stomatitis: Etiology, diagnosis, and treatment. Gen Dent 2002;50:157–166.
15. Ship JA, Chavez EM, Doerr PA, Henson BS, Sarmadi M. Recurrent aphthous stomatitis. Quintessence Int 2000;31:95–112.
16. Scully C, Gorsky M, Lozada-Nur F. The diagnosis and management of recurrent aphthous stomatitis: A consensus approach. J Am Dent Assoc 2003;134:200–207.
17. Dolby AE. Recurrent aphthous ulceration: Effect of sera and peripheral blood lymphocytes upon oral epithelial culture cells. Immunology 1969;17:709–714.
18. Rogers RS, Movius DL, Pierre R. Lymphocyte-epithelial cell interactions in oral mucosal inflammatory disease. Arch Dermatol 1976;67: 599–602.
19. Wright AJ, Ryan FP, Willingham SE, et al. Food allergy or intolerance in severe recurrent aphthous ulceration of the mouth. Br Med J 1986;292:1237–1238.
20. Nolan A, Lamey PJ, Milligan KA, Forsyth A. Recurrent aphthous ulceration and food sensitivity. J Oral Pathol Med 1991;20:473–475.
21. Ferguson MM, Carter JB, Boyle P. An epidemiological study of factors associated with recurrent aphthae in women. J Oral Med 1984; 39:212–217.
22. Wray D, Ferguson JM, Hutcheon AW, Dagg JH. Nutritional deficiencies in recurrent aphthae. J Oral Pathol Med 1978;7:418–423.
23. Eisen D, Lynch DP. Selecting topical and systemic agents for recurrent aphthous stomatitis. Cutis 2001;68:201–206.
24. Miller C. Diagnosis and management of acute disorders of the oral mucosa. In: Falace DA (ed). Emergency Dental Care. Philadelphia: Lea & Febiger, 1995:304–306.
25. Ades AE, Peckhan CS, Dale F, et al. Prevalence of antibodies to herpes simplex virus types 1 and 2 in pregnant women, and estimated rates of infection. J Epidemiol Community Health 1989;43:53–60.
26. Siegel MA. Diagnosis and management of recurrent herpes simplex infections. J Am Dent Assoc 2002;133:1245–1249.
27. Gibson JJ, Hornung CA, Alexander GR, Lee FK, Potts WA, Nahmias AJ. A cross-sectional study of herpes simplex virus types 1 and 2 in college students: Occurrence and determinants of infection. J Infect Dis 1990;162:306–312.
28. Spear PG. Glycoproteins specified by herpes simplex virus. In: Roizman B (ed). The Herpesviruses. New York: Plenum Press, 1983:315–356.

29. Darlington RW, Moss H. Herpesvirus envelopment. J Virol 1968;2:48–55.
30. Rapp F. Virus replication. In: Stringfellow DA (ed). Virology: A Scope Publication. Kalamazoo, MI: Upjohn, 1983:21.
31. Spruance SL, Overall JC, Kern ER, Krueger GG, Pliam V, Miller W. The natural history of recurrent herpes simplex labialis: Complications for antiviral therapy. N Engl J Med 1977;197:69–75.
32. Young SK, Rowe NH, Buchanan RA. A clinical study for the control of facial mucocutaneous herpes virus infections: I. Characterization of natural history in a professional school population. Oral Surg Oral Med Oral Pathol 1976;41:498–507.
33. Corey L, Spear PG. Infection with herpes simplex viruses. N Engl J Med 1986;314:749–757.
34. Reuler JB, Chang M. Herpes zoster: Epidemiology, clinical features and management. South Med J 1984;77:1149–1156.
35. Sklar SH. Herpes zoster, the treatment and prevention of neuralgia with adenosine monophosphate. JAMA 1985;253:1426–1430.
36. Shepp DH, Dandliker PS, Meyer JD. Treatment of varicella-zoster virus infection in severely immunocompromised patients. N Engl J Med 1986;314:208–212.
37. Tyring S. Famiciclovir therapy (famvir) for herpes simplex and herpes zoster infections. Skin Therapy Lett 2001;6:1–2, 5.
38. Tyring SK, Baker D, Snowden W. Valacyclovir for herpes simplex virus infection: Long-term safety and sustained efficacy after 20 years' experience with acyclovir. J Infect Dis 2002;186 (suppl 1):S40–S46.
39. Rowe NH, Shipman C Jr, Drach JC. Herpes simplex virus disease: Implications for dental personnel. J Am Dent Assoc 1984:108:381–382.
40. Raborn GW, McGaw WT, Grace M, Tyrell LD, Samuels SM. Oral acyclovir and herpes labialis: A randomized, double-blind, placebo-controlled study. J Am Dent Assoc 1987;115:38–42.
41. Johnson S. Herpes vaccine effective in animal studies. Advances in dental research. J Am Dent Assoc 1985;111:796.
42. Litalien C, Jacqz-Aigrain E. Risks and benefits of nonsteroidal anti-inflammatory drugs in children: A comparison with paracetamol. Paediatr Drugs 2001;3:817–858.
43. Drage LA, Rogers RS III. Burning mouth syndrome. Dermatol Clin 2003;21:135–145.
44. Guggenheimer J, Moore PA. Xerostomia: Etiology, recognition and treatment. J Am Dent Assoc 2003;134:61–69; quiz 118–119.
45. Wynn RL. The top 50 prescription medications dispensed in pharmacies in 2001. Gen Dent 2002;50:400–404, 406.
46. Grad H, Grushka M, Yanover L. Drug-induced xerostomia: The effects and treatments. J Can Dent Assoc 1985;51:296–300.
47. Binnie W, Wright J. Oral mucosa disease in the elderly. In: Cohen B, Thomson H (eds). Dental Care for the Elderly. London: Heinemann, 1986:40–81.
48. Ship JA, Pillemer SR, Baum BJ. Xerostomia and the geriatric patient. J Am Geriatr Soc 2002;50:535–543.
49. Fox PC, Vander Van PF, Sonies BC, et al. Xerostomia: Evaluation of a symptom with increasing significance. J Am Dent Assoc 1985;110:519–523.
50. Soto-Rojas AE, Kraus A. The oral side of Sjogren syndrome. Diagnosis and treatment. A review. Arch Med Res 2002;33:95–106.
51. Ship JA. Diagnosing, managing, and preventing salivary gland disorders. Oral Dis 2002;8:77–89.
52. Wall GC, Magarity ML, Jundt JW. Pharmacotherapy of xerostomia in primary Sjogren's syndrome. Pharmacotherapy 2002;22:621–629.
53. Gorsky M, Silverman SJ, Chinn H. Burning mouth syndrome: Review of 98 cases. J Oral Med 1987;42:7–9.
54. Grushka M, Epstein JB, Gorsky M. Burning mouth syndrome. Am Fam Physician 2002;65:615–620.
55. Quinn JH. Glossodynia. J Am Dent Assoc 1965;70:1418–1421.
56. Brennan MT, Shariff G, Lockhart PB, Fox PC. Treatment of xerostomia: A systematic review of therapeutic trials. Dent Clin North Am 2002;46:847–856.
57. Guijarro Guijarro B, Lopez Sanchez AF, Hernandez Vallejo G. Treatment of xerostomia. A review. Med Oral 2001;6:7–18.
58. Daniels TE. Evaluation, differential diagnosis, and treatment of xerostomia. J Rheumatol Suppl 2000;61:6–10.
59. Weiss WW, Brenman HS, Katz P, Bennett JA. Use of an electric stimulator for the treatment of dry mouth. J Oral Maxillofac Surg 1986;44:845–850.

11

Pains of Dental Origin

In a survey of 45,711 American households, Lipton et al[1] found that nearly 22% of the general population experienced at least one of five types of orofacial pain in the previous 6 months. The most common type of orofacial pain was toothache, which was reported by 12.2% of the population. Because toothache is so common, it is essential for the clinician who is managing orofacial pain to have a thorough understanding of its clinical presentation. Once the proper diagnosis is established, treatment for pains of dental origin is usually quite reliable.

The teeth are unique structures in that they are visceral tissues that function as part of the musculoskeletal system. This, perhaps, helps to explain some of the enigmatic behavior of dental pain. Tooth pulps serve as isolated organs, each an individual in its own right. The sensory capability of dental pulpal tissue is like that of other visceral structures, and pulpal pain is like other visceral pains. The connection of the tooth to the bone, however, is a true joint and therefore constitutes a musculoskeletal structure. This fibrous joint, called the *periodontal ligament,* is constructed in such a manner as to convert masticatory pressure into traction on the alveolar bone. These joints, termed *gomphoses,* are structurally similar to other fibrous joints in which traction forces predominate. The mechanoreceptors in periodontal ligaments are similar to those of other fibrous joints, although they differ considerably from the proprioceptors found in synovial joint ligaments, tendons, and muscles.[2] Their nerve cell bodies are located in the mesencephalon, along with the other masticatory proprioceptors. They serve to inhibit the action of elevator muscles, which constitutes the driving force of masticatory function.[3–5] The uniqueness of teeth and their alveolar attachment is that visceral structures function as an integral segment of the musculoskeletal system. The sensory behavior, including dental pain, constitutes a mixture of visceral and musculoskeletal characteristics (Fig 11-1).

It should be noted that while sensory input from the face is represented almost exclusively in the subnucleus caudalis, nociceptive signals from the oral cavity have double representation in the subnucleus oralis and caudalis.[6] Periodontal afferent fibers terminate in the rostrally located main sensory trigeminal nucleus. The tooth pulp afferents, however, terminate there, as

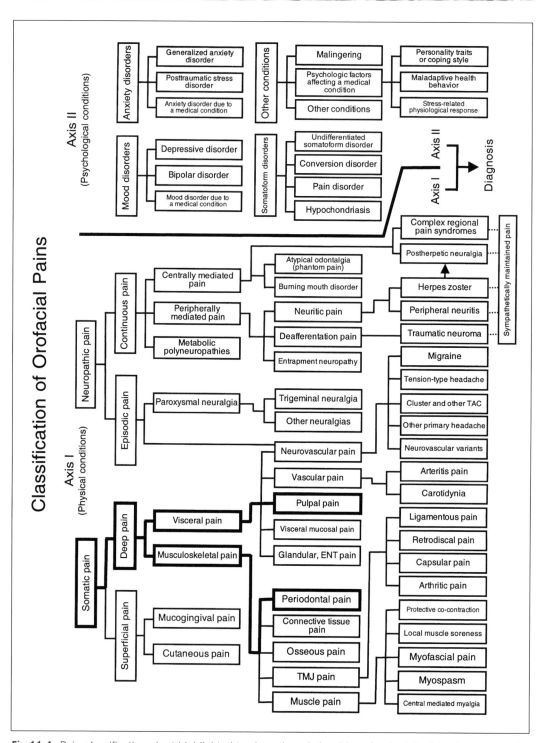

Fig 11-1 Pain classification chart highlighted to show the relationships of pulpal dental pain to other visceral pains and of periodontal dental pain to other musculoskeletal pains.

well as in all three subnuclei of the spinal tract of the trigeminal nucleus complex.[7]

Dentin sensibility is mediated by way of the pulpal nerves. The intradental neural mechanism of this innervation is not yet known. Several theories have been offered: (1) the odontoblast-receptor theory, (2) the direct nerve ending theory, and (3) the hydrodynamic theory.[8] It is known that many if not all nociceptive impulses from human dental pulps are conducted to the trigeminal nucleus by way of sympathetic visceral afferents that leave the head and reach the spinal cord through elements of the cervical sympathetic chain and upper thoracic spinal nerves.[9]

The unique innervation of teeth is pointed out by the report of two cancer patients who had undergone trigeminal tractotomy along with rhizotomy of the 9th and 10th cranial nerves and of several cervical spinal nerves to control intractable face pain. Both patients displayed analgesia or hypalgesia throughout the cutaneous trigeminal distribution; yet they continued to maintain normal sensory response to dental pulp stimulation.[10]

The sensory capabilities of the dental pulp are predominantly but not exclusively nociceptive.[11] The dental pulp also senses thermal stimuli and tingling.[12] It has been determined that, under specially controlled circumstances, pulpal receptors may give rise to nonnociceptive impulses that have some sensory function other than the mediation of painful sensation.[13] It is thought that nonpainful sensations of the pulp are mediated by a distinct population of afferents that are nonnociceptive.[14] The pulp contains both fast and slowly conducting neurons.[15] There is conclusive evidence for the presence of a significant C-fiber population in tooth pulps that can be activated by electrical stimulation.[16] The innervation density of the dental pulp is calculated to be about 15 times that of skin.[17] The mediation of sensory impulses from the dental pulp to the subnucleus caudalis, as well as

to the more rostrally located subnucleus oralis, has been confirmed.[18,19]

The teeth are united to the alveolar bone by fibrous joints, the periodontal ligaments comprising the flexible, fibrous portions. The collagenous fibers that connect the cementum to the alveolar cortex are arranged in an oblique fashion so as to convert the pressures of mastication into traction forces on the bone. The sensory receptors include free nerve endings and mechanoreceptors. When stimulated by pressure on the tooth, the mechanoreceptors exert an inhibitory influence on masticatory elevator muscle action.[20,21] This response is known as the *nociceptive reflex*. It should be noted that sensory innervation of the teeth is strictly ipsilateral.[22] Except for pain emanating from midface structures, sensory manifestations from the oral cavity are not expressed contralaterally or bilaterally.

Behavior of Dental Pains

It should be recognized that dental pains are extremely versatile and have the propensity to mimic nearly any pain disorder. The degree of such pain may vary from mild tenderness to unbearable intensity. Dental pain may be spontaneous, or it may be induced in various ways. It can be intermittent, with periods between attacks that are completely free of pain. It may be continuous but punctuated by lancinating exacerbations that radiate throughout the face and head. The extreme variability of toothache is such that a good rule for any examiner is to consider all pains about the mouth and face to be of dental origin until proven otherwise. An adequate dental examination is the essential first step in the management of all pain disorders involving the teeth, mouth, and face.

In spite of such variability, pains of dental origin present clinical features that categorize them as deep somatic pain. It is on the basis of these features that the examiner is able to clinically classify such pains.

Quality of Pain

The basic background discomfort of odontogenous pain is a dull, depressing quality characteristic of all pain that emanates from deep body structures. This feature should not be confused with pain intensity or its temporal behavior.

Dental pain is usually described as an aching, sometimes throbbing sensation. When mild, it may be felt only as tenderness or soreness. When severe, it may have a burning quality. The basic background aching pain may be punctuated by momentary, repeated lancinating pains that radiate widely. Such effects are not true paroxysms but rather short, sudden exacerbations of otherwise steady pain. Dental pains may occur spontaneously or be induced by a variety of stimuli, such as thermal changes, contact with sweets and other foods and liquids, or by touch or pressure. Dental pains may be momentary or protracted. They may be continuous or intermittent.

Localization

Pain arising solely from the dental pulp is often very poorly localized by the patient. Frequently it is difficult for the patient to determine whether the offending tooth is mandibular or maxillary, much less which tooth is involved. The pain is felt diffusely in the teeth, jaws, face, and head.

Pain arising from the periodontal structures, however, is quite readily localized by the patient, especially when the offending tooth is touched or pressed. This feature may be in addition to otherwise widespread diffuse pain throughout the jaws and face and may require diagnostic manipulation. It is not unusual for the patient to question the validity of locating the offending tooth when he or she feels the pain so diffusely elsewhere. In fact, the patient may be mistaken as to which tooth is being pressed by the examiner. However, localization from periodontal receptors is accurate enough to make this a dependable means of diagnosis.

Localization of odontogenous pain depends on whether the pain emanates solely from pulpal or periodontal sources or from both.

Relationship of Dental Pain to Initiating Stimulus

The relationship between dental pain and noxious stimulation is accurate in that summation effects are not observed. Since pulpal receptors answer all noxious stimulation as pain, there may be considerable variation in threshold levels for different types of stimulation, such as thermal, electrical, and mechanical. Subthreshold stimulation is painless. The apparent delay between application of the irritant and pain reaction is not central summation, as seen in neuralgia, but rather represents the time required for the stimulation to reach threshold level.

Although accurate, the relationship between stimulus and pain reaction is not necessarily proportional. A moderate stimulus may induce pain that is disproportionate to it. Thus, the discomfort incurred does not indicate the seriousness of its cause.

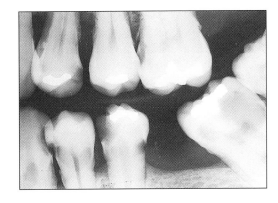

Fig 11-2 Radiograph showing rampant caries and extensive periodontal disease. Such a situation presents several possible causes of odontogenous pain, both pulpal and periodontal.

Types of Dental Pains

Dental pains may have their origin in the dental pulps or in the periodontal structures. These two categories will be discussed separately, since their clinical presentations are different.

Dental Pains of Pulpal Origin

The visceral character of pulpal pain is displayed particularly in its clinical behavior. The pain is of the threshold type, as compared with the graduated response exhibited by musculoskeletal pain. No response occurs until the threshold level is reached. Pulpal pain responds to noxious stimulation that is unrelated to ordinary masticatory movements. It responds to impact, shock, thermal and chemical irritants, and direct exploration, but not to ordinary masticatory function. The pain is often very difficult for the patient to localize.

Pulpal pains may be classified as acute, chronic, recurrent, or mixed with periodontal elements. A basic clinical feature of pulpal pain is that it does not remain the same indefinitely. Generally it resolves, becomes chronic, or proceeds to involve the periodontal structures by direct extension through the apex of the tooth root. Rarely does it remain unchanged for long periods.

Acute pulpal pain

Perhaps the most typical of all visceral pains is *acute pulpal pain*. It is often so difficult for the patient to localize that the patient may not be very helpful in determining the source of the pain. Objective evidence such as deep caries, erosion into the pulp chamber or root canal, or fracture or splitting may immediately identify the offending tooth. If such evidence is lacking, and especially if more than a single tooth might be involved (Fig 11-2), clinical identification of the offending tooth may be difficult, if not impossible.

The cause of acute pulpal pain is noxious stimulation of the pulpal receptors. Normally, the tooth structure protects these nerve endings from superficial stimulation, so that only extreme surface irritation such as electric stimulation or excessive thermal change is sensed as pain. If the tooth structure is breached by splitting, a normal pulp may immediately become painful on contact with saliva or air. This occurs especially when masticatory stress tends to open the split. If the tooth structure is breached by fracture of a submerged metallic filling, pain results from pressure exerted against the pulp and is increased when additional pressure is brought to bear on the filling by biting against it. Until the pulp becomes inflamed, pain from such cause is intermittent.

The pulp tissue responds to injury, whether it be from repeated threshold stimulation of the intact surface, cervical exposure due to gingival recession, repeated irritation of occlusal trauma, breaching of the overlying protective tooth structure due to splitting or fracture, repeated thermal shocks transmitted by metallic fillings, thinning of the overlying tooth structure by erosion or abrasion, traumatic shock, or dental caries. The changes that take place are usually inflammatory. These conditions may be reversible unless congestion occurs and causes pulpal necrosis or gangrene. Once tissue death occurs, extension to the periodontal tissue through the apical foramen of the root almost invariably takes place. This is especially so if the pulpal inflammation is the result of bacterial agents. It should be noted that in multirooted teeth irreversible pulpal changes may occur in one root with reasonably normal pulp tissue surviving in another root. Situations of this type may not occur frequently, but when they do, a confusing symptom picture may result.

It is crucial to understand the pulpal pains that result from such tissue changes. As a rule, the pain threshold of all deep receptors and nerve fibers that mediate pain is lowered by inflammation. Thus, the inflamed dental pulp is hypersensitive to all stimuli, including electric stimulation, thermal shock, probing, and percussion. Pain may be elicited by the application of some or all such stimuli to the tooth. If the tissue change is not too great, application of such stimuli causes pain only for the duration of the noxious stimulation. But if the change is greater, such stimulation may induce a prolonged toothache. As the inflammatory process progresses, spontaneous toothache may occur with no outside provocation.

Acute pulpal pain may range from occasional hypersensitivity caused by sweets and other minor stimulants to spontaneous, violent, throbbing toothache of intolerable intensity that cannot be controlled even with narcotic analgesics. It may be induced by many types of irritants or be wholly spontaneous. It may be increased by both heat and cold or increased by heat and relieved by cold. It may be intermittent or continuous. It may relate to the contact of teeth or to the presence or temperature of foods and beverages. It may be mistaken for sinus headache, sinusitis, earache, neuritis, trigeminal neuralgia, or atypical facial pain. It may induce referred pains, areas of secondary hyperalgesia almost anywhere in the face and head, localized autonomic symptoms, and secondary painful masticatory muscle co-contraction. It may induce a masticatory muscle disorder or be mistaken for temporomandibular joint arthritis. If the pulpal inflammation is great enough to cause severe, continuing toothache, the chance of resolution is extremely low. Under favorable circumstances, resolution does occur. Usually the condition progresses to pulpal necrosis. When this occurs, pain from the pulpal tissue ceases. Such "recovery" from severe toothache should be interpreted as the transition period from pulpal to periodontal involvement. This transition is extremely variable. If the pulpal inflammation is the result of infection, the transition is usually rapid and consists of mixed pulpal and periodontal pains at first, terminating as an acute periodontal abscess (Fig 11-3). If the pulpal inflammation is sterile, all pain may cease, and a painless periapical granuloma or radicular cyst may develop (Fig 11-4). All gradations between these extremes may occur. If a multirooted tooth is involved, one root may exhibit symptoms of acute pulpitis, whereas another may show evidence of pulpal necrosis and periapical abscess (Fig 11-5). When this occurs, the symptom picture can become very confusing.

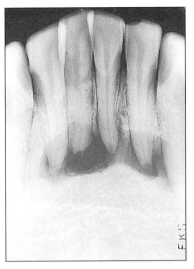

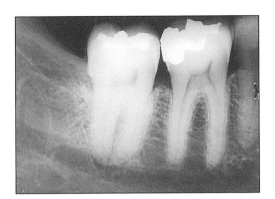

Fig 11-3 Radiograph showing early periapical radiolucent change at the mandibular second molar indicative of periapical abscess. This tooth was split mesiodistally and had elicited recurrent acute pulpal pains on several occasions. As the periapical tissues became involved, both pulpal and periodontal pain could be identified. Early in its clinical course, the first molar was suspected because of its large amalgam restoration.

Fig 11-4 Radiograph showing an extensive apical radiolucency involving the mandibular anterior teeth. The four incisors were slightly discolored and nonresponsive to thermal and electric stimulation. The condition was painless. The history was that of former trauma and acute pulpal pain that soon subsided.

Fig 11-5 Radiograph showing periapical radiolucent change involving the mesial root of the mandibular first molar tooth. Clinical symptoms were those of typical pulpal pain and acute periodontal pain occurring simultaneously in the tooth.

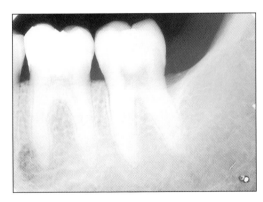

Chronic pulpal pain

Under certain conditions, injured pulpal tissue may progress from an acute to a chronic inflammatory phase and thus undergo changes that proceed neither to resolution nor to necrosis but remain indefinitely as what is usually described as *chronic pulpitis.* The condition that favors this transition is traumatic injury to a young tooth, especially one with an open, expansive root end that is less likely to facilitate conges-

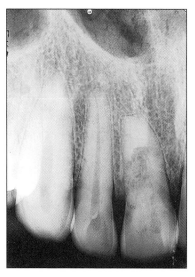

Fig 11-6 Radiograph showing central radiolucency in the maxillary central incisor that is indicative of internal resorption. The tooth had a normal color and responded positively to electric pulp testing but considerably less than the adjacent teeth. The patient was a 32-year-old man. There was history of trauma to his tooth 16 years previously, followed by a "toothache" that promptly subsided. Presently the tooth is asymptomatic.

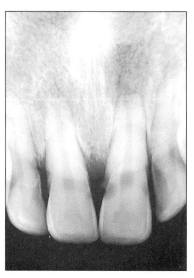

Fig 11-7 Radiograph showing apical and periapical radiolucency of the maxillary central incisors. Both had a normal color and responded positively to electric pulp testing but considerably less so than the adjacent teeth. Both teeth, especially the right incisor, were described as vaguely uncomfortable but not painful.

tion and necrosis of the pulp. Such teeth continue to respond to pulp testing, although they are considerably less responsive than those with normal pulps. Frequently, internal resorption of the tooth occurs (Fig 11-6).

When chronic pulpitis develops, the pain responses change from the extremely variable character of acute pulpal pain to a milder and less variable discomfort, which may not be described as pain at all (Fig 11-7). In fact, the tooth may become asymptomatic unless further injury to it takes place.

Recurrent pulpal pain

Severe acute pulpal pain is rarely recurrent in the true sense because the inflammation usually progresses either to resolution, chronicity, or necrosis. When acute pulpal pain appears to be recurrent, it usually consists of recurring periods of inflammation in a sequential pattern. This may occur when a partially split tooth is opened only by some unusual occlusal stress. Ordinarily, true *recurrent pulpal pain* does not cause a toothache but is sensed as recurrent hypersensitivity. Such conditions are frequently associated with changes in vascular pressure or fluid balance. So-called menstrual toothache and high-altitude toothache fall into this category. The offending tooth is usually slightly inflamed, and the lowered pain threshold becomes symptomatic when the proper environmental conditions prevail. Other instances of recurrent pulpal pain include hypersensitive teeth that are

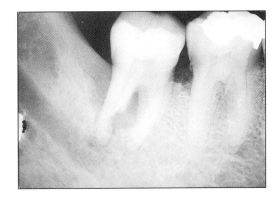

Fig 11-8 Radiograph showing periodontal radiolucency involving the distal root of the mandibular second molar tooth. There is extensive interradicular involvement and deep surface resorption into the mesial aspect of the distal root. Clinically, the tooth had symptoms indicative of a chronic periodontal abscess, with more recent symptoms of acute pulpitis. The tooth was responsive to electric pulp testing.

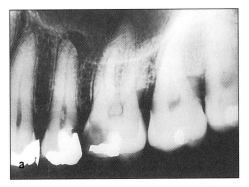
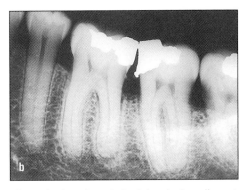

Fig 11-9 Radiographs showing reasonable cause for pulpal and periodontal pain in adjacent teeth. (a) The maxillary second premolar shows periapical radiolucency; the first molar has extensive dental caries. (b) There is evidence of recurrent caries beneath the mesial filling in the mandibular second molar; the distal root of the first molar shows slight but definite periapical involvement.

stimulated to the point of pain by such factors as sweets, thermal changes, and occlusal abuse.

When the transition from pulpal inflammation through necrosis to periapical involvement is rapid, symptoms of both pulpal and periodontal pain may occur. Conversely, when the dental pulp becomes secondarily involved by direct extension from the periodontal structures, mixed symptoms may be evident (Fig 11-8). Also, especially as a result of trauma, both pulpal and periodontal symptoms may occur simultaneously. In all such instances, the cause is usually obvious and the symptoms readily explained. However, a tooth can present with pulpal and periodontal symptoms arising from separate and independent causes, in which case the symptom picture may be confusing. This can occur especially in multirooted teeth. Also, nearby teeth may be simultaneously involved and have symptoms that are misleading to examiner and patient alike (Figs 11-9a and 11-9b).

Obscure causes of pulpal pain

There are several fairly common causes of pulpal pain that are clinically difficult to recognize. Perhaps the most common of these is the mesiodistally split tooth, the

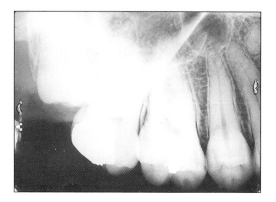

Fig 11-10 Radiograph of an impacted maxillary third molar that had abraded into the root of the second molar. The patient presented with symptoms of acute pulpal pain emanating from the second molar. The tooth was sacrificed. The abraded area involved the nerve canal of the distobuccal root.

margins of which are obscured by adjacent teeth and the presence of which is not radiographically visible. Another common cause is an occlusal filling that is slightly dislodged in a pulpal direction. Recurrent caries obscured both clinically and radiographically by an overlying dental restoration may be the etiologic factor. Still another cause is mechanical abrasion of the root of a tooth due to the presence of an adjacent impacted tooth (Fig 11-10). Abrasions can penetrate the substance of the root until the contents of the root canal are exposed. Another very obscure cause of pulpal involvement is direct extension from a periodontal pocket via an aberrant lateral root canal. Hematogenous infection of the dental pulp has been reported.

All such possibilities should be considered and explored when pain appears to be truly odontogenous but the cause is obscure. Occasionally, direct exploration of the tooth is justified if the pain is severe and the patient is unwilling to wait for natural localization. The risk of opening an innocent dental pulp may be justified to establish a positive diagnosis. This is better than the more radical approach, for example, of extraction of such a tooth on a presumptive diagnosis. At least with the former treatment, endodontic measures can be used to salvage the tooth if a mistake is made.

Identification of pulpal pain

The examiner should suspect pain as being of pulpal origin when it is difficult for the patient to precisely localize it to a certain tooth. A thorough dental examination becomes mandatory. Obvious possible sources of the pulpal pain should be investigated first. This would include such conditions as primary caries, recurrent caries, defective fillings, cervical exposure, erosion, abrasion, split or fractured teeth, and deep or massive dental restorations, as indicated by clinical and radiographic findings. When a suspicious tooth is located, an attempt to induce or increase the pain by noxious stimulation of that tooth by chemical, thermal, mechanical, or electric irritants should be made. If pain is induced by application of heat to the tooth, cold should be applied to see whether the pain is relieved. The examiner should carefully isolate the tooth with celluloid strips when applying thermal or electric irritants to prevent conduction to an adjacent tooth, especially if contacting metallic fillings are present. If the pain can be influenced by local irritation, the tooth should be anesthetized locally to see whether anesthesia promptly and completely arrests the pain and prevents stimulation by applied irritants. If such is the case, the offending tooth has been satisfactorily identified.

Fig 11-11 Radiograph of extensive dental caries involving the maxillary second molar distally. The patient presented with symptoms of acute pulpal pain without evident clinical cause. Although extensive, the caries lesion was obscured clinically by the third molar.

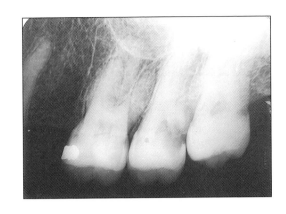

When there are no clues about which tooth is the source of pain (if indeed it is a tooth at all), the examiner is obliged to be suspicious of every tooth on the side on which there is pain, both maxillary and mandibular. Each tooth should be tested by inspection, probing, palpation, percussion, thermal shock, and electric stimulation to determine whether one tooth is considerably more responsive than others. Systematic analgesic blocking should be done, first to determine whether the pain site is maxillary or mandibular and then to more accurately identify the offending tooth or teeth.

Broad conclusions can be drawn as to whether the pain arises from maxillary or mandibular structures. If analgesic blocking fails to arrest the pain promptly and completely for the duration of anesthesia, a conclusion that the pain does not arise from dental structures is justified. If such blocking is accurately effective, the conclusion that the pain is initiated in structures thus anesthetized is usually correct, but it does not necessarily follow that the pain is in fact odontogenous.

If the pain is shown to arise from the dental area but a particular tooth cannot be identified as the offending source, it is wise to wait for pain localization to occur through the process of transition from pulpal to periodontal pain, as previously discussed. Eventually, localized tenderness should identify the proper tooth, probably within a few days or weeks.

Radiographic examination does not identify the source of pulpal pain, other than to give clues as to its cause (Fig 11-11). Electric pulp testing has value when it is performed along with other forms of pulpal stimulation but has very limited value by itself. The history, descriptive characteristics, and clinical behavior are extremely important in the diagnosis of pulpal pain. Recognition of secondary excitatory effects is essential, and the importance of an understanding of how such effects relate to the primary pain source cannot be overemphasized. This is especially true regarding secondary painful muscle spasms.

Dental Pains of Periodontal Origin

Periodontal pain is deep somatic pain of the musculoskeletal type. As such, it is more localized than is pulpal (visceral) pain. It is intimately related to biomechanical (masticatory) function. It responds to provocation proportionately and in graduated increments, rather than as a threshold response like pulpal pain.

The receptors of the periodontal ligament are capable of rather precise localiza-

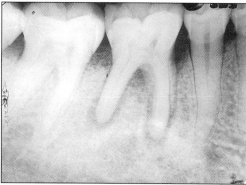

Fig 11-12 Radiograph of the mandibular first molar showing extensive radiolucency around the tooth roots. The tooth was in "traumatic" occlusion.

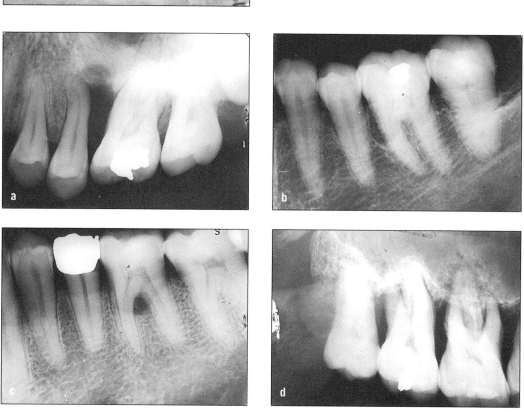

Fig 11-13 Radiographs showing periodontal lesions of various types. (a) Deep periodontal pocket associated with elongation of the maxillary second premolar. (b) Buccally located periodontal lesion involving the mandibular first molar. (c) Interradicular lesion involving the mandibular first molar. (d) Extensive generalized periodontal disease.

tion of the stimulus. Therefore, periodontal pains of all types rarely present any real diagnostic problem, because the proper offending tooth is readily identified. This is true whether the pain is in the apical area of the periodontal ligament (usually designated as *periapical pain*) or in the lateral region of the tooth. This ability of the periodontal receptors to accurately localize the pain source characterizes all periodontal

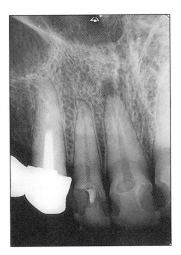

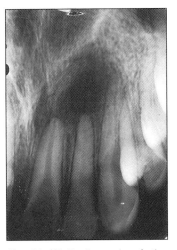

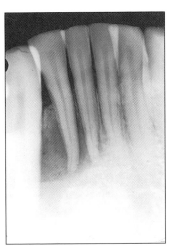

Fig 11-14 Radiograph showing periapical radiolucency involving the maxillary central incisor. This condition followed pulpal inflammation.

Fig 11-15 Radiograph of the maxillary incisor area showing diffuse radiolucency centered around the incisors. The central and lateral incisors had been injured several years before.

Fig 11-16 Radiograph of the mandibular incisor area showing diffuse radiolucency due to a spreading osseous infection.

pains and prevents the uncertainty and mystery associated with acute pulpal pains, as previously discussed.

Such localization is identified by application of pressure to the tooth laterally or axially. Under the load of occlusal pressure during chewing, the tooth feels sore or elongated. The discomfort may sometimes be felt when the biting pressure is released, rather than while it is sustained. Lateral or axial pressure may be applied to the tooth by the examiner as part of the clinical examination.

The causes of periodontal pain are many and varied. It may occur as a primary periodontal inflammatory condition arising from a local cause such as trauma, occlusal overloading (Fig 11-12), or contact with an adjacent embedded tooth. Pain may occur as a result of dental prophylaxis, endodontic treatment, orthodontic therapy, preparation and manipulation of teeth for restoration, inadequate opposing occlusal contact, occlusal interference, overcon-

toured or undercontoured proximal contact points, stresses applied to abutment teeth, and surgical interference of all types. It may result from a spreading inflammatory reaction incidental to nearby trauma or the healing of surgical wounds. It may occur as an acute inflammation of a preexisting chronic periodontal lesion as a result of infection, injury, food impaction, or lowered resistance (Figs 11-13a to 11-13d). It may spread from pulpal inflammation, either directly through the apical root canal to cause a typical periapical abscess (Fig 11-14), or through an aberrant lateral root canal to cause a lateral periodontal abscess. It may occur by direct extension from a nearby inflammatory condition involving an adjacent tooth (Fig 11-15), the maxillary antrum, or a spreading osseous infection (Fig 11-16).

When the periodontal pain involves several teeth, especially opposing teeth, the matter of occlusal overloading should be considered. This may occur with little or no evidence of gross disease. Overloading may occur not only from unusually heavy occlusal contacts during mandibular movements, but also from clenching or bruxism.

With multirooted teeth, one root may be periapically or periodontally involved, while another shows symptoms of pulpal pain. These circumstances can certainly confuse the clinician. Sometimes the location of the electrode of the pulp tester on the tooth may give some indication of the conditions present.[23] Radiographic evidence may add confirmation.

Tooth Pain from Deficient Central Inhibition

All conditions that alter the effectiveness of the endogenous antinociceptive system may permit ordinarily nonnociceptive impulses to be transmitted and felt as pain. As a result, teeth may become unduly sensitive or actually painful. They may hurt when touched, moved, pressed, stressed through occlusal use, or subjected to stimulants such as toothbrushing, flossing, thermal changes, or ingestion of sweets. In such situations, many or all of the teeth may become painful. Multiple toothaches without adequate local dental cause should be a warning sign. When this occurs, it is also common for the patient to complain of allodynia in other surrounding tissues, such as the gingiva, buccal mucosa, muscles, and the temporomandibular joints. Diffuse and generalized pain should always lead the clinician to thoughts of central pain mechanisms.

Secondary Effects of Dental Pain

Because it is of the deep somatic variety, odontogenous pain has the propensity to induce a variety of secondary central excitatory effects. Most acute dental pains have a component of pain that is felt in one or more adjacent teeth of the same arch, in teeth of the opposing arch, or in both. Ordinarily, such heterotopic pain does not cross the midline, except when the site of primary pain is located at or close to the midline. Reference to another major division of the trigeminal nerve usually follows a vertical laminated pattern, as discussed in chapter 4. Referred dental pain is frequently felt as a headache. It may be felt in the orbital and frontal area, in the maxillary sinus region, in the auricular and preauricular areas, or throughout the face. Sometimes, an acute pulpitis will cause pain that radiates throughout the entire face and head, with no subjective localization of the primary site at all. The variable, spontaneous, nonlocalized, and pulsatile qualities of acute pulpal pain together with its secondary effects can imitate almost every known pain disorder of the face and head.

Secondary hyperalgesia is also a common manifestation of dental pain. It may be expressed superficially as an area of sensitive gingiva, skin, or scalp. It may be felt as other tender teeth. Deep secondary hyperalgesia sensed as palpable tenderness may be misdiagnosed as an area of inflammation or muscle tenderness. This is likely to involve the temporal and masseter areas especially.

It is not unusual for dental pain to induce secondary autonomic effects, expressed as nasal congestion, lacrimation, and puffy swelling of the eyelids or other areas of loose facial skin. Such symptoms may be misdiagnosed as sinusitis or cellulitis.

A myalgia originating in muscles innervated by the trigeminal nerve may be induced by dental pain. Such involvement of digastric or mylohyoid muscles may cause symptoms in the floor of the mouth and upper cervical region. If the tensor palatini muscle is involved, palatal soreness, difficulty with swallowing, and eustachian tube symptoms may occur. If the masticatory muscles are involved, a masticatory muscle disorder may result (chapter 12). It should be noted that if such a secondarily induced muscle condition develops into a cycling muscle pain, it becomes wholly independent of the initiating cause and can remain as a separate clinical entity long after the etiologic factor has disappeared. This will be discussed in detail in chapter 12.

Perhaps the most confusing complication of dental pain is the induction of myofascial trigger points in muscles innervated by the trigeminal nerve. Such trigger points tend to remain after the initiating pain has disappeared. As such, they can cause an orofacial complaint for long periods, sometimes in a recurrent, episodic pattern. It should be noted that the zone of reference from such a trigger point frequently is at or near the location of the primary pain that initiated it. Thus, continuing pain at the "toothache site" may be experienced, despite adequate dental therapy for the original cause of pain. Clear diagnostic thinking and skillful use of examination techniques may be required to resolve such issues.

Tender Teeth from Nondental Cause

Stimulation-evoked tooth pain that simulates pain of periodontal origin may occur as the result of deep somatic pain input located elsewhere in the trigeminal area. This manifestation of secondary hyperalgesia is a central excitatory effect. It differs from spontaneous toothache due to referred pain in that it is provoked by manipulation or functional activities. As such, it is localized and can be confused with true odontogenous pain of periodontal origin, from which it should be differentiated.

Secondary hyperalgesia expressed as "tender teeth" is commonplace. It occurs

with pharyngeal and nasal mucosa pains in particular. Similar phenomena, however, occur with other dental pains, especially those of pulpitis.

The differential diagnosis depends chiefly on a failure to find an adequate local dental cause. Confirmation may be done by analgesic blocking of the site of pain. Primary periodontal pain is arrested, while secondary hyperalgesic pain is not.

Toothaches of Nondental Origin

Since dental pain is such a common cause of orofacial pain, the clinician can be easily drawn to this diagnosis. This is especially true when the patient convincingly reports that the pain is felt in a particular tooth. It is a frustrating experience for both the patient and the clinician when toothache continues long after sound dental therapy has been completed. It is not uncommon to hear patients report a history of multiple endodontic procedures followed by an extraction, with no reduction of pain. This type of experience is quite humbling to the dental clinician, who is expected to be successful in managing dental pains. The clinician needs to be aware that some pains felt in the teeth do not originate from the dental structures.

There are many structures of the head and neck that can produce heterotopic pains felt in the teeth. These heterotopic pains occur as secondary effects from central sensitization or excitation of the second-order neurons produced by a constant barrage of nociceptive input from deep structures (see chapter 4). As with any heterotopic pain, this poses a diagnostic problem for the clinician. The patient's chief complaint is toothache, but the origin of the pain lies elsewhere. The clinician must have the diagnostic skills to be able to differentiate the site of pain from the source of pain. As discussed in earlier chapters, heterotopic pains are differentiated by local provocation and by the selective use of local anesthetic. The four clinical rules presented in chapter 8 need to be reviewed here as they relate to toothache. It is extremely important that the dental practitioner is able to adequately differentiate an odontogenic toothache from a nonodontogenic toothache, since therapy demands it. Dentists are likely the only clinicians who can do this and therefore it is basic to helping the patient.

The following four rules will assist the clinician in differentiating primary pain (a dental toothache) from a referred pain (nonodontogenic toothache):

1. Local provocation of the site of pain does not increase the pain. If the toothache is the primary source of pain, then provocation of the toothache should increase the pain (Fig 11-17a), ie, if the clinician places hot or cold on the tooth or has the patient bite on the tooth, one would expect the pain to be increased. This is not the case with a nonodontogenic toothache. Since the source of the toothache is not the same as the site, local provocation of the toothache (the site) will not change the pain. A lack of response to local provocation should make the clinician suspicious of a heterotopic toothache.

2. Local provocation of the source of pain increases the pain, not only at the source but also at the site. When a toothache is suspected to be only a pain site and not a source, the true source needs to be identified to establish the diagnosis and provide effective treatment. Sometimes this can be found relatively easily, such as with myofascial trigger point pain. Once a trigger point is found, it can be provoked and the patient asked if he or she feels the pain anywhere else (Fig 11-17b). Often the patient will report pain not only in the area of palpation (the

trigger point) but also radiating to the site of pain (the tooth). This clinical finding helps confirm that the toothache is a heterotopic pain, and management should be directed to the myofascial pain condition and not the tooth. As will be discussed later in this section, some sources of pain that produce nonodontogenic toothache are not easily located and/or palpated. In these instances, this rule is difficult to clinically demonstrate. Instead, the history should be used to gather this information. Asking the patient to identify any conditions that exacerbate the toothache can be very valuable in identifying the true source of pain. Also, understanding the characteristics of the pain (eg, quality, duration, onset) will give the clinician insight as to the etiology of the pain source (see chapter 7).

3. Local anesthetic blocking of the site of pain does not decrease the pain. Local anesthetic blocking is a very valuable tool in identifying the source of toothache and well within the practice of every dental clinician. When a toothache is the primary source of pain, anesthetizing the tooth will immediately eliminate the pain. When this occurs, the clinician needs to identify the local cause of nociception (pulpal/periodontal) and provide the appropriate dental treatment. However, when local anesthesia fails to eliminate the toothache, heterotopic pain should be suspected (Fig 11-17c). The clinician needs to be careful, however, as to how he or she asks the patient about the pain after anesthesia. Often the therapist will ask the patient if he is "numb." This will not provide the needed information, because of course the patient is numb; the tooth and adjacent soft tissues are anesthetized. The proper question should be, "Now, I know you are numb, but does it still hurt?" This is a different question and more directed to the information needed to make the di-

Fig 11-17 The four important clinical rules that help differentiate odontogenic toothache from nonodontogenic toothache.

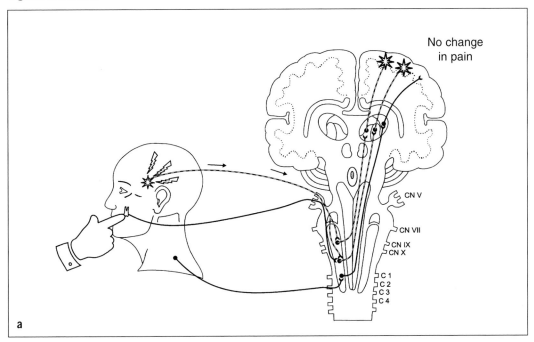

No change
in pain

a

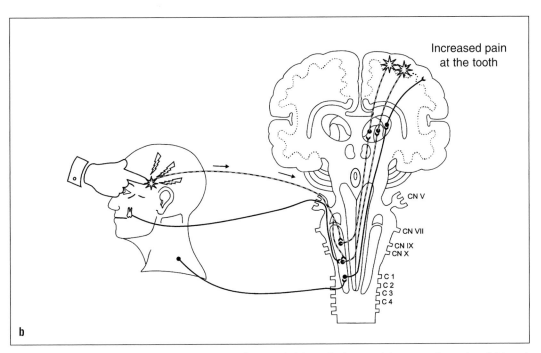

Increased pain
at the tooth

b

Fig 11-17a to 11-17b *(a)* Local provocation of the painful tooth does not increase the pain. *(b)* Local provocation of the source of the pain (a myofascial trigger point in the temporalis muscle) increases the pain, not only at the source but also at the site (increasing the tooth pain).

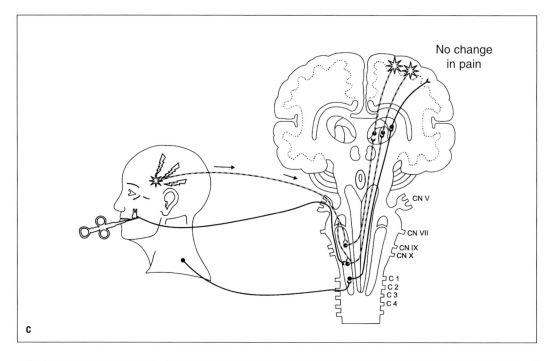

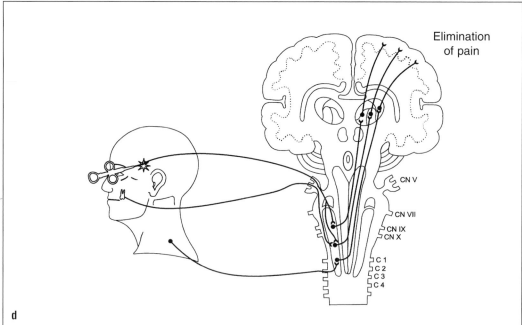

Fig 11-17c to 11-17d (c) Local anesthesia of the site of pain (the painful tooth) does not decrease the pain. (d) Local anesthesia of the source of the pain (the temporalis trigger point) decreases the pain not only at the source but at the site (tooth pain is eliminated).

agnosis. When the patient says "Yes, I am very numb, but it still hurts," the clinician can be certain that the anesthetized tissues are not the structures that need to be treated to resolve the pain. Local anesthesia is basic to differentiating dental pain and should be used whenever there is any question regarding the location of the source of pain.

4. Local anesthetic blocking of the source of the pain decreases the pain at the source as well as the site. When anesthetizing the tooth does not stop the toothache, then the true source of the pain needs to be identified. In instances when the true source is found (as with myofascial trigger points), the source should be anesthetized (trigger point injection). Anesthesia of the true source will eliminate not only the source of pain but also the site (Fig 11-17d), and the toothache will immediately resolve. When this occurs the clinician has identified the true source of the toothache and therapy needs to be directed at treating this source.

Heterotopic toothache is a relatively common finding in a dental practice. Only after the location of the source of pain can effective therapy begin. Although many structures of the face can refer to the teeth, certain structures are more common sources of pain and should be immediately investigated. Common heterotopic toothaches that will be reviewed in this section are: muscular toothache, neurovascular toothache, cardiac toothache, neuropathic toothache, sinus toothache, and psychogenic toothache. Familiarity with the pain characteristics of each of these disorders is an essential key to diagnosis. Each of these pain disorders will be discussed in detail in later chapters. They are mentioned here to remind the clinician that they may be a source of toothache.

Muscular toothache

Although all deep pains in the head and neck have the propensity to induce secondary referred pain felt as toothache, those of muscular origin are the most common. The masseter and temporalis muscles are the chief offenders and not uncommonly refer pain to the teeth. The clinical characteristics of a muscular toothache are as follows:

1. The pain is relatively constant, dull, aching, and nonpulsatile.
2. The pain is not responsive to local provocation of the tooth.
3. Examination reveals the presence of localized firm, hypersensitive bands within the muscle tissues (trigger points).
4. Other heterotopic pains are often reported (eg, "tension-type" headache).
5. The toothache is increased with function of the involved muscle (trigger points).
6. Palpation and provocation of the trigger points increase the toothache.
7. Local anesthesia of the tooth does not affect the toothache.
8. Local anesthesia of the involved muscle (trigger points) reduces the toothache.

A good understanding of the muscular genesis of pain and of the overall behavior of musculoskeletal pain disorders is prerequisite to good management of such toothache complaints (Case 1). Muscle pain disorders will be discussed in detail in chapter 12.

Neurovascular toothache

Migraines, both with and without aura, may cause pain that is felt as a toothache. Usually no management problem arises because such headaches are readily diagnosed, and additional pains about the face and mouth cause little concern on the part of patient or clinician.

Case 1 Heterotopic pain, felt as toothache, referred from the masseter muscle

Chief Complaint   Dull, aching pain felt in the left mandibular teeth, jaw, and ear.

History

A 43-year-old woman presented with mild to severe, variable but continuous, dull, aching pain diffusely located in the left mandibular teeth, jaw, and ear. The pain is usually worse in the early morning and seems to be aggravated by mandibular movement and use. The complaint began about 2 months ago and has been present ever since. During the 2 months that preceded this complaint, endodontic treatment was completed on the mandibular left first premolar, and a fixed partial denture replacing the mandibular left second premolar and first molar was fabricated. This prosthesis was occlusally adjusted several times and then remade. The new denture became loose from the mandibular second molar abutment, and it was at that time the present complaint began. It has continued in spite of recementing the prosthesis, removing the prosthesis, temporarily crowning the abutments, treating the second molar endodontically, and using antibiotics.

There is no history of illness, infection, or trauma. She is medically negative for cause. No medications other than analgesics are presently used.

Examination

Intraoral: There is no clinical or radiographic evidence for the pain. The mandibular left first premolar and second molar have temporary crowns. All left mandibular and maxillary teeth not endodontically treated respond normally to electric pulp testing. There is no hyperalgesia of the teeth or gingiva. There is a slight decrease in the comfortable range of mandibular movement.

> **TMJs:** Well within normal limits clinically and radiographically.
>
> **Muscles:** Acute palpable tenderness in the left masseter muscle.
>
> **Cervical:** Within normal limits.
>
> **Cranial nerves:** Within normal limits.

Diagnostic tests: Local anesthetic blocking of the left mandibular nerve failed to alter the pain. Analgesic blocking of the left masseter muscle arrested the dental, mandibular, and auricular pain completely.

Impression

Deep somatic myofascial pain emanating from the left masseter muscle is producing a central excitatory effect that is being sensed as referred pain in the left mandible and ear. The initiating cause of the myofascial pain appears to relate to the prior dental experience and likely began as protective co-contraction. There is no evidence that the pain arises from dental or oral causes; nor is there any significant masticatory dysfunction.

Diagnosis   Myofascial pain in the left masseter muscle that is producing a left mandibular "muscular toothache."

There are, however, some migraine variants that are not well understood and can pose some difficult diagnostic problems. Neurovascular variants, sometimes called *migrainous neuralgias*, can produce relatively localized pains that present with the clinical characteristic of toothache. Most of these toothaches are mistaken for true odontogenous pains and treated with dental therapies, which fail to resolve the pain. Unfortunately, there are several clinical characteristics that can mislead both patient and practitioner. The following characteristics are common to neurovascular toothache:

1. The pain may be spontaneous, variable, and pulsatile—characteristics that simulate pulpal pain.
2. The pain is usually very intense.
3. The toothache is characterized by periods of total remission between episodes (like migraine pain).
4. The episodes of pain may pose a temporal behavior, appearing at similar times during the day, week, or month.
5. Very frequently, the pain is felt in a maxillary canine or premolar and the patient is so convinced of the source of the toothache that dental treatment may be undertaken without hesitation, even when only minor or no dental cause is found.
6. The pain may actually undergo remission following dental treatment, although recurrence is characteristic with neurovascular pains. The pain may spread to adjacent teeth, opposing teeth, or the entire face.
7. If the pain experience is protracted, it may induce autonomic effects, manifested as nasal congestion, lacrimation, and edema of the eyelids and face, which may be mistaken for sinusitis or dental abscess.
8. The patient reveals a history of other neurovascular disorders (migraine).
9. A trial of an abortive migraine medication (eg, sumatriptan) reduces the toothache (see chapter 16).

The rather typical behavior of neurovascular variants should be well appreciated to prevent unnecessary therapy and the accompanying frustration felt by patient and practitioner alike. Suspicion of the presence of neurovascular pain is the key to diagnosis. Dental treatment, even if it is palliative and quite innocuous, may offer the patient reason to blame the clinician for aggravating the problem, if not actually initiating it (see Case 16).

Neurovascular toothache is actually a neurovascular variant that is felt by the patient in a tooth. It serves to alert the dental profession to an important clinical entity that has been misdiagnosed and mistreated in the past. The absence of other better known clinical characteristics of neurovascular pain can make it difficult to diagnose. The chief indicators that help distinguish this toothache from true odontogenous toothache are *(1)* the absence of adequate local dental cause, *(2)* the tendency for it to be periodic and recurrent, and *(3)* the patient's ability to precisely locate the painful tooth. Confirming evidence consists of identifying the presence of a neurovascular pain disorder by a trial of an abortive migraine medication such as sumatriptan. Diagnostic analgesic blocking may yield confusing data because sometimes it reduces the pain, sometimes it does nothing, and sometimes it may even increase the pain.

Unfortunately, dental therapy often induces a remission of the pain, thereby deluding the clinician into thinking that the condition was in fact a dental one and that a proper treatment has been applied. With recurrence, the clinician may perform additional dental therapy without realizing that it is futile and possibly harmful. The management of this type of pain will be discussed in detail in chapter 16.

Cardiac toothache

Dental practitioners should be particularly aware of the incidence of jaw and tooth

Case 2 Heterotopic pain, felt as toothache, referred from the cardiac muscle

Chief Complaint   Left mandibular pain and toothache.

History

A 61-year-old man presented with mild, continuous but variable, dull, aching pain diffusely located in the left mandible and teeth. Mandibular movement did not increase the pain. The pain was preceded by left shoulder discomfort. The shoulder pain began 3 days ago as a variable, vague but more or less continuous pain. He went to his physician, who diagnosed the complaint as bursitis and initiated some therapy. Two days later, the left "toothache" pain began even though the patient had been edentulous for about 20 years. Thinking the mandibular pain stemmed from the dentures, the physician advised a dental examination. The patient's dentist made a dental radiograph of the left mandibular area and saw part of a deeply impacted third molar. He was then immediately referred to an oral surgeon for removal of the tooth.

No medications are presently being taken, except aspirin for pain.

Examination

Intraoral: A normal appearing edentulous mouth with satisfactory artificial dentures. There is no local hyperemia in the denture-bearing areas. There is no palpable discomfort in the area of the impacted mandibular third molar or in the left submandibular triangle. A panoramic radiograph revealed a deeply impacted mandibular left third molar. This tooth appears to be completely covered with bone, with no coronal radiolucency indicative of dental caries and exhibiting no osseous changes around the tooth. Mandibular functioning is clinically normal in all respects. There is no dental, oral, or masticatory cause for the complaint.

   TMJs: Clinically normal.

   Muscles: Clinically negative for cause of pain.

   Cervical: Within normal limits.

   Cranial nerves: Within normal limits.

Diagnostic tests: Analgesic blocking of the left mandibular nerve did not arrest the pain. Medical consultation advised. A second physician was consulted, who decided the symptoms warranted an electrocardiogram (EKG). The EKG was positive for cardiac ischema with mild cardiac muscle damage. Medical management of the cardiac condition eliminated the left mandibular tooth pain.

Impression

The shoulder pain mistaken for bursitis and the mandibular pain mistaken for "toothache" were not associated with appreciable chest discomfort. It is presumed, therefore, that the primary cardiac muscle pain was not expressed as chest pain and only the secondary central excitatory effects were felt by the patient.

Diagnosis   Myofascial pain in the left masseter muscle that is producing a left mandibular "muscular toothache."

pain that occurs as a secondary manifestation of cardiac pain input.[24,25] Although other clinical evidence of cardiac distress (such as substernal chest discomfort and left arm and neck pain) is usually present, sometimes the dental symptoms may be the only ones of which the patient complains when he comes to the office with what he thinks is a "dental problem."[26] Great care should be exercised in such situations. A lack of adequate dental cause for the pain complaint should always be an alerting sign. Failure of analgesic blocking to arrest the pain promptly and completely is confirming evidence that the primary source of pain is not the tooth (Case 2).

The clinical characteristics of cardiac toothache are as follows:

1. The pain is a deep, diffuse toothache that may sometimes pulsate.
2. The toothache has a temporal behavior that increases with physical exertion or exercise.
3. The toothache is associated with chest pain, anterior neck pain, and/or shoulder pain.
4. The symptoms of the toothache decrease after administration of nitroglycerin tablets.

A complete health history is essential when evaluating this heterotopic toothache. The patient may not share his or her entire medical history, since he or she is in a dental office for tooth pain and currently has no cardiac symptoms. When a cardiac toothache is suspected, an immediate referral to proper medical personal is mandatory.

Neuropathic toothache

Pain felt in a tooth may be the result of a projected or referred pain originating in neural structures. These pains may be either episodic or continuous and are classified in that manner. Each of these neuropathic toothaches will be discussed separately, since their clinical presentations are different.

Episodic neuropathic toothache

Episodic neuropathic toothache is characterized by a sudden, sharp, spontaneous pain felt either in a tooth or radiating to a tooth. It is similar to the pain felt in paroxysmal neuralgia and in fact likely related to such a neuropathic pain disorder. Trigeminal neuralgia or tic douloureux may be triggered from stimulation of the teeth and felt as pain in the teeth. Unfortunately, analgesic blocking arrests the paroxysms of pain and may lead to a mistaken diagnosis of odontogenous pain. Also, dental therapy, especially if a local anesthetic block is used, may induce a remission, thereby leading both patient and clinician to assume that the diagnosis is correct and that a proper treatment has been done. When the condition recurs, additional forms of dental therapy may be employed, thus compounding the mistake (see Case 24). The clinical characteristic of the episodic neuropathic toothache are:

1. The pain is severe, unilateral, lacerating, and shock-like (paroxysmal) and is felt in a tooth.
2. The pain is provoked by relatively innocuous peripheral stimulation of a "trigger zone." The trigger may be the tooth but more commonly is an extraoral site such as the lip or chin. Local anesthetic at the tooth will not reduce the pain unless it is also the trigger (which is very rare).
3. There are pain-free periods between the episodes of pain.
4. Local anesthetic at the trigger will reduce the episodes of paroxysmal pain.

The management of this type of pain will be discussed in detail in chapter 18.

Continuous neuropathic toothache

Some neuropathic toothaches produce a persistent, ongoing, unremitting pain. These pains may be increased by local provocation, such as touching the tooth and surrounding gingiva, which adds confusion to the diagnosis. A key to this diagnosis is the presence of other neurologic complaints, such as hyperesthesia, hypoesthesia, anesthesia, paresthesia, muscular tics, weakness, and paralysis, as well as autonomic and special sense aberrations, depending on the fiber content at the site of neuropathy. The common types of neuropathic conditions that can produce continuous pain felt in a tooth are *neuritic pains* and *deafferentation pains*.

Neuritic pain, sometimes referred to as *neuritis,* arises from an inflammatory response of the nerve. It can occur in the maxillary and mandibular divisions of the trigeminal nerve, which can cause dental pains along with other neurologic symptoms. Neuritis of the superior dental plexus as the result of extension from maxillary sinusitis may cause a toothache in and around one or more maxillary teeth. Such pain is persistent, nonpulsatile, and burning. If the accompanying maxillary sinusitis is asymptomatic, diagnosis may be difficult. The key usually is to recognize accompanying neurologic signs that involve other teeth or nearby structures served by the same nerve (see Case 25). A similar toothache in the mandibular teeth may occur as an expression of neuritis of the inferior alveolar nerve from direct trauma, dental sepsis, or viral infection (see Case 33).

The clinical characteristics of neuritic toothache are as follows:

1. The pain is a persistent, nonpulsatile, often burning pain felt in a tooth.
2. The toothache is accompanied by other neurologic symptoms (eg, paresthesia, dysesthesia, anesthesia).
3. Other teeth may feel "dead" or "strange."
4. The associated gingival tissue may be affected.

5. The onset of the toothache followed an infection or trauma (eg, sinusitis, viral infection, trauma).

The treatment of neuritic pain will be discussed in detail in chapter 17.

Continuous neuropathic pain may also arise from injury to a nerve. The nerve may be injured by gross trauma, tooth pulp extirpation, simple extraction, or major oral surgery. Such pains are called *deafferentation pains* and are often mistaken for a posttraumatic or postoperative complication (see Case 32). Some of these pains may be the result of a neuroma secondary to the nerve trauma.

The clinical characteristics of deafferentation toothache are as follows:

1. The toothache is continuous but often varies in intensity. There are no periods of remission.
2. The most common teeth involved with deafferentation toothache are the maxillary canines and premolars.
3. This condition is most commonly reported in middle-aged women with a history of trauma to the painful region.
4. The pain is not changed by local provocation.
5. The effect of local anesthesia is unpredictable.
6. The toothache is not responsive to dental therapies.

These conditions may be described as a "phantom toothache"[27–29] and have also been described as atypical odontalgia.[30–33]

Atypical odontalgia is a difficult pain condition that most dental practitioners will face sooner or later. The patient will complain of specific tooth pain, yet there will be no local signs of dental pathology. Repeated attempts at dental therapy will fail to resolve the pain. The patient and the clinician will often both become quite frustrated and sometimes desperate. Graff-Radford and Solberg[33] have suggested the

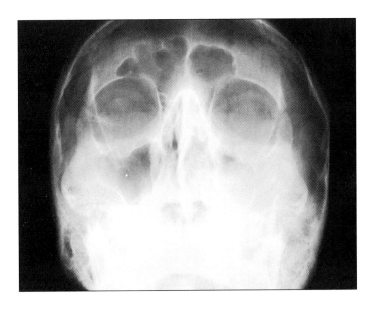

Fig 11-18 Water's view of the maxillary sinus. Note the air/fluid level in the patient's right maxillary sinus. This patient reported right maxillary first molar toothache. (Courtesy of Dr Donald Falace, Lexington, Kentucky.)

following criteria for identification of atypical odontalgia:

1. Pain in a tooth or tooth site
2. Continuous or almost continuous pain
3. Pain persisting more than 4 months
4. No sign of local or referred pain
5. Equivocal results of a somatic block

Although much is still unknown regarding the pathophysiology of atypical odontalgia, it appears that the clinical characteristics fit best in the category of deafferentation pain. As the pain condition becomes chronic, the category likely shifts to a centrally mediated neuropathic pain (chapter 17). As with other deafferentation pain, tricyclic antidepressants can be helpful.[32-35] The treatment of deafferentation pains will be presented in chapter 17.

Sinus or nasal mucosal toothache

Pain arising from the nasal mucosa as the result of viral or allergic rhinitis is prone to be expressed as referred pain throughout the maxilla and maxillary teeth in the form of a toothache. It may also display autonomic signs that are mistaken for symptoms of maxillary sinusitis. The so-called sinus headache may cause management problems because of the tooth pains.

Diagnostically, analgesic blocking by infiltration at the apex of the tooth in question does not arrest the toothache if it is referred from the nasal mucosa. In contrast, topical anesthesia of the nasal mucosa effectively arrests the toothache. Again, suspicion that the dental pain is referred is the key to diagnosis (see Case 19).

The clinical characteristics of sinus or nasal mucosal toothache are as follows:

1. The patient reports a feeling of pressure below the eyes.
2. The pain is increased by application of pressure over the involved sinus.
3. The tooth is sensitive to percussion.
4. The toothache is increased by lowering the head.
5. The toothache is increased by stepping hard on to the heel of the foot (eg, walking down steps).
6. Local anesthesia of the tooth does not eliminate the pain.
7. Diagnosis is confirmed by appropriate imaging of the sinus (Fig 11-18).

Effective treatment of a sinus toothache is accomplished by controlling the infected sinus. These may be accomplished by the appropriate use of antibiotics, decongestants, and/or antihistamines. If the sinus infection does not resolve, referral to an otolaryngologist is indicated.

Psychogenic toothache

On occasion, a patient may report symptoms of toothache that does not appear to fit into any clinical category of orofacial pain. The clinician should always be mindful of somatoform pain disorders. This is a category of mental disorders in which a patient may complaint of a physical condition with the presence of absolutely no physical signs. When this condition is reported as pain in a tooth, it is considered a *psychogenic toothache*. Perhaps this condition is related to a deficiency in the descending inhibitory mechanism or the endogenous antinociceptive system. Somatoform pain disorders felt in the teeth are characterized by the following findings:

1. The pain is reported in many teeth and/or other sites.
2. The pain jumps from tooth to tooth or to other locations.
3. There is a general departure from normal or physiologic patterns of pain.
4. There is a lack of response to reasonable dental treatment.
5. There is an unusual and unexpected response to therapy.
6. The toothache is chronic and often unchanging.
7. The patient presents with chronic pain behavior.
8. There is no identifiable source of pain, and the clinical characteristics do not fit any of the other pain conditions.

Somatoform pain disorders are mental disorders and are best treated by a qualified psychologist or psychiatrist. The dental clinician must identify these disorders so as to avoid unnecessary dental therapies.

Cardinal warning symptoms of nondental toothache

Toothaches of nondental origin require accurate diagnostic identification of the true source of the patient's pain. The most important step toward proper management is for the clinician to be suspicious that the pain is not of dental origin. The cardinal warning symptoms of toothache of nondental origin are as follows:

1. Spontaneous multiple toothaches
2. Inadequate local dental cause for the pain
3. Stimulating, burning, nonpulsatile toothaches
4. Constant, unremitting, nonvariable toothaches
5. Persistent, recurrent toothaches
6. Failure of the toothache to respond to reasonable dental therapy

Differential Diagnosis

Primary deep somatic pain of dental origin should be distinguished diagnostically from nonodontogenous pains that are felt in the teeth and presented as dental complaints. The following nondental sources of toothache should be considered:

1. Heterotopic referred pains and secondary hyperalgesias as secondary effects of deep pain originating in the following somatic structures: musculoskeletal, vascular, cardiac, or sinus mucosa
2. Neuropathic pains, either continuous or episodic
3. Somatoform pain disorders
4. Heterotopic pains of central origin

Therapeutic Options

For the management of primary deep somatic pains of dental origin, the following therapeutic options are available (see chapter 9): *(1)* analgesics for palliative relief, plus counseling; and *(2)* cause-related therapy consisting of accurate location of the true source of pain and proper treatment. Proper treatment of dental pains are either caries control (restorative procedures), endodontic therapy, periodontal therapy, or extraction of the offending tooth.

References

1. Lipton JA, Ship JA, Larach-Robinson D. Estimated prevalence and distribution of reported orofacial pain in the United States. J Am Dent Assoc 1993;124:115–121.
2. Willis RD, DiCosimo CJ. The absence of proprioceptive nerve endings in the human periodontal ligament: The role of periodontal mechanoreceptors in the reflex control of mastication. Oral Surg Oral Med Oral Pathol 1979; 48:108–115.
3. Hannam AG. The response of periodontal mechanoreceptors in the dog to controlled loading of the teeth. Arch Oral Biol 1969;14: 781–791.
4. Anderson DJ, Hannam AG, Matthews B. Sensory mechanisms in mammalian teeth and their supporting structures. Physiol Rev 1970; 50:171–195.
5. Cody EWJ, Lee RWH, Taylor A. A functional analysis of the components of the mesencephalic nucleus of the fifth nerve in the cat. J Physiol (Lond) 1972:226:249–261.
6. Azerad J, Woda A, Albe-Fessard D. Physiological properties of neurons in different parts of the cat trigeminal sensory complex. Brain Res 1982;246:7–21.
7. deLaat A. Reflexes excitable in the jaw muscles and their role during jaw function and dysfunction: A review of the literature. Part II. Central connections of orofacial afferent fibers. J Craniomandib Pract 1987;5:247–253.
8. Krauser JT. Hypersensitive teeth: Part 1. Etiology. J Prosthet Dent 1986;56:153–156.
9. Gross D. Pain and autonomic nervous system. In: Bonica JJ (ed). International Symposium on Pain, vol 4, Advances in Neurology. New York: Raven Press, 1974:93–103.
10. Young RF. Effect of trigeminal tractotomy on dental sensations in humans. J Neurosurg 1982;56:812–818.
11. Sessle BJ. Is the tooth pulp a "pure" source of noxious input? In: Bonica JJ, Liebeskind JC, Albe-Fessard DG (eds). Proceedings of the Second World Congress on Pain, vol 3, Advances in Pain Research and Therapy. New York: Raven Press, 1979:245–260.
12. Mumford JM, Bowsher D. Pain and protopathic sensibility: A review with particular reference to the teeth. Pain 1976;2:223–243.
13. Chatrian GE, Fernandes de Lima JM, Lettich E, Canfield RC, Miller RC, Soso MJ. Electrical stimulation of tooth pulps in humans: II. Qualities of sensation. Pain 1982;14:233–246.
14. McGrath PA, Gracely RH, Dubner R, Heft MW. Nonpain and nonpain sensations evoked by tooth pulp stimulation. Pain 1983;15:377–388.
15. Narhi M, Jyvasjarvi E, Hirvonen T, Huopaniemi T. Activation of heat-sensitive nerve fibers in the dental pulp of the cat. Pain 1982;14: 317–326.
16. Narhi M, Virtanen ASJ, Huopaniemi T, Hirvonen T. Conduction velocities of single pulp nerve fiber units in the cat. Acta Physiol Scand 1982;116:209–213.
17. Rozza AJ, Beuerman RW. Density and organization of free nerve endings in the corneal epithelium of the rabbit. Pain 1982;14:105–120.
18. Nord SG. Responses of neurons in rostral and caudal trigeminal nuclei to tooth pulp stimulation. Brain Res Bull 1976;1:489–492.
19. Vyklicky L, Keller, Jastreboff P, Vyklicky L Jr, Butkhuzi SM. Spinal trigeminal tractotomy and nociceptive reactions evoked by tooth pulp stimulation in the cat. J Physiol (Paris) 1977; 73:379–386.
20. Hannam AG, Matthews B, Yemm R. Receptors involved in the response of the masseter muscle in tooth contact in man. Arch Oral Biol 1970; 15:17–24.
21. Sessle BJ, Schmitt A. Effects of controlled tooth stimulation on jaw muscle activity in man. Arch Oral Biol 1972;17:1597–1607.
22. Wilson S, Fuller PM, Winfrey J. Histochemical evidence for strictly ipsilateral innervation of maxillary canine teeth in cats. Exp Neurol 1980;70:138–145.

23. Mumford JM. Toothache and Related Pain. Edinburgh: Churchill Livingstone, 1973:174–187.

24. Graham LL, Schinbeckler GA. Orofacial pain of cardiac origin. J Am Dent Assoc 1982;104:47–48.

25. Kreiner M, Okeson JP. Toothache of cardiac origin. J Orofac Pain 1999;13:201–207.

26. Batchelder BJ, Krutchkoff DJ, Amara J. Mandibular pain as the initial and sole clinical manifestation of coronary insufficiency: Report of case. J Ant Dent Assoc 1987;115:710–712.

27. Marbach JJ. Phantom tooth pain. J Endod 1978;4:362–371.

28. Marbach J, Hulbrock J, Hohnn C, Segal AG. Incidence of phantom tooth pain: An atypical facial neuralgia. Oral Surg Oral Med Oral Pathol 1982;53:190-193.

29. Marbach JJ. Is phantom tooth pain a deafferentation (neuropathic) syndrome? Part II: Psychosocial considerations. Oral Surg Oral Med Oral Pathol 1993;75:225–232.

30. Rees RT, Harris M. Atypical odontalgia. Br J Oral Surg 1979;16:212–218.

31. Brooke RI. Atypical odontalgia. J Oral Surg 1980;49:196–199.

32. Kreisberg MK. Atypical odontalgia: Differential diagnosis and treatment. J Am Dent Assoc 1982;104:852–854.

33. Graff-Radford SB, Solberg WK. Atypical odontalgia. J Craniomandib Disord Facial Oral Pain 1992;6:260–266.

34. Brooke RI. Atypical odontalgia. Br J Oral Maxillofac Surg 1980;49:196–199.

35. Rees RT, Harris M. Atypical odontalgia: Differential diagnosis and treatment. Br J Oral Surg 1979;16:212–218.

Pains of Muscle Origin

Pains of muscular origin are the most frequent cause of discomfort about the head and neck. Very few humans have escaped this type of pain experience. Since dental pain is the most frequent oral pain, a good rule to follow in diagnosing pains about the face and mouth is initially to assume that it is dental until proved otherwise, then muscular until proved otherwise. The possibility of orofacial pain being of muscular origin should be taken into account with every complaint. Even when the primary cause is not muscular, central excitatory effects tend to be expressed in the muscles, which makes this a frequent complication accompanying other sources of pain.

Muscle pain emanates from the skeletal muscles, tendons, and fascia. Although the exact origin of this type of muscle pain is debated, some authors suggest it is related to vasoconstriction of the relevant nutrient arteries and the accumulation of metabolic waste products in the muscle tissues. Within the ischemic area of the muscle, certain algogenic substances (eg, bradykinins, prostaglandins) are released, causing muscle pain.[1–3]

Muscle pain, however, is far more complex than simple overuse and fatigue. In fact, muscle pain associated with the muscles of mastication does not seem to be strongly correlated with increased activity, such as spasm.[4–8] It is now appreciated that muscle pain can be greatly influenced by central mechanisms,[9,10] as will be discussed later in this chapter.

Muscle pain usually is felt as a nonpulsatile, variable, dull, aching sensation, sometimes with a boring quality. This more constant background discomfort may escalate to or be punctuated by sharper, more severe lancinating pains occurring both spontaneously and in response to stretching, contraction, manipulation, or manual palpation. Sometimes the pain is no more than a feeling of pressure. At other times, it may increase to excruciating intensity. It may be transitory or persistent, constant, intermittent, or recurrent. Its behavior is labile, characterized by suddenness of onset and rapidity of change. It follows no time frame unless it has an inflammatory origin, which is relatively rare. Accompanying dysfunction may be expressed as tightness and weakness, or it may relate to impairment of muscle function, for example, stiffness, rigidity, swelling, or shortening. Pain decreases the biting strength of masticatory

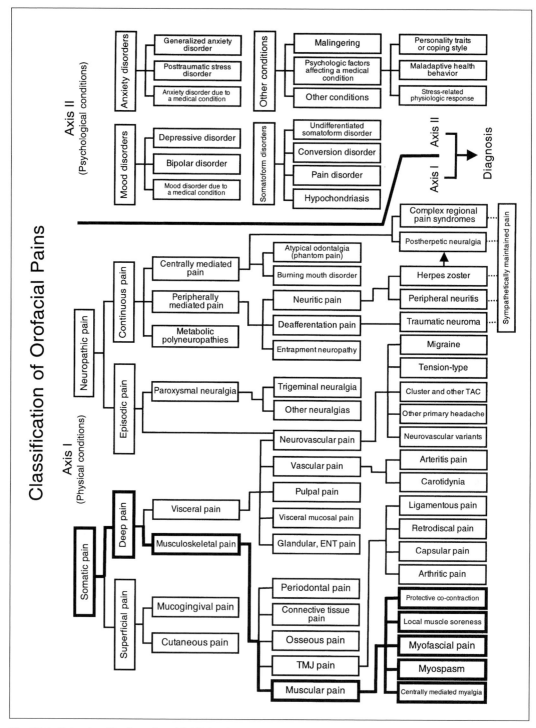

Fig 12-1 Pain classification chart highlighted to show the relationship of muscular pains to other orofacial pain disorders.

muscles by 33% to 50%[11] and induces a feeling of muscular weakness. Muscle pain also impairs the proprioceptive feedback mechanism, thus leading to less precise muscle action.[12] Palpable muscle tenderness and the fact that movement and functioning modify the pain and stiffness are clinical indications of the presence of muscle pain.[13]

Myogenous pains of different types may involve muscles of the mouth, face, and neck, with the symptom complex depending on the kind, number, and location of muscles involved and the degree to which they are affected. The likelihood of secondary central excitatory effects should be considered. When the primary pain remains relatively silent, the secondary referred pain may constitute most of the complaint. Referred pain from muscles can be the source of considerable diagnostic confusion. For example, more or less silent pain arising in the sternocleidomastoid muscle may be felt in and about the ear as earache or as temporomandibular joint (TMJ) pain. Cardiac muscle pain may be referred to the mandible.[14]

Behavior of Muscular Pain

Myogenous pains that emanate from the orofacial structures are classified as musculoskeletal pains of the deep somatic category (Fig 12-1). The general features exhibited by muscle pain include those of deep somatic pain, namely: (1) the pain has a dull, depressing quality; (2) subjective localization is variable and somewhat diffuse; (3) the site of pain may or may not identify the correct location of the source of pain; (4) response to provocation at the site of pain is fairly faithful in incidence and intensity, but not in location; and (5) central excitatory effects often accompany the pain. To these features are added characteristics peculiar to musculoskeletal pain, namely: (1) the pain relates reasonably to the demands of biomechanical function, and (2) manual palpation at the site of pain, or functional manipulation, produces a graduated response of pain that is proportionate to the stimulus.

The stimulation of skeletal muscle tissue induces a dull, aching pain felt deeply and diffusely in a broad region of the muscle. It is mediated by group III (A-delta fiber) and group IV (C-fiber) afferent neurons. A crescendo of intensity indicates some temporal summation.[15] Regardless of the true source of muscle pain, movements that actively stretch the muscle or increase its isometric tension increase the patient's awareness of pain. If passive movement is painful, one or more antagonists should be suspected of containing an abnormally tender muscle region.[16]

The term *temporomandibular disorders* (TMD) refers to a collective term embracing a number of clinical problems that involve the masticatory musculature, the TMJ and associated structures, or both.[17] Pain associated with TMD therefore originates from either muscle or joint sources. This chapter will highlight muscle pain, which is by far the most common type of TMD. TMJ pain will be discussed in the next chapter.

When masticatory muscle pain is present, the patient reports discomfort about the face and mouth that is induced by chewing and other jaw use but is independent of local disease involving the teeth and oral cavity proper.

Types of Masticatory Muscle Pains

Not all masticatory muscle disorders are the same clinically. There are at least five

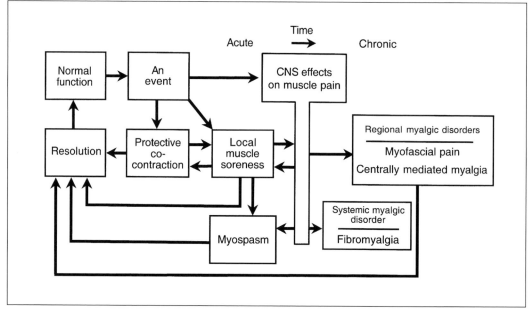

Fig 12-2 A masticatory muscle pain model. This model depicts the relationship between various clinically identifiable muscle pain disorders along with some etiologic considerations. (From Okeson JP. Management of Temporomandibular Disorders and Occlusion, ed 5. St Louis: Mosby, 2003:194. Used with permission.)

different types, and it is important to develop the ability to distinguish among them, because the treatment of each is quite different. The five types are protective co-contraction (muscle splinting), local muscle soreness, myofascial (trigger point) pain, myospasm, and chronic centrally mediated myalgia. A sixth condition known as fibromyalgia also needs to be discussed. The first three conditions (protective co-contraction, local muscle soreness, and myofascial pain) are commonly seen in the dental office. Myospasm and chronic centrally mediated myalgia are seen less frequently. Many of these muscle disorders occur and resolve within a relatively short period of time. When these conditions are not resolved, more chronic pain disorders may result. Chronic masticatory muscle disorders become more complicated, and treatment is generally oriented differently than for acute problems. It therefore becomes important

that the clinician be able to differentiate acute muscle disorders from chronic muscle disorders so that proper therapy can be applied. Fibromyalgia is a chronic myalgic disorder that presents as a systemic musculoskeletal pain problem; it needs to be recognized by the dental practitioner and is best managed by referral to appropriate medical personnel.

Masticatory Muscle Pain Model

To understand the relationship between different muscle pain disorders, a masticatory muscle pain model will be presented (Fig 12-2). Once the model is presented and the clinical characteristics of each subcategory of muscle pain described, the management of each condition will be explained. The model begins with the assumption that the muscles of mastication are healthy and functioning normally. Normal muscle function can be interrupted by certain types of events. If an event is significant, a muscle response occurs, known as *protective co-contraction (muscle splinting)*. In many instances the consequence of the event is minor and the co-contraction quickly resolves, allowing muscle function to return to normal. If, however, protective co-contraction is prolonged, local biochemical and later structural changes can occur, creating a condition known as *local muscle soreness*. This condition may resolve spontaneously with rest or may require treatment.

If local muscle soreness does not resolve, changes in the muscle tissues may develop, resulting in prolonged pain input. This constant deep pain input can affect the central nervous system (CNS), leading to certain muscle responses. Two examples of CNS-influenced muscle pain disorders are *myofascial pain* and *myospasm*. In some instances, the CNS responds to certain events or local conditions by inducing an involuntary contraction, seen clinically as a muscle spasm. Myospasms are not chronic but instead represent a condition of relatively short duration. At one time, myospasm was thought to be the primary condition responsible for myalgia. Recent studies[8,18–21] suggest that true myospasms are not common in patients suffering from masticatory muscle pain.

These masticatory muscle disorders usually present as relatively acute problems and, once identified and treated, the muscle returns to normal function.[22] If, however, these acute myalgic disorders are not recognized or appropriately managed, certain perpetuating conditions can advance the problem into a more chronic myalgic disorder. As the myalgic disorder becomes more chronic, the CNS contributes more to maintaining the condition. Because the CNS is an important factor in this condition, it is referred to as *centrally mediated myalgia*. Chronic centrally mediated myalgia is often very difficult to resolve, and treatment strategies must be changed from those used with the acute myalgic disorders.

Another example of a chronic musculoskeletal pain disorder is *fibromyalgia*. Although this is not primarily a masticatory pain disorder, the dental clinician needs to recognize this condition so as to avoid unnecessary dental therapy. Unlike the other muscle pain disorders, which are regional, fibromyalgia is a widespread, global musculoskeletal pain condition. Dental practitioners need to be aware that the management of these chronic pain disorders is quite different from that of the relatively acute muscle disorders.

To better understand the masticatory muscle pain model, each component of the model will be discussed in detail.

An Event

Normal muscle function can be interrupted by various types of events. These events can arise from either local or systemic factors. Local factors represent any events that acutely alter sensory or proprioceptive input in the masticatory structures, for example, the fracture of a tooth or the placement of a restoration in supraocclusion. Trauma to local structures, such as tissue damage caused by a dental injection, represents another type of local event. Trauma might also arise from excessive or unaccustomed use of masticatory structures, such as chewing unusually hard food or chewing for a long period of time (eg, gum chewing). Opening too wide may strain the ligaments supporting the joint and/or muscles. This may occur as a result of a long dental procedure or even by simply opening too wide (eg, yawning).

Any source of constant deep pain input may also represent a local factor that alters muscle function. This pain input may have its source in local structures such as the teeth, joints, or even the muscles themselves. The source of the pain, however, is not significant, since any constant deep pain, even idiopathic pain, may create a muscle response.

Systemic factors may also represent events that can interrupt normal muscle function. One of the most commonly recognized systemic factors is emotional stress.[23–26] Stress seems to alter muscle function, either through the gamma efferent system to the muscle spindle or by means of sympathetic activity to the muscle tissues and related structures.[27–29] Of course, responses to emotional stress are quite individualized. Therefore, patients' emotional reactions and psychophysiologic responses to stressors may vary greatly. It has been demonstrated that exposure of a subject to an experimental stressor can immediately increase the resting electromyographic (EMG) activity of masticatory muscles.[8,18] This physiologic response provides direct insight about how emotional stress directly influences muscle activity and muscle pain.

Other systemic factors can influence muscle function and are more poorly understood, such as acute illness or viral infections. Likewise, there is a broad category of poorly understood constitutional factors that are unique to each patient. Such factors include immunologic resistance and autonomic balance of the patient. These factors seem to reduce the individual's ability to resist or combat the challenge or demand created by the event. Constitutional factors are likely to be influenced by age, gender, diet, and perhaps even genetic predisposition. Clinicians realize that individual patients often respond quite differently to similar events. It is assumed, therefore, that certain constitutional factors do exist and can influence an individual's response.

At this time these factors are poorly understood and not well defined as they relate to muscle pain disorders.

As with local factors, constant deep pain input can represent a systemic factor that may influence muscle function. Although pain is often felt in local structures, it may not necessarily have its source in these same structures. As mentioned in earlier chapters, pain can be felt not only as a result of peripheral causes, but as a result of a CNS effect.[30] The CNS has the ability to alter pain sensations, both moving toward and away from the cortex.[31,32] If the CNS enhances sensory input, pain may be felt even without organic cause. This pain modulation phenomenon can create a site of pain felt in muscle tissues. One must appreciate, therefore, that this pain modulation phenomenon can represent a systemic event that produces muscle pain and ultimately affect function.

Protective Co-contraction (Muscle Splinting)

The first response of the masticatory muscles to one of the previously described events is *protective co-contraction*. Protective co-contraction is a CNS response to injury or threat of injury. This response has also been called *protective muscle splinting*.[33] It has been described for many years but only recently documented.[34–38] In the presence of an injury or threat of injury, normal sequencing of muscle activity seems to be altered so as to protect the threatened part from further injury. Protective co-contraction can be likened to the co-contraction[39] observed during many normal functional activities, such as bracing the arm when attempting a task with the fingers. In the presence of altered sensory input or pain, antagonistic muscle groups seem to fire during movement in an attempt to protect the injured part. In the masticatory system, for example, a patient experiencing co-contraction will demonstrate an increase in the activity of the elevator muscles during mouth opening.[34,40,41] During closing of the mouth, an increase in activity is noted in the depressing muscles. This co-activation of antagonistic muscles is thought to be a normal protective or guarding mechanism and needs to be recognized by the clinician. Protective co-contraction is not a pathologic condition, although it may lead to muscle symptoms when prolonged.

The etiology of protective co-contraction can be any change in sensory or proprioceptive input from associated structures. An example of such an event in the masticatory system is the placement of a high crown. Protective co-contraction can also be caused by any source of deep pain input or an increase in emotional stress.

Co-contraction is reported clinically as a feeling of muscle weakness directly following some event. There is no pain reported when the muscle is at rest, but use of the muscle usually increases the pain. The patient often presents with limited mouth opening, but when asked to open slowly, he or she can achieve full opening. The key to identifying co-contraction is that it immediately follows an event; therefore, the history is very important. If protective co-contraction continues for several hours or days, the muscle tissue can become compromised and a local muscle problem may develop.

Local Muscle Soreness

Local muscle soreness is a primary, noninflammatory, myogenous pain disorder. It is often the first response of the muscle tissue to prolonged co-contraction. While co-contraction represents a CNS-induced muscle response, local muscle soreness represents a condition that is characterized by changes in the local environment of the muscle tissues. These changes are characterized by the release of certain algogenic substances (ie, bradykinin, substance P, even histamine[42]) that produce pain. These initial changes may be expressed as nothing more than fatigue. Along with protracted co-contraction, other causes of local muscle soreness are local trauma or excessive use of the muscle. When excessive use is the etiology, a delay in the onset of muscle soreness can occur.[43] This type of local muscle soreness is often referred to as *delayed-onset muscle soreness* or *postexercise muscle soreness.*[44]

Since local muscle soreness itself is a source of deep pain, an important clinical event can occur. Deep pain produced by muscle soreness can, in fact, produce protective co-contraction. This additional co-contraction can, in turn, produce more muscle soreness. Therefore, a cycle can be created whereby muscle soreness produces more co-contraction and so on. This condition is called *cyclic muscle pain* and needs to be recognized by the clinician. The important feature of this condition is that the pain condition becomes wholly independent of the original source of pain. If the clinician attempts to continue to treat the original cause, the pain condition will not be resolved. This concept is very often overlooked or not appreciated by the clinician, but it is basic to successful management of muscle pain.

The clinician needs to be aware of the complications that cyclic muscle pain might pose with diagnosis. For example, the medial pterygoid muscle is injured by an inferior alveolar nerve block. This trauma causes local muscle soreness. The pain associated with the soreness in turn produces protective co-contraction. Since protective co-contraction can lead to muscle soreness, a cycle begins. During this cycling, the original tissue damage produced by the injections resolves. When tissue repair is complete, the original source of pain is eliminated; however, the patient may continue to suffer with a cyclic muscle pain disorder. Since the original cause of the pain is no longer part of the clinical picture, the clinician can easily be confused during the examination. The clinician needs to recognize that even though the original cause has resolved, a cyclic muscle pain condition exists and needs to be treated. This condition is an extremely common clinical finding and if not recognized often leads to mismanagement of the patient.

Local muscle soreness presents clinically with muscles that are tender to palpation and reveal increased pain with function. Structural dysfunction is common, and when the elevator muscles are involved, limited mouth opening results. Unlike protective co-contraction, the patient has great difficulty opening any wider. With local muscle soreness, there is actual muscle weakness.[45–47] Muscle strength returns to normal when the muscle soreness is resolved.[46–48]

CNS Effects on Muscle Pain

The muscle pain conditions described to this point are relatively simple, with their origins predominantly in the local muscle tissues. Unfortunately, muscle pain can become much more complex. In many instances, activity within the CNS can either influence or actually be the origin of the muscle pain. This may occur secondary to ongoing deep pain input or altered sensory input, or it may arise from central influences, such as up-regulation of the autonomic nervous system (eg, emotional stress). This occurs when conditions within the CNS excite peripheral sensory neurons (primary afferents), creating the antidromic release of algogenic substances into the peripheral tissues and resulting in muscle pain (ie, neurogenic inflammation) (chapter 4).[10,49–51] These central excitatory effects can also lead to motor effects (primary efferents), resulting in an increase in muscle tonicity (co-contraction).[7,8]

Therapeutically, it is important that the clinician appreciate that the muscle pain now has a central origin. The CNS responds in this manner secondary to: *(1)* the presence of ongoing deep pain input, *(2)* increased levels of emotional stress (ie, an up-regulation of the autonomic nervous system), or *(3)* changes in the descending inhibitory system that lead to a decrease in the ability to counter the afferent input, whether nociceptive or not.

Chronic Myalgic Pain Disorders

Chronic pain disorders need to be recognized as such because therapy demands it. There are many types of chronic pain disorders. One method of classifying these conditions is by the structures that are most involved. A broad term that might be used for muscle problems is *chronic myalgic disorders*. Some of the same disorders discussed as acute myalgic disorders can become chronic when significant perpetuating factors are present (see chapter 9). Myofascial pain, centrally mediated myalgia, and fibromyalgia are considered chronic myalgic disorders. The treatment of these disorders is more complicated, because perpetuating factors and cyclic muscle pain also need to be addressed. Another complicating factor in chronic myalgic disorders is that the area involved in the condition often seems to broaden. In other words, pain that begins in the masseter muscle might spread to involve the temporalis and medial pterygoid muscles and perhaps even later the cervical muscles. Often as pain becomes chronic, it becomes more regional or even global. This, of course, complicates treatment.

Myospasm (tonic contraction myalgia)

Myospasm is a CNS-induced tonic muscle contraction. For many years the dental profession felt that myospasms were the most common source of myogenous pain. More recent studies, however, shed new light on muscle pain and myospasms.

It is reasonable to expect that a muscle in spasm or tonic contraction would reveal a relatively high level of electromyographic activity. Studies, however, do not support the assumption that painful muscles have a significant increase in their EMG output.[4,7,8,19,35] These studies have forced us to rethink the classification of muscle pain and differentiate myospasms from other muscle pain disorders. Although myospasms of the muscles of mastication do occur, this condition is not common; when present it is usually easily identified by clinical characteristics.

The etiology of myospasms has not been well documented. Several factors are likely to combine to promote myospasms. Local muscle conditions certainly seem to foster myospasms. These conditions involve muscle fatigue and changes in local electrolyte balances. Deep pain input may also precipitate myospasms.

Myospasms are easily recognized by the structural dysfunction that is produced. Since a muscle in spasm is contracted, major jaw positional changes result according to the muscle or muscles in spasm. These changes in the position of the jaw create what is known as an *acute malocclusion*. An acute malocclusion is a sudden change in the occlusal condition as a result of a disorder. Since the malocclusion is secondary to a disorder, the clinician should not focus treatment on correcting the malocclusion, but instead on the disorder that has caused the malocclusion. Myospasms are also characterized by very firm muscles, as noted by palpation.

When the inferior lateral pterygoid muscle shortens due to myospastic activity, acute malocclusion results. This is recognized as disclusion of the ipsilateral posterior teeth and premature occlusion of the contralateral anterior teeth. The presence of pain sites within the muscle is identified by functional manipulation: pain is accentuated by maximum intercuspation (stretching the muscle) and by protrusion against resistance (contracting the muscle). It should be noted that pain with clenching of the teeth is relieved by biting ipsilaterally on a tongue blade, because this prevents intercuspation of the teeth and stretches the muscle. Unless acute malocclusion can be identified and pain induced by functional manipulation, a diagnosis of spasm of this muscle is invalid.

Local analgesic blocking of the inferior lateral pterygoid muscle promptly arrests all pain emanating from this source and offers the best clinical means of accurately locating the source of pain.

Regional myalgic disorders

Myofascial pain (trigger point myalgia)

Myofascial pain is a regional myogenous pain condition characterized by local areas of firm, hypersensitive bands of muscle tissue known as *trigger points*. This condition is sometimes referred to as *myofascial trigger point pain*. It is a type of muscle disorder that is not widely appreciated or completely understood, yet it commonly occurs in patients with myalgic complaints. In one study,[52] more than 50% of the patients reporting to a university pain center were diagnosed as having this type of pain.

Myofascial pain was first described by Travell and Rinzler[53] in 1952, yet the dental and medical communities have been slow to appreciate its significance. In 1969, Laskin[54] described the myofascial pain dysfunction (MPD) syndrome as having certain clinical characteristics. Although he borrowed the term *myofascial,* he was not describing myofascial trigger point pain. Instead *MPD syndrome* has been used in dentistry as a general term to denote any muscle disorder (not an intracapsular disorder). Since the term is so broad and general, it is not useful in the specific diagnosis and management of masticatory muscle disorders. MPD syndrome should not be confused with Travell and Rinzler's description, which will be used in this textbook. It is this author's suggestion that if a general term is need to describe muscle pain, the term *masticatory muscle pain* should be used as a generic term for all types of masticatory muscle pain and myofascial pain, unless the condition meets the original description in the medical literature, which will be discussed below.

Myofascial pain arises from hypersensitive areas in muscles called *trigger points.* These very localized areas in muscle tissues and/or their tendinous attachments are often felt as taut bands when palpated, which elicits pain. The exact nature of a trigger point is not known. It has been suggested[1,55] that certain nerve endings in the muscle tissues may become sensitized by algogenic substances that create a localized zone of hypersensitivity.[56] There may be a local temperature rise at the site of the trigger point, suggesting an increase in metabolic demand and/or reduction of blood flow to these tissues.[57] A trigger point is a very circumscribed region in which relatively few motor units seem to be contracting.[58,59] If all the motor units of a muscle contract, the muscle will of course shorten in length. This condition is called *myospasm* and has already been discussed in this chapter. Since a trigger point has only a select group of motor units contracting, no overall shortening of the muscle results, as occurs with myospasm.

The unique characteristic of trigger points is that they are a source of constant deep pain and therefore can produce central excitatory effects (see chapter 4). If a trigger point centrally excites a group of converging afferent interneurons, referred pain will often result, generally in a predictable pattern according to the location of the involved trigger point. The pain is often reported by the patient as headache pain.

The etiology of myofascial pain is complex. Unfortunately, we lack a complete understanding of this myogenous pain condition. It is therefore difficult to be specific concerning all etiologic factors. Travell and Simons have described certain local and systemic factors that seem to be associated, such as trauma, hypovitamintosis, poor physical conditioning, fatigue, and viral infections.[60] Other important factors are likely to be emotional stress and deep pain input.

The most common clinical feature of myofascial pain is the presence of trigger points. Although palpation of trigger points produces pain, local muscle sensitivity is not the most common complaint of patients suffering from myofascial trigger point pain. The most common symptom is usually associated with the central excitatory effects created by the trigger points. In many instances, patients may be aware only of the referred pain and not even acknowledge the trigger points. A perfect example is the patient suffering from myofascial trigger point pain in the trapezius muscle that creates referred pain to the temple region (see Fig 12-9).[61,62] The chief complaint is temporal headache, with very little acknowledgment of the trigger point in the shoulder. This clinical presentation can easily distract the clinician from the source of the problem. The patient will draw the clinician's attention to the site of the pain (the temporal headache) and not the source. The clinician must always remember that for treatment to be effective it must be directed toward the source of the pain, not the site. Therefore, a clinician must always search for the true source of the pain.

Since trigger points can create central excitatory effects,[63-65] it is also important to be aware of all the possible clinical manifestations. As stated in chapter 4, central excitatory effects can appear as referred pain, secondary hyperalgesia, protective co-contraction, or even autonomic responses. These conditions must be considered when evaluating the patient.

An interesting clinical feature of a trigger point is that it may present in either an active or a latent state. In the active state, it produces central excitatory effects. Therefore, when a trigger point is active, a headache is commonly felt. Since referred pain is wholly dependent on its original source, palpation of an active trigger point (local provocation) often increases such pain. Although not always present, when this characteristic appears it is an extremely helpful diagnostic aid. In the latent state, a trigger point is no longer sensitive to palpation and therefore does not produce referred pain. When trigger points are latent, they cannot be found by palpation and the patient does not complain of headache pain. In this case the history is the only data that leads the clinician to make the diagnosis of myofascial pain. In some instances the clinician should consider asking the patient to return to the office when the headache is present so that confirmation of the pattern of pain referral can be verified and the diagnosis confirmed.

It is thought that trigger points do not resolve without treatment. They may in fact become latent or dormant, creating a temporary relief of the referred pain. Trigger points may be activated by various factors,[66] such as increased use of a muscle, strain on the muscle, emotional stress, or even an upper respiratory infection. When trigger points are activated, the headache returns. This is a common finding with patients who complain of regular late afternoon headaches following a very trying and stressful day.

Along with referred pain, other central excitatory effects may be felt. When secondary hyperalgesia is present, it is commonly felt as an increased sensitivity to touching of the scalp. Some patients will even report that their "hair hurts" or that it is painful to brush their hair. Co-contraction is another common condition associated with myofascial pain. Trigger points in the shoulder or cervical muscles can produce co-contraction in the muscles of mastication.[7] If this continues, local muscle soreness in the masticatory muscles can develop. Treatment of the masticatory muscles will not resolve the condition, because its source is the trigger points of the cervicospinal and shoulder muscles. However, treatment of the trigger points in the shoulder muscles will resolve the masticatory muscle disorder. Management may become difficult when muscle soreness has been present for a long time, because it can initiate cyclic muscle pain. In these cases, extending treatment to both the muscles of mastication and the trigger points in the cervicospinal and shoulder muscles will usually resolve the problem.

On occasion, autonomic effects are produced by deep pain input from trigger points. These may result in such clinical findings as tearing or drying of the eyes, or vascular changes (eg, blanching and/or reddening of tissue) may occur. Sometimes the conjunctivae will become red. There may even be mucosal changes that produce nasal discharge similar to an allergic response. The key to determining whether the autonomic effects are related to central excitatory effects or to a local reaction such as allergies is the unilateral appearance. Central excitatory effects in the trigeminal area rarely cross the midline. Therefore, if the deep pain is unilateral, the autonomic effects will be on the same side as the pain. In other words, one eye will be red and the other normal, one nostril draining mucus and the other not. With allergic responses, both eyes or both nostrils will be involved.

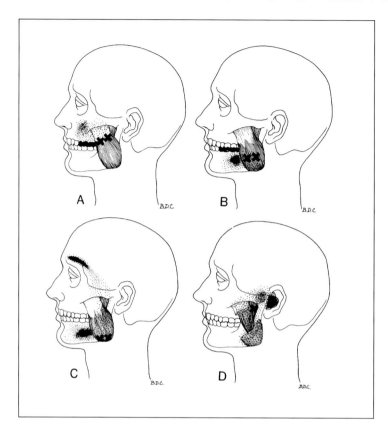

Fig 12-3 Trigger points (**x**) located in various parts of the masseter muscle. Solid black shows essential reference pain zones; stippled areas are spillover pain zones. A = Superficial layer, upper portion; B = superficial layer, midbelly; C = superficial layer, lower portion; D = deep layer, upper part. (From Travell JG, Simons DG. Myofascial Pain and Dysfunction: The Trigger Point Manual. Baltimore: Williams & Wilkins, 1983:220. Used with permission.)

By way of summary, the clinical symptoms reported with myofascial pain are most commonly associated with the central excitatory effects created by the trigger points and not the trigger points themselves. The clinician must be aware of this and find the involved trigger points. When these are palpated, they appear as hypersensitive areas often felt as taut bands within the muscle. There is usually no local pain when the muscle is at rest but some when the muscle is used. Often slight structural dysfunction will be seen in the muscle harboring the trigger points. This is commonly reported as a "stiff neck."

Referral patterns of myofascial pain in the orofacial region.

The clinician treating orofacial pain disorders needs to have a sound understanding of myofascial pain since it is so common in pain populations. The following section will review the most common muscles of the head and neck and the typical referral pattern for each. Familiarity with these patterns can be extremely helpful during history taking, examination, and diagnosis.

Masseter muscle. Trigger points located at sites in the superficial layer of the masseter muscle refer to the posterior mandibular

Fig 12-4 Referred pain patterns from trigger points (**x**) in the temporalis muscle. A = Anterior fibers; B and C = middle fibers; D = posterior fibers. (From Travell JG, Simons DG. Myofascial Pain and Dysfunction: The Trigger Point Manual. Baltimore: Williams & Wilkins, 1983:237. Used with permission.)

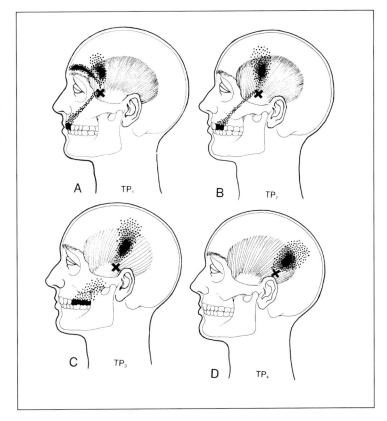

and maxillary teeth, the jaw, and the face (Fig 12-3). Toothache is a common complaint from this source. The deep portion refers to the ear and TMJ area. Earache and preauricular pain thought to be emanating from the joint are common complaints. Moderate restriction of opening associated with ipsilateral deflection of the midline incisal path may be observed. Tinnitus described as a "low roaring noise" may occur from deep masseter trigger points. The muscle is accessible for manual palpation to identify trigger sites.

Temporalis muscle. The reference zone of the temporalis muscle includes all the maxillary teeth and upper portion of the face (Fig 12-4). Headache and toothache (see chapter 11) are the common complaints. A restricted opening is rarely displayed. The muscle is accessible for manual palpation to identify trigger sites.

Medial pterygoid muscle. The reference zone for the medial pterygoid muscle includes the posterior part of the mouth and throat, as well as the temporomandibular and infra-auricular areas (Fig 12-5). Throat and postmandibular (infra-auricular) pain is the common complaint. Eustachian tube symptoms may be displayed. Moderate restriction of the mouth opening associated with contralateral deflection of the midline incisal path may be observed. The muscle is

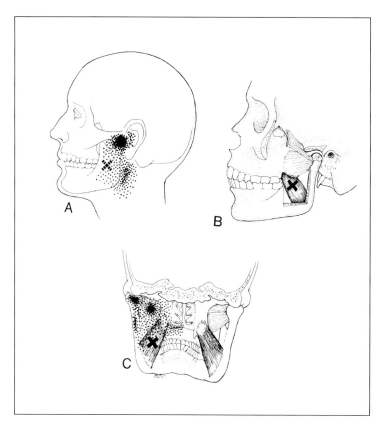

Fig 12-5 Referred pain pattern and location of responsible trigger point (**x**) in the medial pterygoid muscle. A = External areas of pain to which the patient can point; B = anatomic cutaway to show the location of the trigger point; C = coronal section showing internal areas of pain. (From Travell JG, Simons DG. Myofascial Pain and Dysfunction: The Trigger Point Manual. Baltimore: Williams & Wilkins, 1983:250. Used with permission.)

only partially accessible for intraoral manual palpation to identify trigger sites. Functional manipulation therefore may be needed for this purpose: A pain source within the muscle will be accentuated by opening widely (stretching the muscle) and by biting firmly (contracting the muscle).

Inferior lateral pterygoid muscle. The lateral pterygoid muscle has been incriminated as the cause of numerous temporomandibular complaints. This probably stems from a lack of understanding of how the muscle is constructed and what its normal functions are. No doubt, the difficulty of adequately examining the muscle clinically has provided good cover for these incriminations. Several hard facts need to be considered in evaluating the effects of this muscle on masticatory symptoms. It should be understood first that there are two lateral pterygoid muscles: the inferior lateral pterygoid and the superior lateral pterygoid. Only the inferior lateral pterygoid muscle protracts the mandible, and therefore it can act to create acute occlusal disharmony when it is shortened. The superior muscle remains inactive at all times except during power strokes in conjunction with elevator muscle action.[67,68] Even when shortened, the superior lateral pterygoid muscle cannot disrupt joint functioning in the absence of structural joint disease.

The dearth of muscle spindles in the lateral pterygoid muscles reduces the chance of reflex contraction when this muscle is

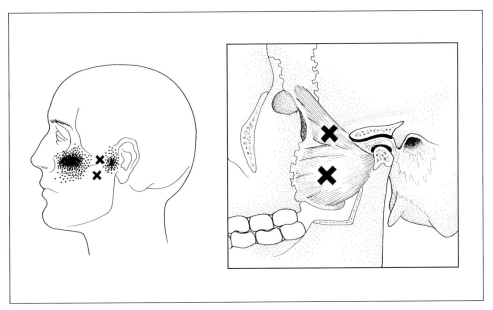

Fig 12-6 Referred pain patterns of trigger points (**x**) in the superior and inferior lateral pterygoid muscles. (From Travell JG, Simons DG. Myofascial Pain and Dysfunction: The Trigger Point Manual. Baltimore: Williams & Wilkins, 1983:261. Used with permission.)

stretched. Then too, this muscle is composed chiefly of slow-twitch fibers[69] that resist fatigue and seldom undergo spastic activity. The prime reason that a diagnosis of this muscle is so difficult is because it is inaccessible for manual palpation.[70] Despite voluminous testimony to the contrary, the possibility of diagnostically accurate manual or instrument palpation of the muscle is remote.[71]

Trigger points in the inferior lateral pterygoid muscle refer to the TMJ area (Fig 12-6). Slight acute malocclusion may be sensed as disclusion of the ipsilateral posterior teeth and premature occlusion of the contralateral anterior teeth (Cases 3 and 4). Since this muscle is inaccessible for palpation, functional manipulation is required to help identify the presence of myofascial pain: A pain source within the muscle will be accentuated by maximum intercuspation (stretching the muscle) and by pro-

truding the jaw against resistance (contracting the muscle).[71]

Superior lateral pterygoid muscle. Trigger points in the superior lateral pterygoid muscle refer to the zygomatic area (Fig 12-6). No dysfunction is observed unless there is extensive deterioration in the TMJ that is sufficient to permit anterior displacement of the articular disc. Diffuse pain in the malar area is the usual complaint. Since this muscle is inaccessible for manual palpation,[70] functional manipulation is required to identify the presence of myofascial pain: A pain source within the muscle will be accentuated by maximum intercuspation (stretching the muscle) and by biting on a separator (contracting the muscle). Opening widely and protruding against resistance do not involve this muscle functionally and therefore are painless.

Case 3 Cycling masticatory muscle pain secondary to chronic ear pain

Chief Complaint Diffuse left side facial pain.

History

A 47-year-old woman presented with mild, continuous, protracted, variable but steady, dull, aching pain diffusely located in the right ear, preauricular area, face, and temple, aggravated by opening widely, chewing food, and clenching the teeth. The pain was also accompanied by acute malocclusion and restricted opening.

The patient had had recurring episodes of earache associated with acute upper respiratory infections for several years. About 3 weeks earlier, she had such an episode with continuous severe earache on the right side. After about 7 days, she noticed her "bite was off," she could not open normally, and she had pain with opening, chewing, and occluding the teeth. This had become progressively worse, even though antibiotic therapy by her ear, nose, and throat (ENT) physician eliminated the ear infection completely. He referred her to her dentist, who recognized the protective co-contraction and occlusal disharmony but declined to adjust the occlusion pending further investigation of the temporomandibular joints. She had no other physical complaints and was taking no medications.

Examination

Intraoral: The teeth are clinically and radiographically normal. There is premature contact of the left anterior teeth and disocclusion of the posterior teeth on the same side of the pain. When she fully occludes the teeth, there is acute pain in the right TMJ area. This is decreased by biting on a tongue blade. Pain also occurs with eccentric biting, forceful lateral and protrusive movements, and opening beyond 10 mm. Opening is restricted to 31 mm, with deflection to the right after 23 mm.

> **TMJs:** Both joints appear structurally normal. The left joint functions normally, but the right condyle appears to be protruded in initial occlusal contact position and fails to move properly with opening efforts.
>
> **Muscles:** There is palpable tenderness in the right masseter and temporal muscles.
>
> **Cervical:** Within normal limits.
>
> **Cranial nerves:** Within normal limits.

Diagnostic tests: Analgesic blocking of the right lateral pterygoid muscle arrested pain induced by fully occluding the teeth and making forceful excursions. Similar blocking of the right masseter and temporal muscles arrested all other pain.

Impression

The masticatory pain is muscular and stems from the right lateral pterygoid, masseter, and temporal muscles only. The acute malocclusion is symptomatic of spasm of the right lateral pterygoid muscle. The limited mouth opening is a result of protective co-contraction of the right masseter and temporal muscles. The myospasm of the right lateral pterygoid occurred by way of muscle co-contraction produced by central excitatory effects induced by primary otalgia. Cyclic muscle pain has occurred.

Diagnosis Masticatory myospasm of the right lateral pterygoid secondary to otalgia. Cycling muscle pain appears to be present.

Case 4 — Masticatory muscle pain expressed as spasm in the lateral pterygoid muscle

Chief Complaint   Right ear and preauricular pain.

History

A 20-year-old woman presented with mild, variable, steady, dull, aching pain diffusely located in the right ear and preauricular area. It was induced by clenching the teeth, chewing, and other jaw use, and lasted variable periods of time. The pains were intermittent and were significantly related to gum chewing, hard biting, and forceful jaw movements. The patient complained that her bite was not very comfortable, with premature contact of the left anterior teeth and disocclusion of the posterior teeth. When she brought the teeth into full occlusion, she felt the acute pain and therefore she avoided this activity.

The complaint began about 2 years ago in sudden recurring episodes, usually lasting only a few days and then disappearing for variable periods of time. The complaint seemed to be worse in the early morning. The present episode began about 6 months ago and has remained the same ever since.

Examination

Intraoral: The teeth are clinically and radiographically negative for pulpal or periodontal pain. An acute malocclusion is evident. There is premature contact of the left anterior teeth, while the posterior teeth do not occlude. When the patient is asked to bring all the teeth into firm occlusion, she experiences pain in the right preauricular area. This can be prevented by biting on a tongue blade to preclude full intercuspation of the teeth. She thinks her occlusion was normal 6 months ago and relates the malocclusion to her present pain complaint.

TMJs: Clinical functioning of the joints is well within normal limits, except for the sensation of malocclusion and the right side pain when she occludes the teeth or moves the jaw forcefully. She opens 45 mm with no deviation or deflection of the incisal path. Protrusive and lateral excursions are adequate and symmetrical. Asking the patient to push the jaw forward against resistance increases the pain. Radiographically, both joints appear to be within normal limits structurally.

Muscles: There is slight palpable muscle tenderness, but the discomfort appears to be very subjective.

Cervical: Within normal limits.

Cranial nerves: Within normal limits.

Diagnostic tests: Analgesic blocking of the right lateral pterygoid muscle immediately arrests the pain complaint.

Impression

The pain is myalgic and arises from the right lateral pterygoid muscle. The malocclusion is acute and relates to muscle spasm.

Diagnosis   Myospasm of the right lateral pterygoid muscle. The cause is presumed to relate to clenching, emotional stress, bruxism, fatigue, etc.

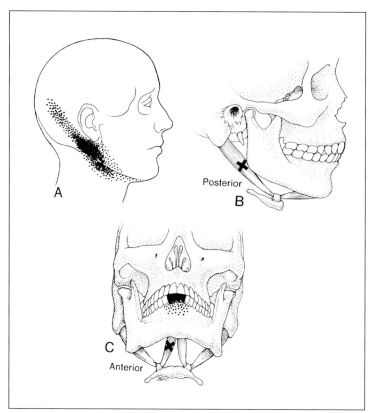

Fig 12-7 Referred pain patterns for trigger points in the digastric muscles. Pain felt behind the angle of the mandible and below the ear (A) is a common referral site for a trigger point (**x**) in the posterior digastric muscle (B). Trigger points (**x**) in the anterior digastric muscles can refer pain to the mandibular teeth (C). (From Travell JG, Simons DG. Myofascial Pain and Dysfunction: The Trigger Point Manual. Baltimore: Williams & Wilkins, 1983:274. Used with permission.)

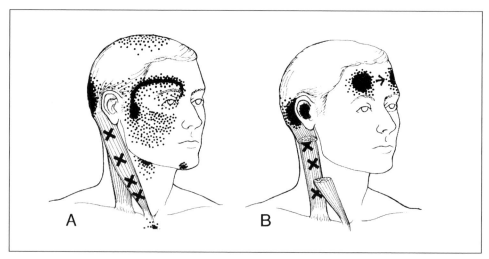

Fig 12-8 Referred pain patterns with locations of corresponding trigger points (**x**) in the sternocleidomastoid muscle. A = Superficial sternal division; B = deep clavicular division. (From Travell JG, Simons DG. Myofascial Pain and Dysfunction: The Trigger Point Manual. Baltimore: Williams & Wilkins, 1983:203. Used with permission.)

Anterior digastric muscle. Trigger points in the anterior belly of the digastric muscle, which is the trigeminal-innervated part, refer pain to the mandibular incisor area (Fig 12-7) (see chapter 11). No dysfunction is observed. This muscle is accessible for manual palpation to identify trigger points.

Sternocleidomastoid muscle. The reference zone from the superficial sternal division of the sternocleidomastoid muscle is throughout the entire face and head (Fig 12-8). A great variety of face pain and headache complaints may arise from this source. The deeper clavicular division refers to the ear, postauricular area, and frontal region. Earache, temporomandibular pain, and frontal headache are common complaints. This muscle is a frequent source of so-called tension-type headache. Postural vertigo may be displayed. The muscle is accessible for manual palpation to identify trigger sites.

Trapezius muscle. The reference zone for trigger points in the upper part of the trapezius muscle is along the posterolateral part of the neck, the postauricular area, the mandibular angle, and the temple (Fig 12-9). This is a major source of so-called tension-type headache. It should be noted that tension-type headache is the result of neither excessive muscular tension nor muscle contraction, because there is no statistically significant difference in the EMG activity between such muscles and non-headache controls.[72,73] This muscle is accessible for manual palpation to identify trigger sites.

Occipitofrontalis muscle. The frontalis portion of the occipitofrontalis muscle refers as frontal headache; the occipital portion refers as lateral cranial and postocular headache (Fig 12-10). This is another major source of tension-type headache. The muscle is accessible for manual palpation to identify trigger sites. The splenius capitis,

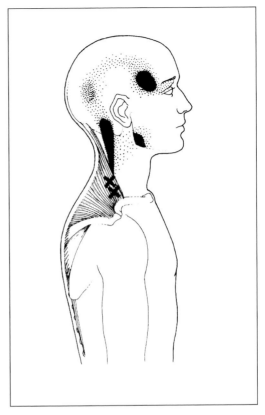

Fig 12-9 Referred pain patterns and location of trigger points (**x**) in upper part of the trapezius muscle. (From Travell JG, Simons DG. Myofascial Pain and Dysfunction: The Trigger Point Manual. Baltimore: Williams & Wilkins, 1983:184. Used with permission.)

splenius cervicis, posterior cervical, and suboccipital muscles are other sources of tension-type headache.[74]

Muscles of facial expression. Trigger points in the orbicularis oculi muscle refer down through the nose and upper lip, those of the zygomaticus major muscle refer upward along the inner canthus of the eye to the mid-forehead, and those in the platysma muscle refer diffusely in the mandibular region (Fig 12-11). These muscles are all accessible for manual palpation to identify trigger sites.

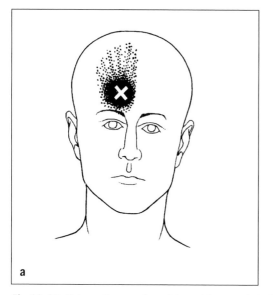
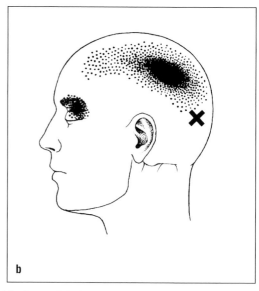

a
b

Fig 12-10 Pain patterns referred from trigger points (**x**) in the occipitofrontalis muscle. A = Frontalis belly; B = occipitalis belly. (From Travell JG, Simons DG. Myofascial Pain and Dysfunction: The Trigger Point Manual. Baltimore: Williams & Wilkins, 1983:291. Used with permission.)

Cervical muscles. It should be noted that myofascial trigger point pain emanating from muscles innervated by cervical spinal nerves often induce heterotopic pain in the orofacial and head regions. Spontaneous referred pain is usually felt as a headache. It is possible, however, that such reference is felt in other structures as an earache, toothache, or masticatory pain. Stimulation-evoked secondary hyperalgesia is also a common form of heterotopic pain that occurs secondary to cervical nociceptive input. Thus, areas of touchy skin or scalp may occur. Frequently, however, deeper areas of palpable tenderness that are accentuated by masticatory function may occur. Such heterotopic manifestation of cervical pain may be mistaken for true masticatory pain. Caution therefore should always be exercised when cervical and masticatory pains are felt concurrently. When this occurs, it behooves the clinician to more completely evaluate the cervical spine.

Such an examination entails observation of the neck contours for deviation or straightening of the neck, rotation or tilting of the head, or elevation of the shoulder (see chapter 8). The mobility of the neck should be tested both actively and passively for range of motion, pain, and crepitation. Tenderness and muscle soreness can be determined by palpation. Sensory evaluation of neck pain sources as identified by dermatome distribution is important on the basis that cervical nerve pain is felt superficially in the shoulder, outer portion of the arm, and hand, whereas thoracic nerve pain is commonly felt in the axillary region and inner part of the arm. Deep tendon reflexes and motor evaluation of the shoulder and arm should be done while keeping in mind that motor innervation of the deltoid, biceps, triceps, and wrist muscles is from the cervical spinal nerves. Last, radial pulse changes with postural maneuvers of the arms should be tested.

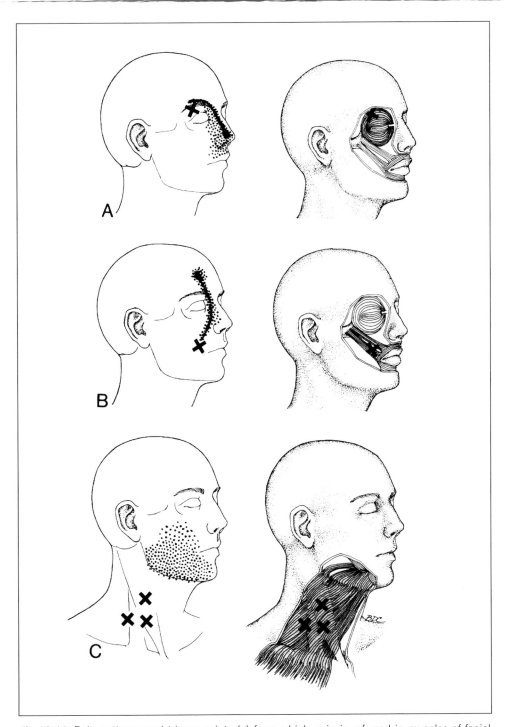

Fig 12-11 Pain patterns and trigger points (**x**) from which pain is referred in muscles of facial expression. A = Orbital portion of orbicularis oculi muscle; B = zygomaticus major muscle; C = platysma muscle. (From Travell JG, Simons DG. Myofascial Pain and Dysfunction: The Trigger Point Manual. Baltimore: Williams & Wilkins, 1983:283. Used with permission.)

Such a clinical examination not only may reveal the presence of pain sources in the neck but also may help to pinpoint which cervical spinal nerves are involved. It should be noted that the upper cervical spinal nerves are more likely sources of pain that refer or spread to the masticatory region than are the lower ones. This examination may produce sufficient evidence to warrant an orthopedic consultation.

Among the neck conditions that the dental practitioner should be familiar with are the following:

1. Chronic cervical myofascial pain
2. Acute cervical strain
3. Osteoarthritis of the cervical spine and intervertebral disc disease
4. Entrapment disorders of the cervical spine, such as scalenus anticus syndrome[75]

Secondary effects of muscle pain include not only reference of pain, as previously discussed, but also the development secondary co-contraction in other muscles, which gives the syndrome a pattern of spreading pain. A cervical strain or whiplash injury may, by central hyperexcitability, induce motor effects in the masticatory muscles. This then leads to a typical masticatory muscle disorder, the symptoms of which may become dominant. As such, the very real masticatory pain disorder may cause the patient to consider this to be the total complaint when in fact it is no more than a secondary effect of the cervical disorder. These types of disorders require astute diagnostic and therapeutic management to avoid failure and chronicity (Case 5).

Persistent cervical sources of deep somatic pain, such as cervical osteoarthritis, are prone to induce central excitatory effects that include heterotopic pain and co-contraction of muscles innervated by cervical, facial, and trigeminal nerves. Thus, a masticatory muscle disorder may be initiated as part of a larger, spreading muscle

pain problem (Case 6). Since cyclic muscle pain can become independent of the initiating cause, such pain represents a separate therapeutic entity. Since the cause is not masticatory, treatment should not be primarily directed toward the masticatory apparatus. Therapy needs to be directed to the original source of pain, in this case, the cervical disorder. Since the masticatory muscle disorder may become independent of the original source, therapy may also need to be directed to this disorder. Treatment of only the masticatory muscle pain, however, will not be successful unless proper cervical treatment is also accomplished. Pain disorders of this type can best be recognized and distinguished from those of true masticatory origin by careful history taking and by a clinical examination that includes the cervical structures.

Tension-type headache

Tension-type headache is characterized by a constant, dull, aching pain felt bilaterally in the temporal and frontal regions and is often described as wearing a tight headband. The International Headache Society considers this a primary headache.[76] This type of headache will be discussed in detail in chapter 16; however, it is mentioned here because the referred pain associated with myofascial pain is often clinically described by the patient as tension-type headache. Previously this type of headache was referred to as a muscular contraction headache or muscle tension headache. More recent studies[77-81] demonstrate that there is no significant increase in EMG activity of these muscles, and therefore these names are not appropriate. Certainly not all tension-type headaches are related to myofascial pain, but many are likely to be secondary to myofascial trigger point pain originating in the head and neck muscles. Sometimes, a vague low-grade muscular discomfort is sensed in the cervical and occipital areas. As just reviewed, pain referred from the frontalis portion of the occipitofrontalis

Case 5 — Myofascial pain of the masticatory muscles secondary to a cervical pain condition

Chief Complaint   Generalized facial pain and headache.

History

A 52-year-old female presented with mild, continuous, protracted, steady, dull, aching pain diffusely located bilaterally in the temporal, preauricular, and occipital areas. The pain was aggravated by head movements, emotional stress, fatigue, and jaw use.

During the past 6 to 7 years, the patient had recurring episodes of bilateral occipital, temporal, and frontal headaches lasting up to 2 to 3 months and occurring at irregular intervals. They were aggravated by head movements, emotional stress, and fatigue and were treated as tension-type headaches by her osteopathic physician. About 8 to 9 months ago, the present episode began, first intermittently, then becoming constant. During recent months, the pains were aggravated by chewing and opening widely and the patient noticed moderate restriction of mouth opening. Her physician therefore recommended a dental examination. She also had neck, hand, arm, and leg complaints but she had been cleared medically and neurologically for cause except minor osteoarthritis of the cervical vertebrae. No medications or therapy presently in use.

Examination

Intraoral: No dental or oral cause for the pain is evident clinically or radiographically. The teeth respond normally to pulp testing. She has bilateral preauricular pain with opening, sustained clenching, and hard biting eccentrically. Her maximum mouth opening is about 34 mm with no deflection. Lateral and protrusive movements are normal. She has moderate joint noise with extended or strained movements only. There is no discernible occlusal disharmony.

   TMJs: Clinically and radiographically normal except for moderate restriction of condylar movement bilaterally with opening.

   Muscles: Palpable tenderness in the masseter, temporal, medial pterygoid, sternocleidomastoid, occipital, and trapezius muscles bilaterally.

   Cervical: Significant pain to palpation of the cervical spine and associated muscles. Restriction of cervical function to rotation and bending.

   Cranial nerves: Within normal limits.

Impression

The masticatory pain and dysfunction appear to be originating from muscular origin and are intimately related to preexisting muscle pain emanating from the cervical musculature bilaterally. From the patient's history, the cervical component preceded the more recent masticatory complaint, and the entire symptom complex is highly suggestive of a cervical myofascial pain disorder that has secondarily involved the masticatory muscles. It is presumed that cervical arthritis is a likely predisposing cause, and this possibility deserves serious investigation on a medical level. There is no identifiable dental, oral, or masticatory cause for the patient's complaint.

Diagnosis   Masticatory myofascial pain expressed in the elevator muscles secondary to a cervical pain condition of undetermined origin.

Case 6 — Masticatory muscle pain expressed as significant co-contraction and cyclic muscle pain

Chief Complaint   Limited mouth opening associated with left face pain.

History

A 67-year-old man presented with mild, continuous, protracted, steady, dull, aching pain diffusely located in the left face, temple, and jaw. The pain was accompanied by marked reduction in mouth opening and aggravated by any attempt to open the mouth or by chewing.

The patient reported to a dentist, who discovered a mandibular left molar with significant decay that had led to a pulpitis. The dentist removed the tooth, but pain persisted in the form of a local osteitis (dry socket). The dentist continued to treat the condition with packing of the socket and medications. After 8 days the dry socket pain resolved, but the generalized facial pain and limited mouth opening persisted.

Examination

Intraoral: Due to the mouth restriction, the teeth cannot be adequately examined. Panoramic radiograph of the mandible shows no unusual bony changes other than the recent extraction site. Opening is restricted to about 20 mm with a slight deflection to the left and accompanied by pain in the left temporal and masseter muscles. Lateral and protrusive movements are only moderately restricted and painful.

TMJs: Both joints appear structurally normal. The restricted condylar movement appears to be the result of an extracapsular restriction associated with pain in the left temporal and masseter muscles.

Muscles: Palpable tenderness in the left temporal and masseter muscles. The left medial pterygoid muscle is not accessible for palpation.

Cervical: Within normal limits.

Cranial nerves: Within normal limits.

Impression

The history, clinical course, and present clinical and radiographic evidence indicate that the present facial pain and limited mouth opening are secondary to the prolonged source of deep pain (pulpitis followed by dry socket). There appears to be a cyclic muscle pain condition that has become independent of the original cause (which has resolved).

Diagnosis   Cyclic muscle pain associated with local muscle soreness and protective co-contraction resulting in limited mouth opening.

muscle is felt as frontal headache, while that from the occipitalis portion is felt as postocular and lateral headache. While pain referred from the sternal division of the sternocleidomastoid muscle is felt diffusely throughout the face and head, referral from the clavicular division is felt as postauricular and frontal headache. The upper trapezius refers pain that is felt as postauricular and temporal headache. The splenius capitis, splenius cervicis, and other posterior cervical and suboccipital muscles may also contribute to tension-type headache.

Tension-type headache mistaken for masticatory pain

It is not unusual for the heterotopic referred pain felt as tension-type headache to be accompanied by secondary hyperalgesia that is felt as discomfort with jaw movements and deep tenderness to manual palpation. The "chewing pain" thus created, which can be "manually palpated" and which is accompanied by "headache," may be misdiagnosed as a masticatory disorder and treated accordingly. This fairly common complaint can be distinguished from true masticatory pain in two ways: there is a lack of masticatory dysfunction, and the discomfort is not arrested by analgesic blocking at the site of pain.

Centrally mediated myalgia (chronic myositis)

Centrally mediated myalgia is a chronic, continuous muscle pain disorder originating predominantly from CNS effects that are felt peripherally in the muscle tissues. This disorder clinically presents with symptoms similar to an inflammatory condition of the muscle tissue and therefore is sometimes referred to as *myositis*. This condition, however, is not characterized by the classic clinical signs associated of inflammation (eg, reddening, swelling). Chronic centrally mediated myalgia results from a source of nociception found in the muscle tissue that has its origin in the CNS (neurogenic inflammation).[82–86]

The most common cause of chronic centrally mediated myalgia is protracted local muscle soreness or myofascial pain. In other words, the longer the patient complains of myogenous pain, the greater the likelihood of chronic centrally mediated myalgia. It should be noted that chronic centrally mediated myalgia is more closely associated with continuity of muscle pain than with actual duration. Many muscle pain disorders are episodic, leaving intermittent periods of no muscle pain. Periodic episodes of muscle pain do not produce chronic centrally mediated myalgia. A prolonged and constant period of muscle pain, however, is likely to lead to chronic centrally mediated myalgia.

On occasion, a bacterial or viral infection can spread to a muscle, producing a true infectious myositis. This condition is not common, but when present needs to be identified and properly treated.

A clinical characteristic of chronic centrally mediated myalgia is the presence of constant, aching myogenous pain. The pain is present during rest and increases with function. The muscles are very tender to palpation, and structural dysfunction is common. The most common clinical feature is the extended duration of the symptoms (Case 7).

Other true inflammatory myogenous pains are fasciitis, tendonitis, and bursitis. *Fasciitis* is an inflammatory condition of the muscle sheath that occurs in conjunction with, and is diagnostically inseparable from, inflammation of the body of the muscle. Although myofascial pain is not inflammatory, it may be designated myofasciitis for administrative or insurance purposes.[74] *Tendonitis* is an inflammatory condition of a tendon or tendon-muscle attachment. Abusive use and trauma are the most frequent causes. Bursae are synovial membrane–lined antifriction structures that

Case 7   Masticatory muscle pain expressed as chronic centrally mediated myalgia

Chief Complaint   Bilateral chronic face pain.

History

A 42-year-old woman presented with a prolonged history of bilateral face pain. The pain began 4 years earlier, associated with the placement of several crowns that were not comfortable. She reported that the crowns were eventually adjusted to fit but the pain continued. The present pain was a bilateral, continuous, dull, aching pain located predominantly in the right and left masseter areas. The pain varied in intensity but was always present. It increased with jaw use and trying to open the mouth wide and decreased with ibuprofen and rest. She also stated that the pain increased during stressful times and her sleep quality was poor. The continuous pain was beginning to take away her energy and her ability to be successful at work. She had had an occlusal appliance and repeated occlusal adjustments that provided little help.

Examination

Intraoral: There is no dental or oral cause for the pain. There is significant pain to palpation of multiple areas of the face, along with some hyperalgesia with light touch. The pain is greatly increased when she attempts to open her mouth wider than 28 mm. Passive stretching of the elevator muscles can achieve an opening of 39 mm. Eccentric movements are normal.

> **TMJs:** Both joints appear to be structurally normal. There is restriction of right condylar movement with maximum opening, interpreted as indicative of myostatic contracture of the elevator muscles.

> **Muscles:** Significant pain to palate the right and left masseter and temporalis muscles.

> **Cervical:** Range of movement is within normal limits, but there is mild to significant pain to palpation of most of the cervical muscles.

> **Cranial nerves:** Within normal limits.

Impression

The continuous, long-standing muscle pain condition began as an adverse response to an acute change in the occlusal condition. The condition continued as a cyclic muscle pain until central changes occurred, making it a centrally mediated pain condition.

Diagnosis   Chronic centrally mediated myalgia.

facilitate muscle movements, especially when bidirectional. A bursa is found at the hamular process of the sphenoid bone to facilitate tensor palatini muscle action. One lies beneath the tongue. Several facilitate muscle action involving the hyoid bone. *Bursitis* is an inflammatory condition of a bursa and usually results from trauma. It may be a manifestation of rheumatoid arthritis.

Chronic systemic myalgic disorders (fibromyalgia)

Chronic systemic myalgic disorders need to be recognized as such because therapy demands it. The word *systemic* is used because the symptoms are reported by the patient to be widespread or global and the etiology appears to be associated with a central mechanism. The treatment of these conditions becomes more complicated, because perpetuating factors and cyclic muscle pain also need to be addressed. A chronic systemic myalgic disorder that the dental practitioner needs to be aware of is *fibromyalgia*. This condition represents a global musculoskeletal pain disorder that can often be confused with an acute masticatory muscle disorder. In the past fibromyalgia has been referred to in the medical literature as *fibrositis*. According to a rheumatologic consensus report,[87] fibromyalgia is a widespread musculoskeletal pain disorder in which tenderness is found in 11 or more of 18 specific tender point sites throughout the body. Fibromyalgia is not a masticatory pain disorder, yet many patients with fibromyalgia are mistreated with TMD therapies.[88] This occurs because 42% of patients with fibromyalgia also report TMD-like symptoms.[88] It must be recognized that several chronic systemic muscle pain conditions can co-exist.[89] When this occurs, the patient may need to be referred to the appropriate medical personnel for each condition.

Muscular Toothache

Heterotopic pain manifested as a spontaneous toothache (referred pain) or palpable tenderness of the teeth (secondary hyperalgesia) may occur as a result of myofascial trigger points in the orofacial musculature (see chapter 11, Case 1). Trigger points in the temporalis muscle may induce pain felt as maxillary toothache. Superficial masseter muscle trigger points cause pain to be felt in the maxillary and mandibular posterior teeth. Trigger points in the anterior digastric muscle refer to the mandibular anterior teeth. Muscle-induced heterotopic tooth pain can be distinguished from odontogenous pain in that there is inadequate local dental cause and the pain is not arrested by analgesic blocking of the tooth.

Referred Pain Mistaken for Masticatory Pain

Heterotopic pain referred to the auricular and preauricular area or from nonmasticatory muscles may be mistaken for pains that emanate from the masticatory apparatus (see Case 18). The source of such pain is myofascial trigger points located in the inferior lateral pterygoid, the medial pterygoid, the deep masseter, or the clavicular division of the sternocleidomastoid muscle. Such pain can be distinguished from true masticatory pain in that it is not accompanied by coincidental symptoms of masticatory dysfunction and it is not arrested by analgesic blocking of the joint proper.

Differentiating Various Masticatory Muscle Pains

Masticatory muscle pain is experienced by the patient as a diffuse, commonly bilateral, complaint. The location of the discomfort felt by the patient may be wholly inaccurate as a means of identifying its source. The overriding painful sensation is usually described as having a dull, aching quality. Spontaneous lancinating pains may occur, shooting to the ear, temple, or face. Such pains may also relate to chewing and opening. Palpable tenderness over the joint is frequently masseteric in origin. Infra-auricular, postmandibular, and pharyngeal discomfort usually originates from the medial pterygoid. Temple discomfort is usually temporal in origin. Earache is usually masseteric in origin. Although secondary referred pains may be felt widely over the auricular, preauricular, infra-auricular, temporal, and facial areas, such pain is rarely described as located in the postauricular, occipital, or cervical areas unless cervical muscles are simultaneously involved. Headache occurs frequently.

Elevator Muscle Pain

Pain of an elevator muscle will often restrict opening movement to the extent of the shortened muscle but does not appreciably restrict protrusive or contralateral excursion, except for that which results from the inhibitory effect of pain. The mandibular incisal path is deflected to the affected side when the masseter or temporalis is shortened unilaterally. It is deflected to the opposite side when the medial pterygoid is shortened unilaterally. Deflection does not occur when both the masseter and medial

pterygoid are shortened unilaterally or with any combination of bilateral muscle shortening. Deflection of protrusive excursion does not occur except that arising from pain inhibition.

Some poorly defined acute malocclusion may occur that is more readily sensed subjectively by the patient than witnessed objectively by the examiner.

Pain originating in the elevator muscles is accentuated when the patient attempts to open the mouth, chew food, or clench the teeth. The clenching pain is not decreased by biting on a tongue blade placed between the teeth on the painful side. Pain with opening is a result of stretching the painful muscle. Pain when chewing food and clenching the teeth is the result of contracting the painful muscle. Eccentric movement of the mandible will not usually increase pain, since this type of movement does not significantly lengthen the elevator muscles.

To summarize, pain originating in an elevator muscle may be felt in and about the ear, temple, and face. The pain increases with opening, chewing food, and clenching the teeth, with the latter pain not being reduced by biting on a tongue blade. The masticatory pain is accompanied by a restriction of opening. Deflection of the incisal path depends on the muscles involved. There is minimal restriction of lateral and protrusive movements except when caused by the inhibitory influence of pain or secondary disc interference. The pain sources are identified by manual palpation and arrested by analgesic blocking of the muscles in a painful spasm.

Inferior Lateral Pterygoid Muscle Pain

Pain originating in the inferior lateral pterygoid muscles may cause an acute malocclusion that is described as premature contact of the anterior teeth on the contralateral side accompanied by bilateral disclusion of the posterior teeth on the ipsilateral side. Local analgesic blocking of the lateral pterygoid will promptly arrest the pain emanating from the muscle and often resolve the acute malocclusion.

Differential Diagnosis

Primary deep somatic musculoskeletal pains that emanate from the musculature of the face and jaws should be distinguished from the following:

1. Odontogenous pains
2. Arthralgic pains that emanate from the TMJs
3. Neurovascular pain disorders
4. Heterotopic referred pains and secondary hyperalgesia arising from other deep somatic pain input
5. Heterotopic projected neuropathic pains
6. Heterotopic pains of central origin
7. Pains of Axis II origin

Therapeutic Options

Since muscle pain is such a common complaint of the orofacial pain patient, the clinician should be very familiar with the management options. As has been stated, not all muscle pain is the same. Therefore in this section, the therapeutic options for each of the muscle categories will be described. Since the muscle model presented depicts a progression of muscle pain disorders, from protective co-contraction to centrally mediated myalgia, a general therapeutic consideration is that if the therapy selected does not resolve the pain complaint, the clinician should consider the next more complicated or chronic muscle condition.

Management of Protective Co-contraction (Muscle Splinting)

It is important for the clinician to remember that protective co-contraction is a normal CNS response, and therefore there is no indication to treat the muscle condition itself. Treatment should instead be directed toward the reason for the co-contraction. When co-contraction results from trauma, definitive treatment is not indicated, since the etiologic factor is no longer present.

When co-contraction results from the introduction of a poorly fitting restoration, definitive treatment consists of altering the restoration to harmonize with the existing occlusion. Altering the occlusal condition to eliminate co-contraction is directed only at the offending restoration and not the entire dentition. Once the offending restoration has been eliminated, the occlusal condition is returned to its preexisting state, which resolves the symptoms.

If the co-contraction is the result of a source of deep pain, then the pain needs to be appropriately addressed. If an increase in emotional stress is the etiology, then appropriate stress management such as physical self regulation (PSR) techniques should be instituted.

When the etiology of protective co-contraction is tissue injury, supportive therapy is often the only type of treatment rendered. It begins with instructing the patient to restrict use of the mandible to within painless limits. A soft diet may be recommended until the pain subsides. Short-term pain medication (eg, nonsteroidal anti-inflammatory drugs [NSAIDs]) may be indicated. Simple PSR techniques can also be initiated. Generally, however, muscle exercises and other physical therapies are not indicated. Co-contraction is usually of short duration, and if the etiologic factors are controlled, symptoms will resolve in several days.

Management of Local Muscle Soreness (Noninflammatory Myalgia)

Since local muscle soreness produces deep pain, which often creates secondary protective co-contraction, cyclic muscle pain is common. Therefore the primary goal in treating local muscle soreness is to decrease sensory input (such as pain) to the CNS. Decrease in sensory input is achieved by the following steps:

1. Eliminate any ongoing altered sensory or proprioceptive input.
2. Eliminate any ongoing source of deep pain input (whether dental or other).
3. Provide patient education and information on self management (PSR). The following four areas should be emphasized:
   a. Advise the patient to restrict mandibular use to within painless limits. Any time use of the mandible causes pain, co-contraction can be re-established. Therefore, the patient should be instructed not to open to the point of pain. A soft diet should be encouraged, along with smaller bites and slower chewing.
   b. The patient should be encouraged to use the jaw within the painless limits so that the proprioceptors and mechanioceptors in the musculoskeletal system are stimulated. This activity seems to encourage a return to normal muscle function.[90] Therefore, careful and deliberate use of the muscle can promote resolution of local muscle soreness. Again, the patient should be encouraged to use the muscles, but only within painless limits; complete

lack of muscle use is not appropriate for patients experiencing local muscle soreness.
   c. The patient should be made aware of the relationship between increased levels of emotional stress and the muscle pain condition. Techniques that reduce stress and promote relaxation should be encouraged.[91]
   d. The patient should be encouraged to reduce any nonfunctional tooth contacts. This begins by asking the patient to become more aware of those subconscious times when the teeth are in contact and then developing techniques to eliminate these contacts (cognitive awareness).[92,93] The patient is instructed to keep the lips together and the teeth apart. Most patients can develop the skills necessary for voluntary disengagement of the teeth during the waking hours.
4. Although patients can often control daytime tooth contacts, most have very little control of nocturnal tooth contacts.[94] When nighttime clenching or bruxing is suspected (early morning pain) it is appropriate to fabricate an occlusal appliance for nighttime use.[95–99] An occlusal appliance is an acrylic resin device that fits over the teeth of one arch and provides precise occlusal contact with the opposing arch (Fig 12-12). A stabilization (centric relation) appliance will provide even occlusal contacts when the condyles are in their anterosuperior position resting on the articular discs against the posterior slopes of the articular eminences (musculoskeletally stable). Eccentric guidance is developed on the canines only. The patient is instructed to wear the appliance at night during sleep and only occasionally during the day if it helps reduce the pain. The part-time use of this type of appliance for local muscle soreness has been demonstrated to be more effective in reducing muscle pain

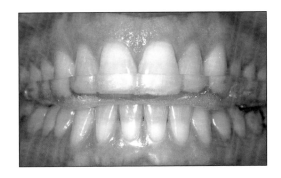

Fig 12-12 An occlusal appliance (stabilization appliance) maybe useful in reducing some muscle pain conditions.

than full-time use.[100] Information on the fabrication of an occlusal appliance can be found in other texts.[101]

The general consideration for managing local muscle soreness is directed toward reducing pain and restoring normal muscle function. In most cases, pain can be controlled easily by the treatments discussed above. However, if pain continues, it can usually be controlled with a mild analgesic such as aspirin, acetaminophen, or an NSAID (eg, ibuprofen). The patient should be encouraged to take the medication regularly so that all pain will be controlled. If the patient takes the medication only occasionally, the cyclic effect of the deep pain input may not be stopped. The patient should be instructed to take the medication every 4 to 6 hours for 5 to 7 days so that the pain is eliminated and the cycle is broken. After this, the patient should no longer need medication.

Manual physical therapy techniques such as passive muscle stretching and gentle massage may also be helpful. Relaxation therapy may also be helpful if increased stress is suspected. On occasion a muscle relaxant[102] may be helpful, even though there is no evidence of any muscle contraction. Muscle relaxants are likely most helpful just before sleep to promote better rest.

Local muscle soreness should respond to therapy in 1 to 3 weeks. When this therapy is not effective, the clinician should consider the possibility of a misdiagnosis. If a re-evaluation of the pain condition reinforces a masticatory muscle disorder, one of the more complicated myalgic disorders should be considered.

Management of CNS-Influenced Conditions

The following four muscle conditions (myospasm, myofascial pain, chronic centrally mediated myalgia, and fibromyalgia) are influenced by activities within the CNS. The clinician's appreciation of the role of the CNS is therapeutically important. Myospasm is an acute local disorder, while myofascial pain and chronic centrally mediated myalgia are more chronic regional disorders. Fibromyalgia is a chronic systemic (global) pain disorder.

Management of myospasms (tonic contraction myalgia)

There are two management considerations for myospasms. The first is directed immediately toward reducing the spasm itself, while the other addresses the etiology.

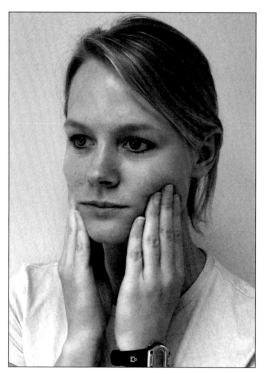

Fig 12-13 Gentle massage of painful muscles accompanied by passive mouth opening to within painful limits can be used to help provide pain relief.

1. Myospasms are best treated by reducing the pain and then passively lengthening or stretching the involved muscle. Reduction of the pain can be achieved by manual massage (Fig 12-13), vapocoolant spray, ice, or even an injection of local anesthetic into the muscle in spasm. Once the pain is reduced, the muscle is passively stretched to full length. If an injection is used—and often it is the most effective way to stop a persistent spasm—2% lidocaine without a vasoconstrictor is recommended.

2. When obvious etiologic factors are present (ie, deep pain input) attempts should be directed toward elimination of these factors so as to lessen the likelihood of recurrent myospasms. When the myospasms are secondary to fatigue and overuse (prolonged exercise), the patient is advised to rest the muscle(s) and re-establish normal electrolyte balance.

On occasion, myospasms can repeatedly occur with no identifiable etiologic factors. When this occurs in the same muscle and the condition is nonresponsive to the above therapies, botulinum toxin A (Botox) injections can be considered. Botulinum toxin A is a neurotoxin that when injected into a muscle causes an irreversible presynaptic blockade of the release of acetylcholine at the motor end plates. The end result is a muscle that can no longer contract (paralysis). This process normally takes 1 to 2 weeks for the effect to be clinically noticeable. Once this has occurred, the neuromuscular end plates react with a collateral sprouting of axons that restores the preexisting condition. In other words, the use of botulinum toxin A appears to be totally reversed in 3 to 4 months. This medication has been used for years for blepharospasm[103] and spasmodic torticollis.[104] More recently it has been used for some masticatory muscle disorders.[105-112] Although the precise indications for botulinum toxin A in the management of TMD is still being debated, certainly the presence of recurrent uncontrolled myospasm (dystonia) is an indication. When this condition exists, the muscle should be injected with botulinum toxin A and the patient should be closely followed. If good success is achieved but the condition returns in 3 to 4 months, the procedure may be repeated.

Often, physical therapy techniques are the key to managing myospasms. Soft tissue mobilization such as deep massage and passive stretching are the two most important immediate treatments. Once the myospasm is reduced, other physical therapies can be helpful in addressing local and systemic factors, such as muscle conditioning exercises and relaxation techniques. Pharmacologic therapy is not usually indicated because of the acuteness of the condition.

Management of myofascial pain (trigger point myalgia)

The treatment of myofascial pain is directed toward the elimination or reduction of etiologic factors. The clinician can accomplish this with the following treatment protocol:

1. Eliminate any source of ongoing deep pain input in an appropriate manner according to the etiology.
2. Reduce the local and systemic factors that contribute to myofascial pain. This treatment is individualized to the patient's needs. For example, if emotional stress is an important part of the disorder, stress management techniques are indicated. When posture or work position contributes to myofascial pain, attempts should be made to improve these conditions. PSR techniques are very useful in managing myofascial pain.
3. If a sleep disorder is suspected, proper evaluation and referral should be made. Often low dosages of a tricyclic antidepressant, such as 10 to 20 mg of amitriptyline before bedtime, can be helpful (see chapter 9).
4. One of the most important considerations in the management of myofascial pain is the treatment and elimination of the trigger points. This is accomplished by painlessly stretching the muscle containing the trigger points. The following techniques can be used to achieve this:
   a. Spray and stretch. One of the most common and conservative methods of eliminating trigger points is with a spray and stretch technique.[66,113] This technique consists of spraying a vapocoolant spray (eg, fluoromethane) on the tissue overlying the muscle with a trigger point and then actively stretching the muscle. The vapocoolant spray provides a burst of cutaneous nerve stimulation that temporarily reduces pain perception in the area. Once the tissue has been sprayed, the muscle is stretched to its full length painlessly (Figs 12-14a and 12-14b). The vapocoolant spray is applied from a distance of approximately 18 inches and in the direction of the referred symptoms. The precise technique for each muscle has been described by Simons et al.[114] This text should be an essential part of the armamentarium of any clinician treating myofascial pain.
   b. Pressure and massage. In some instances massage or manipulation of a trigger point can cause it to be eliminated. Care must be taken, however, not to produce pain. It has been suggested[66] that application of increased pressure to a trigger point also can be an effective eliminating technique. The pressure is increased to approximately 20 pounds and is maintained for 30 to 60 seconds. If this technique produces pain, it must be stopped, since the pain can reinforce cyclic muscle pain.
   c. Ultrasound and electrogalvanic stimulation (EGS). Physical therapy modalities such as ultrasound and EGS can sometimes be useful in managing trigger points. Ultrasound produces deep heat to the area of the trigger point, causing local muscle relaxation.[115] High-voltage EGS rhythmically pulsates the muscle to levels of fatigue, causing muscle relaxation.[116] Although there is little research to verify the efficacy of these techniques, they are generally very conservative and may be useful.
   d. Injection and stretch. Another effective method of eliminating a trigger point is by using injection techniques (Fig 12-15). Most commonly, local anesthetic is injected and the muscle can then be painlessly stretched.[66,117] Although the anesthetic is useful in re-

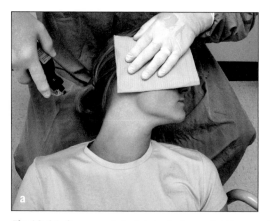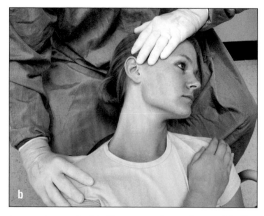

Fig 12-14 Spray and stretch technique. *(a)* Vapocoolant spray is applied to the upper trapezius and to the cervical muscles to eliminate myofascial trigger points. The eyes, nose, mouth, and ear are protected from the spray. *(b)* Immediately following the spray, the muscles are painlessly stretched.

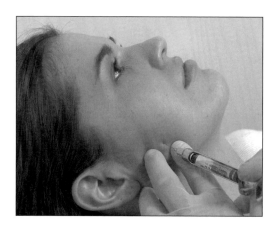

Fig 12-15 Trigger point injection. A trigger point in the right masseter is located, trapped between the fingers, and injected (with a short 27-gauge needle).

ducing pain,[7] it is apparently not the most critical factor in eliminating the trigger point.[118,119] Rather, the mechanical disruption of the trigger point by the needle seems to provide the therapeutic effect.

Local anesthetic is used for two reasons: First, it eliminates the immediate pain, allowing full painless stretching of the muscle. Second, it is diagnostic; in other words, once a trigger point is anesthetized, not only is the local pain reduced, but the referred pain is also eliminated. Thus the clinician can gain valuable information regarding the source of referred pain. For example, the anesthetic injection of a trigger point in the sternocleidomastoid will immediately eliminate a referred temporal headache and enable identification of the true source of the headache pain. The immediate shutdown of pain relates to the interruption of the central excitatory effects produced by the deep pain (the trigger point). This suppression of pain appears to be in part related to the endorphin system.[120]

When local anesthetic injections are indicated, 1% procaine appears to be the least myotoxic. However, this medication is no longer packaged for use in dental syringes; thus, when a dental syringe is used, 2% lidocaine is appropriate. A vasoconstrictor should not be used for muscle injections. A long-acting anesthetic such as bupivacaine (Marcaine) is not indicated for muscle injections because of increased myotoxicity, especially when used with steroids.[121] Only a small amount of lidocaine is needed to treat a trigger point. One dental Carpule is adequate for two or even three points, depending on the size of the muscle being injected. A half Carpule is indicated for a trapezius trigger point; less than a third is adequate for a temporalis trigger point.

Trigger point injections may be an appropriate treatment for myofascial pain when it is found that the injections provide the patient with prolonged relief, even after the anesthetic effect has resolved. Repeated injections may be indicated if the period of pain relief continues to become longer between each injection. If trigger point injections fail to provide any prolonged pain relief, there is no indication to repeat the procedure.

As with any injection, the five rules described in chapter 8 should always be followed. The anatomic considerations and injection technique for each muscle are described by Simons et al,[66] and their text should be consulted by clinicians interested in treating myofascial pain with trigger point injections.

5. Pharmacologic therapy such as a muscle relaxant can be helpful, but it will not usually eliminate the trigger points. A medication such as cyclobenzaprine (Flexeril; 10 mg at bedtime) can often reduce pain, but the trigger points still need to be treated as discussed above. Muscle relaxants help convert an active trigger point into a latent or dormant trigger point but may not necessarily eliminate it. Analgesics may also be helpful in interrupting the cyclic effect of pain.

6. Posture is another possible contributor in some patients to myofascial pain.[57] Muscles that are maintained at shortened length tend to develop trigger points more than others. Daily stretching to full length can be beneficial in maintaining them pain free. This is especially true in the neck and shoulder region. Regular exercise should always be encouraged.[60,122]

Management of centrally mediated myalgia (chronic myositis)

The clinician needs to recognize the condition of chronic centrally mediated myalgia, since the outcome of therapy will not be as immediate as when treating local muscle soreness. Neurogenic inflammation of muscle tissue, and the chronic central sensitization that has produced it, often takes time to resolve. When the diagnosis of chronic centrally mediated myalgia is established, the clinician should discuss with the patient the expected results and time table. The patient should be informed that reduction of symptoms is initially slow and not dramatic. Patients need to be aware of this so as to minimize disappointment in treatment results. As etiologic factors are controlled, neurogenic inflammation will resolve and symptoms will slowly decrease.

As is true with local muscle soreness, four general treatment strategies are followed in the patient with chronic centrally mediated myalgia. However, although somewhat similar, they are not identical. In fact, therapy for local muscle soreness will often aggravate chronic centrally mediated myalgia. Therefore, if the clinician is treating local muscle soreness and the symptoms become greater, it is likely that the condition is actually chronic centrally mediated myalgia. The following regimen should then be used:

1. Restrict mandibular use to within painless limits. Using painful muscles only aggravates the condition. The patient should keep the jaw immobile, as needed to reduce pain. A soft diet is initiated, along with slower chewing and smaller bites. There may be indications to use a liquid diet if functional pain cannot be controlled. The liquid diet should be maintained long enough to allow pain reduction so that the patient can return to a soft diet without pain.

2. Avoid exercise and/or injections. Since the muscle tissue is inflamed, any use initiates pain. The patient should rest the muscles as much as possible. Local anesthetic injections should be avoided since they traumatize already inflamed tissues. Local anesthetic blocking in chronic centrally mediated myalgia will often cause a marked increase in pain after the anesthetic has been metabolized. This clinical feature may help establish the diagnosis.

3. Disengage the teeth. As with local muscle soreness, the management of chronic centrally mediated myalgia is assisted by disengaging the teeth both voluntarily and involuntarily. Voluntary disengagement is accomplished by the PSR techniques discussed in chapter 9. Involuntary disengagement of the teeth (nocturnal bruxism) is achieved by a stabilization appliance in the same manner as with local muscle soreness.

4. Begin taking an anti-inflammatory medication. Since local muscle tissue is inflamed, it is quite appropriate to prescribe an anti-inflammatory. An NSAID, such as ibuprofen, is a good choice and should be given on a regular basis (eg, 600 mg four times daily) for 2 weeks so blood levels are sufficiently elevated to achieve a clinical effect. Irregular doses taken only as needed will not achieve the desired effect. Ibuprofen is also analgesic, and it can thus help reduce cyclic muscle pain that can propagate chronic centrally mediated myalgia. As previously discussed, the patient should be questioned for any history of stomach complaints and monitored for any gastric irritation symptoms during the course of the medication. If these symptoms are present, a cyclooxygenase inhibitor should be considered (see chapter 9).

Early in the treatment of chronic centrally mediated myalgia, physical therapy modalities should be used cautiously, since any manipulation can increase the pain. Sometimes moist heat can be helpful (Fig 12-16). For other patients, ice seems to be more helpful. The patients will clearly relate which is best for them. As the symptoms begin to resolve, ultrasound therapy and gentle stretching can begin. If pain is increased by the therapy, the intensity should be decreased.

Since the treatment of chronic centrally mediated myalgia often takes time, two distinct conditions can develop: hypotrophic changes and myostatic contracture. These occur as a result of the lack of use of the elevator muscles (temporalis, masseter, medial pterygoid). Once the acute symptoms have resolved, activity of the muscles should slowly begin. Some gentle isometric jaw exercise will be effective for increasing the strength and use of the muscles (Figs 12-17a and 12-17b). Passive stretching is also helpful in regaining the original length of the elevators. Remember, the treatment of chronic centrally mediated myalgia is a slow process and it cannot be rushed. If physical therapy is introduced too quickly, the chronic centrally mediated myalgia can worsen.

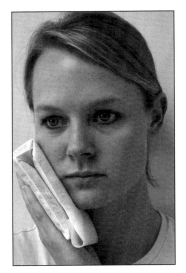 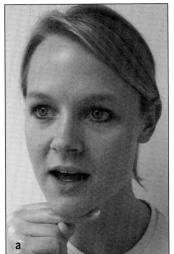 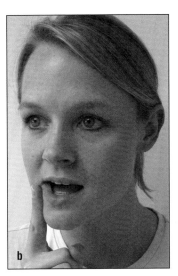

Fig 12-16 Moist heat can be used to reduce muscle pain.

Fig 12-17 Gentle isometric jaw exercises are helpful for increasing the strength of hypotrophic muscles. *(a)* The objective is to resist the mouth-opening movement slightly. *(b)* The patient moves the jaw laterally while resisting the movement with the fingers. This is done for 3 to 5 seconds in an opening, a right, and a left lateral movement, as well as in a protrusive movement. The exercises are repeated throughout the day.

Management of chronic systemic myalgic disorders (fibromyalgia)

Since the knowledge of fibromyalgia is limited, treatment should be conservative and directed toward the etiologic and perpetuating factors. The clinician should remember that fibromyalgia is not a primary masticatory muscle disorder. The dental practitioner, therefore, should not assume the role of primary therapist. Instead, he or she must be able to recognize fibromyalgia and make the proper referral. When significant masticatory symptoms are present, the dental clinician should manage these symptoms along with a team of health professionals. Other health professionals that can help manage this problem are rheumatolo-

gists, rehabilitative therapists, psychologists, and physical therapists.[123] The following general treatments should be considered:

1. When other masticatory muscle disorders also exist, therapy should be directed toward these disorders.
2. Any perpetuating conditions that continue to aggravate the symptoms should be properly addressed.
3. NSAIDs seem to be of some benefit with fibromyalgic symptoms and should be administered in the same manner as for chronic centrally mediated myalgia.
4. If a sleep disturbance is identified, it should be addressed. Low dosages of a tricyclic antidepressant such as 10 to 50 mg of amitriptyline at bedtime can be

helpful in reducing symptoms associated with fibromyalgia.[124,125] The mechanism is thought to be related to an improvement in the quality of sleep.[124-126] Cyclobenzaprine (Flexeril; 10 mg at bedtime) may also be helpful to assist in sleep and reduce pain.[127,128]

5. If depression is present, it should be managed by appropriate health professionals.

Physical therapy modalities and manual techniques can be helpful for the patient with fibromyalgia. Techniques such as moist heat, gentle massage, passive stretching, and relaxation training can be the most helpful. Also, muscle conditioning can be an important part of treatment. A mild and well-controlled general exercise program such as walking or light swimming can be very helpful in lessening the muscle pain associated with fibromyalgia.[122,129] Care should be taken to develop an individual program for each patient.

References

1. Mense S, Meyer H. Bradykinin-induced sensitization of high-threshold muscle receptors with slowly conducting afferent fibers [abstract]. Pain 1981;(suppl 1):S204.
2. Keele KD. A physician looks at pain. In: Weisenberg M (ed). Pain: Clinical and Experimental Perspectives. St Louis: Mosby, 1975:45–52.
3. Layzer RB. Muscle pain, cramps and fatigue. In: Engel AG, Franzini-Armstrong C (eds). Myology. New York: McGraw-Hill, 1994:1754–1786.
4. Lund JP, Widmer CG. Evaluation of the use of surface electromyography in the diagnosis, documentation, and treatment of dental patients. J Craniomandib Disord Facial Oral Pain 1989;3:125–137.
5. Lund JP, Widmer CG, Feine JS. Validity of diagnostic and monitoring tests used for temporomandibular disorders [see comments]. J Dent Res 1995;74:1133–1143.
6. Paesani DA, Tallents RH, Murphy WC, Hatala MP, Proskin HM. Evaluation of the reproducibility of rest activity of the anterior temporal and masseter muscles in asymptomatic and symptomatic temporomandibular subjects. J Orofac Pain 1994;8:402–406.
7. Carlson CR, Okeson JP, Falace DA, Nitz AJ, Lindroth JE. Reduction of pain and EMG activity in the masseter region by trapezius trigger point injection. Pain 1993;55:397–400.
8. Curran SL, Carlson CR, Okeson JP. Emotional and physiologic responses to laboratory challenges: Patients with temporomandibular disorders versus matched control subjects. J Orofac Pain 1996;10:141–150.
9. Mense S. Considerations concerning the neurobiological basis of muscle pain. Can J Physiol Pharmacol 1991;69:610–616.
10. Mense S. Nociception from skeletal muscle in relation to clinical muscle pain. Pain 1993;54:241–289.
11. Molin C. Vertical isometric muscle forces of the mandible. A comparative study of subjects with and without manifest mandibular pain dysfunction syndrome. Acta Odontol Scand 1972;30:485–499.
12. Nielsen IL, Ogro J, McNeill C, Danzig WN, Goldman SM, Miller AJ. Alteration in proprioceptive reflex control in subjects with craniomandibular disorders. J Craniomandib Disord 1987;1:170–178.
13. Wolff HG. Headache and Other Head Pain, ed 2. New York: Oxford University Press, 1963.
14. Kreiner M, Okeson JP. Toothache of cardiac origin. J Orofac Pain 1999;13:201–207.
15. Ochoa JL, Torebjork HE. Pain from skin and muscle [abstract]. Pain 1981;11(suppl 1):87.
16. MacDonald AJR. Abnormally tender muscle regions and associated painful movements. Pain 1980;8:197–205.
17. Okeson J. Orofacial Pain: Guidelines for Classification, Assessment, and Management. Chicago: Quintessence, 1996.
18. Carlson CR, Okeson JP, Falace DA, Nitz AJ, Curran SL, Anderson D. Comparison of psychologic and physiologic functioning between patients with masticatory muscle pain and matched controls. J Orofac Pain 1993;7:15–22.
19. Yemm R. A neurophysiological approach to the pathology and aetiology of temporomandibular dysfunction. J Oral Rehabil 1985;12:343–353.

20. Schroeder H, Siegmund H, Santibanez G, Kluge A. Causes and signs of temporomandibular joint pain and dysfunction: An electromyographical investigation. J Oral Rehabil 1991;18:301–310.

21. Flor H, Birbaumer N, Schulte W, Roos R. Stress-related electromyographic responses in patients with chronic temporomandibular pain. Pain 1991;46:145–152.

22. Linton SJ, Hellsing AL, Andersson D. A controlled study of the effects of an early intervention on acute musculoskeletal pain problems. Pain 1993;54:353–359.

23. Sternbach RA. Pain and "hassles" in the United States: Findings of the Nuprin pain report. Pain 1986;27:69–80.

24. Selye H. Stress Without Distress. Philadelphia: Lippincott, 1974:32.

25. Schiffman EL, Fricton JR, Haley D. The relationship of occlusion, parafunctional habits and recent life events to mandibular dysfunction in a non-patient population. J Oral Rehabil 1992;19:201–223.

26. McCreary CP, Clark GT, Merril RL, Flack V, Oakley ME. Psychological distress and diagnostic subgroups of temporomandibular disorder patients. Pain 1991;44:29–34.

27. Grassi C, Passatore M. Action of the sympathetic system on skeletal muscle. Ital J Neurol Sci 1988;9:23–28.

28. Passatore M, Grassi C, Filippi GM. Sympathetically-induced development of tension in jaw muscles: The possible contraction of intrafusal muscle fibres. Pflugers Arch 1985;405:297–304.

29. McNulty WH, Gevirtz RN, Hubbard DR, Berkoff GM. Needle electromyographic evaluation of trigger point response to a psychological stressor. Psychophysiology 1994;31:313–316.

30. Wall PD, Devor M. Sensory afferent impulses originate from dorsal root ganglia as well as from the periphery in normal and nerve injured rats. Pain 1983;17:321–339.

31. Melzack R, Wall PD. Pain mechanisms: A new theory. Science 1965;150:971–979.

32. Wall PD. The gate control theory of pain mechanisms: A reexamination and restatement. Brain 1978;101:1–18.

33. Bell WE. Normal craniomandibular function. In: Temporomandibular Disorders: Classification, Diagnosis, Management, ed 3. Chicago: Year Book, 1990:60–61.

34. Ashton-Miller JA, McGlashen KM, Herzenberg JE, Stohler CS. Cervical muscle myoelectric response to acute experimental sternocleidomastoid pain. Spine 1990;15:1006–1012.

35. Lund JP, Donga R, Widmer CG, Stohler CS. The pain-adaptation model: A discussion of the relationship between chronic musculoskeletal pain and motor activity. Can J Physiol Pharmacol 1991;69:683–694.

36. Lund JP, Olsson KA. The importance of reflexes and their control during jaw movements. Trends Neurosci 1983;6:458–463.

37. Finger M, Stohler CS, Ash MM Jr. The effect of acrylic bite plane splints and their vertical dimension on jaw muscle silent period in healthy young adults. J Oral Rehabil 1985;12:381–388.

38. Stohler CS, Ash MM. Excitatory response of jaw elevators associated with sudden discomfort during chewing. J Oral Rehabil 1986;13:225–233.

39. Smith AM. The coactivation of antagonist muscles. Can J Physiol Pharmacol 1981;59:733–747.

40. Stohler CS. Clinical perspectives on masticatory and related muscle disorders. In: Sessle BJ, Bryant PS, Dionne RA (eds). Temporomandibular Disorders and Related Pain Conditions. Seattle: IASP Press, 1995:3–29.

41. Stohler CS, Ashton-Miller JA, Carlson DS. The effects of pain from the mandibular joint and muscles on masticatory motor behaviour in man. Arch Oral Biol 1988;33:175–182.

42. Watanabe M, Tabata T, Huh JI, et al. Possible involvement of histamine in muscular fatigue in temporomandibular disorders: animal and human studies. J Dent Res 1999;78:769–775.

43. Christensen LV, Mohamed SE, Harrison JD. Delayed onset of masseter muscle pain in experimental tooth clenching. J Prosthet Dent 1982;48:579–584.

44. Abraham WM. Factors in delayed muscle soreness. Med Sci Sports 1977;9:11–20.

45. Bakke M, Michler L. Temporalis and masseter muscle activity in patients with anterior open bite and craniomandibular disorders. Scand J Dent Res 1991;99:219–228.

46. Tzakis MG, Dahlstrom L, Haraldson T. Evaluation of masticatory function before and after treatment in patients with craniomandibular disorders. J Craniomandib Disord Facial Oral Pain 1992;6:267–272.

47. Sinn DP, de Assis EA, Throckmorton GS. Mandibular excursions and maximum bite forces in patients with temporomandibular joint disorders. J Oral Maxillofac Surg 1996;54:671–679.

48. High AS, MacGregor AJ, Tomlinson GE. A gnathodynamometer as an objective means of pain assessment following wisdom tooth removal. Br J Maxillofac Surg 1988;26:284–291.

49. Mense S. The pathogenesis of muscle pain. Curr Pain Headache Rep 2003;7:419–425.

50. Gonzales R, Coderre TJ, Sherbourne CD, Levine JD. Postnatal development of neurogenic inflammation in the rat. Neurosci Lett 1991;127:25–27.

51. Levine JD, Dardick SJ, Basbaum AI, Scipio E. Reflex neurogenic inflammation. I. Contribution of the peripheral nervous system to spatially remote inflammatory responses that follow injury. J Neurosci 1985;5:1380–1386.

52. Fricton JR, Kroening R, Haley D, Siegert R. Myofascial pain syndrome of the head and neck: A review of clinical characteristics of 164 patients. Oral Surg Oral Med Oral Pathol 1985;60:615–623.

53. Travell JG, Rinzler SH. The myofascial genesis of pain. Postgrad Med 1952;11:425–434.

54. Laskin DM. Etiology of the pain-dysfunction syndrome. J Am Dent Assoc 1969;79:147–153.

55. Simons DG, Travell J. Myofascial trigger points, a possible explanation [letter]. Pain 1981;10:106–109.

56. McMillan AS, Blasberg B. Pain-pressure threshold in painful jaw muscles following trigger point injection. J Orofac Pain 1994;8:384–390.

57. Simons DG, Travell JG, Simons LS. General overview. In: Travell & Simons' Myofascial Pain and Dysfunction: The Trigger Point Manual, ed 2. Baltimore: Williams & Wilkins, 1999:11–93.

58. Fricton JR, Auvinen MD, Dykstra D, Schiffman E. Myofascial pain syndrome: Electromyographic changes associated with local twitch response. Arch Phys Med Rehabil 1985;66:314–317.

59. Hubbard DR, Berkoff GM. Myofascial trigger points show spontaneous needle EMG activity. Spine. 1993;18:1803–1807.

60. Simons DG, Travell JG, Simons LS. Perpetuating factors. In: Travell & Simons' Myofascial Pain and Dysfunction: The Trigger Point Manual, ed 2. Baltimore: Williams & Wilkins, 1999:178–235.

61. Giunta JL, Kronman JH. Orofacial involvement secondary to trapezius muscle trauma. Oral Surg Oral Med Oral Pathol 1985;60:368–369.

62. Wright EF. Referred craniofacial pain patterns in patients with temporomandibular disorders. J Am Dent Assoc 2000;131:1307–1315.

63. Simons DG. The nature of myofascial trigger points. Clin J Pain 1995;11:83–84.

64. Hoheisel U, Mense S, Simons DG, Yu XM. Appearance of new receptive fields in rat dorsal horn neurons following noxious stimulation of skeletal muscle: A model for referral of muscle pain? Neurosci Lett 1993;153:9–12.

65. Hong CZ, Simons DG. Pathophysiologic and electrophysiologic mechanisms of myofascial trigger points. Arch Phys Med Rehabil 1998;79:863–872.

66. Simons DG, Travell JG, Simons LS. Apropos of all muscles. In: Travell & Simons' Myofascial Pain and Dysfunction: The Trigger Point Manual, ed 2. Baltimore: Williams & Wilkins, 1999:94–177.

67. McNamara JAJ. The independent functions of the two heads of the lateral pterygoid muscle. Am J Anat 1973;138:197–205.

68. Mahan PE, Wilkinson TM, Gibbs CH, Mauderli A, Brannon LS. Superior and inferior bellies of the lateral pterygoid muscle EMG activity at basic jaw positions. J Prosthet Dent 1983;50:710–718.

69. Eriksson PO. Muscle-fiber composition of the human mandibular locomotor system. Swed Dent J 1982;20(suppl 12):8–44.

70. Johnstone DR, Templeton M. The feasibility of palpating the lateral pterygoid muscle. J Prosthet Dent 1980;44:318–323.

71. Thomas CA, Okeson JP. Evaluation of lateral pterygoid muscle symptoms using a common palpation technique and a method of functional manipulation. Cranio 1987;5:125–129.

72. Martin PR, Mathews AM. Tension headaches: Psychophysiological investigation and treatment. J Psychosom Res 1978;22:389–399.

73. Sutton EP, Belar CD. Tension headache patients versus controls: A study of EMG parameters. Headache 1982;22:133–136.

74. Travell JG, Simons DG. Myofascial Pain and Dysfunction: The Trigger Point Manual. Baltimore: Williams & Wilkins, 1983:103–164.

75. Finneson BE. Diagnosis and Management of Pain Syndromes. Philadelphia: Saunders, 1969.

76. Headache Classification Subcommittee of the International Headache Society. The International Classification of Headache Disorders. Cephalalgia 2004;24(suppl 1):9–160.

77. Carlson CR, Okeson JP, Falace DA, Nitz AJ, Curran SL, Anderson DT. Comparison of psychologic and physiologic functioning between patients with masticatory muscle pain and matched controls. J Orofacial Pain 1993;7:15–22.

78. Schroeder H, Siegmund H, Santibanez G, Kluge A. Causes and signs of temporomandibular joint pain and dysfunction: An electromyographical investigation. J Oral Rehabil 1991;18:301–331.

79. Yemm R. A neurophysiological approach to the pathology and aetiology of temporomandibular dysfunction. J Oral Rehabil 1985;12:343–353.

80. Lund JP, Widmer CG. Evaluation of the use of surface electromyograph in the diagnosis, documentation and treatment of dental patients. J Craniomandib Disord Facial Oral Pain 1989; 3:125–137.

81. Lund JP, Donga R, Widmer CG, Stohler CS. The pain-adaptation model: A discussion of the relationship between chronic musculoskeletal pain and motor activity. Can J Physiol Pharmacol 1991;69:683–694.

82. Bowsher D. Neurogenic pain syndromes and their management. Br Med Bull 1991;47: 644–666.

83. LaMotte RH, Shain CN, Simone DA, Tsai EF. Neurogenic hyperalgesia: Psychophysical studies of underlying mechanisms. J Neurophysiol 1991;66:190–211.

84. Sessle BJ. The neural basis of temporomandibular joint and masticatory muscle pain. J Orofac Pain 1999;13:238–245.

85. Simone DA, Sorkin LS, Oh U, et al. Neurogenic hyperalgesia: Central neural correlates in responses of spinothalamic tract neurons. J Neurophysiol 1991;66:228–246.

86. Wong JK, Haas DA, Hu JW. Local anesthesia does not block mustard-oil–induced temporomandibular inflammation. Anesth Analg 2001; 92:1035–1040.

87. Wolfe F, Smythe HA, Yunus MB, et al. The American College of Rheumatology 1990 Criteria for the Classification of Fibromyalgia. Report of the Multicenter Criteria Committee [see comments]. Arthritis Rheum 1990;33:160–172.

88. Korszun A, Papadopoulos E, Demitrack M, Engleberg C, Crofford L. The relationship between temporomandibular disorders and stress-associated syndromes. Oral Surg Oral Med Oral Pathol Oral Radiol Endod 1998;86:416–420.

89. Aaron LA, Burke MM, Buchwald D. Overlapping conditions among patients with chronic fatigue syndrome, fibromyalgia, and temporomandibular disorders [see comments]. Arch Intern Med 2000;160:221–227.

90. Bell WE. Masticatory muscle disorders. In: Temporomandibular Disorders: Classification, Diagnosis and Management. Chicago: Year Book, 1990:280–284.

91. Turk DC, Zaki HS, Rudy TE. Effects of intra-oral appliance and biofeedback/stress management alone and in combination in treating pain and depression in patients with temporomandibular disorders. J Prosthet Dent 1993; 70:158–164.

92. Rosen JC. Self-monitoring in the treatment of diurnal bruxism. J Behav Ther Exp Psychiatry 1981;12:347–350.

93. Bornstein PH, Hamilton SB, Bornstein MT. Self-monitoring procedures. In: Ciminero AR, Calhoun KS, Aams HE (eds). Handbook of Behavioral Assessment. New York: Wiley, 1986: 176–222.

94. Pierce CJ, Gale EN. A comparison of different treatments for nocturnal bruxism. J Dent Res 1988;67:597–601.

95. Solberg WK, Clark GT, Rugh JD. Nocturnal electromyographic evaluation of bruxism patients undergoing short-term splint therapy. J Oral Rehabil 1975;2:215–223.

96. Clark GT, Beemsterboer PL, Solberg WK, Rugh JD. Nocturnal electromyographic evaluation of myofascial pain dysfunction in patients undergoing occlusal splint therapy. J Am Dent Assoc 1979;99:607–611.

97. Yap AU. Effects of stabilization appliances on nocturnal parafunctional activities in patients with and without signs of temporomandibular disorders. J Oral Rehabil 1998;25:64–68.

98. Kurita H, Kurashina K, Kotani A. Clinical effect of full coverage occlusal splint therapy for specific temporomandibular disorder conditions and symptoms. J Prosthet Dent 1997;78: 506–510.

99. Kreiner M, Betancor E, Clark G. Occlusal stabilization appliances: Evidence of their efficacy. J Am Dent Assoc 2001;132:700–777.

100. Wilkinson T, Hansson TL, McNeill C, Marcel T. A comparison of the success of 24-hour occlusal splint therapy versus nocturnal occlusal splint therapy in reducing craniomandibular disorders. J Craniomandib Disord Facial Oral Pain 1992;6:64–69.

101. Okeson JP. Occlusal appliance therapy. In: Management of Temporomandibular Disorders and Occlusion. St Louis: Mosby-Year Book, 2003:507–536.

102. VanHelder WP. Medical treatment of muscle soreness [editorial; comment]. Can J Sport Sci 1992;17:74.

103. Manni E, Bagolini B, Pettorossi VE, Errico P. Effect of botulinum toxin on extraocular muscle proprioception. Doc Ophthalmol 1989;72: 189–198.

104. Roser M, Cornelius CP, Topka H. New techniques in maxillofacial surgery: Local injection treatment with botulinum toxin A. Mund Kiefer Gesichtschir 1998;2(suppl 1):S121–124.

105. Cheshire WP, Abashian SW, Mann JD. Botulinum toxin in the treatment of myofascial pain syndrome. Pain 1994;59:65–69.

106. Freund B, Schwartz M, Symington JM. The use of botulinum toxin for the treatment of temporomandibular disorders: Preliminary findings. J Oral Maxillofac Surg 1999;57:916–920.

107. Freund B, Schwartz M, Symington JM. Botulinum toxin: New treatment for temporomandibular disorders. Br J Oral Maxillofac Surg 2000;38:466–471.

108. Daelen B, Thorwirth V, Koch A. Treatment of recurrent dislocation of the temporomandibular joint with type A botulinum toxin. Int J Oral Maxillofac Surg 1997;26:458–460.

109. Ivanhoe CB, Lai JM, Francisco GE. Bruxism after brain injury: Successful treatment with botulinum toxin-A. Arch Phys Med Rehabil 1997;78:1272–1273.

110. Moore AP, Wood GD. The medical management of masseteric hypertrophy with botulinum toxin type A. Br J Maxillofac Surg 1994;32:26–28.

111. Moore AP, Wood GD. Medical treatment of recurrent temporomandibular joint dislocation using botulinum toxin A. Br Dent J 1997;183:415–417.

112. Sankhla C, Lai EC, Jankovic J. Peripherally induced oromandibular dystonia. J Neurol Neurosurg Psychiatry 1998;65:722–728.

113. Jaeger B, Reeves JL. Quantification of changes in myofascial trigger point sensitivity with the pressure algometer following passive stretch. Pain 1986;27:203–210.

114. Simons DG, Travell JG, Simons LS. Head and neck pain. In: Travell & Simons' Myofascial Pain and Dysfunction: The Trigger Point Manual, ed 2. Baltimore: Williams & Wilkins, 1999:237–483.

115. Zohn DA, Mennell JM. Musculoskeletal Pain: Diagnosis and Physical Treatment. Boston: Little, Brown, 1976:126.

116. Bonica JJ. Management of myofascial pain syndromes in general practice. JAMA 1957;164:732–738.

117. Pippa P, Allegra A, Cirillo L, Doni L, Rivituso C. Fibromyalgia and trigger points. Minerva Anesthesiol 1994;60:281–283.

118. Hong CZ. Lidocaine injection versus dry needling to myofascial trigger point. The importance of the local twitch response. Am J Phys Med Rehabil 1994;73:256–263.

119. Scicchitano J, Rounsefell B, Pilowsky I. Baseline correlates of the response to the treatment of chronic localized myofascial pain syndrome by injection of local anaesthetic. J Psychosom Res 1996;40:75–85.

120. Fine PG, Milano R, Hare BD. The effects of myofascial trigger point injections are naloxone reversible. Pain 1988;32:15–20.

121. Guttu RL, Page DG, Laskin DM. Delayed healing of muscle after injection of bupivicaine and steroid. Ann Dent 1990;49:5–8.

122. McCain GA. Role of physical fitness training in fibrosis/fibromyalgia syndromes. Am J Med 1986;81(suppl 3A):73–77.

123. Bennett RB, Campbell S, Burckhardt C. A multidisciplinary approach to fibromyalgia management. J Musculoskeletal Med 1991;8:21–32.

124. Carette S, McCain GA, Bell DA, Fam AG. Evaluation of amitriptyline in primary fibrositis. A double-blind, placebo-controlled study. Arthritis Rheum 1986;29:655–659.

125. Goldenberg DL, Felson DT, Dinerman H. A randomized, controlled trial of amitriptyline and naproxen in the treatment of patients with fibromyalgia. Arthritis Rheum 1986;29:1371–1377.

126. Goldenberg DL. A review of the role of tricyclic medications in the treatment of fibromyalgia syndrome. J Rheumatol Suppl 1989;19:137–139.

127. Reynolds WJ, Moldofsky H, Saskin P, Lue FA. The effects of cyclobenzaprine on sleep physiology and symptoms in patients with fibromyalgia. J Rheumatol 1991;18:452–454.

128. Hamaty D, Valentine JL, Howard R, Howard CW, Wakefield V, Patten MS. The plasma endorphin, prostaglandin and catecholamine profile of patients with fibrositis treated with cyclobenzaprine and placebo: A 5-month study. J Rheumatol Suppl 1989;19:164–168.

129. Granges G, Littlejohn GO. A comparative study of clinical signs in fibromyalgia/fibrositis syndrome, healthy and exercising subjects. J Rheumatol 1993;20:344–351.

Temporomandibular Joint Pains

Masticatory pain that emanates from the temporomandibular joints (TMJs) is called *masticatory arthralgia* (Fig 13-1). Arthralgic pains can arise only from pain-sensitive structures of the joint and its ligaments. Normally, the pressure-bearing articular surfaces as well as the articular disc are noninnervated and therefore are incapable of initiating sensory response of any kind, including nociception. Proprioceptive input needed for functional guidance does not come from the articular surfaces but from proprioceptors located in the ligaments and muscles. Pain from the TMJs can therefore emanate from the associated soft tissue structures of the joint or the osseous tissues themselves. Pain emanating from the osseous structures usually only occurs after loss of the fibrous articular surface of the joint. When this occurs, it is commonly referred to as *osteoarthritis*. Not all joint pains, however are osteoarthritis. When the soft tissues of the joint produce pain, the condition is classified according to the tissues involved (eg, retrodiscitis, capsulitis).

Behavior of TMJ Pains

Pains that emanate from the structures of the TMJ are of the deep somatic category. As such, they display the clinical characteristics of deep somatic pain. Additionally, they are of the musculoskeletal type and therefore display the features that identify such pains, namely *(1)* the pain is intimately related to masticatory function, and *(2)* the degree of pain is proportionate to the amount of function or manual palpation.

It should be noted that most arthralgia is related to functional abuse and trauma, which may be accompanied by inflammation. Thus, arthralgia frequently displays clinical characteristics of inflammatory pain that are influenced by the location, degree, and phase of inflammation present. Such pains exhibit features that depend on local provocation and functional manipulation, as well as on the extent and confinement of inflammatory exudate. As long as joint pain occurs intermittently, it remains

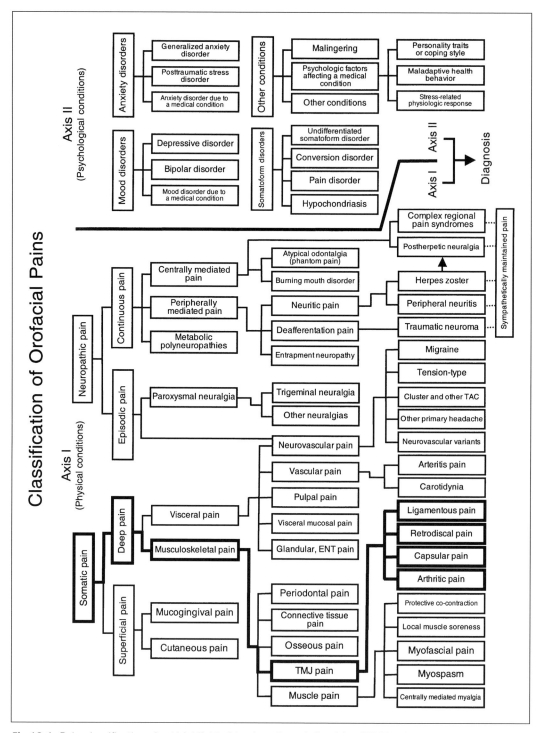

Fig 13-1 Pain classification chart highlighted to show the relationship of TMJ pains to other orofacial pain disorders.

diffusely localized to the joint region and does not initiate secondary central excitatory effects. If arthralgia becomes continuous, however, a variety of secondary effects may become evident, such as referred pain that may be felt as headache, secondary hyperalgesia expressed as areas of deep palpable tenderness, and co-contraction activity in the masticatory musculature.

Normal Anatomy and Function of the TMJ

The TMJ represents the articulation of the mandible to the temporal bone of the cranium (Figs 13-2a and 13-2b). The bony components of the joint are separated by a structure composed of dense fibrous connective tissue, called the *articular disc*. Like any mobile joint, the integrity and limitations of the joint are maintained by ligaments. Ligaments are composed of collagenous fibers that have specific lengths. As in all mobile joints, ligaments do not actively participate in the function of the joint. Ligaments act as guide wires to restrict certain movements (border movements) while allowing other movements (functional movements). If joint movements consistently function against ligaments, the length of the ligaments can become altered. Ligaments have a poor ability to stretch; therefore, when this occurs, they often permanently elongate. This elongation creates a change in joint biomechanics and can lead to certain clinical changes that will be discussed later.

The TMJ is capable of both hinging and gliding movements and therefore is known as a *ginglymoarthrodial* joint. For a simplified understanding of the mechanics of this extremely complex joint, let us separate it into two distinct joints. The lower joint is made up of the condyle and disc, which are at-

tached to each other by ligaments. This combined structure is referred to as the *condyle-disc complex*. The condyle-disc complex allows rotational movement between the disc and the condyle. The upper joint is formed by the articulation of the condyle-disc complex with the glenoid fossa. It is between these structures that translation occurs as the condyle-disc complex moves out of the fossa during opening.

Careful examination of the condyle and disc reveals that the disc is attached to the condyle both medially and laterally by the discal collateral ligaments (Fig 13-3). These ligaments allow rotation of the disc across the articular surface of the condyle in an anterior and posterior direction while restricting medial and lateral movements. The range of anterior and posterior rotation of the disc is also restricted by ligaments. The inferior retrodiscal lamina limits anterior rotation of the disc on the condyle, whereas the anterior capsular ligament limits posterior rotation of the disc (see Fig 13-2b).

The morphology of the disc is extremely important. It is thinnest in the intermediate zone, thicker in the anterior border, and thickest in the posterior border. The condyle articulates on the intermediate zone of the disc and is maintained in this position by constant interarticular pressure provided by the elevator muscles (masseter, temporalis, and medial pterygoid). Although the pressure between the condyle, disc, and fossa can vary according to the activity of the elevator muscles, some pressure is always maintained to prevent separation of the articular surfaces. If contact between the articular surfaces is lost, a condition of dislocation exists (dislocation means separation of the articular surfaces).

Posterior to the disc are the retrodiscal tissues. These tissues are highly vascularized and well innervated. Anterior to the condyle-disc complex are the superior and inferior lateral pterygoid muscles. The inferior pterygoid muscle inserts on the neck of

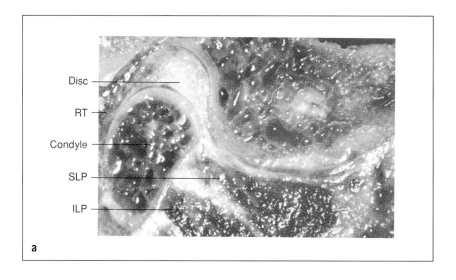

a

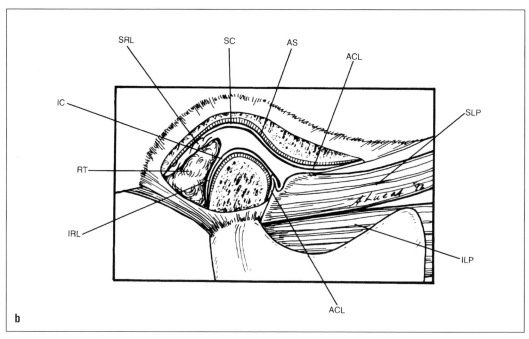

b

Fig 13-2 The TMJ. *(a)* Lateral view; *(b)* diagram showing the anatomic components. RT = retrodiscal tissues; SLP and ILP = superior and inferior lateral pterygoid muscles; SRL = superior retrodiscal lamina (elastic); SC and IC = superior and inferior joint cavities; AS = articular surface; ACL = anterior capsular ligament (collagenous); IRL = inferior retrodiscal lamina (collagenous). The discal (collateral) ligaments have not been drawn. (From Okeson JP. Management of Temporomandibular Disorders and Occlusion, ed 5. St Louis: Mosby-Year Book, 2003:10. Used with permission.)

Fig 13-3 The TMJ (anterior view). The following are identified: AD = articular disc; CL = capsular ligament; IC = inferior joint cavity; LDL = lateral discal ligament; MDL = medial discal ligament; SC = superior joint cavity. (From Okeson JP. Management of Temporomandibular Disorders and Occlusion, ed 5. St Louis: Mosby-Year Book, 2003:14. Used with permission.)

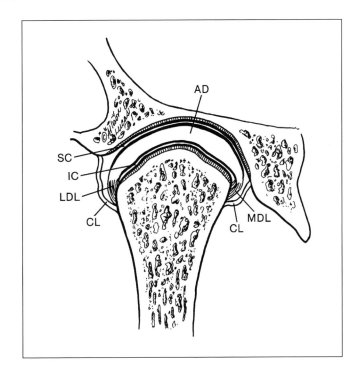

the condyle, whereas the superior lateral pterygoid muscle inserts on both the neck of the condyle and the articular disc. Although the inferior lateral pterygoid is active with the depressing muscles (mouth opening), the superior lateral pterygoid muscle has been shown to be active in conjunction with the elevator muscles (mouth closing).[1,2] The superior lateral pterygoid muscle appears to be a stabilizing muscle for the condyle-disc complex, especially during unilateral chewing.[3]

When the condyle-disc complex translates down the articular eminence (mouth opening), the disc rotates posteriorly on the condyle (Fig 13-4). The superior surface of the retrodiscal tissues is unlike any other structure in the joint. The superior retrodiscal lamina is composed of loose connective tissue and elastin fibers that allow the condyle-disc complex to translate forward without damage to the retrodiscal tissues. In the closed mouth position, the superior retrodiscal tissues are passive and have very little influence on disc position. During full mouth opening, however, the superior retrodiscal lamina is fully stretched and produces a posterior, retractive force on the disc. It is important to remember that this is the only structure in the TMJ capable of providing a retractive force on the articular disc.

During opening and closing, the disc and condyle move together, not because of ligamentous attachments, but because of two fundamental features: the morphology of the disc and interarticular pressure (pressure between the articular surfaces). Because some degree of interarticular pressure is always present, the condyle maintains itself on the thinnest intermediate zone of the disc. The thicker anterior and posterior borders of the disc force it to translate with the condyle during mouth opening and closing. It is the disc's morphology, therefore, that requires it to move with the condyle. If there is an alteration in interar-

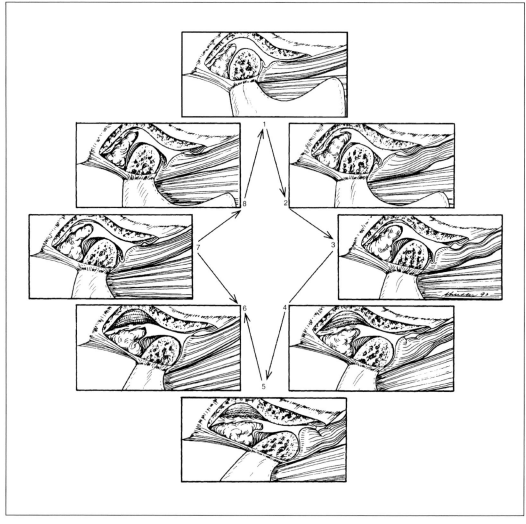

Fig 13-4 Normal functional movement of the condyle and disc during the full range of opening and closing. Note that the disc is rotated posteriorly on the condyle as the condyle is translated out of the fossa. The closing movement is the exact opposite of opening. (From Okeson JP. Management of Temporomandibular Disorders and Occlusion, ed 5. St Louis: Mosby-Year Book, 2003:26. Used with permission.)

ticular pressure or a change in the morphology of the disc, condyle-disc movement can be altered. This, in fact, begins the biomechanical changes associated with many intracapsular symptoms.

Normally, the thinnest portion of the disc is centered on the condyle when the interarticular space is minimal, as during maximum intercuspation. Biting on one side against a bolus of food depresses the condyle on the ipsilateral side and widens the articular space. When this occurs, the disc is rotated anteriorly by the superior lateral pterygoid muscle, which contracts in conjunction with elevator muscle action. Thus, the thicker posterior part of the disc firmly fills the articular disc space, and adequate stability of the joint is maintained. Then, as the teeth bite through the bolus and the space narrows accordingly, the disc contour causes it to rotate posteriorly, thereby bringing the thinner portion of the disc back into position. It becomes fully centered when maximum intercuspation is accomplished. As the resting position is assumed, the space increases, with compensating rotation of the disc anteriorly as the result of muscle tonus in the resting superior lateral pterygoid muscle. This permits synovial fluid to bathe the surfaces from which it was expelled by pressure during the biting effort.

Subtle but essential disc rotary movement is constantly going on. This is in addition to that necessary for keeping the upper surface of the disc in proper contact with the eminence during translatory movement, as well as for gross separation of the jaws for opening. The more steeply inclined the articular eminence, the greater the disc movement required for condylar translation.[4]

Types of TMJ Pains

Arthralgic pain that emanates from a nonarticular structures of the TMJ must arise from structures that are innervated, namely, the collateral discal ligaments, the retrodiscal tissue, and the joint capsule itself, which includes the strong temporomandibular (lateral) ligament that reinforces its lateral wall.[4] Therefore, depending on the structure from which the pain emanates, nonarticular temporomandibular arthralgia may be identified as ligamentous pain, retrodiscal pain, or capsular pain—or some combination of the three. Arthritis comprises a fourth source of arthralgia that may be identified as arthritic pain.

The ligamentous structures of the joint are innervated for proprioceptive function.

They therefore are particularly responsive to such biomechanical factors as pressure, traction, stress, strain, torque, and movement. If such mechanical influence becomes noxious, pain results.[5] It should be noted that both proprioceptive and nociceptive responses are dependent upon the presence of normal neural structures.[6] As ligamentous deterioration takes place, the proprioceptive response and the pain diminish. It is a paradox that decreasing pain emanating from such structures may be indicative of a worsening condition of the ligaments from which it arises. It is important that this be kept in mind when evaluating the seriousness of joint pains. It should also be noted that proprioceptive responses are answered by skeletal muscle activity. Muscle co-contraction is a normal protective reaction of muscles in response to altered proprioceptive input. Therefore, muscle pain of the protective co-contraction type may accompany noxious biomechanical forces that affect the joint. Again, such response depends on normal innervation of the ligamentous structures of the joint. Acute muscle effects are indicative of normally functioning proprioceptors and therefore identify a lesser degree of deterioration in the ligaments. As deterioration takes place due to continued functional abuse and trauma, such muscle effects are less likely to occur.

It should be recognized that masticatory pain emanates from masticatory muscles, from pain-sensitive structures of the TMJs, or from both. Effective therapy depends on accurate identification of the pain source. It is therefore of considerable importance that the clinician should not only distinguish myalgia from arthralgia, but the type of myalgia or arthralgia must be correctly identified (see chapter 12 for a description of the diagnostic categories of muscle pain disorders). Arthralgia emanating from the TMJs may be classified as ligamentous pain, retrodiscal pain, capsular pain, and/or arthritic pain.

Ligamentous Pain

Pain originating from the ligamentous attachments of the condyle-disc complex may present as a range of conditions, some of which can be viewed as a continuum of progressive events. They occur secondary to changes in the relationship between the articular disc and the condyle. These conditions are often referred to as *disc-interference disorders* or *internal derangement disorders.*

If the morphology of the disc is altered and the discal ligaments become elongated, the disc is then permitted to slide (translate) across the articular surface of the condyle. This type of movement is not present in the healthy TMJ. Its degree is determined by changes that have occurred in the morphology of the disc and the degree of elongation of the discal ligaments.

Assume for the purposes of this discussion that the discal ligaments become elongated. (Ligaments can be only elongated—they cannot be stretched. Stretch implies extension that is followed by a return to the original length. Ligaments do not have elasticity and therefore, once elongated, generally remain at that length.) In the normal closed-joint position and during function, interarticular pressure still allows the disc to position itself on the condyle, and no unusual symptoms are noted. However, alteration in the morphology of the disc accompanied by elongation of the discal ligaments can change this normal functioning relationship. In the resting closed-joint position, the interarticular pressure is very low. If the discal ligaments become elongated, the disc is free to move on the articular surface of the condyle. Since in the closed-joint position the superior retrodiscal lamina does not provide much influence on disc position, tonicity of the superior lateral pterygoid will encourage the disc to assume a more forward position on the condyle. The forward movement of the disc will be limited by the length of the discal ligaments, the inferior retrodiscal lamina,

and the thickness of the posterior border of the disc. As this area is thinned, the disc may be displaced more in the anteromedial direction. Since the superior retrodiscal lamina provides little residence in the closed-joint position, the medial and anterior position of the disc is maintained. As the posterior border of the disc becomes thinned, it can be displaced further into the discal space, so that the condyle becomes positioned on the posterior border of the disc. This condition is known as *functional disc displacement* (Figs 13-5a to 13-5c). Most persons report functional displacements of the disc initially as a momentary altered sensation during movement, but not usually as pain. Pain may occasionally be experienced when the person bites (a power stroke) and activates the superior lateral pterygoid. As this muscle pulls, the disc is displaced further, and tightness in the already elongated discal ligament can produce joint pain.

With the disc in this more forward and medial position, function of the joint can be somewhat compromised. As the mouth opens and the condyle moves forward, a short distance of translatory movement can occur between the condyle and the disc until the condyle once again assumes its normal position on the thinnest area of the disc (intermediate zone). Once it has translated over the posterior surface of the disc to the intermediate zone, interarticular pressure maintains this relationship, and the disc is again carried forward with the condyle through the remaining portion of the translatory movement. After the full forward movement is completed, the condyle begins to return and the stretched fibers of the superior retrodiscal lamina actively assist in returning the disc with the condyle to the closed-joint position. Again, the interarticular pressure maintains the articular surface of the condyle on the intermediate zone of the disc by not allowing the thicker anterior border to pass between the condyle and the articular eminence.

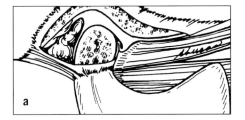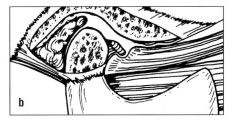

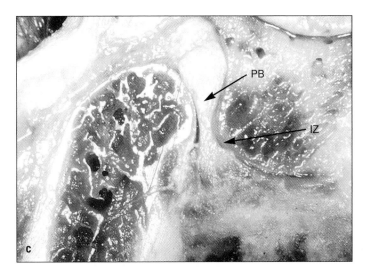

Fig 13-5 *(a)* Normal position of the disc on the condyle in the closed-joint position. *(b)* Functional displacement of the disc. Note that its posterior border has been thinned and the discal and inferior retrodiscal ligaments are elongated, allowing activity of the superior lateral pterygoid to displace the disc anteriorly (and medially). *(c)* Note that in this specimen the condyle is articulating on the posterior band of the disc (PB) and not on the intermediate zone (IZ). This depicts an anterior displacement of the disc. (From Okeson JP. Management of Temporomandibular Disorders and Occlusion, ed 5. St Louis: Mosby-Year Book, 2003:207. Used with permission.)

Once in the closed-joint position, again the disc is free to move according to the demands of its functional attachments. The presence of muscle tonicity will again encourage the disc to assume its most anteromedial position allowed by the discal attachments and its own morphology. One can imagine that if muscle hyperactivity was present (as with bruxism), the superior lateral pterygoid would have even a greater influence on the disc position.

The important feature of this functional relationship is that the condyle translates across the disc to some degree when movement begins. This type of movement does not occur in the normal joint. During such movement the increased interarticular pressure may prevent the articular surfaces from sliding across each other smoothly. The disc can stick or be bunched slightly, causing an abrupt movement of the condyle over it into the normal condyle-disc relationship. Often, a clicking sound accompanies this movement. Once the joint has clicked, the normal relationship of the disc and condyle is re-established, and this relationship is maintained during the rest of the opening movement. During closing of the mouth, the normal relationship of the disc and condyle is maintained because of interarticular pressure. However, once the mouth is closed and the interarticular pressure is lower, the disc can once again be displaced forward by tonicity of the superior lateral pterygoid muscle. In many instances, if the displacement is slight and the interarticular pressure is low, no click is noted during this redisplacement. This single click observed during opening movement represents the very early stages of disc-derangement disorder or what is also called internal derangement.

If this condition persists, a second stage of derangement can arise. As the disc is more chronically positioned forward and medially by muscle action of the superior lateral pterygoid and normal opening and closing, the discal ligaments can be further elongated. Continued forward positioning of the disc also causes elongation of the inferior retrodiscal lamina. Accompanying this breakdown is a continued thinning of the posterior border of the disc, which permits the disc to be positioned more anteriorly, resulting in a more posterior positioning of the condyle on the posterior border.[7] The morphologic changes of the disc at the area where the condyle rests can create a second click during the later stages of condylar return, just prior to reaching the closed-joint position. This closing click is called the *reciprocal click*[8] (Fig 13-6).

The opening click can occur at anywhere during that movement, depending on disc-condyle morphology, muscle pull, and the pull of the superior retrodiscal lamina. The closing click almost always occurs very near the closed or intercuspal position.

It should be remembered that the longer the disc is anteriorly displaced, the more the superior retrodiscal lamina are being elongated. If this condition is maintained for a prolonged period, the elasticity of the superior retrodiscal lamina can break down and be lost. It is important to remember that the superior retrodiscal lamina is the only structure that can apply retractive force on the disc, even though the retractive force is very minimal in the closed-mouth position. Once this force is lost, there is no mechanism to retract the disc posteriorly.

Some authors[9] debate the role of the superior lateral pterygoid muscle on the anterior medial displacement of the disc. Although this would appear to be the obvious influencing factor, certainly other features need to be considered. Tanaka[10,11] has identified a ligamentous attachment of the medial portion of the condyle-disc complex to the medial wall of the fossa. If this ligament were tightly bound, forward movement of the condyle could create a tethering of the disc to the medial. Tanaka[12] has also identified that the retrodiscal tissues are tightly attached in the medial aspect of the posterior fossa, but not in the lateral aspect. This might suggest that the lateral aspect of the disc can be more easily displaced then the medial, allowing the direction of the disc displacement to be more anteromedial. There are likely other factors that have not yet been described. Further investigation in this area is needed.

With this in mind, we can now begin a discussion of the next stage of disc derangement. Remember that the longer the disc is displaced anteriorly and medially, the greater will be the thinning of its posterior border and the more the lateral discal ligament and inferior retrodiscal lamina will be elongated. Also, protracted anterior displacement of the disc leads to a greater loss of elasticity in the superior retrodiscal lamina. The more the shape of the disc changes to accommodate the pull of the muscle and the position of the condyle, the greater the likelihood that the disc will be forced through the discal space, collapsing

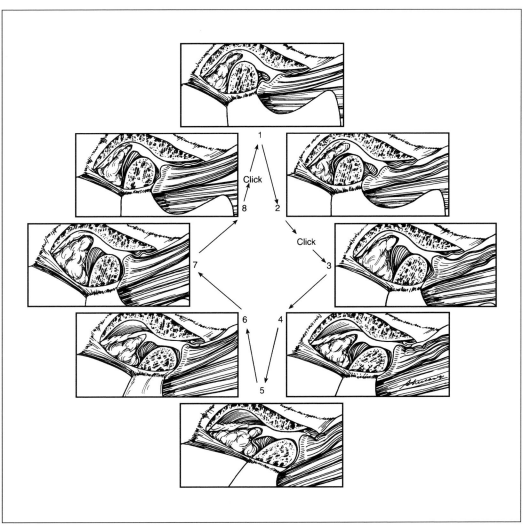

Fig 13-6 Reciprocal click. Between positions 2 and 3, a click is felt as the condyle moves across the posterior border of the disc. Normal condyle-disc function occurs during the remaining opening and closing movement until the closed-joint position is approached. Then a second click is heard as the condyle once again moves from the intermediate zone to the posterior border of the disc (between positions 8 and 1). (From Okeson JP. Management of Temporomandibular Disorders and Occlusion, ed 5. St Louis: Mosby-Year Book, 2003:210. Used with permission.)

the joint space behind. In other words, if the posterior border of the disc becomes more thinned, the disc can move even more anteromedially and actually pass completely through the discal space. When this occurs, interarticular pressure will collapse the discal space, trapping the disc in the forward position. Then the next full translation of the condyle is inhibited by the anterior and medial position of the disc. The person feels the joint being locked in a limited closed position. Since the articular sur-

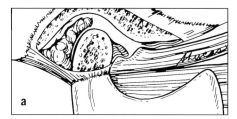
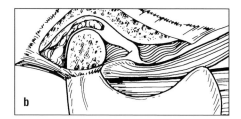
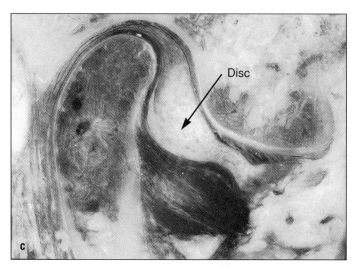

Fig 13-7 *(a)* Functionally displaced disc; *(b)* functionally dislocated disc. Note that in the functionally dislocated disc the joint space has narrowed and the disc is trapped anteriorly (and medially). *(c)* Note that in this specimen the disc is functionally dislocated anterior to the condyle. (From Okeson JP. Management of Temporomandibular Disorders and Occlusion, ed 5. St Louis: Mosby-Year Book, 2003:212. Used with permission.)

faces have actually been separated, this condition is referred to as a *functional dislocation* of the disc (Figs 13-7a to 13-7c).

As already described, a functionally displaced disc can create joint sounds as the condyle moves across the disc during normal translation of the mandible. If the disc becomes functionally dislocated, the joint sounds are eliminated, since the condyle no longer moves onto the disc. This can be helpful information in distinguishing a functional displacement from a functional dislocation.

Some persons with a functional dislocation of the disc are able to move the mandible in various lateral directions to accommodate the movement of the condyle over the posterior border of the disc, and the locked condition is resolved. If the lock occurs only occasionally and the person can resolve it with no assistance, it is referred to as a *functional dislocation with reduction* (Fig 13-8). The patient will often report that the jaw "catches" when opening wide. This condition may or may not be painful depending on the severity and duration of the lock

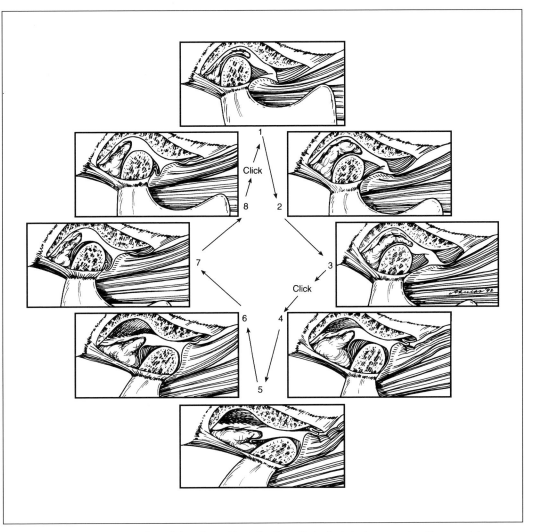

Fig 13-8 Functional dislocation of the disc with reduction. Note that during opening the condyle passes over the posterior border of the disc onto the intermediate area of the disc, thus reducing the dislocated disc. This may be felt as a "catching" sensation and is often associated with reciprocal clicking. (From Okeson JP. Management of Temporomandibular Disorders and Occlusion, ed 5. St Louis: Mosby-Year Book, 2003:213. Used with permission.)

and the integrity of the structures in the joint. If it is acute, with a short history and duration, joint pain may only be associated with elongation of the joint ligaments (such as trying to force the jaw open). As episodes of catching or locking become more frequent and chronic, ligaments break down and innervation is lost. Pain becomes associated less with ligaments and is related more to forces placed on the retrodiscal tissues.

The next stage of disc derangement is known as *functional disc dislocation without reduction*. This condition occurs when the

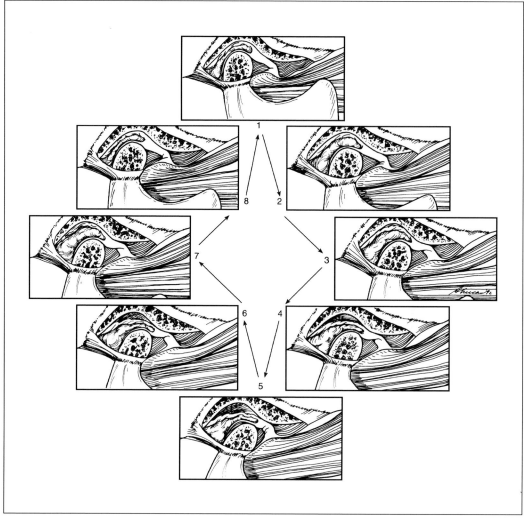

Fig 13-9 Closed lock. Note that the condyle never assumes a normal relationship on the disc but instead causes the disc to move forward ahead of it. This condition limits the distance it can translate forward. (From Okeson JP. Management of Temporomandibular Disorders and Occlusion, ed 5. St Louis: Mosby-Year Book, 2003:214. Used with permission.)

person is unable to return the dislocated disc to its normal position on the condyle. The mouth cannot be open maximally because the position of the disc does not allow full translation of the condyle (Fig 13-9). Typically, the initial opening will be only 25 to 30 mm interincisally, which represents mostly the rotational movement of the joint. The person usually is aware of which joint is involved and can remember the occasion that led to the locked feeling. Since usually only one joint becomes locked, a distinct pattern of mandibular movement is observed clinically. The joint with the functionally dislocated disc without reduction does not allow complete translation of its condyle, whereas the other joint functions normally. Therefore, when the patient attempts to open wide, the midline of the mandible is deflected to the affected side. Also, the patient is able to perform a normal lateral movement to the affected side (the condyle on the affected side only rotates). However, when movement is attempted to the unaffected side, the full range of eccentric movement is not achieved (the condyle on the affected side cannot translate past the anterior functionally dislocated disc). The dislocation without reduction is also known as a *closed lock*. Patients may report pain when the mandible is moved to the point of limitation, but pain is not always associated with this condition.[13]

If the closed lock continues, the condyle is chronically positioned on the retrodiscal tissues. These tissues are not anatomically structured to accept force. Therefore, as force is applied, there is a great likelihood that the tissues will break down.[14] With this breakdown comes tissue inflammation. This disorder will be discussed in the next category of TMJ pains.

Any condition or event that leads to elongation of the discal ligaments or thinning of the disc can cause these derangements of the condyle-disc complex disorders. Certainly one of the most common factors is trauma. Two general types of trauma need to be considered: macrotrauma and microtrauma.

Macrotrauma

Macrotrauma is considered any sudden force to the joint that can result in structural alterations. The most common structural alterations affecting the TMJ are elongation of the discal ligaments. Macrotrauma can be sub-divided into two types: direct trauma or indirect trauma.

Direct trauma

There is little question that significant direct trauma to the mandible, such as a blow to the chin, can instantly create an intracapsular disorder. If this trauma occurs when the teeth are separated (open-mouth trauma), the condyle can be suddenly displaced from the fossa. This sudden movement of the condyle is resisted by the ligaments. If the force is great, the ligaments can become elongated, which may compromise normal condyle-disc mechanics. The resulting increased looseness can lead to discal displacement and to the symptoms of clicking and catching. Unexpected macrotrauma to the jaw (as might be sustained during a fall or in a motor vehicle accident) may lead to discal displacement and/or dislocation.[15–25]

Macrotrauma can also occur when the teeth are together (closed-mouth trauma). If trauma occurs to the mandible when the teeth are together, the intercuspation of the teeth maintains the jaw position, resisting joint displacement. Closed-mouth trauma is therefore less injurious to the condyle-disc complex. This reduction of potential injury becomes obvious when one examines the incidence of injury associated with athletic activity. Athletes who wear soft protective mouth appliances have significantly fewer jaw-related injuries than those that do not.[26,27] It would be wise, therefore, if facial trauma were expected, to have a soft appliance in place or at least hold the teeth tightly in the intercuspal position. Unfortunately, most direct macrotrauma is unexpected (ie, motor vehicle accident) and therefore the teeth are separated, commonly resulting in injury to the joint structures.

Closed-mouth trauma is not likely to be without some consequence. Although ligaments may not be elongated, articular surfaces can certainly receive sudden traumatic loading.[28] This type of impact loading may disrupt the articular surface of the condyle, fossa, or disc, which may lead to alterations in the smooth sliding surfaces of the joint, causing roughness and even sticking during movement. This type of trauma therefore may result in adhesions, which will be addressed later in this chapter.

Direct trauma may also be iatrogenic. Any time the jaw is overextended, elongation of the ligaments can occur. Patients are more at risk for this type of injury if they have been sedated, reducing normal joint stabilization by the muscles. A few common examples of iatrogenic trauma are intubation procedures,[29,30] third molar extraction procedures, and a long dental appointment. In fact, any extended wide opening of the mouth (eg, a yawn) has the potential of elongating the discal ligaments.[15] The medical and dental professions need to be acutely aware of these conditions so as not to create a disc-derangement problem that might last the patient's lifetime.

Indirect trauma

Indirect trauma refers to injury that may occur to the TMJ secondary to a sudden force, but not one that occurs directly to the mandible. The most common type of indirect trauma reported is associated with a cervical extension/flexion injury (whiplash injury).[17,23,31,32] Although the literature reflects an association between whiplash injury and symptoms of TMJ disorders, the data are still lacking regarding the precise nature of this relationship.[33,34]

Recent computer modeling suggests that certain motor vehicle injuries do not produce a TMJ flexion-extension event similar to that seen in the neck.[35,36] In support, human volunteers in motor vehicular crash tests fail to show jaw movement during a rear-end impact.[37] Therefore, there is little compelling evidence at this time to support the concept that indirect trauma commonly results in quick movement of the condyle within the fossa, creating a soft tis-

sue injury similar to that seen in the cervical spine.[38,39] This is not to say that this type of injury could never occur—only that it is likely very rare.

If this statement is true, why then are TMJ symptoms so commonly associated with cervical spine injuries?[17,23,32] The answer to this question lies in the understanding of heterotopic symptoms (chapter 4). The clinician always needs to be mindful that constant deep pain input originating in the cervical spine commonly creates heterotopic symptoms in the face.[40] These heterotopic symptoms may be referred pain (sensory) and/or co-contraction of masticatory muscles (motor). Kronn[32] reported that patients who experienced recent whiplash injuries have a greater incidence of TMJ pain, limited mouth opening, and masticatory muscle pain on palpation than a matched group of controls. All of these symptoms can be explained as heterotopic symptoms associated with deep pain input from the cervical spine. The clinical significance of understanding this concept is enormous, since it dictates therapy. As will be discussed in future chapters, when these circumstances occur, therapy extended to the masticatory structures will have little effect on resolving the cervical deep pain input. Primary emphasis needs to be directed to the cervical injury (the origin of the pain).

Microtrauma

Microtrauma refers to any small force that is repeatedly applied to the joint structures over a long period of time. As discussed earlier in this chapter, the dense fibrous connective tissues that cover the articular surfaces of the joints can well tolerate loading forces. In fact, these tissues need a certain amount of loading to survive, since loading forces drive synovial fluid in and out of the articular surfaces, passing with it nutrients coming in and waste products going out. If, however, loading exceeds the functional limits of the tissue, irreversible changes or damage can result. When the functional limitation has been exceeded, the collagen fibrils become fragmented, resulting in a decrease in the stiffness of the collagen network. This allows the proteoglycan-water molecules to swell and flow out into the joint space, leading to a softening of the articular surface. This softening is called *chondromalacia*.[41] This early stage of chondromalacia is reversible if the excessive loading is reduced. If, however, the loading continues to exceed the capacity of the articular tissues, irreversible changes can occur. Regions of fibrillation can begin to develop. resulting in focal roughening of the articular surfaces.[42] This alters the frictional characteristics of the surface and may lead to sticking of the articular surfaces, causing changes in the mechanics of condyle-disc movement. Continued sticking and/or roughening leads to strains on the discal ligaments during movements and eventually disc displacements.[41]

Another consideration regarding loading is the hypoxia/reperfusion theory. As previously stated, loading of the articular surfaces is normal and necessary for health. However, on occasion the forces applied to the articular surfaces can exceed the capillary pressure of the supplying vessels. If this pressure is maintained, hypoxia can develop in the structures supplied by the vessels. When the interarticular pressure is returned to normal, there is a reperfusion phase. It is thought that during this reperfusion phase, free radicals are released into the synovial fluid. These free radicals can rapidly break down the hyaluronic acid that protects the phospholipids that line the joint surfaces and provide important lubrication.[43-46] When the phospholipids are lost,[47] the articular surfaces joint no longer slide frictionless leading to breakdown. The resulting "sticking" can also lead to disc displacement. Free radicals are also associated with hyperalgesic states and can therefore produce a painful joint.[48,49]

Microtrauma can result from joint loading associated with muscle hyperactivity, such as bruxism or clenching.[50,51] This may be especially true if the bruxing activity is intermittent and the tissues have not had an opportunity to adapt. It is likely that if the bruxing is long-standing, the articular tissues have adapted to the loading forces and changes will not be seen. In fact, in most patients, gradual loading of the articular surfaces leads to a thicker, more tolerant articular tissue.[52-54]

Another type of microtrauma results from mandibular orthopedic instability. Orthopedic stability in the masticatory system exists when the stable intercuspal position of the teeth is in harmony with the musculoskeletally stable position of the condyles.[55] When this condition does not exist, microtrauma to the joint structures can result. This trauma occurs not when the teeth are initially brought into contact, but only during loading of the masticatory system by the elevator muscles. Once the teeth are in the intercuspal position, elevator muscle activity loads the teeth and the joints. Since the intercuspal position represents the most stable position for the teeth, loading is accepted by the teeth without consequence. If the condyles are also in a stable relationship in the fossae, loading occurs with no adverse effect to the joint structures. If, however, loading occurs when a joint is not in a stable relationship with the disc and fossa, unusual movement can occur in an attempt to gain stability. This movement is often a translatory shift between disc and condyle and can lead to elongation of the discal ligaments and thinning of the disc. Remember that the amount and intensity of the loading greatly influence whether the orthopedic instability will lead to a disc-derangement disorder. Bruxing patients with orthopedic instability, therefore, are more likely to create problems than non-bruxers with the same occlusion.

An important question that arises in dentistry is: "What occlusal conditions are

Case 8 Temporomandibular arthralgia originating in the retrodiscal tissues

Chief Complaint   Right TMJ pain.

History

A 45-year-old woman presented with mild to severe, intermittent, steady, dull, aching pain diffusely located in the right preauricular area. The pain was induced by clenching the teeth and lasted from a few minutes to an hour or longer. The pain was accompanied by sensations of interference and disc noise especially associated with occluding the teeth firmly.

The complaint began about 6 months ago. One day while chewing, she bit down firmly and sensed a locking of the right joint. As she opened, it popped very loudly and she felt severe, sharp pain in the TMJ area. The noise and pain have occurred with firmly occluding the teeth ever since. She reports that for several years prior to this, she had noisy TMJs with chewing. She presently has no complaint of restriction of mandibular movements or any recent alteration in her "bite." She is taking no medications of any kind.

Examination

Intraoral: Clinical examination fails to identify any dental or oral cause for the pain except for the orthopedic instability provided by the occlusal condition, as indicated by sensing premature contact of the right premolars, a feeling of increased pressure on those teeth in the fully occluded position, and some movement from primary contact to the full occlusal position. She feels right preauricular pain when she clenches the teeth, and this is accompanied by a "binding sensation." As she releases the teeth, moderate right disc noise is heard. All this is readily prevented by biting on a tongue blade. Otherwise, masticatory functioning is clinically normal.

TMJs: Both joints present clinical evidence of changes in the articular disc positions. When the condyles are positioned by bilateral manual manipulation into the musculoskeletally stable position, the teeth do not occlude soundly. When the patient is asked to fully close the teeth together, a 3-mm shift forward and to the left is noted.

Muscles: No palpable tenderness in the masticatory muscles. All functioning appears to be well within normal limits.

Cervical: Within normal limits.

Cranial nerves: Within normal limits.

Impression

The patient presents with an orthopedically unstable relationship between the stable occlusal position and the orthopedically stable position for the joints. Over the years, this instability, coupled with chewing and other loading factors, has resulted in alteration in normal condyle/disc function, leading to the joint sounds. A few months ago, she accidentally impinged the right disc with sufficient force to injure its attachments to the condyle, thus causing the symptoms of acute retrodiscitis.

Diagnosis   Acute retrodiscitis of the right TMJ, as a result of intrinsic injury.

commonly associated with disc derange-ments?" It has been suggested that when an occlusal condition causes a condyle to be positioned posterior to the musculoskele-tally stable position, the posterior border of the disc can be thinned.[56] A common oc-clusal condition that has been suggested to provide this environment is the skeletal Class II deep bite, which may be further aggravated when a division 2 anterior rela-tionship also exists.[57–60] One needs to be aware, however, that not all patients with Class II malocclusions present with disc-derangement disorders. Some studies show no relationship between Class II malocclu-sion and these disorders.[61–71] Other studies show no association between the horizon-tal and vertical relationship of the anterior teeth and disc-derangement disorders.[72–74] The important feature of an occlusal condi-tion that leads to disc-derangement disor-ders is the lack of joint stability when the teeth are tightly occluded. It is likely that some Class II malocclusions provide joint stability, while others do not. Another fac-tor that must be considered is the amount and duration of joint loading. Perhaps joint loading is more damaging with certain Class II malocclusions. It becomes obvious that no simple relationship exists. It is vi-tally important, however, that when ortho-pedic instability exists it be identified as an etiologic factor; successful management may depend on prompt alteration of the damaging relationship (Case 8).

The following are clinical symptoms by which ligamentous pain can be recognized:

1. The pain occurs intermittently in con-junction with clinically evident disc in-terference of some type.
2. Pain that occurs in conjunction with condylar translatory movements relates specifically to one of the following etio-logic groups of disc-interference disor-ders[4]:
   a. Excessive passive interarticular pres-sure

b. Structural incompatibility between the sliding parts
   c. Degeneration of the articular surfaces
   d. Impaired disc-condyle complex
3. Protective muscle co-contraction may be displayed.
4. Dysfunction in the form of interference during mandibular movements is char-acteristic. If such interference is sufficient to arrest condylar movement, dysfunc-tion in the form of restricted range of motion is displayed.
5. Ordinarily, central excitatory effects are not seen. (If the ligaments become in-flamed, the clinical characteristics of capsular pain will be displayed. Then, secondary effects may become evident.)

Retrodiscal Pain

The retrodiscal tissues are located posterior to the articular disc and extend back to the posterior wall of the joint capsule. As previ-ously mentioned, these tissues are com-posed of highly vascularized, loose connec-tive tissue. The inferior retrodiscal lamina is composed of collagenous tissue and serves as a ligament that restricts anterior rota-tion of the disc on the condyle and delin-eates the inferior synovial sac between the articular disc and the mandibular condyle posteriorly. The superior retrodiscal lamina is composed of elastic tissue and serves not as a ligament but as a retractive force on the articular disc when the condyle is translated forward. At the closed-mouth occluded po-sition, however, both laminae are relaxed and exert no traction on the disc. The supe-rior retrodiscal lamina delineates the supe-rior synovial sac between the articular disc and the tympanic plate posteriorly. The retrodiscal tissue is sometimes referred to as the posterior attachment of the disc.

Both retrodiscal laminae are surfaced with synovial membrane. The vascularity of the retrodiscal tissue is a major source of synovial fluid to both compartments of the joint. This tissue is structured so that full and extensive translatory movements of the condyle do not interfere with the continuous flow of nutrients and metabolic exchange supplying the nonvascularized articular surfaces and articular disc. The retrodiscal tissue is innervated, as is other loose connective tissue, with somatic and visceral afferents, including nociceptors, and with visceral efferents to the blood vessels.[6] It has little or no proprioceptive capability; its chief function is nutritional.

The vital retrodiscal tissue is not subject to injury under normal conditions of mandibular function. If condylar encroachment does occur, inflammation may take place. This is marked by extensive swelling, extravasation of inflammatory fluid into the synovial spaces, and pain, especially when the condyle presses against the swollen tissue during maximum intercuspation. Trauma to the mandible can therefore induce an acute retrodiscitis. Such a condition causes an acute malocclusion in the resting occluded position due to swelling of the retrodiscal tissue and excessive intracapsular fluid. The pain that occurs when the teeth are firmly occluded may be reduced considerably by biting against a separator that prevents intercuspation of the teeth. There may be some accentuation of pain when forceful ipsilateral excursions are made (Case 9).

It should be noted that retrodiscitis displays symptoms that may be misdiagnosed as inferior lateral pterygoid muscle pain or as disc attachment (ligamentous) pain due to orthopedic instability that occurs when the teeth are clenched in maximum intercuspation. It is important that these conditions be differentiated because the treatment is not the same. Inferior lateral pterygoid muscle pain is identified by increased pain with resisted protrusive effort. Disc attachment pain due to orthopedic instability displays no acute malocclusion in the resting occluded position. It should be noted, how-

ever, that radiographically these three conditions may appear much the same. Radiographic evidence therefore should not be accepted as conclusive unless it is confirmed by clinical symptoms.

The possibility of acute retrodiscitis should be considered in traumatic incidents that involve the mandible, both with and without osseous fracture (Case 9). The symptoms may be misdiagnosed as a mandibular fracture when none exists. Therapy should also take into consideration the possibility of hemarthrosis, which presents the chance of adhesions between the disc and temporal fossa (fibrosis ankylosis) or between the disc and condyle.

An insidious chronic form of retrodiscitis may occur as the result of functional encroachment of the condyle on the retrodiscal tissue due to orthopedic instability that displaces the condyle posteriorly when the teeth are firmly clenched in maximum intercuspation. The resultant deterioration in the discal ligaments, the disc proper, and the temporomandibular ligament permits condylar encroachment on the retrodiscal tissue. Such a condition comes on slowly, so that inflammatory changes sufficient to elicit symptoms usually do not occur. Such condylar encroachment involves the inferior retrodiscal lamina first, then the body of retrodiscal tissue. This usually leaves the vital superior retrodiscal lamina to function within normal limits. As metaplasia converts the retrodiscal loose connective tissue into a denser fibrotic tissue, the decreased vascularity may affect the metabolism of the synovial fluid. This may further complicate the already difficult problem of functional displacement of the articular disc upon which the retrodiscal condition is superimposed. If the matter of functional displacement proceeds to the point of anterior dislocation of the articular disc, biting pressure of the condyle against the remaining unprotected retrodiscal tissue may induce retrodiscal pain.

Case 9   Acute retrodiscitis secondary to trauma

Chief Complaint   Left TMJ area pain.

History

A 46-year-old woman presented with mild, intermittent, steady, dull, aching pain diffusely located in the left preauricular area induced by clenching the teeth and accompanied by acute malocclusion, described as premature contact of the right anterior teeth with disclusion of the posterior teeth unless forced into full occlusion.

The complaint began a week ago following an automobile accident in which she sustained a heavy blow to the right chin. Radiographs failed to identify a mandibular fracture. Because of the acute malocclusion, the oral surgeon was suspicious of an unidentified fracture and placed arch bars and inter-arch elastics to bring the teeth into normal occlusion. In doing so, however, pain increased until it became intolerable, and he was forced to remove the maxillomandibular elastics and refer the patient for a TMJ examination. Only ibuprofen was being taken for the pain.

Examination

Intraoral: There is no dental or oral cause for the complaint other than the obvious acute malocclusion. Deep tenderness in the left joint is sensed with heavy manual palpation, and this increases considerably with forced occlusion of the teeth. There is slight discomfort with maximum opening and extended lateral and protrusive movements, and the patient senses a feeling of muscular weakness with these movements as well as with attempting to fully occlude the teeth. The pain produced by forcing the teeth into occlusion is prevented by biting on a tongue blade on the same side as the pain. There is no discomfort with eccentric biting or with manually straining the mandible as long as the teeth are slightly separated.

> **TMJs:** Both joints appear to be structurally normal on radiograph. The left condyle is displaced anteriorly in primary occlusal contact position, interpreted as a possible result of inflammatory swelling of the left retrodiscal tissues.

> **Muscles:** There is no marked palpable tenderness in any masticatory muscle and no muscular dysfunction of any kind.

> **Cervical:** Within normal limits.

> **Cranial nerves:** Within normal limits.

Diagnostic tests: Analgesic blocking of the left lateral pterygoid muscle did not arrest the pain or acute malocclusion, confirming that it is not of muscular origin.

Impression

It is presumed that the blow on the chin forced the left condyle posteriorly and traumatized the retrodiscal tissues. The ensuing retrodiscitis produced swelling that displaced the condyle forward, causing the acute malocclusion.

Diagnosis   Acute retrodiscitis of the left TMJ, traumatically induced.

This would disappear as further metaplasia of the tissue takes place.

It should be noted that, since the retrodiscal tissue is not responsive proprioceptively, protective muscle co-contraction may not occur. Also, the pain is frequently intermittent and may not induce secondary central excitatory effects. Acute retrodiscitis from trauma, however, may induce referred pain and secondary co-contraction of the masticatory muscles.

The following are clinical symptoms by which acute retrodiscal pain can be recognized:

1. The pain is accentuated by clenching the teeth in maximum intercuspation.
2. Such pain is decreased by biting against a separator that prevents intercuspation of the teeth, thus reducing forces to the retrodiscal tissues.
3. The pain is accentuated by forced ipsilateral excursive movement of the mandible.
4. Pain is not induced by resisted protrusion of the mandible.
5. Dysfunction may be displayed as acute malocclusion in the resting occluded position.
6. Secondary central excitatory effects may be displayed.

Capsular Pain

Capsular pain results from inflammation of the synovial and fibrous capsules, referred to as *synovitis* and *capsulitis,* respectively. To distinguish between the two is difficult if not impossible clinically. Pain occurs when the inflamed capsule is stretched by translatory movement of the condyle. It is accentuated therefore by protrusion, contralateral excursion, and opening widely. There is palpable tenderness directly over the condyle and on occasion fluctuant swelling as well. Although acute capsulitis may cause restriction in the outer ranges of condylar movement due to swelling, most masticatory dysfunction results only from the inhibitory influence of pain.

Synovitis causes swelling due to effusion within the joint cavity, discomfort with joint movements, and alteration of the synovial fluid. The increase in intracapsular fluid may induce a measure of acute malocclusion. In more chronic form, gelatinization of the synovial fluid may alter joint movements and cause some stiffness, especially after periods of inactivity. This may be accompanied by peculiar joint sounds. Such symptoms usually decrease as normal activity is resumed. Synovitis may result from localized trauma, abusive use, toxemias, specific infection, or as an allergic response. It frequently occurs as a manifestation of arthritis.

Capsulitis may result from acute trauma or from intrinsic strains that injure the capsular ligament (Case 10). A frequent cause has to do with inflammatory conditions of the discal ligaments and the temporomandibular ligament as a result of orthopedic instabilities between the stable intercuspal position and the stable joint position. This disharmony can result in positioning of the condyle away from its most stable loaded position and into the capsular ligament(s). Bruxism combined with such orthopedic instability is an important activating factor. Capsulitis may result from habits that entail excessive mandibular movements and from abusive joint hypermobility.

Inflammatory conditions of the capsule may cause varying degrees of capsular fibrosis that may restrict the outer ranges of condylar movement. Ordinarily, capsular fibrosis is entirely painless. However, if the condition is exacerbated by excessive condylar movement, acute capsulitis may result (Case 11).

Since capsular pain is more or less continuous, some secondary central excitatory effects may be induced. This may be mani-

Case 10   Temporomandibular arthralgia expressed as capsular pain

Chief Complaint   Left TMJ area pain.

History

A 20-year-old woman presented with mild, continuous, protracted, steady, dull, aching pain diffusely located in the left preauricular area, described as deep tenderness to pressure over the left condyle, that increased considerably with opening beyond 30 mm as well as with extended protrusive and contralateral excursions. There were no complaints of restricted mandibular movements, interference with movements, or acute malocclusion.

The complaint began about 3 weeks earlier following a volleyball accident in which she received a sharp blow on the left mandible. She thought her mouth was partly open at the time. The blow was painful, and after 24 hours the left TMJ became acutely sore and slightly swollen. All jaw use was painful and difficult for several days. Then the pain subsided to the present level. When the complaint persisted, she consulted her dentist, who promptly referred her for a TMJ examination. No medications are presently being taken.

Examination

Intraoral: There is no dental or oral cause for the pain nor any evidence of injury to the dentition. She has deep tenderness to pressure over the left condyle. The discomfort increases with all condyle movements that tend to stretch the capsule. She has a feeling of muscular weakness with these movements and they may be slightly inhibited by pain, but there is no identifiable orthopedic instability or masticatory dysfunction.

TMJs: Both joints are radiographically normal structurally and functionally, except for a slight decrease in distance of translatory movement in the left joint, interpreted as the effect of pain inhibition.

Muscles: There is no palpable tenderness in any masticatory muscle and no muscular dysfunction.

Cervical: Within normal limits.

Cranial nerves: Within normal limits.

Diagnostic tests: Analgesic blocking of the left lateral pterygoid muscle did not arrest the pain, confirming that the discomfort was not muscular.

Impression

By history, clinical course, and the present behavioral characteristics of the complaint, it is presumed that the left capsular ligament was traumatized by the blow, causing acute immobilizing capsulitis, which has not subsided to a subacute nonimmobilizing stage.

Diagnosis   Subacute capsulitis of the left TMJ, traumatically induced.

Case 11   Capsular pain arising from inflamed capsular fibrosis

Chief Complaint   Left TMJ area pain.

History

A 46-year-old woman presented with mild to severe recurring episodes of continuous, protracted, steady, dull, aching pain diffusely located in the left preauricular area, induced by forceful or prolonged opening of the mouth, and aggravated by jaw use.

The complaint appeared to relate to moderate restriction of opening (about 32 mm interincisal distance), which dated from a childhood injury. The present pain complaint began about 6 months ago following extensive dental treatment that required extended and prolonged opening of the mouth. This was immediately followed by soreness in the left joint area and acute pain when opening fully. The episodes of discomfort depended on the amount and type of force used to open the mouth beyond her "normal" range. Her physician had treated her with systemic as well as local injections of corticosteroid medications, with only transitory benefit. He then advised "correction of her bite" by her dentist. The dentist saw no reason for occlusal alteration and referred her for a TMJ examination.

Examination

Intraoral: Three first molar teeth are missing and the spaces are moderately closed, leaving considerable loss of vertical support, but there is no significant orthopedic instability. She feels sharp pain in the left TMJ area with opening beyond 28 mm and dull tenderness with protrusive and contralateral movements. Opening is restricted to 32 mm with slight deflection to the left. Protrusive and contralateral movements appear to be adequate.

TMJs: Both joints appear to be structurally normal. There is restriction of left condylar movement that is interpreted as capsular, presumed to be the result of preexisting capsular fibrosis or contracture, probably of traumatic origin.

Muscles: Essentially negative for cause of pain.

Cervical: Within normal limits.

Cranial nerves: Within normal limits.

Impression

Capsular fibrosis appears to be responsible for the left condylar movements. When strained by excessive and prolonged opening, often associated with dental treatment, the capsule became inflamed, and episodes of capsulitis have continued ever since.

Diagnosis   Painful adhesions that restrict condyle movements (capsular fibrosis).

fested as referred pain, including headache, areas of heterotopic deep palpable tenderness, and secondary co-contraction of the masticatory muscles.

The following are clinical symptoms by which capsular pain can be recognized:

1. There is palpable tenderness directly over the condyle.
2. There is occasional palpable fluctuant swelling over the joint proper.
3. The pain is accentuated by translatory movements that stretch the capsule.
4. There is no increase in pain by clenching the teeth, nor is there any alteration in pain while biting against a separator.
5. Dysfunction occurs in the form of restricted mandibular movement, especially in extended ranges. Most restriction is caused by the inhibitory influence of pain. Joint stiffness and strange joint sounds may occur during the first few movements following periods of inactivity. Acute malocclusion may occur as the result of increased intracapsular fluid.
6. Secondary central excitatory effects may be displayed.

Arthritic Pain

Inflammation of the articular surfaces of the joint is termed *inflammatory arthritis.* Normally, these surfaces are nonvascularized, so that an inflammatory reaction cannot occur. They are also noninnervated, so that painful sensation cannot be felt. For the joint surfaces to become inflamed, fundamental arthropathic change must occur. Such change may be the result of trauma, which is termed *traumatic arthritis.* It can occur as a result of the proliferation of inflamed synovial membrane onto the articular surfaces, which is termed *rheumatoid arthritis.* It can occur as a result of degeneration of the avascular fibrous tissue that normally constitutes the articular surfaces.

When degenerative changes proceed until this tissue no longer is protective, the underlying innervated and vascularized osseous tissue may become exposed to the effects of movement, attrition, and articular pressures, thus becoming inflamed. This is termed *degenerative joint disease* or *osteoarthritis.*

Inflamed articular surfaces are the source of persistent though variable arthralgia. The patient usually reports a persistent, dull, aching pain that is aggravated by jaw movement. The irritation of occlusal pressure usually increases the discomfort, but sometimes the pressure of clenching the teeth temporarily relieves the pain. Usually, pain is increased by chewing food and by all movements that press upon, rub, or irritate the inflamed articular surfaces.

If the inflammation is acute and widespread, the capsule may become involved so that symptoms of capsulitis are added—ie, pain with movements, swelling of the joint, and palpable tenderness over the joint proper. Lesser degrees of inflammation may be accompanied by little or no gross dysfunction, other than interference with mandibular movements that are expressed as discal noise and sensations of altered movements. As acute inflammation occurs and functioning of the joint is decreased due to pain inhibition, inflammatory exudate, or secondary muscle effects, the earlier noninflammatory dysfunction symptoms may decrease or subside. This effect is presumably the result of the restraint of condylar movements. If intracapsular edema occurs, some sensation of acute malocclusion may be sensed. This is described as premature occlusion of the teeth on the opposite side. If osseous resorption decreases the vertical height of the mandibular ramus, some occlusal disharmony may be sensed; this is described as overstressing of the ipsilateral posterior teeth during maximum intercuspation. When such occlusal disharmony is advanced, clinical evidence of a progressive anterior open bite may result (Fig 13-10).

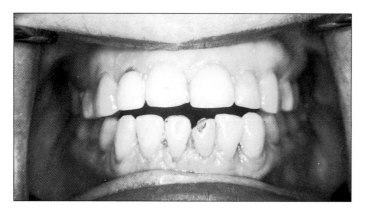

Fig 13-10 Progressive anterior open bite resulting from osseous changes in the TMJs as a result of advanced rheumatoid arthritis in a 49-year-old woman. (From Bell WE. Management of TMJ problems. In: Goldman HM, Gilmore HW, Royer RQ, et al (eds). Current Therapy in Dentistry, vol 4. St Louis: Mosby, 1970:172. Used with permission.)

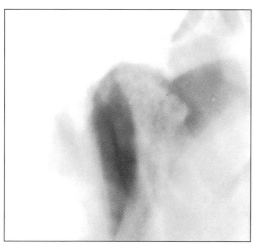

Fig 13-11 Radiograph of the TMJ of a patient with rheumatoid arthritis. Note the gross flattening of the condyle.

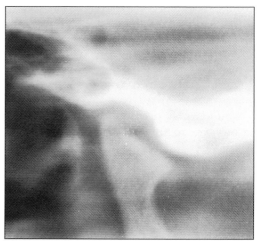

Fig 13-12 Radiograph of a TMJ with advanced rheumatoid arthritis. (Courtesy of Dr Jay Mackman, Radiology and Dental Imaging Center of Wisconsin, Milwaukee, Wisconsin.)

Radiographic evidence of osteoarthritis may be variable. Prior to gross structural change, rheumatoid arthritis may present some loss of definition of the osseous articular surfaces that is suggestive of diffuse surface resorption bilaterally (Fig 13-11). Although not diagnostic, this appearance is sufficient to warrant medical investigation of the possibility of rheumatoid arthritis. Advanced rheumatoid arthritis may present with dramatic resorption of bone (Fig 13-12). Such changes do not necessarily relate functionally to the clinical symptoms. Fibrous ankylosis may be identified. The inhibitory effect of pain also may be recorded as restricted range of motion.

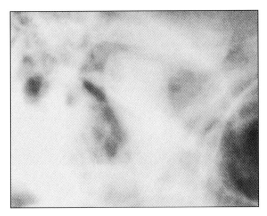

Fig 13-13 Radiograph of a TMJ undergoing degenerative change expressed as flattening and paralleling of the osseous surfaces.

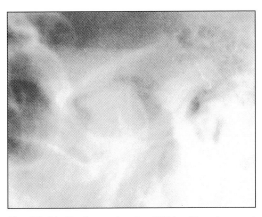

Fig 13-14 Radiograph of a TMJ with advanced degenerative joint disease. Note the flattened articular surfaces and anterior lipping of the condylar surface.

Fig 13-15 Radiographic appearance of osseous change in the left TMJ resulting from advanced osteoarthritis in a 45-year-old woman. The right joint is not affected.

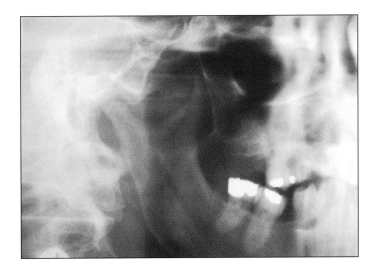

Osteoarthritis may show little or no radiographic evidence in the early phase. As degenerative changes in the osseous surfaces occur, alterations in contour may become evident radiographically. These changes may be identified as flattened, parallel surfaces (Fig 13-13); anterior lipping (Fig 13-14); loss of definition indicative of active osseous resorption (Fig 13-15); or gross change in condylar form (Fig 13-16). It is important to note that radiographic changes in the contour of the condyle and/or fossa do not necessarily correlate with pain. It appears that, for many patients, osteoarthritic changes do not progress throughout their lifetime. Therefore

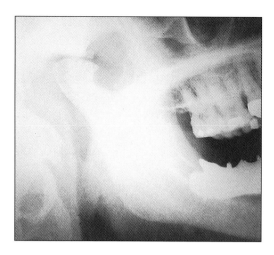

Fig 13-16 Radiograph of a TMJ exhibiting marked lipping of the condyle.

the bony changes can persist long after adaptation of the osseous structures. Once adaptive changes have occurred and the joint structures have stabilized, the condition is called *osteoarthrosis*. This will be discussed in more detail later in this chapter.

Traumatic arthritis may present similar radiographic changes. In addition, some evidence of former trauma such as malposition following fracture may be seen. Other changes are condylar hyperplasia and malformation (Figs 13-17 and 13-18).

In acute inflammatory arthritis, intracapsular edema may be sufficient to cause an acute malocclusion. This condition appears clinically as a loss of posterior occlusal contact on the ipsilateral side. If inflammatory swelling immobilizes the joint, restriction of condylar movements will be observed both clinically and radiographically. Restriction of condylar movement due to disc dislocation and the inhibitory influence of pain may also be observed (Case 12).

The following are clinical symptoms by which arthritic pain can be recognized:

1. There is usually some degree of capsular pain, along with other symptoms of synovitis/capsulitis.
2. The pain is accentuated by biting pressure, fast movements, and forced movements.
3. The pain is decreased by biting against a separator on the ipsilateral side.
4. The pain is increased by biting against a separator on the contralateral side.
5. Dysfunction is expressed as restricted movement, interference during movements, and acute malocclusion. Restricted movement may be the result of inflammatory swelling, capsular inflammation, altered synovial fluid function, and the inhibitory influence of pain (muscle co-contraction). Interference during movement results from damaged articular surfaces or condyle-disc complex impairment. Acute malocclusion may be the result of increased intracapsular fluid or osseous change.

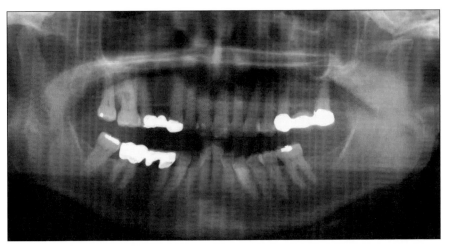

Fig 13-17 Panoramic radiograph revealing left TMJ osteoarthritic changes. The condyle was subjected to macrotrauma 4 years earlier. (Courtesy of Dr Jay Mackman, Radiology and Dental Imaging Center of Wisconsin, Milwaukee, Wisconsin.)

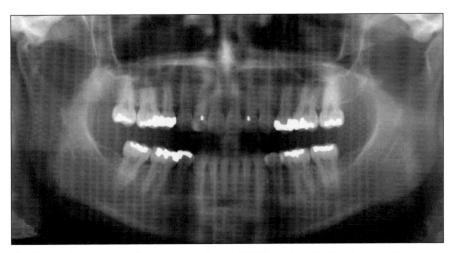

Fig 13-18 Panoramic radiograph revealing right TMJ osteoarthritic changes. There has been significant erosion of the condylar head. (Courtesy of Dr Jay Mackman, Radiology and Dental Imaging Center of Wisconsin, Milwaukee, Wisconsin.)

Periarticular inflammation

Periarticular inflammation that envelops the joint may cause swelling, pain, and immobilization of the joint, the severity of symptoms depending on the degree, extent, location, and phase of the inflammatory reaction. Both rheumatoid arthritis and hy-

peruricemia may so involve the TMJs. When periarticular inflammation occurs without other obvious local cause, the examiner should consider the possibility of these causes (Case 13).

Periarticular inflammation may occur as a result of trauma or by direct extension from another contiguous inflammatory

Case 12 Temporomandibular arthralgia expressed as degenerative joint disease or osteoarthritis

Chief Complaint Right TMJ area pain.

History

A 61-year-old man presented with mild to severe continuous, protracted, steady, dull, aching, and throbbing pain diffusely located in the right preauricular area. The pain was accompanied by tenderness and slight swelling over the TMJ and marked restriction of all jaw movements. The pain was aggravated by clenching the teeth, opening, chewing, and talking. Recently the patient reported a change in his occlusion.

The complaint began after an episode of extraordinary chewing about 2 weeks ago. Prior to that, the right joint was asymptomatic. For a few days, he noticed mild stiffness and vague discomfort in the right TMJ, gradually increasing in severity. After a week, the localized pain, fixation of the joint, and the sensation of acute malocclusion occurred. These symptoms had remained much the same ever since. Antibiotics prescribed by his physician had not controlled the complaint. No medications are presently in use other than simple analgesics.

Examination

Intraoral: The teeth and mouth are clinically and radiographically negative for cause of pain, except that there is subjective acute malocclusion described as a sensation of premature contact of the left canines with slight disocclusion of the right posterior teeth. The pain increases when he attempts to fully occlude the teeth. This is reduced by insertion of a tongue blade on either side to prevent intercuspation. There is very slight swelling over the right condyle and acute palpable tenderness both directly over the condyle and intra-aurally. Pain increases with all joint movements and a feeling of muscular weakness is described when he moves the mandible. Mouth opening is restricted to about 26 mm and deflects to the right. Protrusion is restricted and deflects to the right. Left lateral excursion is only 2 mm.

> **TMJs:** The left joint appears to be normal. The right joint presents radiographic evidence of degenerative changes.
>
> **Muscles:** Essentially negative except for minor tenderness and weakness, presumed to represent the inhibitory influence of pain.
>
> **Cervical:** Some restriction to head flexion and extension but not related to present complaint. He reports a history of cervical arthritis that is being managed by his physician.
>
> **Cranial nerves:** Within normal limits.

Impression

Radiographic evidence of preexisting degenerative changes of the right condyle. The acute activating cause was related to the extraordinary chewing episode. As a result, acute inflammatory changes of the joint have occurred, resulting in the acute malocclusion.

Diagnosis Degenerative joint disease with acute inflammatory arthritis of the right TMJ.

Case 13 Temporomandibular arthralgia expressed as arthritic pain secondary to hyperuricemia

Chief Complaint   Right TMJ pain.

History

A 70-year-old man presented with mild, continuous, variable, steady, dull, aching pain diffusely located in the right TMJ area and aggravated by all joint use. There was localized tenderness to touch and pressure directly over the lateral pole of the joint.

The complaint began about 8 weeks ago as very mild tenderness over the right joint and minor discomfort with jaw movements. Some stiffness of the joint was noticed, especially in the early mornings. The discomfort had gradually increased until the last 2 weeks, when the pain became great enough to interfere with normal chewing and talking. Increasing restriction of mouth opening and pain with opening was noticed. During the last 2 weeks he had also noticed some soreness in the little finger and the big toe. He sought aid from his physician, who in turn referred him for a TMJ examination. He presently is receiving an NSAID but no other forms of therapy.

Examination

Intraoral: Several missing mandibular posterior teeth were replaced satisfactorily with a partial denture. The remaining teeth are clinically and radiographically negative for any cause for the pain. No occlusal instability is identified. There is pain with lateral and protrusive movements as well as opening beyond 23 mm. Left lateral movement is restricted. Protrusive movement is restricted and deflects to the right. Opening is restricted to about 30 mm and deflects to the right.

TMJs: Both joints appear to be structurally within normal limits and the left joint appears to function normally. The right joint presents restricted condylar movement, interpreted as a result of periarticular and capsular inflammation plus the effect of pain inhibition.

Muscles: There is moderate palpable tenderness in the right masseter muscle. All other muscles are normal to palpation.

Cervical: Within normal limits.

Cranial nerves: Within normal limits.

Diagnostic tests: Serum uric acid: 8.9 mg/dL.

Impression

The right TMJ appears to be acutely inflamed, presumably as a result of hyperuricemia involving the periarticular and capsular structures of the joint. There is moderate secondary muscle pain emanating from the right masseter muscle.

Diagnosis   Periarticular and capsular inflammation of the right TMJ, due presumably to hyperuricemia.

process, such as otitis media. Under such circumstances the cause should be so obvious as to present no diagnostic problem. If the injury or infection penetrates the capsule, acute inflammatory or infectious arthritis may follow, and the condition may terminate as a chronic mandibular hypomobility.

In periarticular inflammation, the joint appears normal radiographically except for possible restriction of translatory movement. This is a result either of the presence of inflammatory exudate or of the inhibitory influence of inflammatory pain.

Painful chronic mandibular hypomobilities

As the result of periarticular and articular inflammation, scar tissue may form around the joint, in the fibrous capsule, or between the joint surfaces, depending on the location of the inflammatory process. Such fibrosis, contracture, or adhesions restrict condylar movements, depending on the location and extent of cicatrization. As long as the mandibular movements do not exceed the limitations thus imposed, these conditions usually remain painless. As such, they are classified as *chronic mandibular hypomobilities*. If the adhesions are injured by straining or applying force to move the mandible beyond such limitation, the adhesions may become inflamed and painful.

Painful fibrous ankylosis presents with clinical symptoms of acute inflammatory arthritis. It will be noted that when the acutely painful condition resolves, clinical and radiographic evidence of preexisting fibrous ankylosis remains (Case 14).

Painful growth disorders

Most growth problems involving the TMJs are painless and therefore do not come within the scope of this text. However, if the lack of structural harmony between the condyle and fossa, between the two joints bilaterally, or between the joints and the dentition becomes sufficient to interfere seriously with normal functioning, painful conditions may arise. Pain in such instances would probably relate to intrinsic trauma, with symptoms of capsulitis, retrodiscitis, or inflammatory arthritis, depending on what structures are inflamed. Radiographic evidence of malformation may confirm the diagnosis.

Rarely do malignant tumors involve the TMJs. The characteristic feature is slow, progressive immobilization of the joint without apparent cause and is usually painless at first. The early clinical and radiographic features suggest fibrous ankylosis. It is usually the progressiveness of the condition and finally pain with all joint use that lead the examiner to believe that the condition is something other than a simple chronic mandibular hypomobility (Case 15).

Case 14   Temporomandibular arthralgia expressed as arthritic pain secondary to inflamed fibrous ankylosis

Chief Complaint   Left TMJ pain and mouth opening restriction.

History

A 34-year-old woman presented with mild, continuous, intermittently severe, variable, dull, aching pain diffusely located in the left preauricular area. The pain was induced by forceful opening and excursive movements and accompanied by restricted movement of the left mandibular condyle.

The complaint followed a motor vehicle accident about 18 months earlier in which the patient sustained multiple fractures of the mandible, one through the left condylar process. Soreness and restricted movement of the left joint persisted after treatment of the fractures and had been present ever since. The pain was related chiefly to efforts to open the mouth. Physiotherapy, muscle relaxants, and corticosteroid injection therapy had failed to give much benefit. The patient was therefore referred for evaluation of the TMJs. No medications are presently being used.

Examination

Intraoral: No dental or oral cause for the complaint is evident clinically or radiographically. There is palpable tenderness over the left condyle but no pain described in resting or in any occlusal positions. There is a stable occlusal condition. All pain appears to occur with movements that tend to induce translation of the left condyle beyond about 22 mm. The severity of pain relates directly to the degree of attempted movement. Protrusion movement deflects the mandible to the left. Right lateral excursion is 2 mm. Maximum opening is 24 mm and deflects the mandible to the left.

> **TMJs:** Both joints appear to be structurally normal. Radiographs reveal a restriction of left condylar movement that is interpreted as representing fibrous ankylosis.
>
> **Muscles:** Essentially negative.
>
> **Cervical:** Within normal limits.
>
> **Cranial nerves:** Within normal limits.

Impression

Fibrous ankylosis of the left TMJ appears to have developed as a posttraumatic sequela. As the adhesions matured, continued efforts to execute normal left condylar movements induced inflammation, making them painful.

Diagnosis   Painful adhesions that immobilize the left mandibular condyle (fibrous ankylosis).

Case 15 · Temporomandibular arthralgia expressed as arthritic pain secondary to an invasive malignant tumor

Chief Complaint   Left ear, TMJ, and temple pain.

History

A 54-year-old woman presented with mild to severe continuous, variable, protracted, steady, dull, aching pain diffusely located in the left ear and preauricular area, spreading to the temple, face, and submandibular triangle, aggravated by opening 13 mm, and accompanied by restricted mandibular movements.

The complaint began about 4 years ago with no history of injury. It began insidiously as left eustachian blockage, followed soon by restriction of opening to about 25 mm. ENT therapy was ineffective. Three years ago her dentist made an occlusal splint to "correct the bite." After 2 to 3 months, mild pain began and had gradually increased ever since. After a year, the splint was discarded. About a year ago, surgery on the opposite ear was followed by an increase in the pain and trismus. Six months ago, she was given a general anesthetic and the muscles were stretched, without any benefit. Recent muscle relaxant therapy and a corticosteroid injection into the left joint had not been beneficial.

Examination

Intraoral: There is no dental or oral cause for her complaint. The left face and ear pain increases with opening beyond 13 mm. There is no palpable tenderness over the left condyle. Opening is restricted to 18 mm with deflection to the right (suggestive of medial pterygoid myospasm). Protrusion deflects to the left. There is almost no right lateral excursion movement.

TMJs: Both joints appear structurally normal. There is marked restriction of the left condylar movement, interpreted as being indicative of fibrous ankylosis.

Muscles: There is only very slight palpable tenderness in the left temporal and masseter muscles. The medial pterygoid cannot be palpated due to the restricted opening.

Cervical: Within normal limits.

Cranial nerves: The left side of the face exhibits marked anesthesia and paresthesia. Motor function is normal for both CN V and CN VII.

Diagnostic tests: Analgesic blocking of the left medial pterygoid muscle via the sigmoid notch arrested about 75% of the pain but did not alter the dysfunction.

A 4-day trial therapy of passive stretching of the medial pterygoid muscle was not effective. The patient was referred for comprehensive evaluation by a neurologist. Magnetic resonance imaging confirmed a diagnosis of carcinoma in the left nasopharynx invading the periarticular structures of the left TMJ.

Impression

In retrospect, no doubt the invasive neoplasm caused the symptoms, which were clinically and radiographically interpreted as fibrous ankylosis complicated by spasm of the left medial pterygoid muscle.

Diagnosis   Immobilization of the left TMJ due to an invasive malignant tumor.

Diagnostic Considerations

To plan effective therapy, accurate identification of the pain source is needed. Masticatory pains constitute a major segment of orofacial pain complaints. Frequently, the complaint consists of both myalgic and arthralgic components, which should be differentiated. Primary and secondary pains also must be distinguished. This may require considerable diagnostic effort. However, the more accurately it is done, the less complex the management problem and the more predictable the treatment.

Intermittent Arthralgia

Intermittent arthralgic pains relate primarily to the effect of biomechanical abuse. As such, little or no secondary referred pain, secondary hyperalgesia, or muscle co-contraction results. The pain remains relatively "clean-cut." It is diffusely localizable to the joint region and responds rather faithfully to manual palpation and functional manipulation. Acute intermittent arthralgic pain may induce protective co-contraction of the masticatory muscles. This may occur bilaterally. It should be noted, however, that protracted muscle co-contraction may develop into local muscle soreness that, if persistent, may become inflammatory. Thus, it is important to eliminate such pains before complications develop, or else therapy must be instituted for the muscle condition as well.

Intermittent arthralgic pains may cause a change in muscle activity patterns. It is hypothesized that latent memory traces may persist after neural stimulation; thus, repeated stimulation may induce altered habitual patterns of muscle activity. It is presumed that such muscle engram change is responsible for deviations in the midline incisal path during opening-closing movements. (*Deviation* refers to an alteration in the opening pathway away from midline that returns again with further opening to the centered position.) This may also account for such anomalies as avoidance closure movements, slides from the centric to the maximum intercuspal position, as well as various habitual jaw movements and mannerisms. Time and repetition are required. Acute and changing conditions do not cause such effects; they induce muscle co-contraction instead.

Inflammatory Arthralgia

When the condition that induces arthralgic pain becomes inflammatory, continuity of input results, along with the propensity to induce secondary central excitatory effects. Thus, inflammatory arthralgia (retrodiscal pain, capsular pain, and arthritic pain) may be complicated by a variety of secondary effects, such as referred pains including headache, secondary hyperalgesia displayed as superficial touchy spots or areas of deep palpable tenderness, or secondary muscle symptoms. Careful differentiation between primary sources of pain input and the secondary effects of deep somatic pain is essential to accurate diagnosis and effective management. It should be noted that, while muscle co-contraction may be induced by deep pain input, it may soon develop local muscle soreness, which in turn becomes painful. This pain can then induce continued co-contraction and a cycling mechanism can begin. This cycling condition is known as *cycling muscle pain*. As such, it may become wholly independent of the initiating cause, thus requiring a separate therapeutic effort for resolution (see chapter 12).

Arthralgia of Nonmasticatory Origin

From the dental standpoint, it is important to distinguish between arthralgia of masticatory origin, which can reasonably be expected to respond to proper masticatory therapy, and arthralgia of nonmasticatory origin, which may require medical therapy, surgical intervention, or both. Arthralgias from hyperuricemia and rheumatoid arthritis are essentially medical problems, for which treatment of the masticatory apparatus would be secondary and supplemental. Infections, traumatic arthritis, and temporomandibular involvement from adjacent pathosis may require considerable interdisciplinary attention. Chronic mandibular hypomobilities and growth disorders are usually surgically treated problems.

Neuropathic Pain Felt in the Joint

Neuropathic pain may emanate from a traumatic neuroma that has developed secondary to a lacerating injury or surgery of the joint. Such pain displays the clinical characteristics of neuropathic pain rather than deep somatic pain. This may especially be the source of pain after multiple surgeries to the TMJ. The clinician needs to be aware of this possible source of pain, because too often the surgeon may assume that the surgical repair has failed and plan another surgery. Repeated surgeries only increase the likelihood of more neuropathic pain and should be avoided whenever possible (see Case 32).

Referred Pain Felt in the Joint Area

True arthralgia that emanates from the TMJ must be differentiated from heterotopic pain that is felt in the joint area. As discussed in chapter 12, myogenous pain may be referred to the joint. This is especially true of myofascial trigger point pain involving the sternocleidomastoid, masseter, medial pterygoid, and lateral pterygoid muscles (see Case 18). Referred pain from any source within the vast trigeminal distribution may also be felt in the joint area. The salivary glands are known sources of such reference (see Case 17).

Eagle Syndrome

Eagle syndrome[75–78] may be confused with TMJ pain because it typically induces a sensation of persistent raw throat, pain and difficulty with swallowing, and pain associated with neck movement and referred to the auricular/TMJ areas. The condition results from elongation of the styloid process or calcification of the stylohyoid ligament. The elongated styloid process may encroach on the carotid artery, causing carotid arteritis. The resulting carotodynia may refer pain through the face to the ophthalmic area. Encroachment on the carotid artery is said to cause faintness or syncope when the head is turned from side to side.[79]

Glossopharyngeal Neuralgia

A neuropathic pain that may be confused with TMJ pain is glossopharyngeal neuralgia. This paroxysmal neuralgia is triggered by stimulation of receptors in the pharyngeal mucosa. It is associated therefore with talking as well as with jaw and throat movements incidental to chewing and swallowing. The pain usually is felt deeply in the post-mandibular and infra-auricular area. It presents the clinical characteristics of neuropathic rather than deep somatic pain and is temporarily arrested by topical anesthesia of the pharyngeal mucosa (see Case 25).

Differential Diagnosis

The primary deep somatic musculoskeletal pains that emanate from the TMJs should be distinguished diagnostically from the following conditions:

1. Masticatory myalgia
2. Odontogenous pains
3. Arthralgia of nonmasticatory origin, such as rheumatoid arthritis and hyperuricemia
4. Adjacent inflammatory and neoplastic conditions, such as pseudoankylosis and Eagle syndrome
5. Heterotopic referred pains and secondary hyperalgesias felt in the temporomandibular or preauricular area as secondary effects of other deep pain input
6. Heterotopic projected neuropathic pains, especially glossopharyngeal neuralgia
7. Somatoform pain disorders
8. Heterotopic pains of central origin

Therapeutic Options for Disc-Interference Disorders

During the past 20 years, the dental profession has proposed a variety of different approaches to the management of intracapsular pain conditions. Since these pain conditions are common, a specific discussion of these therapies is in order. Disc-interference or internal derangement disorders actually represent a continuum of the pain conditions that have already been discussed. Early in these disorders, disc-attachment pain is the predominant complaint. Later, capsulitis and synovitis are common. As the disc is further displaced, retrodiscal pain becomes the predominant feature. Finally, the articular surfaces are affected, resulting in osteoarthritis. This discussion is therefore appropriate for many of the pain conditions discussed in this chapter.

The rationale for any therapy begins with a thorough understanding of the disease and its natural course. As a general rule, diseases that are progressive and destructive need to be treated quickly and aggressively. Diseases that are nonprogressive and characterized by reparative processes can often be treated more palliatively and observed over time. The rationale for the management of intracapsular disorders begins with an understanding of the natural course of these disorders. The clinician must appreciate, however, that in the practice of dentistry the natural course of the disease can be misinterpreted. Patients most often seek care when pain and/or dysfunction becomes great. When the clinical examination reveals signs and symptoms associated with disc-interference disorders, the condition is easily interrupted as progressive and in need of aggressive treatment. Well-controlled, longitudinal studies are the only reliable method of evaluating the natural course of these disorders as well as the effects of therapy on the disorder's outcome. Although these studies are the most difficult to accomplish, we are most fortunate to have a few studies that shed light on these common disorders.

In the examination of the long-term effects of dysfunction on the TMJs, certain stages need to be identified for assessment purposes. There are three clinical stages that have been commonly used.[80] The first stage is that of disc displacement with reduction. This stage is characterized by joint clicking with movement but no radiographic signs of any abnormalities in the condyle or articular eminence. The second stage is that of disc displacement without reduction. This stage is characterized by a sudden restriction in mouth opening and a loss of joint sounds during movement. Radiographic changes may or may not be present during this stage, depending upon the chronicity of the disorder. The third stage is that of permanent disc displacement with osteoarthritic changes, as depicted by radiographic assessment.

It appears that long-term studies support the concept that many patients seem to progress through these three stages.[81-86] Initially it would appear that these disorders are progressive and need to be aggressively treated. However, a careful look at these studies reveals that the final stage of the disorder is not often painful or debilitating. In fact, in one longitudinal study, patients with internal derangements who were observed for 30 years were found to be no different than a control group in most evaluation parameters.[86] The greatest differences that existed between these groups were that the patients experienced a slight reduction in mouth opening compared to the controls and that the patients expressed a greater concern that if they opened widely the joint would hurt.[80] However, there was no difference in the general musculoskeletal complaints of the patients and the controls in this study. Another significant difference was in the radiographic evidence of bony changes that had commonly occurred in the internal derangement group. These changes, however, were not necessarily correlated with pain nor often even with dysfunction.[81-84] This would suggest an adaptive condition clinically known as osteoarthrosis.

These long-term studies leave the impression that the natural course of disc-interference disorders or internal derangements is toward disc displacement without reduction and osteoarthritic changes. This is not always the case, however, as depicted by long-term studies that do not show consistent progression of clicking joints to disc dislocation without reduction.[87-94] Therefore, long-term studies suggest that internal derangements may be progressive, but even when they are, for many patients they seem to be rather self-limiting, resulting in no significant disability. An understanding of the natural course of these disorders allows the clinician to assume the most appropriate role as therapist. If these disorders are self-limiting for most patients, then one might question any need for aggressive therapy. Instead, the role of the therapist should be one that assists the patient through the symptomatic phase of the disorder while the tissues adapt. Palliative therapy is often the most appropriate therapy, especially early in the disorder. However, some patients may suffer greatly through this disorder, and therefore, more assistance may be needed for these patients. The aggressiveness of the therapy should be escalated only when more palliative therapy fails to control symptoms and the patient's quality of life decreases markedly.

Since tissue adaptation seems to play a major role in the natural course of these disorders, treatment should be oriented toward promoting a joint condition that is most likely to repair or adapt.[95] An important part of this therapy is directed toward reducing mechanical loading of the articular surfaces. Four types of therapies should be initially considered for each patient with a symptomatic internal derangement disorder. These therapies are patient education, physical therapy, pharmacologic therapy, and occlusal appliance therapy.

Patient Education

It is very important that each patient understands the mechanism that is causing his or her disorder. There are several important reasons for this education. The first relates to the nature of internal derangements. Since these disorders have a significant biomechanical component, the well-informed patient can play a significant role in therapy. The patient should be instructed to decrease loading of the joint as much as possible. Softer foods, slower chewing, and smaller bites should be promoted. The patient should be told, when possible, not to allow the joint to click. The mechanics of some joints allow certain movements to occur with minimal dysfunction. When possible, these movements should be encouraged, while painful movements should be discouraged.

Each clinician treating internal derangement disorders should have a model or well-drawn illustration of the TMJ in the office so that the patient can visualize the mechanical dysfunction. This will not only help the patient understand the condition but also subtly inform the patient that the disorder is common and one of which the clinician is well informed. This understanding will enhance the patient's confidence in the doctor, which will likely help the patient through the adaptive phase of the disorder. The patient should also be informed of the natural course of the disorder so that reasonable expectations can be met. It is important that the patient be told that in many instances this condition is self-limiting; however, the pain and dysfunction may be present for a considerable period of time. The patient should be told of the therapies that will be used, and if they are not satisfactory, the clinician can offer more aggressive therapy. If more aggressive therapies are needed, the patient should always take part in the decision-making process. It is important that the patient realizes that the disorder is not an aggressive, tissue-destructive

disease such as cancer. This information will likely decrease anxiety and stress, promoting a better environment for healing.

In those patients with a disc displacement without reduction, the patient should be shown, with a model or illustration, the reason for limitation in mouth opening. The patient should be instructed not to attempt to force the mouth open, especially when pain is present. Instead the patient should be told that with time, the mouth will return to a more normal opening. If the patient attempts to force the mouth open too soon, tissues may be damaged and repair delayed. Once the condition has become relatively asymptomatic, the patient should then be encouraged to attempt to return back to a more normal opening, as discussed in the next section.

Physical Therapy

Physical therapy modalities can be helpful in managing some of the symptoms associated with disc-interference disorders. These therapies can be divided into two broad types: those that reduce pain and those that improve function.

Physical therapy for pain

In instances when pain is significant, application of moist heat or ice over the joint region can often be helpful. Thermotherapy utilizes heat as a prime mechanism and is based on the premise that heat increases circulation to the applied area. Surface heat is applied by laying a hot, moist towel over the symptomatic area.[96] Placement of a hot water bottle over the towel will help maintain the heat. This combination should remain in place for 10 to 15 minutes, not to exceed 30 minutes. An electric heating pad may be used, but care must be taken not to leave it unattended.

Like thermotherapy, coolant therapy has proven to be a simple and often effective method of reducing pain. Ice should be applied directly to the symptomatic joint and/or muscles and moved in a circular motion without pressure to the tissues. The patient will initially experience an uncomfortable feeling that will quickly turn into a burning sensation. Continued icing will result in a mild aching and then numbness.[97] When numbness begins, the ice should be removed. The ice should not be left on the tissues for longer than 5 to 7 minutes. After a period of warming, a second application may be desirable. It is thought that during warming there is an increase in blood flow to the tissues, which assists in tissue repair.

A common coolant therapy utilizes a vapor spray. Two of the most common sprays used are ethyl chloride and fluoromethane. Vapocoolant spray is applied to the desired area from a distance of 18 inches for approximately 5 seconds. After the tissue has been rewarmed, the procedure can be repeated. Care must be taken not to allow the spray to contact the eyes, ears, nose, or mouth (a towel should be placed to protect these areas). Vapocoolant sprays do not penetrate tissue like ice and therefore it is likely that the reduction in pain is more associated with the stimulation of cutaneous nerve fibers that in turn shut down the smaller pain fibers (the C fibers). This type of pain reduction is likely to be of short duration.

The clinician should suggest both heat and cold modalities to the patient, since the results can be very individual. The patient should determine the most effective modality for his or her pain. Both these modalities are very conservative and can be used as often as the patient feels is necessary.

Other physical therapy modalities that have been investigated are iontophoresis, phonophoresis, and cold laser. Iontophoresis is a technique by which certain medications are introduced into the tissues without affecting any other organs. With iontophoresis, the medication is placed in a pad and the pad is placed over the involved joint. Then a low electrical current is passed through the pad, driving the medication into the tissue.[98] Local anesthetics and anti-inflammatories are common medications used with iontophoresis.[99,100] If the medication is driven into the tissues with ultrasound therapy, the modality is known as phonophoresis.[101]

In recent years, the cold or soft laser has been investigated for wound healing and pain relief. Presently it is not considered to be a routine physical therapy modality, but it is included in this section for completeness. Most studies on the cold laser report on its use in chronic musculoskeletal, rheumatic, and neurologic pain conditions.[102-105] It is thought that cold laser accelerates collagen synthesis, increases vascularity of healing tissues, decreases the number of microorganisms, and decreases pain. Several case studies have been published in which cold laser therapy has been used on persistent TMJ pain.[106-108] Although the results of the studies investigating iontophoresis, phonophoresis, and cold laser have been somewhat favorable, the studies generally lack controls and adequate sample sizes. More investigations will be needed to better understand their effectiveness.

Physical therapy to improve function

Early in a disc-interference disorder or osteoarthritis, pain may cause the patient to restrict joint function. Although this can be helpful at first, restricting joint function can lead to chronic hypomobility and muscle atrophy. A few passive exercises can be helpful in returning the jaw to normal function. The patient should be instructed to gently open the mouth to resistance and close. The jaw should then be moved eccentrically. Early in the process of healing, these exercises should not produce any significant pain. Later, as tissue adaptation progresses, the exercises should become more active, so that the patient can regain a normal range of movement.

Passive distraction of a joint can increase mobility as well as inhibit the activity of muscles that pull across the joint (elevator muscles). Distraction of the TMJ is accomplished by placing the clinician's thumb in the patient's mouth over the mandibular second molar area on the side to be distracted. With the cranium stabilized by the other hand, the clinician places downward force on the molar with the thumb (Fig 13-19). Distraction for relaxation of muscles does not require translation of the joint but merely involves unloading in the closed-joint position. The distraction should be maintained for several seconds and then released. It can be repeated several times. When joint mobility is the problem, distraction should be combined with manual translation of the joint.

Joint distraction has been suggested as a method of reducing a disc that has become permanently displaced.[109] Although this technique may provide some immediate success, few studies have evaluated the long-term success. For management of an acute disc dislocation without reduction (less than a week), the technique should be attempted. If the clinician successfully reduces the disc, an anterior positioning appliance is indicated (discussed later in this chapter). Discs that have been displaced for more than several weeks are very difficult to reduce and the distraction procedure will likely fail. If the disc cannot be reduced, a stabilization appliance is indicated merely to reduce loading forces in the joint associated with bruxing activity (also discussed later in this chapter).

Pharmacologic Therapy

Pharmacologic therapy can be an effective adjunct in managing symptoms associated

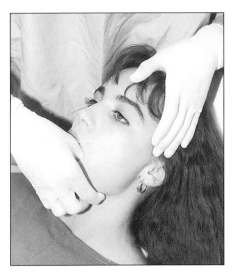

Fig 13-19 Manual distraction of the TMJ may be helpful in improving joint mobility.

with an intracapsular disorder. Patients should be aware that medication will not likely offer a solution or cure to the problem. However, medication in conjunction with appropriate physical therapy and definitive treatment does offer the most complete approach to many problems. The two most common types of medications used for internal derangement disorders are analgesics and anti-inflammatories.

Analgesic medications

Analgesic medications can often be an important part of supportive therapy for many intracapsular disorders. Control of pain is not only appreciated by the patient, but it also reduces the likelihood of other complicating pain disorders such as muscle co-contraction,[110] referred pain,[111] and central sensitization.[112] The nonsteroidal anti-inflammatory drugs (NSAIDs) are very helpful for most intracapsular pains. Included in this category are aspirin, acetaminophen, and ibuprofen. Ibuprofen (ie, Motrin, Advil, Nuprin) has proven to be very effective in reducing musculoskeletal pains. A common dosage of 600 to 800 mg three times a day will often reduce pain and stop the cyclic effects of the deep pain input. There are numerous other NSAIDs, and if ibuprofen does not reduce the pain another should be tried, since individual patients may respond differently to these medications. Continued use may result in stomach irritation, so the patient should be questioned about prior stomach problems before use and monitored closely during treatment. It is suggested that these medications be taken with meals to lessen the likelihood of stomach irritation.

When a patient reports stomach upset or a history of such, a cyclooxygenase 2 (COX_2) inhibitor should be considered. As discussed in chapter 9, COX_2 inhibitors often result in reduced adverse gastrointestinal side effects.[113-115] Examples of COX_2 inhibitor drugs are celecoxib (Celebrex), rofecoxib (Vioxx), and valdecoxib (Bextra).

Anti-inflammatory medications

When inflammatory conditions are present, anti-inflammatories can be helpful in altering the course of the disorder. These agents suppress the body's overall response to the irritation. Anti-inflammatory agents can be administered orally or by injection.

Oral NSAIDs have already been discussed under the category of analgesics. When taken on a regular basis, these medications are quite useful in the management of inflammatory joint disorders. Aspirin or ibuprofen can serve in this capacity while providing an analgesic effect. Many other oral NSAIDs are available. It should be remembered that these drugs do not immediately achieve good blood levels and therefore should be taken on a regular schedule for a minimum of 1 to 2 weeks. The general health and condition of the patient must always be considered before these (or any) medications are prescribed; and, as is often

the case, it may be necessary to consult the patient's primary physician regarding the advisability of such drug therapy.

Injection of an anti-inflammatory such as hydrocortisone into the joint has been advocated[116-120] for the relief of pain and restricted movements. A single intra-articular injection seems to be somewhat helpful in older patients; however, less success has been observed in patients under age 25.[118] Although a single injection is occasionally helpful, it appears[121,122] that multiple injections may be harmful to the structures of the joint and should be avoided. Therefore the intra-articular anti-inflammatory agents should be used only in selected cases.

Occlusal Appliance Therapy

During the past 30 years, the dental profession's attitude toward management of internal derangements has changed greatly. This is especially true with regard to the use of occlusal appliances. In the early 1970s Farrar[123] introduced the anterior mandibular positioning appliance. This appliance provided an occlusal relationship that required the mandible to be maintained in a forward position. This type of appliance was an attempt to position the condyle back on the disc ("recapture the disc"). It was originally suggested that this appliance be worn 24 hours a day for as long as 3 to 6 months.

Clinicians quickly discovered that the anterior mandibular positioning appliance was useful in reducing painful joint symptoms.[124,125] When this appliance successfully reduced symptoms, a major treatment question was then asked: What next? Some clinicians believed that the mandible needed to be permanently maintained in this forward position. Dental procedures were suggested to create an occlusal condition that maintained the mandible in this therapeutic relationship. However, accomplishing this task was never a simple dental procedure. Others felt that once the discal ligaments were repaired, the mandible should be returned to its normal position in the fossa (the musculoskeletally stable position) and the disc would still remain in proper position (recaptured). Although one approach was more conservative than the other, neither has been supported by long-term data.

In early short-term studies,[92,124,126-130] the anterior positioning appliance proved to be much more effective in reducing intracapsular symptoms than the more traditional centric relation (stabilization) appliance. This, of course, led the profession to believe that returning the disc to its proper relationship with the condyle was an essential part of treatment. The greatest insight regarding the appropriateness of a treatment modality, however, is gained from long-term studies. Forty patients with various derangements of the condyle-disc complex were evaluated 2$^1/_2$ years after anterior positioning therapy and performance of a step-back procedure.[131] No patients received any occlusal alterations. It was reported that 66% of the patients still had joint sounds, but only 25% were still experiencing pain. If the criteria for success in this study were the elimination of both pain and joint sounds, then success was achieved in only 28% of patients. Other long-term studies[90,126] have reported similar findings. If the presence of asymptomatic joint sounds is not a criterion for failure, however, then the success rate for anterior positioning appliances rises to 75%. The issue that must be addressed, therefore, is the clinical significance of asymptomatic joint sounds.

As already stated, joint sounds are very common in the general population. In many cases[132,133] it appears that they are not related to pain or decreased joint mobility. If all clicking joints always progressed to more serious disorders, then this would be a good indication to treat each and every joint that clicked. However, the presence of unchanging joint sounds over time indicates that the structures involved can adapt to less than optimum functional relationships.

Long-term studies reveal that anterior positioning appliances are not as effective as once thought. They appear to be helpful in reducing pain in 75% of patients, but joint sounds appear to be much more resistant to therapy. The fact that these sounds persist over time does not necessarily indicate the presence of a progressive disorder. These studies do, however, give insight as to how the joint responds to anterior positioning therapy. In many patients, advancing the mandible forward for a time prevents the condyle from articulating with the highly vascularized, well-innervated retrodiscal tissues. This is the likely explanation for an almost immediate reduction of intracapsular pain. During the forward positioning, the retrodiscal tissues undergo adaptive and reparative changes.[134] These tissues can then become fibrotic[135-142] and avascular (Fig 13-20).

We know now that discs are not generally recaptured by anterior positioning appliances.[143] Instead, as the condyle returns to the fossa, it moves posteriorly to articulate on the adapted retrodiscal tissues. If these tissues have adapted adequately, loading occurs without pain. The condyle now functions on the newly adapted retrodiscal tissues, although the disc is still anteriorly displaced. The result is a painless joint that may continue to click with condylar movement. At one time the dental profession believed that the presence of joint sounds indicated treatment failure. Long-term follow-up studies have given the profession new insight regarding success and failure. We, like our orthopedic colleagues, have learned to accept that some dysfunction is likely to persist once joint structures have been altered. Controlling pain, while allowing joint structures to adapt, appears to be the most important role of the therapist.

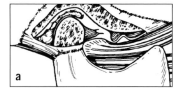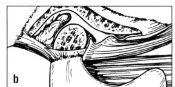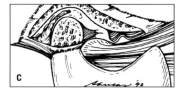

Fig 13-20 *(a)* An anteriorly displaced disc with the condyle articulating on the retrodiscal tissues, producing pain. *(b)* An anterior positioning appliance is placed in the mouth to bring the condyle forward off of the retrodiscal tissues onto the disc. This relationship lessens the loading of the retrodiscal tissues, which decreases the pain. *(c)* Once the tissues have adapted, the appliance is removed, allowing the condyle to assume the original musculoskeletally stable position. The condyle now functions on adaptive fibrotic tissues, resulting in a painless functioning joint, but because the disc is still displaced, clicking may be present. (From Okeson JP. Management of Temporomandibular Disorders and Occlusion, ed 5. St Louis: Mosby-Year Book, 2003:338.)

It should be noted that a few long-term studies[129,144] do support the concept that permanent alteration of the occlusal condition can be successful in controlling most major symptoms. However, such treatment requires extensive dental therapy, and one must question the need for it when natural adaptation appears to work well for most patients. Reconstruction of the dentition or orthodontic therapy should be reserved only for those patients who present with a significant orthopedic instability.

The use of anterior positioning appliance therapy is not without adverse consequences. A certain percentage of patients who wear these appliances develop a posterior open bite. This may be the result of a reversible, myostatic contracture of the inferior lateral pterygoid muscle. When this condition exists, a gradual relengthening of the muscle can be accomplished by slowly stepping the condyle back to the more musculoskeletally stable (anterosuperior) position in the fossa. This can be accomplished by gradually adjusting the appliance to allow the condyle to return to the musculoskeletally stable position, by slowly decreasing use of the appliance, or both. The de-

gree of myostatic contracture that develops is likely to be proportional to the length of time the appliance has been worn. As already mentioned, when these appliances were first introduced, it was suggested that they be worn 24 hours a day for 3 to 6 months. The philosophy now is to reduce the wearing time as much as possible so as to limit the adverse effects on the occlusion. For many patients, full-time use is not necessary to reduce symptoms. When possible, the patient should wear the appliance only at night to protect the retrodiscal tissues from heavy loading (bruxism). If the symptoms can be controlled without wearing the appliance during the day, myostatic contracture will be avoided.

For some patients with a disc-interference disorder, a more traditional stabilization (centric relation) appliance can reduce symptoms. This is the appliance of choice since the risk of altering the occlusion is minimized. It should also be noted that both of these appliances should provide full-arch coverage so as to prevent tooth eruption.

If symptoms persist with only nighttime use of the appliance, the patient may need to wear it more often. Daytime use may be necessary for a few weeks. As soon as the patient becomes symptom-free, the use of the appliance should be gradually reduced. If reduction of use creates a return of symptoms, either there has not been adequate time for tissue repair or significant orthopedic instability is present. It is best to assume that inadequate time for tissue repair is the reason for return of symptoms. The anterior positioning appliance should therefore be reinstituted and more time given for tissue repair.

When repeated attempts to eliminate the appliance fail to control symptoms, orthopedic instability should be suspected. When this occurs, the appliance should be gradually reduced, allowing the condyle to return to the musculoskeletally stable (anterosuperior) position. Once the condyles are in the musculoskeletally stable position, the occlusal condition should be assessed for orthopedic stability. Orthopedic instability is not a common finding, but when it is present, dental therapy may be indicated.

If the disc is permanently displaced without reduction, an anterior positioning appliance is contraindicated. This type of appliance will likely only aggravate the anteriorly positioned disc. Patient education, physical therapy, and medications are the best methods of promoting adaptation of the permanently displaced disc. If the patient is suspected to perform significant bruxing or clenching, a stabilization appliance is indicated to reduce loading of the retrodiscal tissues during sleep. A lack of adaptation is usually accompanied by pain. When nonsurgical therapies fail to adequately reduce symptoms over a reasonable period of time, surgical considerations are indicated.

Other Therapeutic Options

1. Muscle therapy (see chapter 12) for interrelated muscle symptoms.
2. Cause-related therapy consisting of the identification and treatment of etiologic factors and contributing conditions. This applies especially to preexisting etiologic occlusal disharmonies, abusive use and habits, and bruxism.[55,145-148]
3. Medical management for appropriate arthritic conditions such as rheumatoid arthritis and hyperuricemia.
4. Surgical consultation for painful conditions, including recalcitrant degenerative arthritis, chronic mandibular hypomobilities, and growth disorders of the joint.
5. Medical consultation.

References

1. McNamara JA. The independent functions of the two heads of the lateral pterygoid muscle, Am J Anat 1973;138:197–205.
2. Gibbs CH, Mahan PE, Wilkinson TM, Mauderli A. EMG activity of the superior belly of the lateral pterygoid muscle in relation to other jaw muscles. J Prosthet Dent 1984;51:691–702.
3. Okeson JP. Functional anatomy and biomechanics of the masticatory system. In: Management of Temporomandibular Disorders and Occlusion. St Louis: Mosby–Year Book, 2003: 3–27.
4. Bell WE. Normal craniomandibular structure. In: Temporomandibular Disorders: Classification, Diagnosis, Management, ed 3. Chicago: Year Book, 1990:35–103.
5. DuBrul EL. Sicher's Oral Anatomy. St Louis: Mosby, 1980:174–209.
6. Thilander B. Innervation of the temporomandibular joint capsule in man. Trans R Sch Dent 1961;7:1.

7. Westessen PL, Bronstein SL, Liedberg J. Internal derangement of the temporomandibular joint: Morphologic description with correlation to joint function. Oral Surg Oral Med Oral Pathol 1985;59:323–331.

8. Farrar WB, McCarty WL. The TMJ dilemma. Alabama Dent Assoc 1979;63:19–26.

9. Wilkinson T. The relationship between the disk and the lateral pterygoid muscle in the human temporomandibular joint. J Prosthet Dent 1988;60:715–724.

10. Tanaka TT. Advanced Dissection [videotape]. San Diego: T. T. Tanaka, 1989.

11. Tanaka TT. TMJ Microanatomy, An approach to current controversies [videotape]. San Diego: T. T. Tanaka, 1992.

12. Tanaka TT. Head, Neck and TMD Management. San Diego: Clinical Research Foundation, 1989.

13. Roberts CA, Tallents RH, Espeland MA, Handelman SL, Katzberg RW. Mandibular range of motion versus arthrographic diagnosis of the temporomandibular joint. Oral Surg Oral Med Oral Pathol 1985;60:244–251.

14. Isberg A, Isacsson G, Johansson AS, Larson O. Hyperplastic soft-tissue formation in the temporomandibular joint associated with internal derangement. Oral Surg Oral Med Oral Pathol 1986;61:32–38.

15. Harkins SJ, Marteney JL. Extrinsic trauma: A significant precipitating factor in temporomandibular dysfunction. J Prosthet Dent 1985;54:271–272.

16. Moloney F, Howard JA. Internal derangements of the temporomandibular joint. III. Anterior repositioning splint therapy. Aust Dent J 1986;31:30–39.

17. Weinberg S, Lapointe H. Cervical extension-flexion injury (whiplash) and internal derangement of the temporomandibular joint. J Oral Maxillofac Surg 1987;45:653–656.

18. Pullinger AG, Seligman DA. Trauma history in diagnostic groups of temporomandibular disorders. Oral Surg Oral Med Oral Pathol 1991;71:529–534.

19. Westling L, Carlsson GE, Helkimo M. Background factors in craniomandibular disorders with special reference to general joint hypermobility, parafunction, and trauma. J Craniomandib Disord 1990;4:89–98.

20. Pullinger AG, Seligman DA. Association of TMJ subgroups with general trauma and MVA. J Dent Res 1988;67:403.

21. Pullinger AG, Monteriro AA. History factors associated with symptoms of temporomandibular disorders. J Oral Rehabil 1988;15:117–124.

22. Skolnick J, Iranpour B, Westesson PL, Adair S. Prepubertal trauma and mandibular asymmetry in orthognathic surgery and orthodontic paients. Am J Orthod Dentofac Orthop 1994;105:73–77.

23. Braun BL, DiGiovanna A, Schiffman E, et al. A cross-sectional study of temporomandibular joint dysfunction in post-cervical trauma patients. J Craniomandib Disord Facial Oral Pain 1992;6:24–31.

24. Burgess J. Symptom characteristics in TMD patients reporting blunt trauma and/or whiplash injury. J Craniomandib Disord 1991;5:251–257.

25. De Boever JA, Keersmaekers K. Trauma in patients with temporomandibular disorders: Frequency and treatment outcome. J Oral Rehabil 1996;23:91–96.

26. Seals RR Jr, Morrow RM, Kuebker WA, Farney WD. An evaluation of mouthguard programs in Texas high school football. J Am Dent Assoc 1985;110:904–909.

27. Garon MW, Merkle A, Wright JT. Mouth protectors and oral trauma: A study of adolescent football players. J Am Dent Assoc 1986;112:663–665.

28. Luz JGC, Jaeger RG, de Araujo VC, de Rezende JRV. The effect of indirect trauma on the rat temporomandibular joint. Int J Oral Maxillofac Surg 1991;20:48–52.

29. Knibbe MA, Carter JB, Frokjer GM. Postanesthetic temporomandibular joint dysfunction. Anesth Prog 1989;36:21–25.

30. Gould DB, Banes CH. Iatrogenic disruptions of right temporomandibular joints during orotracheal intubation causing permanent closed lock of the jaw. Anesth Analg 1995;81:191–194.

31. Barnsley L, Lord S, Bogduk N. Whiplash injury; A clinical review. Pain 1994;58:283–307.

32. Kronn E. The incidence of TMJ dysfunction in patients who have suffered a cervical whiplash injury following a traffic accident. J Orofac Pain 1993;7:209–213 [erratum 1993 Summer; 7(3):234].

33. Goldberg HL. Trauma and the improbable anterior displacement. J Craniomandib Disord Facial Oral Pain 1990;4:131–134.

34. McKay DC, Christensen LV. Whiplash injuries of the temporomandibular joint in motor vehicle accidents: Speculations and facts. J Oral Rehabil 1998;25:731–746.

35. Howard RP, Hatsell CP, Guzman HM. Temporomandibular joint injury potential imposed by the low-velocity extension-flexion maneuver. J Oral Maxillofac Surg 1995;53:256–262.

36. Howard RP, Benedict JV, Raddin JH Jr, Smith HL. Assessing neck extension-flexion as a basis for temporomandibular joint dysfunction [see comments]. J Oral Maxillofac Surg 1991;49: 1210–1213.

37. Szabo TJ, Welcher JB, Anderson RD, et al. Human occupant kinematic response to low speed rear-end impacts. In: Society of Automotive Engineers (eds). Occupant Containment and Methods of Assessing Occupant Protection in the Crash Environment. Warrendale, PA: Society of Automotive Engineers, 1994:SP-1045.

38. Heise AP, Laskin DM, Gervin AS. Incidence of temporomandibular joint symptoms following whiplash injury. J Oral Maxillofac Surg 1992; 50:825–828.

39. Probert TCS, Wiesenfeld PC, Reade PC. Temporomandibular pain dysfunction disorder resulting from road traffic accidents—An Australian study. Int J Oral Maxillofac Surg 1994; 23:338–341.

40. Okeson JP. Functional neuroanatomy and physiology of the masticatory system. In: Management of Temporomandibular Disorders and Occlusion. St Louis: Mosby Year Book, 2003:29–66.

41. Stegenga B. Temporomandibular Joint Osteoarthrosis and Internal Derangement: Diagnostic and Therapeutic Outcome Assessment. Groningen, The Netherlands: Drukkerij Van Denderen, 1991:500.

42. Dijkgraaf LC, de Bont LG, Boering G, Liem RS. The structure, biochemistry, and metabolism of osteoarthritic cartilage: A review of the literature. J Oral Maxillofac Surg 1995;53:1182–1192.

43. Nitzan DW, Nitzan U, Dan P, Yedgar S. The role of hyaluronic acid in protecting surface-active phospholipids from lysis by exogenous phospholipase A(2). Rheumatology (Oxford) 2001;40:336–340.

44. Nitzan DW. The process of lubrication impairment and its involvement in temporomandibular joint disc displacement: A theoretical concept. J Oral Maxillofac Surg 2001;59:36–45.

45. Nitzan DW, Marmary Y. The "anchored disc phenomenon": A proposed etiology for sudden-onset, severe, and persistent closed lock of the temporomandibular joint. J Oral Maxillofac Surg 1997;55:797–802; discussion 802–803.

46. Zardeneta G, Milam SB, Schmitz JP. Iron-dependent generation of free radicals: Plausible mechanisms in the progressive deterioration of the temporomandibular joint. J Oral Maxillofac Surg 2000;58:302–308; discussion 309.

47. Dan P, Nitzan DW, Dagan A, Ginsburg I, Yedgar S. H_2O_2 renders cells accessible to lysis by exogenous phospholipase A2: A novel mechanism for cell damage in inflammatory processes. FEBS Lett 1996;383:75–78.

48. Milam SB, Zardeneta G, Schmitz JP. Oxidative stress and degenerative temporomandibular joint disease: A proposed hypothesis. J Oral Maxillofac Surg 1998;56:214–223.

49. Aghabeigi B, Haque M, Wasil M, Hodges SJ, Henderson B, Harris M. The role of oxygen free radicals in idiopathic facial pain. Br J Oral Maxillofac Surg 1997;35:161–165.

50. Israel HA, Diamond B, Saed Nejad F, Ratcliffe A. The relationship between parafunctional masticatory activity and arthroscopically diagnosed temporomandibular joint pathology. J Oral Maxillofac Surg 1999;57:1034–1039.

51. Nitzan DW. Intraarticular pressure in the functioning human temporomandibular joint and its alteration by uniform elevation of the occlusal plane. J Oral Maxillofac Surg 1994;52: 671–679.

52. Milam SB, Schmitz JP. Molecular biology of temporomandibular joint disorders: Proposed mechanisms of disease. J Oral Maxillofac Surg 1995;12:1448–1454.

53. Monje F, Delgado E, Navarro MJ, Miralles C, Alonso DH Jr. Changes in temporomandibular joint after mandibular subcondylar osteotomy: An experimental study in rats. J Oral Maxillofac Surg 1993;51:1221–1234.

54. Shaw RM, Molyneux GS. The effects of induced dental malocclusion on the fibrocartilage disc of the adult rabbit temporomandibular joint. Arch Oral Biol 1993;38:415–422.

55. Okeson JP. Causes of functional disturbances in the masticatory system. In: Management of Temporomandibular Disorders and Occlusion. St Louis: Mosby–Year Book, 2003:149–189.

56. Isberg A, Isacsson G. Tissue reactions associated with internal derangement of the temporomandibular joint. A radiographic, cryomorphologic, and histologic study. Acta Odontol Scand 1986;44:160–164.

57. Wright WJ Jr. Temporomandibular disorders: Occurrence of specific diagnoses and response to conservative management. Clinical observations. Cranio 1986;4:150–155.

58. Seligman DA, Pullinger AG. Association of occlusal variables among refined TM patient diagnostic groups. J Craniomandib Disord 1989;3:227–236.

59. Solberg WK, Bibb CA, Nordstrom BB, Hansson TL. Malocclusion associated with temporomandibular joint changes in young adults at autopsy. Am J Orthod 1986;89:326–330.

60. Tsolka P, Walter JD, Wilson RF, Preiskel HW. Occlusal variables, bruxism and temporomandibulae disorder: A clinical and kinesiographic assessment. J Oral Rehabil 1995;22:849–956.

61. Williamson EH, Simmons MD. Mandibular asymmetry and its relation to pain dysfunction. Am J Orthod 1979;76:612–617.

62. DeBoever JA, Adriaens PA. Occlusal relationship in patients with pain-dysfunction symptoms in the temporomandibular joint. J Oral Rehabil 1983;10:1–7.

63. Brandt D. Temporomandibular disorders and their association with morphologic malocclusion in children. In: Carlson DS, McNamara JA, Ribbens KA (eds). Developmental Aspects of Temporomandibular Joint Disorders, no 16, Craniofacial Growth Series. Ann Arbor, MI: University of Michigan Press, 1985:279–291.

64. Thilander B. Temporomandibular joint problems in children. In: Carlson DS, McNamara JA, Ribbens KA (eds). Developmental Aspects of Temporomandibular Joint Disorders, no 16, Craniofacial Growth Series. Ann Arbor, Michigan: University of Michigan Press, 1985:89–102.

65. Bernal M, Tsamtsouris A. Signs and symptoms of temporomandibular joint dysfunction in 3 to 5 year old children. J Pedod 1986;10:127–140.

66. Nilner M. Functional disturbances and diseases of the stomatognathic system. A cross-sectional study. J Pedod 1986;10:211–238.

67. Stringert HG, Worms FW. Variations in skeletal and dental patterns in patients with structural and functional alterations of the temporomandibular joint: A preliminary report. Am J Orthod 1986;89:285–297.

68. Gunn SM, Woolfolk MW, Faja BW. Malocclusion and TMJ symptoms in migrant children. J Craniomandib Disord 1988;2:196–200.

69. Dworkin SF, Huggins KH, LeResche L, Von KM, Howard J, Truelove E, Sommers E. Epidemiology of signs and symptoms in temporomandibular disorders: Clinical signs in cases and controls. J Am Dent Assoc 1990;120:273–281.

70. Glaros AG, Brockman DL, Acherman RJ. Impact of overbite on indicators of temporomandibular joint dysfunction. J Craniomandib Pract 1992;10:277–281.

71. McNamara JA Jr, Seligman DA, Okeson JP. Occlusion, orthodontic treatment, and temporomandibular disorders: A review. J Orofac Pain 1995;9:73–90.

72. Ronquillo HI, Guay J, Tallents R, Katzberg R, Murphy W, Proskin H. Comparison of internal deranagements with condyle-fossa relationship, horizontal and vertical overlap, and angle class. J Craniomandib Disord Facial Oral Pain 1988;2:137–140.

73. Pullinger AG, Seligman DA, Solberg WK. Temporomandibular disorders. Part II: Occlusal factors associated with temporomandibular joint tenderness and dysfunction. J Prosthet Dent 1988;59:363–367.

74. Pullinger AG, Seligman DA. Overbite and overjet characteristics of refined diagnositic groups of temporomandibular disorder patients. Am J Orthod Dentofac Orthop 1991;100:401–415.

75. Eagle WW. Elongated styloid process: Further observations and a new syndrome. Arch Otolaryngol Head Neck Surg 1948;47:630–640.

76. Eagle WW. Symptomatic elongated styloid process. Arch Otolaryngol Head Neck Surg 1949;49:490–503.

77. Breault MR. Eagle's syndrome: Review of the literature and implications in craniomandibular disorders. J Craniomandib Pract 1986;4:323–337.

78. Lawrence FR, Cornielson E. Eagle's syndrome. J Oral Maxillofac Surg 1962;40:307–309.

79. Correll RW, Wescott WB. Eagle's syndrome diagnosed after history of headache, dysphagia, otalgia, and limited neck movement. J Am Dent Assoc 1982;104:491–492.

80. de Leeuw R, Boering G, Stegenga B, de Bont LGM. Temporomandibular joint osteoarthrosis: Clinical and radiographic characteristics 30 years after nonsurgical treatment: A preliminary report. J Craniomand Pract 1993;11:1524.

81. Boering G. Arthrosis deformans van het kaakgewricht (thesis). Groningen, The Netherlands: University of Groningen, 1966.

82. Boering G, Stegenga B, de Bont LGM. Temporomandibular joint osteoarthritis and internal derangement. Part I: Clinical course and initial treatment. Int Dent J 1990;40:339–346.

83. Rasmussen OC. Clinical findings during the course of temporomandibular arthropathy. Scand J Dent Res 1981;89:283–288.

84. Rasmussen OC. Temporomandibular arthropathy. Int J Oral Surg 1983;12:365–397.

85. Stegenga B, de Bont LGM, Boering G. Osteo-arthrosis as the cause of craniomandibular pain and dysfunction: A unifying concept. J Oral Maxillofac Surg 1989;47:249–256.

86. Nickerson JW, Boering G. Natural course of osteoarthrosis as it relates to internal derangements of the temporomandibular joint. Oral Maxillofac Surg Clin North Am 1989;1:27–45.

87. Bush FM, Carter WH. TMJ clicking and facial pain. J Dent Res 1983;62(special issue):304.

88. Greene CS, Turner C, Laskin D. Long-term outcome of TMJ clicking in 100 MPD patients. J Dent Res 1982;61(special issue):218.

89. Greene CS, Laskin D. Long-term status of TMJ clicking in patients with myofascial pain and dysfunction. J Am Dent Assoc 1988;117:461–465.

90. Lundh H, Westesson PL, Kopp S. A three-year follow-up of patients with reciprocal temporomandibular joint clicking. Oral Surg Oral Med Oral Pathol 1987;63:530–533.

91. Magnusson T. Five-year longitudinal study of signs and symptoms of mandibular dysfunction in adolescents. J Craniomandib Pract 1986;4:338–344.

92. Okeson JP. The long-term treatment of disc-interference disorders. J Prosthet Dent 1988;60:611–616.

93. Magnusson T, Egermark I, Carlsson GE. A longitudinal epidemiologic study of signs and symptoms of temporomandibular disorders from 15 to 35 years of age. J Orofac Pain 2000;14:310–319.

94. Egermark I, Carlsson GE, Magnusson T. A 20-year longitudinal study of subjective symptoms of temporomandibular disorders from childhood to adulthood. Acta Odontol Scand 2001;59:40–48.

95. de Leeuw R, Boering G, Stegenga B, de Bont LGM. TMJ osteoarthrosis and internal derangement 30 years after nonsurgical treatment. J Orofacial Pain 1994;8:18–24.

96. Nelson SJ, Ash MM. An evaluation of a moist heat pad for the treatment of TMJ/muscle pain dysfunction. J Craniomandib Pract 1988;6:355–359.

97. Satlerthwaite JR. Ice massage. Pain Manage 1989;2:116–121.

98. Lark MR, Gangarosa LP. Iontophoresis: An effective modality for the treatment of inflammatory disorders of the temporomandibular joint and myofascial pain. J Craniomandib Pract 1990;8:108–119.

99. Gangarosa LP. Iontophoresis in Dental Practice. Chicago: Quintessence, 1983.

100. Gangarosa LP, Ikeshima A, Morihana A, et al. Ionotophoresis (IONTO) of lidocaine (Lido) into the TMJ of rabbits [abstract]. J Dent Res 1991;70(special issue):444.

101. Kleinkort JA, Wood F. Phonopheresis with one percent versus ten percent hydrocortisone. Phys Ther 1985;55:1320–1324.

102. Kleinkort JA, Foley R. Laser acupuncture. Its use in physical therapy. Am J Acupuncture 1984;12:51–56.

103. Synder-Mackler L, Bork CE. Effect of helium-neon laser irradiation on peripheral sensory nerve latency. Phys Ther 1988;68:223–225.

104. Walker J. Relief from chronic pain from low-power laser irradiation. Neurosci Lett 1983;43:339–344.

105. Bliddal H, Hellesen C, Ditlevsen P, Asselberghs J, Lyager L. Soft laser therapy of rheumatoid arthritis. Scand J Rheumatol 1987;16:225–228.

106. Hanson TL. Infrared laser in the treatment of craniomandibular arthrogenous pain. J Prosthet Dent 1989;61:614–617.

107. Palano D, Martelli M, et al. A clinic statistical investigation of laser effect in the treatment of pain and dysfunction of the temporomandibular joint (TMJ). Medical Laser Report 1985;(No 2):21–26.

108. Bezuur NJ, Habets LLMH, Hansson TL. The effect of therapeutic laser treatment in patients with craniomandibular disorders. J Craniomandib Disord Facial Oral Pain 1988;2:83–86.

109. Okeson JP. Treatment of temporomandibular joint disorders. In: Management of Temporomandibular Disorders and Occlusion. St Louis: Mosby–Year Book, 2003:437–489.

110. Okeson JP. Treatment of masticatory muscle disorders. In: Management of Temporomandibular Disorders and Occlusion. St Louis: Mosby–Year Book, 2003:413-435.

111. Bell WE. Normal craniomandibular structure. In: Orofacial Pains, Classification, Diagnosis, and Management, ed 3. Chicago: Year Book, 1990:67–75.

112. Woolf CJ, Thompson SWN. The induction and maintenance of central sensitization is dependent on N-methyl-D-aspartic acid receptor activation: Implications for the treatment of post-injury pain hypersensitivity. Pain 1991;44:293–300.

113. Crossley HL, Bergman SA, Wynn RL. Non-steroid anti-inflammatory agents in relieving dental pain: A review. J Am Dent Assoc 1983; 106:61–64.

114. Sheridan P. Flurbiprofen as an alternative pain suppressor to standard analgesic therapy. J Am Dent Assoc 1986;113:671.

115. Guilbaud G, Iggo A, Tegner R. Sensory changes in joint-capsule receptors of arthritic rats: Effect of aspirin. In: Fields HL, Dubner R, Cervero F (eds). Proceedings of the Fourth World Congress on Pain: Seattle, vol 9, Advances in Pain Research and Therapy. New York: Raven Press, 1985:81–89.

116. Henny FA. Intra-articular injection of hydrocortisone into the temporomandibular joint. J Oral Surg 1954;12:314–319.

117. Toller PA. Osteoarthritis of the mandibular condyle. Br Dent J 1973;134:233–231.

118. Toller PA. Non-surgical treatment of dysfunctions of the temporomandibular joint. Oral Sci Rev 1976;7:70–85.

119. Kopp S, Carlsson GE, Haraldson T, Wenneberg B. Long-term effects of intra-articular injections of sodium hyaluronate and corticosteroids on temporomandibular joint arthritis. J Oral Maxillofac Surg 1987;45:929–935.

120. Wenneberg B, Kopp S, Grondahl HG. Long-term effect of intra-articular ingections of a glucocorticosteroid into the TMJ: A clinical and radiographic 8-year follow-up. J Craniomandib Disord Facial Oral Pain 1991;5:11–18.

121. Poswillo DE. Experimental investigation of the effects of intra-articular hydrocortisone and high condylectomy on the mandibular condyle. Oral Surg Oral Med Oral Pathol 1970;30: 161–173.

122. Zarb GA, Spech JE. The treatment of mandibular dysfunction. In Zarb GA, Carlsson GE: Temporomandibular Joint: Function and Dysfunction. St Louis: Mosby, 1979:373–389.

123. Farrar WB. Differentiation of temporomandibular joint dysfunction to simplify treatment. J Prosthet Dent 1972;28:629–636.

124. Anderson GC, Schulte JK, Goodkind RJ. Comparative study of two treatment methods for internal derangements of the temporomandibular joint. J Prosthet Dent 1985;53:392–397.

125. Gazit E, Lieberman M, Eini R, et al. Prevalence of functional disturbances in 10–18 year old Israeli school children. J Oral Rehabil 1984;11: 307–317.

126. Moloney F, Howard JA. Internal derangements of the temporomandibular joint. III. Anterior repositioning splint therapy. Aust Dent J 1986;31:30–39.

127. Burns R, McKinney J, Chase D, et al. Occlusal splint therapy for treatment of internal derangements: Retrospective study. J Dent Res 1983;62(special issue):304.

128. Lundh H, Westesson PL, Kopp S, Tillstrom B. Anterior repositioning splint in the treatment of temporomandibular joints with reciprocal clicking: Comparison with a flat occlusal splint and an untreated control group. Oral Surg Oral Med Oral Pathol 1985;60:131–136.

129. Lundh H, Westesson PL, Jisander S, Eriksson L. Disk-repositioning onlays in the treatment of temporomandibular joint disk displacement: Comparison with a flat occlusal splint and with no treatment. Oral Surg Oral Med Oral Pathol 1988;66:155–162.

130. McGowan P, McKinney J, Chase D, Anderson D. Treatment of anterior disc displacement with Jankelson Myosplint: retrospective study [abstract]. J Dent Res 1983;62(special issue):304.

131. Okeson JP. Long-term treatment of disk-interference disorders of the temporomandibular joint with anterior repositioning occlusal splints. J Prosthet Dent 1988;60:611–616.

132. Heikinheimo K, Salmi K, Myllarniemi S, Kirveskari P. Symptoms of craniomandibular disorders in a sample of Finnish adolescents at the ages of 12 and 15 years. Eur J Orthod 1989;11:325–331.

133. Vincent SD, Lilly GE. Incidence and characterization of temporomandibular joint sounds in adults. J Am Dent Assoc 1988;116:203–206.

134. Bay R, Timmis D, Helme E, Sharawy M. Histopathology of human TMJ disc perforation after anterior repositioning splint therapy. J Dent Res 1989;68(special issue):1004.

135. Akerman S, Kopp S, Rohlin M. Histological changes in temporomandibular joints from elderly individuals. Acta Odontol Scand 1986;44: 231–239.

136. Baldioceda F, Bibb C, Pullinger A. Morphologic variability in the human TMJ disc and posterior attachment [abstract]. J Dent Res 1989;68(special issue):229.

137. Blaustein DI, Scapino RP. Remodeling of the temporomandibular joint disk and posterior attachment in disk displacement specimens in relation to glycosaminoglycan content. Plastic Reconstr Surg 1986;78:756–764.

138. Hall MB, Brown RW, Baughman RA. Histologic appearance of the bilaminar zone in internal derangement of the temporomandibular joint. Oral Surg Oral Med Oral Pathol 1984;58:375–381.

139. Salo L, Raustia A, Pernu H, Virtanen K. Internal derangement of the temporomandibular joint: A histochemical study. J Oral Maxillofac Surg 1991;49:171–176.

140. Scapino RP. Histopathology associated with malposition of the human temporomandibular joint disc. Oral Surg Oral Med Oral Pathol 1983;55:382–397.

141. Solberg WK, Hansson TL, Nordstrom B. The temporomandibular joint in young adults at autopsy: A morphologic classification and evaluation. J Oral Rehabil 1985;12:303–321.

142. Solberg WK, Nordstrom BB, Hanson TL. Malocclusion associated with temporomandibular joint changes in young adults at autopsy. Am J Orthod Dentofacial Orthop 1986;89:326–330.

143. Kirk WS. Magnetic resonance imaging and tomographic evaluation of occlusal appliance treatment for advanced internal derangement of the temporomandibular joint. J Oral Maxillofac Surg 1991;49:9–12.

144. Tallents RH, Katzberg RW, Machen DJ, Roberts CA. Use of protrusive splint therapy in anterior disk displacement of the temporomandibular joint: A 1 to 3 year follow-up. J Prosthet Dent 1990;63:336–341.

145. Friedman MH, Weisberg J. Temporomandibular Joint Disorders: Diagnosis and Treatment. Chicago: Quintessence, 1985.

146. Gelb HE. Clinical Management of Head, Neck and TMJ Pain and Dysfunction. Philadelphia: Saunders, 1985.

147. Morgan DH, House LR, Hall WP (eds). Diseases of the Temporomandibular Apparatus. St Louis: Mosby, 1982.

148. Sarnat BG, Laskin DM (eds). The Temporomandibular Joint, ed 4. Springfield, IL: Thomas, 1992.

chapter 14

Other Musculoskeletal Pains

For purposes of description, pains that emanate from musculoskeletal structures of the mouth and face have been divided into separate groups: periodontal and odontogenous pains (chapter 11), pains of muscular origin (chapter 12), temporomandibular joint pains (chapter 13), and other musculoskeletal pains of the mouth and face. All such musculoskeletal pains display the clinical characteristics of deep somatic pain, of which they constitute a major subdivision. In addition, they display features that identify them as being of musculoskeletal origin, namely, the pain relates reasonably to the demands of biomechanical function, and manual palpation (or functional manipulation) induces a graduated response. The other musculoskeletal pains of the face and mouth include osseous pains, periosteal pains, and soft connective tissue pains (Fig 14-1). It should be noted that osseous structures and soft connective tissue are generally less proprioceptively innervated and therefore may not be intimately related to biomechanical function. Pain originating from these structures is often more difficult for the patient to localize and less likely to induce muscle effects.

Osseous Pains

Pains that emanate from the bony structures of the mouth and face, exclusive of the periodontal structures and the temporomandibular joints, constitute another subdivision of musculoskeletal pain. Pains from this source are predominantly inflammatory as a result of injury, infection, or surgical intervention.

Osseous pains are more constant than myogenous pains, and they typically follow an inflammatory time frame. They usually differ from cellulitic pains in that, initially, pain alone dominates the complaint. Osseous pains also show less evidence of other inflammatory symptoms. Because of the rigid, unyielding structure of the tissues involved, inflammatory swelling may not be observed until the surrounding structures become involved. During this phase, the pain relates especially to three factors: (1) the susceptibility of inflamed osseous tissue to environmental noxious irritation, such as mechanical encroachment, movement of fractured or injured parts, and contact with saliva; (2) the confinement of in-

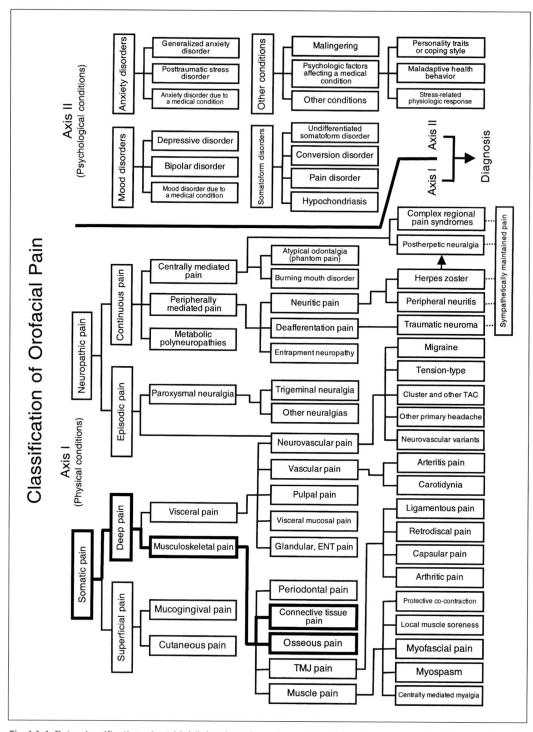

Fig 14-1 Pain classification chart highlighted to show the relationship of osseous and soft connective tissue pains to other orofacial pain disorders.

flammatory exudate; and *(3)* the type and virulence of the contaminating organism. The pain level usually drops rapidly as these factors are obtunded by natural resolution or therapy. Final relief of pain follows a protracted inflammatory time frame. There is minimal dysfunction other than that resulting from the inhibitory influence of pain. However, secondary factors, such as muscle co-contraction, local muscle soreness, myospasm, or cellulites, may contribute to some dysfunction.

By definition, *osteitis* denotes inflammation of bone involving the haversian spaces, canals, and medullary spaces.[1(p1332)] Acute septic osteitis is usually designated as *osteomyelitis*. The inflammatory reaction occurs in the soft tissues confined within the rigid osseous compartments, a condition that in some ways simulates pulpal inflammation. Congestion within such rigidly confined areas may cause pain out of proportion to that experienced when such confinement is not present. This may give the pain a throbbing quality. It induces necrosis by pressure against the unyielding walls. Thus, the inflammatory condition spreads through the bone by following the paths of least resistance.

When the cortex is penetrated, the inflammatory process is considerably less confined, and the intensity of the pain decreases. Subperiosteal spreading occurs with surface swelling and pain, which is readily identifiable by manual palpation. Subperiosteal spreading may proceed until a barrier is reached, such as a muscle attachment. At that point it may rupture through, and the inflammation may spread to the overlying soft tissues. Confined acute subperiosteal inflammation may be extremely painful due to sensitivity of the periosteum to pain.[2]

When confinement is released by rupture or surgical drainage, the pain intensity drops dramatically, and the throbbing quality disappears. In turn, cellulitic involvement accompanies the osteitis, and further spreading takes place along natural barriers such as the fascial planes. The degree of pain again is determined largely by confinement imposed by the relationship of the anatomic features to the quantity of exudate and degree of purulence. Tissues offering little resistance to swelling provide less intense pain, whereas tissues that tightly contain the inflammatory process increase the pain level and incidence of throbbing. Surface rupture and fistulization (or surgical drainage) reduce pain intensity, and the throbbing usually disappears.

It should be evident therefore that the pain behavior is determined by several factors, including the type of injury, virulence and behavioral characteristics of the invader, resistance of the host, and anatomic conditions imposed at the site of inflammation. Nonseptic inflammatory conditions are less painful. Chronicity may cause the pain to disappear entirely or to remain as only low-grade tenderness. Accompanying cellulitis, regional lymphadenitis, and systemic symptoms are valuable clues to the progress and resolution of all such inflammatory conditions.

Dry-Socket Pain

A frequent osteitic involvement of the mouth is *acute dental alveolitis* or the so-called dry socket that follows tooth extraction. This condition is the result of inflammation of remnants of the periodontal ligament and cortical bone of the alveolus. Since they are components of a fibrous joint, these structures are richly innervated with both mechanoreceptors and nociceptors. They therefore have the propensity to initiate reactive muscle effects and considerably more nociceptive response than do other osseous structures. Protective muscle co-contraction and secondary central excitatory effects are frequent complications. Referred pain involving many teeth, spots of touchy gingiva or skin, areas of deep palpable tenderness, and secondary masticatory muscle soreness may be displayed. Dry-socket pain may also initiate a myofascial trigger point pain mechanism especially affecting the masseter and temporalis muscles. The referred pain from such trigger points may be felt at or near the site that initiated the mechanism. It therefore may be mistaken for continuing primary pain from the extraction site. Accurate differentiation between primary pain input and its secondary effects is essential for effective management.

Since confinement usually is not present, spreading of infection from the dental alveolus into the deeper osseous tissue is rare. If deep-seated infection or excessive surgical trauma complicates the problem, osteomyelitis may result. As soon as the exposed surface becomes covered with granulation tissue, the pain subsides, and healing usually proceeds uneventfully.

Osseous pains of inflammatory origin should be differentiated from other less common pains, such as those that stem from cysts and tumors. Radiographic evidence is essential with most osseous lesions.

Periosteal Pains

The periosteum, in contrast to bone, is richly innervated with sensory receptors. It is particularly sensitive to pressure and impact stress. The mechanoreceptors in periosteal tissue supply proprioceptive input for underlying bony structures. Noxious stimulation of the periosteum therefore has a high potential to induce reactive muscle effects and nociception. The pain that emanates from the periosteum is disproportionately greater than the initiating noxious stimulus.

Inflammatory conditions of the periosteum are commonplace. Periosteitis may

occur as a primary osseous condition following injury or superficial infection. Acute suppurative periosteitis may be painful. Subperiosteal spreading occurs with involvement of the surface cortical layer of bone, which is relatively insensitive to pain.[2] If it penetrates more deeply, osteomyelitis may develop. Periosteitis is frequently encountered in the mouth because of the vulnerability presented by prominent bony contours and exostoses. Edentulous ridges are vulnerable.

Injury or infection that penetrates sufficiently to involve the periosteum and osseous cortex may occur as a result of dental appliances and accidental injuries from such causes as toothbrushing, coarse, abrasive foods, burns, and objects held in the mouth. The tongue may rub through and expose prominences, especially along the mandibular internal oblique ridge. If the overlying tissues are thin, full-thickness ulceration including the periosteum may occur, with the cortical bone becoming exposed. The pain arises chiefly from the margins of the ulcer. Since there is no confinement, spreading beneath the periosteum and into the cancellous bone is limited, and the condition usually remains localized. Elimination of the cortical bone by "back resorption" may be slow and healing delayed.

Periosteitis may arise from contiguous obscure dental sepsis and involve the adjacent bony structure extensively. Formation of such subperiosteal abscesses may be accompanied by deeper osteomyelitic and superficial cellulitic development, thus presenting a rather complex clinical problem that generates considerable pain. Muscle attachments that penetrate the periosteum and attach directly to the bone form barriers to subperiosteal spreading. An intimate knowledge of such attachments is extremely valuable to the examiner.[3]

Chronic forms of periosteitis may become troublesome management problems but do not present a diagnostic challenge as far as pain is concerned. Local tenderness evident to manual palpation and other clinical signs usually make the diagnosis simple.

Soft Connective Tissue Pains

Pain that emanates from the soft connective tissue structures of the mouth and face constitutes a major subdivision of musculoskeletal pain. Pains from these structures are predominantly inflammatory and relate to other signs of inflammation by which the source of pain may be identified.

Soft connective tissue pain is considerably more constant than muscle pain, and it usually follows an inflammatory time frame. When the inflammatory exudate is confined, the pain develops a pulsatile quality and increases in intensity. When evacuated by penetration, rupture, or surgical drainage, pain intensity drops dramatically, and the pulsatile quality disappears. Dysfunction is the result chiefly of inflammatory swelling.

By definition, *cellulitis* denotes inflammation of cellular tissue, especially purulent inflammation of loose connective tissue.[1(p328)] Most purulent inflammatory conditions involving the deeper soft tissues of the face and mouth are designated as cellulitis. Specific terms may designate certain types and locations of cellulitic involvement. The intensity of pain depends largely on the acuity, rate of spreading, distension of tissues, and confinement of inflammatory exudate. Manual palpation gives essential information, as do concomitant regional lymphadenitis and systemic effects. Spreading follows the fascial planes.

Acute cellulitis is usually evident from the swelling and pain, and no diagnostic problem occurs as long as the inflammation is located in accessible regions. When this condition involves the sublingual area, its location relative to the mylohyoid muscle largely determines its clinical features and behavior. *Supramylohyoid cellulitis* lifts the tongue and interferes with speech and swallowing. *Inframylohyoid cellulitis* causes external swelling in the submental and submandibular areas and may impede respiration if it encroaches on the glottis. *Palatal cellulitis* causes swelling that interferes with speech and swallowing. In the buccal regions, it usually causes external swelling of the face that spreads readily to the eyelids. Confinement, spreading, and location of the swelling relate to the anatomic arrangement of facial muscles and to the anchorage of fascial barriers. Cellulitis in the pterygomandibular space causes trismus as a result of medial pterygoid muscle involvement. Similar inflammation adjacent to the masseter muscle does likewise. Cellulitis in the infratemporal fossa area causes characteristic facial swelling above the zygoma and trismus as a result of temporal muscle involvement.

Subacute cellulites and chronic cellulitis are less dramatic and may present diagnostic problems of differentiation from cysts and tumors.[4] The history and clinical course, plus manual palpation and surgical aspiration, are the usual means of establishing the diagnosis.

Pain of cellulitic origin should be differentiated from muscle pain, vascular pain, and glandular pain. Other conditions that may initiate soft connective tissue pain are cysts and tumors, both benign and malignant.

Differential Diagnosis

The primary deep somatic musculoskeletal pains that emanate from the osseous, periosteal, and soft connective tissue structures of the orofacial area should be distinguished diagnostically from the following conditions:

1. Odontogenous pains
2. Orofacial myalgia and arthralgia
3. Neoplastic and cystic pains
4. Vascular, neurovascular, and other visceral pains
5. Heterotopic referred pains and secondary hyperalgesias resulting from other deep pain input
6. Heterotopic projected neuropathic pains
7. Somatoform pain disorders
8. Heterotopic pains of central origin

Therapeutic Options

For the management of primary deep somatic musculoskeletal pains that emanate from osseous, periosteal, and soft connective tissue structures, the following therapeutic options are available (see chapter 9):

1. Analgesics for palliative relief, reduction of functional demands, and counseling
2. Cause-related therapy consisting of the identification and treatment of etiologic factors and contributing conditions and general medical and surgical supportive care, including antibiotics, anti-inflammatory agents, and deep heat therapy

References

1. Dorland's Illustrated Medical Dictionary, ed 30. Philadelphia: Saunders, 2003.
2. Wolff HG, Wolf S. Pain, ed 2. Springfield, IL: Thomas, 1958.
3. DuBrul EL. Sicher's Oral Anatomy. St Louis: Mosby, 1980.
4. Kaplan JN, Cummings CW. Pain in the ear, midface, and aerodigestive tract. In: Bonica JJ (ed). The Management of Pain. Malvern, PA: Lea & Febiger, 1990:769–783.

15

Visceral Pains

Primary deep somatic pain emanates from either the musculoskeletal structures or the visceral structures of the body. Musculoskeletal pain derives from the structures that give physical form and stability to the body as well as provide for the biomechanical functions that accomplish posture, locomotion, and other useful working movements. Visceral pain derives from components of the supply and maintenance system that subserve the musculoskeletal structures. The visceral system has to do with oxygen supply, nutrition, metabolism, detoxification, and elimination of waste products. It is composed of organs of many different types, glandular structures, and a network of different kinds of vessels to transport substances throughout the body. Whereas sensation emanating from the musculoskeletal structures relates to more or less conscious volitional biomechanical functions, sensation initiated in visceral structures is largely unconscious and serves to facilitate ongoing automatic metabolic functioning of the body. Pain of musculoskeletal origin therefore relates to biomechanical function as a graduated response, while pain of visceral origin commands attention only to warn that all is not well within. The clinical symptoms displayed by the two kinds of deep somatic pain are sufficiently different to make them identifiable. This is of considerable importance diagnostically.

In addition to the clinical characteristics of deep somatic pain, all such visceral pains display features by which they may be recognized: first, the pains are of threshold type and do not yield graduated responses, and second, the pains are influenced very little by biomechanical function. Visceral pains are usually not accompanied by distinctive evidence of dysfunction other than that induced by the inhibitory influence of pain. Cervero[1] described visceral pain as being accompanied frequently by generalized increased excitability of the central nervous system (CNS), which is expressed as general discomfort, tenderness of the skin, skeletal muscle spasms, and autonomic reflexes. He confirmed that visceral pain was mediated by visceral afferents in sympathetic nerves.

Behavior of Visceral Pains

The mechanism of visceral pain has been described by several authors.[2–9] Ordinarily, sensory information transmitted by afferent neurons of the visceral nervous system remains well below conscious levels. It serves to monitor the involuntary muscle action of vessels, glands, and organs. It reports unusual sensation occurring in the lining membranes of organs and cavities. It helps regulate the automatic functioning of the body by supplying the CNS with a constant inflow of information. When such sensation becomes noxious, pain is felt. Visceral afferent fibers of both the sympathetic and parasympathetic type are known to mediate pain.[8] Visceral pain usually has a distinct stinging or burning quality. It is said that protracted visceral pain[9] tends to provoke vasomotor effects, local edema, and trophic changes.

It appears that conscious visceral sensation is normally of a very low order of intensity, since the visceral afferents have high-threshold receptors. However, the presence of inflammation may reduce this threshold considerably so that conscious pain becomes evident with little added provocation. For example, the stomach yields minimal sensation other than when it is very empty or very full. But an inflamed gastric mucosa causes the normal stomach contents to excite painful sensation, usually described as heartburn.

Visceral pain in the maxillofacial region is not rare. Esophagitis and pharyngitis have the dull, diffuse, burning quality of visceral pain. Pain in the nasal and ostium maxillare mucosa has a similar burning quality.[3,10] The major salivary glands as well as the numerous glands of the lymphatic system, the skin, and the mucous membranes are other sources of this type of pain.

Some pains arising in the maxillofacial region are mediated by sympathetic afferent fibers that do not enter the CNS via any cranial or cervical nerve sensory root. Rather, these visceral fibers leave the orofacial structures and pass through the cervical sympathetic chain and finally enter the CNS via the sensory roots of the upper thoracic spinal nerves. Head and neck pains mediated by this route cannot be arrested by division of any or all cranial and cervical spinal sensory roots. Such pains are arrested by analgesic blocking of the stellate ganglion, through which such afferents pass, even though they undergo no synapse prior to reaching the CNS.[9,11,12]

Analgesic blocking of the stellate ganglion does not necessarily arrest some of these vascular pains. This strongly suggests that the cranial parasympathetics constitute the mediating pain pathway. No parasympathetic afferent fibers pass through the dorsal root of the trigeminal nerve. Rather, they leave this nerve and enter the CNS via the seventh and ninth cranial nerve dorsal roots. Thus, division of the trigeminal sensory root will not arrest pains from the trigeminal area that are mediated by parasympathetic afferent fibers.

Visceral pain input tends to provoke central excitatory effects. Referred pains, secondary hyperalgesias, and localized autonomic effects may accompany visceral pains. Sometimes they dominate the symptom picture and constitute the patient's complaint. The so-called sinus headache typifies this clinical behavior.

For purposes of description, visceral pains have been separated into three groups: pulpal odontogenous pains, vascular pains of the mouth and face, and other visceral pains, including those of mucosal, glandular, ocular, and auricular origin. Pulpal pains have already been reviewed in chapter 11. Since vascular pains are a common and important type of pain originating from the orofacial structures, an entire chapter will be devoted to them (chapter 16). This chapter will review visceral pains that have their origin in mucosal tissues of the pharynx, nose, and paranasal sinuses. This chapter will also review pains from glandular, ocular, and auricular structures (Fig 15-1).

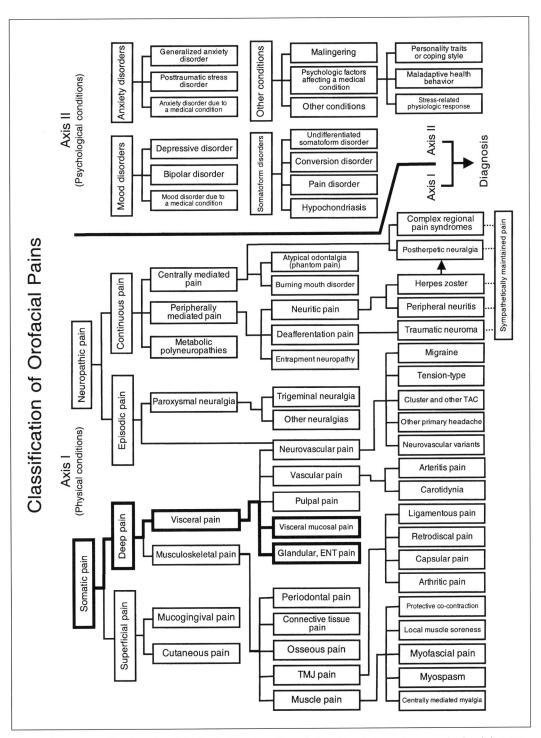

Fig 15-1 Pain classification chart highlighted to show the relationship of visceral mucosal, glandular, ocular, and auricular pains to other orofacial pain disorders.

Pains Emanating from Visceral Mucosa

While pain emanating from the oral muco-gingival tissues is exteroceptive in character and displays clinical characteristics of the superficial somatic type, pain from other mucosal structures of the face is definitely interoceptive in character and exhibits the clinical characteristics of deep pain of the visceral type. This refers particularly to the mucosal linings of the pharynx, the nasal cavity, and the paranasal sinuses.

Ordinarily, sensory perception of visceral mucosa linings remains below conscious levels. This rule applies especially to the more deeply situated structures. The closer such tissues are located to external environmental sources of stimulation, however, the more responsive they are to all stimuli and the more conscious such sensation becomes. For example, the nasal mucosa is more sensitive to low-level stimulation than is the pharyngeal mucosa, while that of the esophagus is less reactive. The fine sensibility of nasal mucosa applies also to the ostium maxillare, but the lining membrane of the maxillary sinus remains resistant to all stimuli. The external portion of esophageal mucosa is highly responsive to stimuli of threshold intensity, but the more deeply situated portion is nearly insensible to all noxious stimuli. It should be noted that there is a transitional zone where the oral mucogingival tissue joins the pharyngeal mucosa, and symptoms of both superficial somatic and deep visceral pain categories may be displayed.

An appreciation of the different types and degrees of sensibility of the lining membranes of the oral, nasal, and pharyngeal structures is needed to understand the nociceptive sensations that emanate from these tissues.

The normal inflow of sensation from visceral mucosa serves to regulate automatic functioning. Several reflex mechanisms are recognized: irritation of the nasal mucosa excites the sneeze reflex, the pharyngeal mucosa initiates the swallowing and gag reflexes, upper esophageal mucosa may induce esophageal spasm, and irritation of the upper tracheal and laryngeal mucosa stimulates the cough reflex. When mucosal stimulation becomes noxious, burning pain is felt.[3,5-8,10,13] It is said that continuing visceral pain tends to provoke vasomotor effects, local edema, and trophic changes.[9] The normally high threshold level of sensibility is lowered in the presence of inflammation so that nociceptive impulses may be generated by otherwise nonnociceptive stimuli.

Nociceptive pathways from orofacial mucosal structures likely involve afferent elements of both the somatic and the visceral nervous systems. Somatic afferents are mediated by the fifth, seventh, and ninth cranial nerves. Parasympathetic visceral afferents are mediated by the seventh and ninth cranial nerves only. As noted earlier, sympathetic visceral afferents do not enter the CNS by way of cranial nerves but travel the cervical sympathetic chain to enter through the upper thoracic spinal nerves.

Like other forms of deep pain, visceral mucosa pain tends to initiate central sensitization or excitatory effects. Many times, the secondary symptoms predominate, while the primary pain input remains silent or goes unnoticed. Some orofacial pain disorders are expressed almost exclusively as secondary central excitatory effects. Caution should be exercised in differentiating such effects from the true source of primary input.

Pharyngeal Mucosa Pain

Inflammatory conditions of the pharyngeal mucosa expressed as a sore throat point out the marked difference between nociceptive conditions involving the oral mucogingival tissues and the visceral mucosa of the pharynx. While the pharyngeal mucosa is quite susceptible, the oral lining membranes are resistant.

Nonspecific pharyngitis

Ordinary pharyngitis is usually viral in origin and occurs in conjunction with nasal and laryngeal symptoms. Pain on swallowing is characteristic. Central excitatory effects include referred pain, especially with swallowing. The reference zone is usually deep in the ear, and the pain is sensed as sharp and lancinating. Secondary hyperalgesia may be felt as a deep palpable tenderness in the throat, larynx, neck, or face or as superficial touchiness of the facial skin or scalp. Secondary autonomic symptoms may include puffy swelling of the eyelids, lacrimation, and nasal secretion. Sneeze and cough reflexes are active. Referred headache is common.

Streptococcal pharyngitis

Streptococcal pharyngitis is typified by sore throat, fever, acutely inflamed pharyngeal mucosa, and referred pains including headache. Cervical and submandibular lymphadenitis is present. Laryngitis, coughing, and nasal congestion are not the result of the streptococcal infection; when present, other etiologic agents coexist. Definitive diagnosis rests on laboratory examination to identify the group A beta-hemolytic organism.

Tonsillitis

Tonsillitis is an acute inflammation of the palatine tonsils that results usually from viral and/or bacterial infection.[14] Severe pain on swallowing, fever, malaise, headache, and regional lymphadenopathy are common. A differential diagnosis includes diphtheria, Vincent angina, and infectious mononucleosis, each of which requires laboratory examination for identification.

Diagnostic considerations

Pharyngeal mucosa pain should be differentiated from Eagle syndrome, glossopharyngeal neuralgia, geniculate neuralgia, and Ramsay Hunt syndrome. Eagle syndrome is characterized by an elongated styloid process or calcification of the stylohyoid ligament. The symptoms are persistent raw throat, ear pain, and pain and difficulty with swallowing. The pain is often increased with head movement, and limited jaw movement may be present.[15-17] Glossopharyngeal neuralgia is typical neuropathic pain of the paroxysmal neuralgia type that is triggered by throat movement incidental to swallowing, talking, and chewing food. Geniculate neuralgia is an extremely rare neuropathic pain of the paroxysmal neuralgia type that is felt as sharp lancinating pain within the depths of the ear. It is triggered by touching the external ear canal or by movement of the auricle.[8] Ramsay Hunt syndrome is herpes zoster of the nervus intermedius portion of the seventh cranial nerve. It is felt as ongoing burning pain deep in the ear and is accompanied by herpetic lesions in the external auditory canal and sometimes on the soft palate as well.

Nasal Mucosa Pain

Pain that emanates from the nasal mucosa is typically a dull, burning sensation that exhibits the clinical characteristics of visceral mucosa pain. Pain arising from the external lining of the nasal alae exhibits features of the superficial somatic category. When the deeper nasal mucosa is irritated as a result of viral or bacterial infection or as an expression of allergic rhinitis, typical deep visceral pain along with a variety of central excitatory effects may occur spontaneously or with the normal passage of air through the nose. The primary pain may go

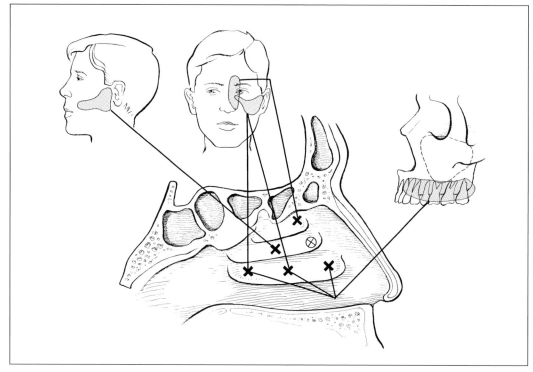

Fig 15-2 Stimulation of points on turbinates (**x**), cause referred pain to be felt in all maxillary teeth as well as in the face. (From Wolff HG. Headache and Other Head Pain, ed 2. New York: Oxford University Press, 1963. Used with permission.)

unnoticed because of the predominance of secondary effects such as referred pain, secondary hyperalgesia, and autonomic symptoms.

Primary pain in the inferior turbinate area has secondary reference zones that include all the ipsilateral maxillary teeth and areas of the face (Fig 15-2). Pain from the region of the ostium maxillare induces referred pain in the maxillary molar teeth and on the face (Fig 15-3).[3,10,18] The referred pain may be sensed as a spontaneous toothache (Case 16). Secondary hyperalgesia may be felt as tender teeth or areas of touchy gingiva. Pain emanating from the nasal mucosa may induce referred pain

throughout the entire upper part of the face. It may be sensed as a headache. Secondary hyperalgesia may be felt as areas of deep palpable tenderness in the upper portion of the face or as superficial touchy areas of skin, scalp, or mucogingival tissue.

Central excitatory effects are frequently expressed as autonomic symptoms. This includes puffy swelling of the eyelids and other loose facial tissue, injection of the conjunctivae, lacrimation, nasal secretion, and nasal congestion. When such symptoms occur in conjunction with diffuse maxillary pain, the condition is usually thought to be the result of maxillary sinusitis. When complicated by a spontaneous maxillary

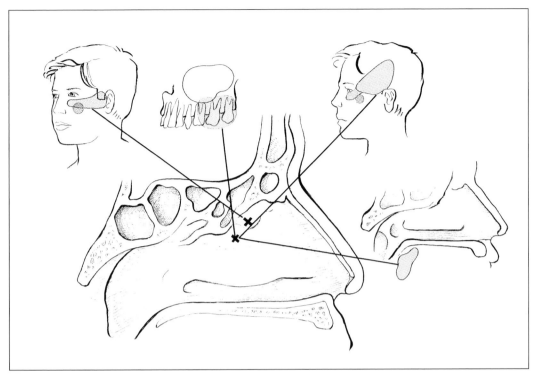

Fig 15-3 Stimulation of the ostium maxillare causes referred pain to be felt in the maxillary molar teeth and in the face. The **X**s represent areas near the ostium that, when painful, can cause pain referred to the areas connected by the lines. (From Wolff HG. Headache and Other Head Pain, ed 2. New York: Oxford University Press, 1963. Used with permission.)

toothache or tender teeth (see chapter 11), the condition may cause doctor and patient alike to think that it constitutes a dental problem, a sinus problem, or both. Not finding adequate dental cause, the dental clinician may refer the patient for ear, nose, and throat (ENT) evaluation or vice versa.

When the referred pain is sensed as a headache, the condition is popularly known as sinus headache. This is especially so when allergic rhinitis is the precipitating cause.

Upper respiratory infections

Upper respiratory infections frequently involve the nasal and pharyngeal mucosa as well as that of the larynx and upper part of the trachea. The inflammatory reaction is of the serous type that produces serous exudate on the surface. When the nasal mucosa is inflamed, the secondary effects of referred pain, secondary hyperalgesia, or autonomic symptoms may be displayed throughout the maxillary region and upper part of the face. Such symptoms frequently include aching or tender teeth. The differential diagnosis depends on distinguishing between the primary pain and its secondary effects. Application of a topical anesthetic to the nasal mucosa will arrest a spontaneous referred toothache but will not arrest stimulus-evoked tenderness of the teeth,

Case 16 — Heterotopic pain felt as toothache and referred from an inflamed nasal mucosa (so-called sinus headache)

Chief Complaint — Nonlocalizable maxillary toothache.

History

A 56-year-old man presented with mild to severe, continuous but recurrent episodes of steady, dull, aching pain diffusely located bilaterally in the upper face and described as maxillary "toothache" that spreads to the zygomatic and orbital areas. The pain was accompanied by sensations of stopped-up ears and nose, swelling of the eyelids, tenderness of the scalp, and discomfort in the masseter and temporal areas with chewing. The episodes were irregular and fairly frequent, lasting from a few hours to 1 or 2 days. The pain was increased with lowering of the head position. He sometimes reported a mandibular toothache as well.

The complaint began about 2 to 3 years earlier and had been recurrently present ever since in spite of treatment by dentists, oral surgeons, internists, otolaryngologists, orthopedists, and neurosurgeons for dental disease, chronic sinusitis, temporomandibular arthropathy, nasal obstruction, neuralgia, and Ménière syndrome, all without success. The TMJs had been injected with corticosteroid many times, without much relief. Presently he takes hydrocodone almost daily for the pain.

Examination

Intraoral: Clinically and radiographically negative for cause of pain.

> **TMJs:** Clinically and radiographically normal.

> **Muscles:** Palpable tenderness in the masseter and temporal muscles bilaterally and discomfort with firm contraction of these muscles but no masticatory dysfunction of any kind.

> **Cervical:** Within normal limits.

> **Cranial nerves:** Within normal limits.

Diagnostic tests: An application of topical anesthetic to nasal passages significantly reduced all pain to the maxillary teeth. Some muscle pain remained. Allergic rhinitis was confirmed by allergist. The patient was referred to another otolaryngologist for evaluation of sinus disease.

Impression

No dental, oral, or masticatory cause was responsible for the complaint. It appears that all pains and muscle effects are expressions of central excitation that arise from the nasal mucosa as a result of deep somatic nasal mucosa pain due chiefly to allergic rhinitis. Once the rhinitis pain has been controlled, successful withdrawal from the narcotic should be carefully monitored.

Diagnosis — So-called "sinus toothache" resulting from expression of allergic rhinitis.

which is a heterotopic expression of secondary hyperalgesia. Analgesic blocking of the tooth may reduce but does not arrest the symptoms of secondary hyperalgesia. (Note that if the tooth were the primary source of pain, analgesic blocking would arrest it.)

With such conditions, the question may arise as to whether it represents a complication of maxillary sinusitis. The symptoms as described do not emanate from maxillary sinusitis, except insofar as the ostium maxillare, nasal mucosa, or both are involved by direct extension from the antrum. The lining membrane of the maxillary sinus does not initiate appreciable secondary excitatory effects of any kind. Determination of whether the antrum is truly involved in such conditions requires radiography and other specific examining techniques.

Paranasal Sinus Pain

Inflammatory conditions of the maxillary antrum and other paranasal sinuses are generally misunderstood. The syndrome of symptoms usually thought to be clinically indicative of sinusitis is chiefly secondary autonomic and sensory effects induced by primary pain emanating from the nasal mucosa, as previously described. Whether such symptoms occur in conjunction with antral disease depends chiefly on patency of the ostium maxillare. Inflammatory exudate that accumulates in the antral cavity remains below the opening of the antrum into the middle meatus of the nose as long as the head is erect. Bending forward, however, permits the fluid to wash over the pain-sensitive tissue around the ostium, thus eliciting pain. If the ostium is open, antral inflammation can spread to the nasal mucosa and thereby initiate the symptoms described previously. If the ostium is closed by swollen membrane or mucous polyps, the maxillary sinus may remain essentially nonsymptomatic. This is because the lining membrane is nearly insensible to pain. This is altered very little even when the sinus is inflamed.[10] Contrary to popular belief, pain is not a highly characteristic symptom of paranasal sinusitis, and chronic sinusitis seldom gives rise to facial pain or a headache.[19] Waltner[20] stated that in his experience no more than 20% of patients treated for sinus disease had any disease of the sinus at all. Chronic obstructive sinusitis exhibits symptoms of fullness or pressure, but not pain or headache, unless the nasal mucosa is conjointly affected.[21]

The question may arise whether the teeth and the maxillary sinus are affected in a common disease process. Sinusitis, of course, can result from dental sepsis, just as antral disease can spread to involve teeth. A determination, however, of which is the primary source cannot be made from the clinical symptoms alone. If the cause of the sinusitis is dental, adequate clinical and radiographic evidence of the dental sepsis should be forthcoming. If the teeth are secondarily involved by direct extension of prior antral disease, the dental pain will be sensed initially as periodontal in type, with pulpal pain coming later. This, it should be noted, is the reverse of what takes place in the usual temporal sequence of pain of odontogenic origin.

Referred spontaneous toothache and secondary hyperalgesia involving the teeth and mouth do not arise as a result of antral inflammation. There is, however, a condition that does cause tooth pain. This is neuritic neuralgia that occurs as a result of inflammation of elements of the superior alveolar plexus by direct extension of antral inflammation. The neuritic symptoms occur in the peripheral distribution of the affected nerve. Thus, any ipsilateral maxillary tooth can be painful. The quality and character of the pain, however, are that of the neuritic type of neuropathic pain (see chapter 17). It is also accompanied by other

Case 17 — Heterotopic pain felt as preauricular pain and referred from an inflamed submandibular gland

Chief Complaint   Left TMJ and facial pain.

History

A 38-year-old man presented with mild, continuous, protracted, steady, dull, aching pain located diffusely in the left preauricular and facial area, which was aggravated by chewing and opening widely but without any accompanying masticatory dysfunction.

The complaint began about a year ago as intermittent pain in the left face. It continued to increase in frequency and severity until about 6 months ago. It was constant but variable. During the last 6 weeks it had become severe enough to seek medical aid. His ENT physician found nothing wrong with the ear and advised a dental examination. His dentist removed the mandibular left third molar, injected the left TMJ with a corticosteroid, and then prescribed a narcotic analgesic, all without benefit. He then referred him to another dentist, who fabricated an occlusal appliance that seemed to aggravate the complaint. He was then referred for a temporomandibular disorder examination. No medications are presently being taken.

Examination

Intraoral: Although the patient is missing three of the first molar teeth, the remaining teeth are clinically and radiographically negative for cause of pain. No occlusal instabilities are noted. All jaw movements are adequate in amplitude and symmetric. Tongue movements are normal. There is no palpable tenderness except in the left submandibular triangle, where an indurated mass is felt and acute pain is elicited on firm palpation. An occlusal radiograph revealed a large, irregular, calcific mass in the region of the left submandibular salivary gland, and this was seen also in the left lateral oblique film of the mandible. This mass was interpreted to represent massive sialolithiasis. Manipulation of the left submandibular gland seemed to increase the left facial and preauricular pain.

TMJs: Normal structurally and functionally.

Muscles: Negative for pain and dysfunction.

Cervical: Within normal limits.

Cranial nerves: Within normal limits.

Impression

The patient's masticatory discomfort appears to be a secondary manifestation of primary pain arising from the left submandibular gland, presumably from the sialolith observed radiographically. The primary pain apparently is largely inhibited except when stimulated by firm manual palpation. Normal mandibular movements seem sufficient to induce impulses that are felt as referred pain in the left preauricular area and face.

Diagnosis   Masticatory pain referred from primary sources in the submandibular gland.

sensory symptoms that may go unnoticed. These include hyperesthesia, hypoesthesia, paresthesia, and anesthesia of other maxillary teeth, the adjacent gingiva, or the tissues around the infraorbital foramina. To confirm the diagnosis, clinical or radiographic evidence of preexisting antral disease is needed. Positive confirmation can be made by surgical aspiration of the maxillary sinus (see Case 26).

Glandular Pains

Primary visceral pain that emanates from glandular structures of the mouth and face is not uncommon. A diagnostic problem may occur, especially when heterotopic pains, secondary muscle co-contraction, autonomic symptoms, or a combination of these are displayed. The source of such pain includes the major salivary glands, the mucous and sebaceous glands, the lacrimal and oil glands, and especially the lymph glands.[10]

Most glandular pain is inflammatory and therefore relates to infection, trauma, or sialolithiasis. Cystic degeneration or tumor formation may be present. Lymphadenitis results primarily from infection. Infectious mononucleosis and neoplasia are other possible causes. The major salivary glands are subject to the irritating effects of mineral deposits and retrograde infection through the ducts that communicate with the oral cavity. Distension and compression may accentuate the pain. Salivary gland pain usually increases at mealtime and therefore may be associated with mastication. Submandibular salivary gland pain is frequently accentuated by chewing and swallowing movements. It may be mistaken for masticatory pain (Case 17).

Because most painful glands are inflammatory, the pain can be localized quite well by manual palpation and by the presence of other signs of inflammation. Secondary central excitatory effects may complicate the symptom picture. Occasionally, heterotopic pains constitute the entire complaint. Careful diagnostic identification of the pain source is important. Lymphadenopathy, especially of the low-grade or chronic type, may be mistaken for a cyst or tumor.

Ocular Pains

Primary pains emanating from the nonmuscular structures of the orbit are mediated by the trigeminal nerve. Ocular muscle pain displays the clinical characteristics of musculoskeletal pain, while pain from the eye proper is chiefly visceral in type. All such pains should be diagnosed and managed by a competent ophthalmologist.

Heterotopic pain felt in the eye is frequently of muscle origin. Eye pain is usually accompanied by a headache. Although retro-orbital pain is sometimes attributed to masticatory causes, it is usually referred from nonmasticatory muscles. The occipital portion of the occipitofrontalis, the splenius cervicis, and the sternocleidomastoid muscles are the chief sources of such pain. It occurs frequently in conjunction with tension headache. Careful diagnostic identification of the pain source is needed to avoid therapeutic errors.

Auricular Pains

Since the ear is innervated by several different cranial and cervical nerves, the symptom of earache can be quite misleading. Primary pain emanating from the ear may

Case 18 — Heterotopic pain felt as preauricular pain due to a trigger point affecting the sternocleidomastoid muscle

Chief Complaint   Left ear pain.

History

A 46-year-old man presented with intermittent short periods of mild to severe, steady, dull, aching pain diffusely located in the left ear and preauricular area, lasting a few minutes each time, and vaguely related to head and jaw movements.

The complaint began about 2 years ago following a severe upper respiratory infection and was initially diagnosed as otitis media. The periods of increased discomfort had been such that he sought only medical attention for his "bad ear." Recently, he went to an ENT physician, who found the ear to be normal and suggested it to be a "bite problem." His dentist was unable to find any cause and returned him to the physician, who then prescribed therapy for "neuralgia" without benefit. He was then returned to his dentist to "take care of this TMJ problem" and was promptly referred for a TMD examination. Presently he is taking no medications.

Examination

Intraoral: There is no apparent dental or oral cause of pain. The occlusal condition is stable and within normal limits. All mandibular functioning is well within normal limits. No discomfort of any kind is elicited by mandibular movements.

TMJs: Both joints are clinically and radiographically normal.

Muscles: The masticatory muscles are entirely negative for cause of pain or dysfunction. There is palpable tenderness in the midbody of the left sternocleidomastoid muscle which, when pressure is firmly applied, causes acute pain to be felt in the left ear and preauricular area.

Cervical: Bending and rotation of the head seems to increase the pain felt in the ear.

Cranial nerves: Within normal limits.

Diagnostic tests: Analgesic blocking of the left sternocleidomastoid muscle trigger point arrested all local tenderness as well as the induced ear and preauricular pain.

Impression

The present pain complaint does not originate from masticatory, dental, or oral cause. It appears to be referred pain arising from stimulation of the painful myofascial trigger point in the left sternocleidomastoid muscle.

Diagnosis   Preauricular nonmasticatory pain referred from myofascial pain originating in the sternocleidomastoid muscle.

arise from different causes and be mediated by different nociceptive pathways. All such complaints should be diagnosed and managed by a competent otolaryngologist.

External auditory canal pain is of considerable interest to the dental practitioner. Such pain is usually inflammatory and causes heterotopic symptoms in the face as well as deep in the ear and throat. Since it usually is accentuated by swallowing, it may be mistaken for masticatory pain or glossopharyngeal neuralgia. Otitis externa may be mistaken for temporomandibular joint arthralgia. One point of difference, however, is that ear pain is accentuated by movement of the auricle.

Since it is common practice to palpate the mandibular condyle through the external auditory canal, consideration should be given to the condition of the ear prior to inserting the finger. It should be inspected visually with a speculum and direct light if an otoscope is not available.

Earache, like headache and retro-orbital pain, is frequently a heterotopic manifestation of deep somatic pain located elsewhere. Frequent sources of such pain are the deep masseter and the clavicular portion of the sternocleidomastoid muscle (Case 18). Earache may be referred from inflamed dental pulps and from the pharyngeal mucosa. Such ear pain is a dominant symptom of a sore throat. Preauricular pain is frequently referred from the lateral pterygoid muscle.

Ear pain such as that of otitis media has the propensity to induce a variety of central excitatory effects, including co-contraction of masticatory muscles, thus often producing a restriction in the range of mandibular movement. In this sense the clinician can easily mistake the condition for a temporomandibular disorder. Careful diagnosis as to etiology is therefore essential for effective management of the condition. If the ear pain is protracted, the cycling nature of muscle pain may perpetuate the muscle disorder long after the initiating deep pain input has disappeared. Such a complaint would then constitute a true masticatory muscle disorder requiring treatment (see chapter 12).

Since ear pains and masticatory pains have an intimate interrelationship, it is important that the pain source be accurately identified prior to definitive therapy by either dentist or otolaryngologist.

Differential Diagnosis

Primary deep somatic pains arising from visceral structures of the orofacial area other than blood vessels should be distinguished diagnostically from the following conditions:

1. Odontogenic pains of pulpal origin
2. Vascular and neurovascular pain disorders
3. Eagle syndrome and carotodynia
4. Primary pains of musculoskeletal, neoplastic, or cystic origin
5. Heterotopic referred pains and secondary hyperalgesias arising from other deep pain input
6. Heterotopic projected neuropathic pains
7. Somatoform pain disorders
8. Heterotopic pains of central origin

Therapeutic Options

For the management of primary deep somatic pains that emanate from visceral structures of the orofacial area other than blood vessels, the following therapeutic options are available (see chapter 9).

1. Analgesics for palliative relief and counseling
2. Medications such as antihistamines, decongestants, antimicrobials, vasoconstrictors, and cough suppressants
3. Vaporizers for nasopharyngeal mucosa complaints
4. Referral for specialized medical care of the eye, ear, nose, and throat
5. General supportive medical care

References

1. Cervero F. Visceral pain [abstract]. Pain 1987; 31(suppl 4):1.
2. Bonica JJ, Procacci P. General considerations of acute pain. In: Bonica JJ. The Management of Pain. Philadelphia: Lea & Febiger, 1990:161–169.
3. Dalessio DJ, Silberstein SD. Wolff's Headache and Other Head Pain, ed 6. New York: Oxford University Press, 1993.
4. Procacci P, Zoppi M. Pathophysiology and clinical aspect of visceral and referred pain. In: Bonica JJ, Lindblom U, Iggo A (eds). Proceedings of the Third World Congress on Pain, vol 5, Advances in Pain Research and Therapy. New York, NY: Raven Press, 1983:643–658.
5. Wolff HG, Wolf S. Pain, ed 2. Springfield, IL: Thomas, 1958.
6. Wall PD, Melzack R. Textbook of Pain. New York: Churchill Livingston, 1984:309–392.
7. Finneson BE. Diagnosis and Management of Pain Syndromes. Philadelphia: Saunders, 1969.
8. Abram SE. Sympathetic pain. In: Raj PP (ed). Practical Management of Pain. Chicago: Year Book, 1986:209–214.
9. Gross D. Pain and autonomic nervous system. In: Bonica JJ (ed). International Symposium on Pain, vol 4, Advances in Neurology. New York: Raven Press, 1974:93–103.
10. Procacci P, Zoppi M. Pathophysiology and clinical aspects of visceral and referred pain. In: Bonica JJ, Lindblom U, Iggo A (eds). Proceedings of the Third World Congress on Pain, vol 5, Advances in Pain Research and Therapy. New York: Raven Press, 1983:643–658.
11. Moore DC. Stellate Ganglion Block. Springfield, IL: Thomas, 1954.
12. Verrill P. Sympathetic ganglion lesions. In: Wall PD, Melzack R (eds). Textbook of Pain. New York: Churchill Livingston, 1984:581–584.
13. Bonica JJ. The Management of Pain. Malvern, PA: Lea & Febiger, 1990:168–169.
14. Steyer TE. Peritonsillar abscess: Diagnosis and treatment. Am Fam Physician 2002;65:93–96.
15. Lawrence FR, Cornielson E. Eagle's syndrome. J Oral Maxillofac Surg 1982;40:307–309.
16. Correll RW, Wescott WB. Eagle's syndrome diagnosed after history of headache, dysphagia, otalgia, and limited neck movement. J Am Dent Assoc 1982;104:491–492.
17. Prasad KC, Kamath MP, Reddy KJ, Raju K, Agarwal S. Elongated styloid process (Eagle's syndrome): A clinical study. J Oral Maxillofac Surg 2002;60:171–175.
18. Hummel T, Mohammadian P, Marchl R, Kobal G, Lotsch J. Pain in the trigeminal system: Irritation of the nasal mucosa using short- and long-lasting stimuli. Int J Psychophysiol 2003; 47:147–158.
19. Mahan PE, Alling CC. Facial Pain. Philadelphia: Lea & Febiger, 1991:311–322.
20. Waltner JG. Otolaryngeal sources of pain. J Am Dent Assoc 1955;51:417–419.
21. Druce HM, Slavin RG. Sinusitis: Critical need for further study. J Allergy Clin Immunol 1991; 88:675–677.

Vascular and Neurovascular Pains

Primary deep somatic pain of the visceral type may arise from the pulps of the teeth (see chapter 11) or from other visceral structures described in chapter 15 (mucosa of the pharynx, nose, and paranasal sinuses, from the glandular, ocular, or auricular structures). Probably some of the most common sources of visceral face pain, however, are the vascular and neurovascular structures.

Behavior of Vascular and Neurovascular Pains

Vascular pain can be a very debilitating condition for many patients. The distinctive feature of vascular pain is its primary pulsatile or throbbing quality. The pulsations match the heartbeat and no doubt stem from the cardiac systoles. The greater the amplitude of vascular dilation, the more pronounced the throbbing quality of the pain. This quality may be very slight at times and may be masked by coexisting muscle pain. The pulsatile feature of vascular pain is not always present but is usually present during exacerbations. Between such peaks of discomfort, the pulsations may diminish in intensity or be imperceptible.

The throbbing quality of true vascular pain must be distinguished from other throbbing pains. Inflammatory pains, especially those confined in such a way that the pulsating vessels in the inflamed area cause noxious stimulation, can have a throbbing quality. Examples of such inflammatory pains frequently encountered by the dental practitioner are pulpitis, osteitis, periosteitis, and confined cellulitis. Usually differentiation can be made on the basis of other clinical signs of inflammation. Some neoplastic lesions have a pulsatile quality.

For the purpose of discussion in this text, vascular pains will be divided into two categories: those pains that actually have their origin in the vascular tissues (vascular pains) and those vascular pains initiated by neurovascular mechanisms (neurovascular pains). This division is made because etiologies, diagnosis, and therapies are different. Since the etiology of neurovascular pains are related to neural mechanisms, these pains are also related to the category of episodic neuropathic pains.

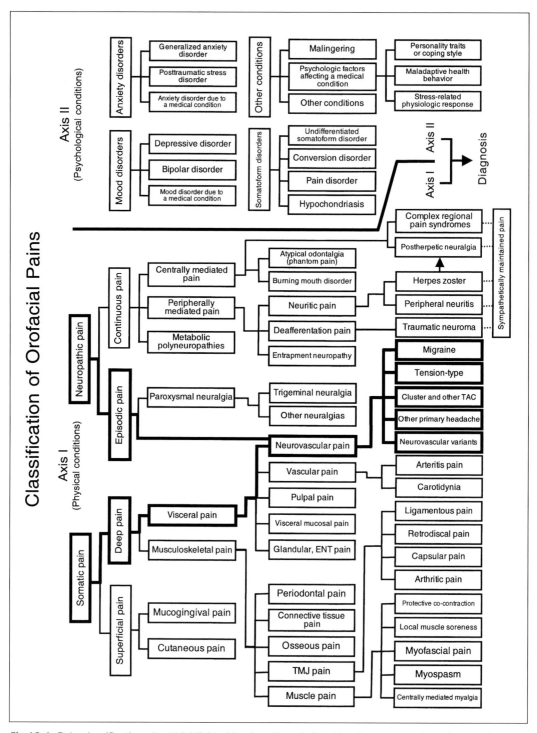

Fig 16-1 Pain classification chart highlighted to show the relationship of neurovascular pains to other orofacial pain disorders.

Neurovascular Pains of the Mouth and Face

Probably the most commonly known neurovascular pain in the mouth and face is migraine. Until recently migraine pain has not been well understood. Early on Wolff[1] explored these pains in depth, and his investigations indicated that pain occurred as a result of the dilation of arteries, which distort and noxiously stimulate the sensory receptors and afferent fibers in the vascular and perivascular tissues. When a vasoconstricting medication such as ergotamine tartrate reduced the dilation and amplitude of pulsation of such arteries, the pain decreased. He also demonstrated that pressure on the carotid artery diminished the pain. However, it has now been demonstrated that migraine pain does not always relate to cerebral blood flow or vessel dilation.[2] With these findings and other research investigations, the profession has had to reevaluate the prevailing thoughts regarding the mechanisms of neurovascular pain. It is now believed that the vascular changes that have been observed to be associated with the pain are merely a result of the condition and not the actual cause of the pain. The actual mechanism appears to be more closely related to a neurogenic phenomenon, and thus the term *neurovascular pain.*

Neurovascular pains are a group of visceral pain disorders that are generally characterized by episodic pains accompanied by neurologic, gastrointestinal, and psychologic changes (Fig 16-1). These pains are commonly unilateral with varying duration and can greatly debilitate the patient. The International Headache Society[3] classifies these neurovascular pains as primary headaches. They are divided into the following categories: *(1)* migraine, *(2)* tension-type headache, *(3)* cluster headache and other trigeminal autonomic cephalalgias, and *(4)* other primary headaches (Table 16-1). In this text a fifth group will be included, called neurovascular variants.

Migraine

Clinical characteristics

Migraine is a severe type of headache that affects approximately 16% of the population. It is more commonly found in women, affecting 25%, while only 8% of men seem to be affected. The male-to-female ratio is 1:3.[4] The lifetime prevalence of migraine is 93.8% in men and 99.25% in women. Prevalence of migraine in the previous year is 6% in men and 15% in women. Of migraine patients, 15% report having a migraine headache between 8 and 10 days per year, while 9% report having the pain more than 14 days per year. Eighty-five percent of migraine sufferers report the headache as severe.

Migraine has a significant impact on the US economy associated with loss of work. Migraineurs required 3.8 bedrest days for men and 5.6 days for women each year, resulting in a total of 112 million bedridden days. Migraine costs American employers about $13 billion a year because of missed workdays and impaired work function; close to $8 billion was directly attributed to missed workdays.[5,6]

It appears that there exists a predisposition to migraine pain, making some people more susceptible to this condition than others.[7] Earlier studies suggest that migraine susceptibility is related to genetic factors. These studies[8-12] report that between 50% and 60% of migraine patients have parents who also experience migraines. In one study by Dalsgaard-Nielsen,[13] 90 of 100 women with migraine had an immediate family member who also experienced migraine. Although this evidence is strong, some[14] have

Table 16-1 The International Headache Society's Classification for Primary Headaches*

1. Migraine
  1.1 Migraine without aura
  1.2 Migraine with aura
 	
2. Tension-type headache
  2.1 Infrequent episodic tension-type headache
    2.1.1 Associated with pericranial muscle tenderness
    2.1.2 Not associated with pericranial muscle tenderness
  2.2 Frequent episodic tension-type headache
    2.2.1 Associated with pericranial muscle tenderness
    2.2.2 Not associated with pericranial muscle tenderness
  2.3 Chronic episodic tension-type headache
    2.3.1 Associated with pericranial muscle tenderness
    2.3.2 Not associated with pericranial muscle tenderness
	3. Cluster headache and other trigeminal autonomic cephalalgias
	  3.1 Cluster headache
	    3.1.1 Episodic cluster headache
	    3.1.2 Chronic cluster headache
	  3.2 Paroxysmal hemicrania
	    3.2.1 Episodic paroxysmal hemicrania
	    3.2.2 Chronic paroxysmal hemicrania
	  3.3 Short-lasting unilateral neuralgiform headache attack with conjunctival injection and tearing (SUNCT)
	
	4. Other primary headaches
	  4.1 Primary stabbing headache
	  4.2 Primary cough headache
	  4.3 Primary exertional headache
	  4.4 Primary headache associated with sexual activity
	  4.5 Hypnic headache
	  4.6 Primary thunderclap headache
	  4.7 Hemicrania continua
	  4.8 New daily-persistent headache (NDPH)

*Numbers correspond to the International Headache Code.[3]

questioned whether this relationship is actually inherited or environmentally influenced.

Migraine most often develops in the first three decades of life. The episodes may occur at any time of the day or night but most frequently on arising in the morning. The pain onset is usually gradual, peaking and then subsiding. The pain episode commonly lasts 4 to 72 hours in adults and 2 to 4 hours in children.[15] The headache is unilateral in 60% of the cases and consistently occurs on the same side of the head in only 20% of the patients.[16] The pain can vary greatly from mild to very intense.[17] When mild, the pain may be constant and described by the patient as tight or band-like. At this level, the headache takes on the clinical characteristics of a tension-type headache (tension-type headache will be discussed later in this section). When the headache is severe, it will assume a throbbing quality that may move from one part of the head to another, even radiating down to the neck and shoulder. The pain is commonly aggravated by physical activity or simple head movement.[18] Scalp tenderness occurs in two thirds of the patients during or after the headache.

The migraine attack can be divided into four phases[19]: the premonitory phase, the aura, the headache itself, and the postdrome.

The *premonitory phase* (sometimes called the *prodrome*) is the period of time that occurs hours or even days before the headache

Table 16-2 Symptoms Associated with the Premonitory Phase (Prodrome) of Migraine*

Psychologic	Neurologic	General
Depression	Photophobia	Stiff neck
Hyperactivity	Difficulty concentrating	Food cravings
Euphoria	Phonophobia	Cold feeling
Talkativeness	Dysphasia	Anorexia
Irritability	Hyperosmia	Sluggishness
Drowsiness	Yawning	Diarrhea or constipation
Restlessness		Thirst
		Urination
		Fluid retention

*From Silberstein S, Saber J, Freitag F. Migraine: Diagnosis and treatment. In: Silberstein S, Lipton R, Dalessio D (eds). Wolff's Headache and Other Head Pains, ed 7. New York: Oxford University Press, 2001:124.

is felt. The premonitory phase occurs in about 60% of migraineurs.[20] It can consist of mental, neurologic, and general symptoms that relate to autonomic and constitutional factors (Table 16-2). Mental symptoms may include depression, euphoria, irritability, restlessness, mental slowness, hyperactivity, fatigue, and drowsiness. Neurologic symptoms may include photophobia, phonophobia, and hyperosmia. Other general symptoms may include stiff neck, sluggishness, increased thirst, increased urination, anorexia, diarrhea, constipation, fluid retention, and food cravings.

Two types of migraine prodromes have been described: *nonevolutive,* which precedes the attack by up to 48 hours, and *evolutive,* which starts approximately 6 hours before the attack, gradually increasing in intensity and culminating in the attack. Amery et al[21] have suggested that a dopaminergic mechanism may be responsible for the prodrome.

The migraine *aura* is a complex of focal neurologic symptoms that immediately precedes the headache. The aura usually develops in 5 to 20 minutes and lasts less than 1 hour. Up to 20% of migraine suffers experience an aura before the headache.[22,23] The aura is commonly characterized by visual, sensory, or motor phenomena and may even include language and brainstem disturbances. The visual symptoms are the most common phenomena associated with aura. These symptoms are reported by 99% of patients who have an aura.[24] Visual symptoms can be characterized by sensations of unformed flashes of light before the eyes (photopsia); the partial loss of sight (scotoma); or a zigzagging, flashing, colored phenomena that migrates across the visual field (teichopsia). The classic visual aura symptom is called the *fortification scotoma.* This is reported as colored, pulsating, jagged lines that begin as a small paracentral arc. Over the course of 15 to 30 minutes, the angulated boundary enlarges and progresses toward the temporal visual field, leaving a scotoma in its wake. The time course and evolution of this visual phenomenon is thought to correspond to a slow, spreading wave of depression over the surface of the occipital cortex.

Sensory symptoms may also be associated with the aura. Paresthesia is the most common sensory symptom and occurs in about one third of the migraineurs with aura. Paresthesias may start with numbness in the hand, migrating up the arm, and them jumping to involve the face, lips, and tongue.[25] Motor effects may present (in about 18% of patients with aura) as focal fatigue or difficulty with speech. On occasion, the patient may have difficulty understanding language.

As stated earlier, not all patients who experience migraine headaches report an aura before their pain begins. Migraine therefore can be divided into two types: *migraine with aura* and *migraine without aura*. Earlier terminology referred to migraine with aura as *classic migraine* and migraine without aura as *common migraine*. At this time it appears that these two headaches originate by the similar mechanisms and therefore are likely to represent variations of the same condition.

The clinical characteristics of the migraine headache pain have been reviewed in an earlier section. Suffice it to say here that the pain is characterized by throbbing, moderate to severe, often debilitating pain. Sixty percent of the time the headache is unilateral. The patient will often report photophobia, phonophobia, and osmophobia, and will seek a dark, quiet room.[26,27] The pain is aggravated by routine physical activity and sometimes even simple head movements. Some patients report lightheadedness and vertigo.[28] Anorexia is common and food cravings may occur. Nausea is typical and vomiting is frequent.[29] Almost 70% of all migraineurs report that vomiting has occurred during an attack, with one third reporting that they routinely vomit during major attacks. These same migraineurs report that the symptoms interfere with their ability to take oral migraine mediations. Some patients may have nasal stuffiness during the migraine attack, followed in some by profuse nasal secretion as the attack terminates.[30]

During the *postdrome*, after the headache pain has terminated, the patient will feel very tired, listless, and generally washed out. The patient may also be irritable and lack the ability to concentrate. Muscle weakness and aching are common. Anorexia and food cravings can occur.[31] Some individuals may feel unusually refreshed or euphoric after an attack.

Pathophysiologic features

Understanding the pathophysiology of migraine begins with a reminder that the brain is a visceral organ and, like all visceral organs, has a pain-signaling mechanism. Like most other structures of the head, the trigeminal nerve carries nociceptive input from the innervated intracranial structures to the brainstem by way of the trigeminal spinal tract nucleus. This system of neural innervation of the intracranial structures is called the trigeminovascular system.

It is interesting to note that not all brain structures are innervated with nociceptors. The cortex, for example, appears to be without nociception. All of the supratentorial pain-sensitive structures, such as the meninges and intracranial vessels, are innervated by the trigeminovascular system.[32] Pain sensation from the posterior fossa structures is carried centrally by the vagus nerve, the upper three cervical nerves, and the trigeminal nerve. It becomes obvious that the trigeminal nerve is an extremely important nerve involved in migraine pain.

The trigeminovascular system can be stimulated by both neural (electrical) and chemical activators (neurotransmitters) (Figs 16-2a and 16-2b). Once activated, a cascade of events can take place that results in migraine pain. It appears at this time that mechanism of neurogenic inflammation is a significant contributor to migraine. When stimulated, the C-fibers in the trigeminal nerve antidromically release tachykinins, such as substance P and calcitonin gene-related peptide (CGRP) into the dural and meningeal blood vessels (Fig 16-2c). These substances cause the degranulation of mast cells releasing histamine, thus causing vasodilatation and plasma extravasation into the tissues (Fig 16-2d). The release of substance P also results in inflam-

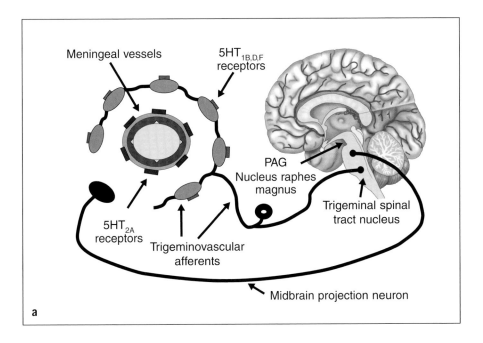

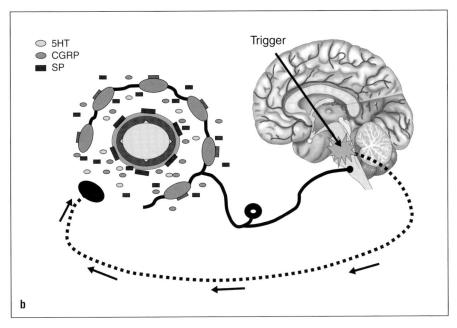

Fig 16-2 Graphic depiction of the neurophysiology of migraine. *(a)* The important anatomic structures involved in producing the migraine include the trigeminal spinal tract nucleus in the brainstem, the midbrain 5HT projection neurons, and the meningeal vessel innervated by the primary afferent neuron. PAG = periaqueductal gray matter. *(b)* A trigger is initiated in the brainstem that causes the antidromic release of neuroactive chemicals such as substance P, CGRP, and 5HT into the tissues of the meningeal vessel.

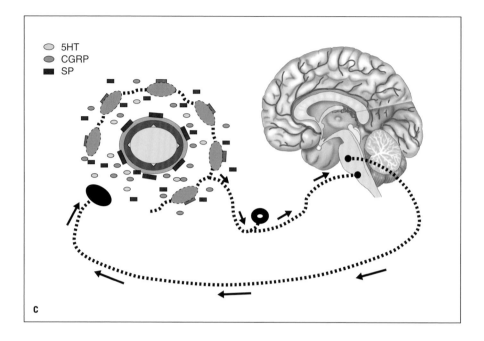

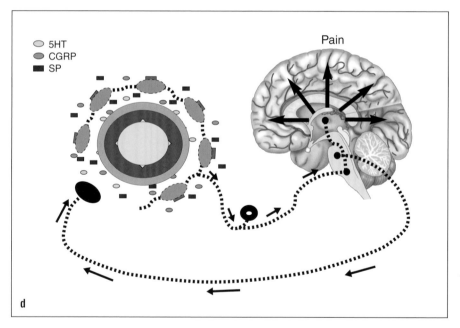

Fig 16-2 (cont) *(c)* The neuroactive chemicals excite receptors in the area, producing a nociceptive response that is carried by the primary afferent neuron back centrally to the brainstem. *(d)* The primary afferent nociceptive input is carried to the higher centers, eliciting the intense pain felt as migraine. Associated with the neurogenic inflammation is plasma extravasation and dilation of the meningeal vessel. (Adapted from Moskowitz MA. Neurogenic versus vascular mechanisms of sumatriptan and ergot alkaloids in migraine. Trends Pharmacol Sci 1992;13:307–311.)

mation and swelling of the blood vessel walls. To further compounding this condition is the release of serotonin (5-hydroxytryptamine [5HT]) from the platelets. Although serotonin in the brainstem is generally an inhibitory neurotransmitter, in the peripheral structures it has excitatory effects. The release of serotonin, therefore, seems to play a significant role in this condition.[33–38] This local inflammation and the resultant sensitization of polymodal nociceptors by substance P are thought to cause the pain associated with migraine.[39]

It is interesting to note that the action of histamine in initiating attacks of neurovascular pain applies only to migraineurs and not to nonmigraine subjects.[40] It has also been shown that attacks of migraine without aura display an increase in electromyographic (EMG) activity in pericranial muscles.[41,42] Masticatory muscle pains occur frequently with migraine headaches. They usually do not constitute a clinical complaint, however, because of the limited duration. Most migraine sufferers know that discomfort is a part of the headache problem and give it no thought. Therapeutic mistakes in this regard are usually those of the doctor who mistakenly attributes the headaches to a dental or masticatory cause. Moss[43,44] reported that migraine without aura and migraine with aura appear to be dissimilar phenomena etiologically. Migraine without aura is largely muscular pain and responds to muscular relaxation techniques.[45] Clinically, there appears to be some common pathophysiology between neurovascular headaches and tension-type headaches.[46] It is likely that the underlying central factors stem from a common cause. Currently, it is believed that central factors, complex as they are, exercise a dominant role in neurovascular pain disorders.

A major advancement in the understanding of migraine has come with studies of the 5HT receptors.[47] There are at least five serotonin receptor subtypes (5HT$_{1A}$, 5HT$_{1C}$, 5HT$_{1D}$, 5HT$_2$, and 5HT$_3$) that have been implicated in the pathophysiology of migraine. The 5HT$_{1D}$ receptors are widespread in the human brain. Studies suggest these receptors are involved in the constriction of cerebral blood vessels and arteriovenous anastomoses.[48] It has also been found that 5HT$_{1D}$ receptor agonists can block trigeminovascular neurogenic inflammation but will not prevent inflammation caused by systemic substance P.[49] The 5HT$_{1A}$ receptor has been shown to mediate serotonin-induced contractions of the basilar artery in dogs.[48] Additionally, 5HT$_{1A}$ receptor agonists inhibit raphe cell firing.[48] The 5HT$_2$ receptor has been shown to mediate smooth muscle contraction in many vascular beds. Serotonin, probably via 5HT$_2$ receptors, can stimulate production of prostacyclin and other products of arachidonic acid metabolism in smooth muscle cells. Theoretically, 5HT$_2$ antagonists are able to inhibit serotonin from inducing an arachidonic acid–derived inflammatory state. It quickly becomes evident that an understanding of the function of these receptors can open pharmacologic avenues of therapies for the management of migraine pain. This aspect will be discussed further in the section on management.

To assume that only the primary afferents in the trigeminal nerve are involved in migraine pain is likely to be quite naïve. The autonomic nervous system, as well as several brainstem structures, also affect cranial vessel function and have been implicated in migraine pain. The parasympathetic fibers arise in the superior salivatory nucleus of the brainstem and accompany the facial nerve to traverse the sphenopalatine ganglion and otic ganglion, onto the intracranial vessels, including the internal carotid artery. The parasympathetic fibers are thought to contribute to migraine by the release of substances such as acetylcholine, vasoactive intestinal polypeptide, and peptide histidine isoleucine. Sympathetic fibers ascend from the superior cervical ganglion to form a plexus in the walls of both the internal and external carotid arteries. These sympathetic fibers can contribute to migraine by the release of norepinephrine, neuropeptide Y, and peptide YY.

Located in the wall of the fourth ventricle in the upper pons is the locus ceruleus. This nucleus is made up of cells that contain the highest concentration of noradrenaline in the brain. It receives afferent fibers from the cortex, amygdala, hypothalamus, reticular formation, raphe, vestibular nucleus, and tractus solitarius. All these areas relate to the internal and external sensory stimuli or to the affective state. The locus ceruleus also projects out to the thalamus, geniculate nuclei, facial nerve nucleus, and the trigeminal spinal tract nucleus. It has been found in monkeys that stimulation of the locus ceruleus decreases cerebral blood flow and increases vascular permeability.[50] Not only can the locus ceruleus directly affect intracranial vessels, but it can cause the release of norepinephrine from the adrenal gland by its connection with the intermediolateral cell column of the thoracic cord. This norepinephrine, along with 5HT-releasing factor, causes a platelet release reaction. Free 5HT released from the platelets increases the sensitivity of vascular receptors, thus augmenting the afferent inflow through the trigeminal nerve and increasing the cascade of events leading to the migraine pain.

Studies that investigate cerebral blood flow during migraine attacks reveal a decrease in flow during certain phases of the attack. Several studies[51,52] have demonstrated that in the early stages of migraine there may be patchy areas of increased cerebral blood flow just prior to a systematic decrease in blood flow. Diminution of the flow starts in the occipital region and extends forward as a "spreading oligemia."[51] This wave of oligemia progresses over the cortex at a rate of 2.2 mm/min and stops short of the central and lateral sulci. The spreading oligemia typically begins before the patient notices any local neurologic symptoms, reaching the sensorimotor area only after the appropriate symptoms have started and outlasting these symptoms. Oligemia lasts for several hours and is followed by delayed hyperemia. The headache usually starts while the cerebral blood flow is diminished.

This spreading oligemia seems to follow a pattern that was first described by Laeo in 1944.[53] Laeo observed in animal brains a pattern of activity that seems to slowly progress as a wave over the cortex, starting in the posterior region and migrating anteriorly at a rate of 3 mm/min. This phenomenon was known as the "spreading depression of Laeo" and is likely to be associated with the wave of decreased blood flow just described.

It appears that the focal neurologic symptoms associated with migraine are accompanied by diminished cortical perfusion of the appropriate part of the opposite cerebral hemisphere. On some occasions, a wave of hypoperfusion may advance slowly over the cortex in association with a slow march of visual or other neurologic symptoms. However, this is not always the case. It is not possible to deduce with certainty from current techniques whether constriction of the cortical microcirculation precedes or follows diminution in cortical neuronal activity. Adams et al[54] found that stimulation of the locus ceruleus at frequencies that reduced cerebral blood flow in the cat had no consistent effect on the resting discharge of neurons in the visual cortex, suggesting that an important action of this brain stem area was constriction of the microcirculation. It is clear that cortical blood flow does not always dictate the presence or absence of headache, but dilation of the middle cerebral artery and possibly other intracranial arteries may certainly contribute to the perception of pain.

To summarize its pathophysiology, migraine is a neurovascular pain disorder that appears to be related to a trigeminovascular reflex involving both peripheral and central mechanisms. Stimulation of the trigemino-vascular reflex by either excessive afferent or central input can create excessive discharge of part of the spinal tract nucleus of the trigeminal nerve and its thalamic connections. This discharge produces a neurogenic inflammation of the primary afferents that innervate the intracranial vessels, resulting in an antidromic release of excitatory neurotransmitters. This begins a cascade of events that produces the migraine pain. Accompanying this trigeminovascular reflex activity is the effect of the locus ceruleus on the cerebral cortex that initiates cortical oligemia, possibly spreading depression. This activity could account for the migrainous aura that often occurs prior to the headache. The end result is a complex interaction between the brainstem, cranial nerves, and the cranial blood vessels, with the afferent impulses from the latter intensifying pain perception through the trigeminovascular system. It is reasonable to assume that patients with unstable trigeminovascular reflexes are more susceptible to migraine disorders.

Certainly the neurochemistry of migrane is very complex. A summary of this neurochemistry is presented in Fig 16-3.

Precipitating factors (triggers)

The combination of trigeminal nerve input, along with the parasympathetic, sympathetic, and brain function activities makes up what has been suggested to be a *trigeminovascular reflex* that is responsible for migraine pain.[55] It has been found that a number of different factors can activate this reflex and precipitate a migraine attack. Factors that stimulate the cascade of events leading to migraine are called triggers.

Some common triggers are listed in Table 16-3. Some common triggers are foods that contain nitrites[56] (eg, hot dogs) or monosodium glutamate[57]; red wines[58]; or any type of alcohol.[56] Sometimes changes in normal sleep patterns—either too little sleep, or too much—can trigger a migraine.[59] Work shift changes or even jet lag may be responsible. In other cases, environmental conditions may be triggering factors. Bright or flashing lights, weather changes, pungent odors, or high altitudes may trigger a migraine.[60] Hormonal changes can also trigger migraines; menstrual migraine attacks are linked to the period of menses in 60% of women and exclusively to this period in 14%.[61] Migraines may worsen in the first trimester of pregnancy but significantly improve during later pregnancy. This is thought to relate to high levels of estrogen during this time.[10,62] Other common triggers are emotional stress and anxiety. This may be especially true of the poststress letdown period.[30,63,64]

Diagnostic considerations

In 2003 the International Headache Society (IHS) revisited and updated their original Classification for Headaches[3] (see Table 16-1). Since this is the most universally accepted classification for headache, it will be used in this chapter. Each type of headache will be accompanied by the IHS classification number. If more details are needed for any specific diagnostic category, the original classification should be reviewed.[3]

Since the main purpose of this text is to provide information on a wide variety of orofacial pain conditions, all headaches will not be included. There are a number of excellent texts[65,66] dedicated solely to headache, including the IHS Classification, that should be reviewed for a more thorough review of all headaches. This text will include the most common headaches.

Migraine without aura (IHC 1.1)
Migraine without aura is a recurring headache disorder manifesting in attacks lasting 4 to 72 hours. Typical characteristics of the headache are unilateral location, pulsating quality, moderate or severe intensity, aggravation by routine physical activity, and as-

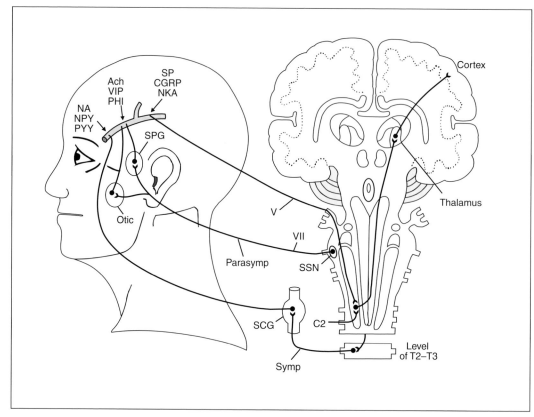

Fig 16-3 The central pain pathways and neurotransmitters with afferent and efferent pathways in the trigeminovascular system. Vascular afferents are carried by the trigeminal nerve (V) and descend into the trigeminal spinal tract to synapse with the second-order neuron in the nucleus caudalis. Input from the cervical neurons (C2) also synapses in the region and can influence ascending input onto the thalamus. Sympathetic nerve fibers (Symp) leave the spinal cord at the level of T2 and T3 to join the sympathetic cervical chain to ascend to the superior cervical ganglion (SCG). Sympathetic fibers then leave the ganglion to innervate the cranial vessels. The parasympathetic neurons (Parasymp) leave the superior salivatory nucleus (SSN) and travel by way of the facial nerve (VII) to the sphenopalatine ganglion (SPG) and the otic ganglion (Otic). From these ganglions, the parasympathetic fibers move on to the cranial vessels. Each type of neuron is responsible for the release of neurotransmitters that can play an active role in neurovascular pain disorders. Abbreviations for these neurotransmitters are: *Afferent*: substance P (SP), calcitonin gene-related peptide (CGRP), neurokinin A (NKA); *parasympathetic*: acetylcholine (Ach), vasoactive intestinal polypeptide (VIP), peptide histidine isoleucine (PHI); *sympathetic*: norepinephrine (noradrenaline, NA), neuropeptide Y (NPY), peptide YY (PYY). (Adapted from Goadsby PJ, Zagami AS, Lambert GA. Neural processing of craniovascular pain: A synthesis of the central structures involved in migraine. Headache 1991;31:365–371.)

sociation with nausea, photophobia, and phonophobia.

The IHS[3] has developed the following specific criteria that must be fulfilled for the diagnosis of migraine without aura (International Headache Code [IHC] 1.1):

1. At least five headache attacks fulfilling criteria 2 to 4 listed below.
2. The headache attack lasts 4 to 72 hours (untreated or unsuccessfully treated).
3. The headache has at least two of the following characteristics: unilateral location, pulsating quality, moderate to severe intensity, or aggravated by or causing avoidance of routine physical exercise.
4. During the headache at least one of the following occurs: nausea and/or vomiting, photophobia, or phonophobia.
5. The headache cannot be attributed to any other disorder.

Migraine with aura (IHS 1.2)

Migraine with aura is a recurring headache disorder manifesting with attacks of reversible focal neurologic symptoms that usually gradually develop over 5 to 20 minutes and last for less than 60 minutes. The headache with features of migraine without aura usually follows the aura symptoms. Less common are headaches that lack the migrainous features or no headache at all (ie, the patient experiences the aura only).

The following specific criteria must be fulfilled for the diagnosis of migraine with aura (IHC 1.2)[3]:

1. At least two headache attacks fulfilling criteria 2 to 4 listed below.
2. An aura consisting of at least one of the following but no motor weakness: *(1)* fully reversible visual symptoms including positive features (eg, flickering lights, spots, or lines) and/or negative features (eg, loss of vision); *(2)* fully reversible sensory symptoms including positive features (eg, pins and needles) and/or

Table 16-3 Common Migraine Triggers*
Diet
Hunger
Alcohol
Additives (eg, nitrites, monosodium glutamate)
Certain foods (eg, chocolate, aged cheese)
Chronobiologic
Sleep (too much or too little)
Change in schedule
Hormonal changes, eg, menstruation
Environmental factors
Light (eg, bright, flashing, glaring)
Odors (eg, perfume, cigarette smoke)
Altitude (eg, airplane travel)
Weather changes
Head and neck pain
Temporomandibular disorders or TMD pain
Cervical myofascial pain
Toothache
Physical exertion
Exercise
Sexual activity
Stress and anxiety
Increased exposure to emotional stress
Letdown after a stressful period
Head trauma

*Adapted from Silberstein S, Saber J, Freitag F. Migraine: Diagnosis and treatment. In: Silberstein S, Lipton R, Dalessio D (eds). Wolff's Headache and Other Head Pains, ed 7. New York: Oxford University Press, 2001:136.

negative features (eg, numbness); *(3)* fully reversible dysphasic speech disturbance.
3. At least two of the following characteristics: *(1)* homonymous visual symptoms and/or unilateral sensory symptoms; *(2)* gradual development of at least one aura over 5 minutes or more and/or different aura symptoms occurring in succession

over 5 minutes or more; *(3)* each symptom lasts longer than 5 minutes but not longer than 60 minutes.

4. The headache fulfills the criteria 2 to 4 for migraine without aura (IHC 1.1).
5. The headache cannot be attributed to any other disorder.

Management considerations

The general management of migraine with or without aura can be divided into three categories: patient education and trigger avoidance, nonpharmacologic methods, and pharmacologic methods. Pharmacologic methods can be subdivided into those drugs that abort the migraine and those that prevent the migraine.

Patient education and trigger avoidance

Patients who experience migraine headaches need to understand basic information regarding their pain condition. They need to know that even though the pain is very severe, it is still benign and not an aggressive tumor such as cancer. (Of course, if other neurologic symptoms are present, additional tests need to be ordered to rule out any aggressive diseases.) Assuring the patient that the pain is not life-threatening often assists them in coping with the pain attacks. Probably the most important aspect of education, however, is in having the patient identify any triggering factors that initiate the migraine attack. Often patients may have no appreciation for triggers. If the patient can identify a trigger, then proper avoidance can be instituted. The best way to identify triggers is to ask your patient to maintain a pain diary. The patient should keep a record of any and all headaches, along with the circumstances that were present prior to or during the onset. With time, the patient is often able to identify factors that are associated with the headache. Once these factors are identified, effort is made to avoid them, so that the number of episodes of migraine may be reduced. Factors that relate to diet can usually be quickly controlled. Sometimes environmental factors such as light, weather changes, and pungent odors may be more difficult to avoid. Other factors such as fatigue, sleep patterns, and stress need to be identified and addressed appropriately. Nothing is more satisfying to the patient than his or her own ability to control the number of migraine attacks. This, of course, can only occur with patient education.

Nonpharmacologic methods

Migraine patients should be encouraged to maintain a regular schedule of events through their day. Changes in routine should be avoided since they may precipitate attacks.[64] Migraine patients should be encouraged to participate in regular exercise, good health practices, regular mealtimes, and good sleep hygiene. The patient should go to sleep and arise at the same times each day. This same schedule should be maintained even on the weekends, when often the individual can sleep longer. Migraine attacks frequently begin in the last hour of sleep when the regular sleep duration has been lengthened.

Other nonpharmacologic methods of managing migraines are relaxation training,[67-69] biofeedback,[70] hypnosis, cognitive-behavioral therapy,[71-75] and sometimes even formal psychotherapy. These therapies are oriented toward stress management by decreasing the autonomic nervous system responsiveness.

Pharmacologic methods

Pharmacologic management of migraine with and without aura can be divided into two types: medications that are used to abort a migraine at its start and medications that are used to prevent migraine attacks. The choice of which type of management approach to use lies in the frequency of the migraine attacks. As a general rule, migraine attacks that occur less than once a week are managed with abortive medications so that treatment is provided during the onset of the attack. If migraine attacks occur more than once a week, the patient should be managed with preventive medications.

Abortive medications. In a small number of patients, analgesic medications such as aspirin, acetaminophen, and nonsteroidal anti-inflammatory drugs (NSAIDs, eg, ibuprofen) can be useful in aborting migraine. When these medications are helpful, they should be used because of their low toxicity and side effects. Unfortunately, these medications are not usually effective once a migraine has begun.

A standard class of medications that have been used for migraine are the ergotamine derivatives. The ergotamines are known vasoconstrictors and for years were thought to counter the effects of vasodilation associated with the migraine. The importance of constricting cranial vessels during a migraine attack has been less of a concern recently, since it is now thought that the vasodilation is a result of the neurogenic inflammation and not the actual cause of the headache. Cafergot (ergotamine tartrate and caffeine) is an example of this class of medications that still has some use in migraine. Dihydroergotamine (DHE) is one of the more popular of this class of drugs[76,77] and is still used as an abortive agent. DHE can be administered either intravenously,[78] intramuscularly,[79] or subcutaneously.[80] Today the most common form of DHE is probably an intranasal formulation[81] called Migranal.

In recent years the triptans have been found to have significant effects on the 5HT receptors that are closely linked to the pathophysiology of migraine. The first to reach the American market was sumatriptan (Imitrex). It was first packaged in a subcutaneous injectable form[82] so the patient could administer the drug him or herself at the onset of the attack. Imitrex was demonstrated to be quite effective in aborting the

migraine attack. Sumatriptan is also available in oral tablets[83] or intranasally.[84] The effectiveness and ultimate popularity of sumatriptan opened the market to many other triptans. Today the clinician has a variety of triptans from which to choose for the migraine sufferer. Some of these choices are zolmitriptan (Zomig), rizatriptan (Maxalt), naratriptan (Amerge), eletriptan (Relpax), frovatriptan (Frova), and almotriptan (Axert). Many of these are available in a variety of dosage forms, such as oral tablets, sublingual tables, nasal sprays, or subcutaneous injections. These triptans have become the mainstay for migraine abortive therapy.

Both the triptans and DHE seem to work at the $5HT_{1D}$ and the $5HT_{1A}$ receptor sites to block the trigeminovascular neurogenic inflammation associated with migraine. Generally speaking, medications that act as $5HT_{1D}$ and the $5HT_{1A}$ agonists decrease neurogenic inflammation and are therefore abortive medications. Medications that have antagonist activity at the $5HT_2$ and the $5HT_{1C}$ receptor sites provide prophylactic migraine activity.[85]

Preventive medications. Frequent migraine attacks are best managed with medications that, when taken regularly, decrease the likelihood of the next attack.[86,87] As just mentioned, these medications seem to provide antagonist activity at the $5HT_{1D}$ and the $5HT_{1A}$ receptors. One group of such medications is the beta-adrenergic agents (beta blockers).[88] Medications such as propranolol (Inderal), metoprolol (Lopressor), timolol (Blocadren), nadolol (Corgard), and atenolol (Tenormin) reduce the attack frequency in migraine patients with and without aura.[89,90] Along with the beta blocker effect on the 5HT receptors, they also act centrally to inhibit the central beta receptors and decrease the vigilance enhancing adrenergic pathways.

Another group of medications used to prevent migraine attacks are the calcium-channel blockers.[91] These medications were originally developed as a cardiovascular agent but were later found to be useful in preventing migraines. Not only do these medications act on the 5HT receptors, but they also inhibit contraction of vascular smooth muscle, inhibit prostaglandin formation, and prevent hypoxia of cerebral neurons. The most common calcium-channel blockers used in migraine are nifedipine (Procardia), verapamil (Calan, Isoptin), diltiazem (Cardizem), and nimodipine (Nimotop).

Another group of prophylactic migraine medications are the serotonin antagonists. The most common used is methysergide (Sansert). Methysergide is a semisynthetic ergot $5HT_2$ receptor antagonist that displays affinity for the $5HT_1$ receptor. Its chronic administration blocks the development of neurogenic inflammation.[49] However, methysergide can induce retroperitoneal fibrosis and pleural and heart valve fibrosis with an estimated incidence of 1 in 5,000 treated patients. Therefore, it should be reserved for severe cases in which other migraine preventive drugs are not effective.[92]

Still another group of prophylactic migraine medications are the tricyclic antidepressants. These medications have proven to be most helpful in the management of many chronic pain disorders at dosages that are far below antidepressive levels. The tricyclic antidepressants increase the availability of synaptic serotonin and norepinephrine by inhibiting its reuptake. They also seem to down-regulate the $5HT_2$ receptors and decrease beta receptor density. Some of the more common tricyclic antidepressants used for prevention of migraine are amitriptyline (Elavil, Endep), nortriptyline (Pamelor), doxepin (Sinequan), desipramine (Norpramin), and protriptyline (Vivactil). Preventive dosages for migraines may be as little as 25 to 50 mg at bedtime. This dosage is not thought to have any antidepressant effects.

Many of the drugs used to manage migraine have significant side effects, especially on the cardiovascular system. Although most are quite safe in a healthy patient, the medically compromised patient may experience significant problems that will need to be properly managed. Before any medication is used, the clinician should be well informed of the patient's medical condition and have a good understanding of the medication that will be used. When any question arises, appropriate medical personnel should be consulted.

Tension-Type Headache

Clinical characteristics

Tension-type headache is a very common source of head pain. The headache is described as a dull, nonpulsating pain. Often patients will use the terms *tightness*, *pressure*, or *soreness*. Some will describe the feeling of a tight "headband" compressing their head as if they were wearing a tight cap. Most tension-type headaches are of mild or moderate intensity, rarely becoming debilitating as with migraine. In 90% of the cases the pain is felt bilaterally.[93] The typical location of tension-type headache is in the occipital, parietal, temporal, and frontal regions.[94]

In a cross-sectional population study of 740 adult subjects, 74% had experienced tension-type headache within the previous year, while as many as 31% of the same population had more than 14 days of this type of headache during the previous year.[93] In one study, the lifetime prevalence of tension-type headache was 69% in men and 88% in women. Prevalence of tension-type headache in the previous year was reported at 63% for men and 86% for women. The differences according to sex were significant, with a male-to-female ratio of 4:5 in tension-type headache.[95]

Friedman et al[96] found a positive family history in 40% of the tension-type headache patients compared to 70% in the migraine patients.

Most tension-type headaches are episodic lasting an average of 12 hours. The duration can vary greatly from 30 minutes to 72 hours.[94] The onset of the headaches is usually between 20 and 40 years of age.[96] If the headaches last more than 15 days a month, the condition is considered to be a *chronic tension-type headache.* Nausea and vomiting are rare with episodic tension-type headache. However, with chronic tension-type headache, the pain can become moderate to severe, and nausea and vomiting have been reported.[94] Phonophobia and photophobia can also be associated with severe chronic tension-type headache but are rare with episodic tension-type headache.[93,94]

Pathophysiologic features

Although tension-type headache is the most common headache experienced by humans, its pathophysiology remains unclear. Part of the problem may be that tension-type headache, as a type of primary headache, likely has a central etiology mechanism. However, there are many other disorders that result in headache that present with the same clinical characteristics of tension-type headache. For example, trigger points associated with myofascial pain (see chapter 12) result in a headache at the referred site that will be clinically described by the patient as a tension-type headache. This type of headache is secondary to the myofascial condition and therefore should not be classified as a tension-type headache. When the headache is secondary to another disorder, the primary disorder should be used to classify the headache. This type of classification properly identifies the primary disorder, thereby focusing proper direction of treatment for the headache.

For many years it was thought that tension-type headache was directly related to muscle tension. In fact, for years this headache was referred to as *muscle-contraction headache* or *muscle-tension headache.* More recently it has been demonstrated that although some muscle tenderness is commonly present, increased levels of EMG activity are not always associated with the condition.[97] Some studies[98,99] do suggest that tension-type headache patients have an increased EMG response to emotional stressors as compared to controls. It has been suggested, however, that this increase in EMG activity may not be the cause of the pain but in fact a response to the pain.[100] Although muscle pain may sometimes play a role in tension-type headache, it is not always present. The etiology of tension-type headache as a primary headache is likely to relate to the interaction of significant central factors, especially the limbic structures. Emotional stress, anxiety, and depression seem to present causal relationships with tension-type headaches.[101-104] Olesen and Schoenen[46,105] have proposed a model that describes tension-type headaches occurring as a result of an interaction between changes in the descending inhibitory system, which controls nociceptive brainstem neurons, and peripheral input coming from myofascial and vascular sources. The input from each of these sources combines to influence the characteristics of the headache. Significant myofascial input may produce the referred tension-type headache[106] described in chapter 12. Greater input from vascular sources may reflect a headache more similar to migraine. Significant input from the limbic structures (eg, anxiety, depression) may greatly affect descending inhibitory function and produce a more chronic tension-type headache.

Some researchers believe that migraine and tension-type headache are two different presentations of the same pathophysiologic mechanism. Perhaps migraine represents a pain condition with a significant vascular input, while tension-type headache represents a pain condition with more myofascial input. Careful patient interviews will often reveal that many patients experience both of these headaches. Commonly they will report a tension-type headache for several hours or days and then develop a migraine. Once the migraine has resolved, the tension-type headache will linger for a few more hours or days. This pain condition is referred to as a *mixed headache*. Mixed headaches are common and reflect a unified pain mechanism.

Precipitating factors

As just mentioned, factors that influence either the limbic, myofascial, or vascular structures can be important in precipitating a tension-type headache. It is for this reason that tension-type headache needs to be included in this chapter as well as in the chapter on muscle pains (see chapter 12). Obvious precipitating factors are emotional stress, anxiety, depression, and myofascial pain. There are also other factors that influence or cause tension-type headaches. Some of these are daily hassles,[107,108] unphysiologic working position, muscle strains,[109] sleep deprivation,[108,110] severe snoring,[111] weather changes,[108,112,113] and menstruation.[112,114] Chronic tension-type headache can also be induced by analgesic abuse. Patients who have overused or abused drugs, even over-the-counter analgesics, can have what is called a "rebound headache" when the medication is withdrawn.[115-118] These patients need to be educated to the problem, which may seem foreign at first. Then they must be slowly withdrawn from their medications.

There is some evidence that masticatory muscle activity may play a role in some tension-type headaches.[119] Masticatory muscle disorders seem to be related to tension-type headaches in a number of studies.[120-124] Tension-type headaches can sometimes be precipitated by clenching the teeth or introduction of a high occlusal contact.[125] Although this relationship is not clear, the

dental clinician needs to be aware of any increased masticatory muscle activity that may be contributing to a tension-type headache. When this is suspected, proper therapy to reduce muscle activity should begin.

Diagnostic considerations

Since tension-type headache is so common and its frequency so variable, the IHS decided to classify this headache according to frequency, which would ultimately determine the need for treatment. The following are the specific criteria determined by the IHS that must be fulfilled for the specific diagnosis of tension-type headache (IHC 2.0).[3]

Infrequent episodic tension-type headache (IHC 2.1)
1. Fewer than one headache occurs per month (averaging fewer than 12 per year) and fulfilling criteria 2 to 4 below.
2. The headache lasts from 30 minutes to 7 days.
3. The headache has at least two of the following characteristics: bilateral location, pressing/tightening (nonpulsating) quality, mild or severe intensity, lack of aggravation by routine physical activity such as walking or climbing stairs.
4. Both of the following conditions are met: no nausea or vomiting (anorexia may occur), and either phonophobia or photophobia, but not both.
5. The headache is not attributed to any other disorder.

Since some tension-type headaches are associated with pericranial muscle tenderness, the IHS felt it was important to subdivide these headaches into two groups according to this feature. If the tension-type headache is accompanied by muscle tenderness to manual palpation, it is classified as IHC 2.1.1. If no muscle tenderness is noted, it is classified as IHC 2.1.2.

Frequent episodic tension-type headache (IHC 2.2)

1. At least 10 episodes of headache occur at least once a month but not more than 15 days per month (averaging more than 12 and fewer than 180 days per year) and fulfilling criteria 2 to 4 below.
2. The headache lasts from 30 minutes to 7 days.
3. The headache has at least two of the following characteristics: bilateral location, pressing/tightening (nonpulsating) quality, mild or severe intensity, lack of aggravation by routine physical activity such as walking or climbing stairs.
4. Both of the following conditions are met: no nausea or vomiting (anorexia my occur), and either phonophobia or photophobia, but not both.
5. The headache is not attributed to any other disorder.

If frequent episodic tension-type headache is accompanied by muscle tenderness to manual palpation, it is classified as IHC 2.2.1. If no muscle tenderness is noted, it is classified as IHC 2.2.2.

Chronic tension-type headache (IHC 2.3)

Often, unsuccessfully managed episodic tension-type headache will evolve to a chronic tension-type headache, with daily or very frequent episodes of headache lasting minutes to days. The pain is typically bilateral, pressing, or tightening in quality and of mild to moderate intensity, and it does not worsen with routine physical activity. There may be mind nausea, phonophobia, or photophobia.

1. The headache occurs on an average of more than 15 days per month for more than 3 months (more than 180 days per year) and fulfilling criteria 2 to 4 below.
2. The headache lasts hours, or it may be continuous.
3. The headache has at least two of the following characteristics: bilateral location, pressing/tightening (nonpulsating) quality, mild or severe intensity, lack of aggravation by routine physical activity such as walking or climbing stairs.
4. Both of the following conditions are met: no more than one of photophobia, phonophobia, or mild nausea is present, and neither moderate or severe nausea nor vomiting are present.
5. The headache is not attributed to any other disorder.

If chronic tension-type headache is accompanied by muscle tenderness to manual palpation, it is classified as IHC 2.3.1. If no muscle tenderness is noted, it is classified as IHC 2.3.2.

Chronic tension-type headache often evolves over time from episodic tension-type headache. This may be referred to as new daily-persistent headache (IHC 4.8). If medication overuse is suspected, the chronic tension-type headache may be referred to as medication overuse headache (IHC 8.2).

Management of tension-type headache

Patients suffering from long-lasting chronic tension-type headaches can be very difficult to treat. This is especially true when the disorder is complicated by medication overuse, comorbid psychiatric disease, low frustration tolerance, and physical and emotional dependence.[126,127] Like many pain disorders, management of tension-type headache begins with patient education. The sufferer needs to know about those factors that are aggravating the condition as well as those that might be helpful in relieving symptoms. It is often helpful to have the patient maintain a headache diary, so that factors that are not always easily identified might be recognized. The patient should be encouraged to decrease intake of caffeine (coffee, tea, soft drinks) and alcohol, as well as any medications that have been chronically used for the headache. The patient should be informed that elimination of these substances may at first increase the frequency and intensity of the headaches. After 1 to 2 weeks, the withdrawal effects should subside.

Since emotional stress often plays an important role in tension-type headache, the patient should be assessed for any significant stressors. This is, of course, a difficult task, since one's perception, and response to stress is very individual. When significant stressors are identified, corrective behaviors or, when possible, avoidance should be encouraged. Stress management skills can be important therapies with tension-type headache. Relaxation training and biofeedback techniques[103,104,128] can also be very helpful. The patient must be willing to take the time to work with these therapies. This will only happen if the clinician educates the patient about their importance and the patient is willing to actively participate in the treatment. Success in managing tension-type headaches often resides in the hands of the patient. If a major depression disorder or anxiety disorder is present, these conditions need to be managed by the proper medical personnel.

Judicious use of mild analgesics may be needed, but the patient should be aware of the potential complications. NSAIDs are often helpful, especially if the patient has not been using them previously. When a previous NSAID has been used occasionally, the patient should change to another. Often low dosages of a cyclic antidepressant, such as amitriptyline, can be helpful in managing the headache. When tricyclic antidepressants are used, they are best taken before bedtime because of their sedative effects. These effects are often beneficial when a coexisting sleep disorder is present. When a mixed headache is present, antimigraine medications may be useful, as described earlier.

When the tension-type headache is secondary to another disorder, therapy needs to be extended to that disorder. For example, when the headache is associated with a masticatory muscle disorder, the muscle disorder needs to be managed.[129] Headache upon awaking may be related to nocturnal bruxism. In such instances, an occlusal appliance that is directed toward reducing bruxism can be very helpful. This appliance is best worn only at night, when the bruxism occurs. During the day the patient should be taught cognitive awareness so that he or she becomes aware of the bruxing or clenching habit and subsequently learns to stop it. The dental practitioner should be aware that not all morning headaches are caused by bruxism. A good history and dental examination should be completed before an appliance is fabricated.

Often tension-type headache is a heterotopic pain originating in the cervical muscles. When a cervical myofascial pain disorder is present, treatment should be oriented toward resolving this disorder. Physical therapy modalities such as spray and stretch can be helpful. Heat, ultrasound, and deep massage may also be used. On occasion, trigger point injections may be therapeutic. These therapies are reviewed in chapter 12.

Recent evidence suggests that chronic tension-type headache may respond to botulinum toxin injections.[130-134] There are even data that suggest botulinum toxin may be useful in managing migraine.[135-138] The precise mechanism by which botulinum toxin provides pain relief is unknown. It is logical to assume that pain associated with muscle contraction would be reduced by the paralytic effect of the toxin in skeletal muscles. However, as has already been discussed, many of these chronic headache conditions, both tension-type and migraine, have no associated muscle condition. It is hypothesized that the botulinum toxin may be broken down and transported centrally to not only to inhibit acetylcholine release but also to act as a blocking action in the parasympathetic nervous system.[137]

The injection technique for headache has not been well defined at this time. Some researchers suggest that specific standard sites should be injected for all headache patients.[139] Other researchers[140] advocate that the botulinum toxin be injected into the painful muscles, which may vary from patient to patient. No technique has been found to be superior at this time. Typically, a total of 50 to 100 units are injected into multiple sites in the head and neck muscles.

Cluster Headache and other Trigeminal Autonomic Cephalalgias

Cluster headache and other trigeminal autonomic cephalalgias (TAC) are a group of headache disorders that are characterized not only by the headache but also by their prominent cranial parasympathetic autonomic features. Experimental and human functional imaging suggests that these syndromes activate a normal human trigeminal-parasympathetic reflex with clinical signs of secondary cranial sympathetic dysfunction. There are three relatively distinct presentations of trigeminal autonomic cephalalgias: cluster headache, paroxysmal hemicrania, and short-lasting unilateral neuralgiform headaches with conjunctival injection and tearing (SUNCT). The IHS has developed specific criteria for each, and they will be reviewed separately in this section.

Cluster headache

Clinical characteristics
Probably the most common headache in this class is the cluster headache. Cluster headache has also been referred to as *migrainous neuralgia, Raeder's syndrome, spheno-palatine neuralgia, ciliary neuralgia, histamine cephalalgia,* and *Sluder's headache.* It affects more men than women, at a ratio of 6:1. Although most patients begin experiencing headache between the ages of 20 and 50 years (mean of 30 years), the disorder may begin as early as the first decade and as late as the eighth decade. It was originally thought that cluster headache did not appear to have a significant hereditary factor. Kudrow[141] reported that only 18 out of 495 cluster patients reported a family history of the disorder. Migraine headache occurred no more frequently among the cluster headache population than among random populations.[142] More recently, however, studies reveal a slight hereditary factor, but not nearly as significant as that for migraine.[143,144]

The pain of cluster headache commences quickly, without warning, and reaches a crescendo within 2 to 15 minutes. It is often excruciating in intensity and is deep, nonfluctuating, and explosive in quality. Only occasionally is it pulsatile, which is not typical of neurovascular pains. Approximately 10% to 20% of sufferers will report superimposed paroxysms of stabbing, ice pick–like pains in the periorbital region that last for a few seconds and may occur once or several times in rapid succession. The pain usually begins in, around, or above one eye or the temple. It is always unilateral and generally affects the same side in every episode.

A unique clinical feature of cluster headache and other trigeminal autonomic cephalalgias is the accompanying autonomic symptoms. All of the autonomic features are transient, usually lasting only for the duration of the attack. Lacrimation and conjunctival injection are the most common local signs of autonomic involvement, being present in more than 80% of patients. Nasal stuffiness or rhinorrhea is experienced by 68% to 76% of patients during attacks. These symptoms are usually ipsilateral to the pain but may on rare occasions occur on both sides. Forehead sweating, facial flushing, and edema are rare.

Focal neurologic symptoms as seen in migraine are very uncommon in patients with cluster headache; however, on occasion patients may experience typical photopsia, teichopsia, facial paresthesia, and vertigo at the time of the attack.

The attacks last from 30 minutes to 2 hours in about 75% of the cases. A patient will experience a group or cluster of these headaches as frequently as six per day or as infrequently as once a week. These attacks will cycle for 4 to 8 weeks, and then 90% of patients experience a pain-free period of remission. This pain behavior is how the disorder received its name. Most patients experience one or two bouts of the pain each year, but some may be pain-free for years.

Periodicity is a characteristic feature in 85% of the cases, meaning that the pain occurs at the same time of the day. About 75% of the attacks occur between 9 PM and 10 AM.[145] A common time to experience the pain is between 1 and 2 AM,[146] with the patient waking up with the paroxysms of pain in 50% of the cases, usually within 2 hours of falling asleep.[147] Another common time period for the onset of cluster headache seems to be 1 to 3 PM.

Pathophysiology

In earlier studies it was suggested that cluster headaches resulted from a dilation of the external carotid artery.[148] Because of the retro-orbital pain, investigators have more recently looked at the possibility of changes in the internal carotid artery. Ekbom and Greitz[149] found a segmental luminal narrowing of the ipsilateral internal carotid artery in the region of the carotid canal, as well as a significant dilation of the ipsilateral ophthalmic artery. Along with these changes is an increase in the cerebral blood flow in the central, basal, and parietotemporal regions during the attack.[150] Further investigations have revealed that, as with migraine, these vascular changes may be

the result of this pain disorder and not actually the cause. It is now thought that these vascular changes are related to an autonomic nervous system dysfunction.[151,152] This sympathetic activity is responsible for the ipsilateral lacrimation, nasal drainage, lid drooping, pupillary change, and conjunctival injections seen during the attack.

It appears that histamine may play a significant role in pathophysiology of cluster headache. The level of histamine found in the blood is greatly increased during the attack.[153,154] As with migraine, the increased level of histamine is related to mast cell degranulation in the area of the involved vessels.

The interesting clockwork periodicity phenomena of cluster headache may also shed light on its pathophysiology. Cluster headache may be the result of a central nervous system discharge in the region of the hypothalamus containing the posterior cells that regulate autonomic functions and anterior nuclei that serves as the major circadian pacemaker in mammals.[155] The "biologic clock" is serotonergically modulated and is connected anatomically to the eye.[156] Perhaps cluster headache is the result of an antidromic discharge of this biologic "pacemaker."[157]

Precipitating factors

A common triggering factor in cluster headache is alcohol. This trigger is present in approximately 50% of patients. Patients who are sensitive to alcohol note that drinking alcohol will trigger an attack 70% to 80% of the time they are exposed. The attacks are triggered within 5 to 45 minutes after ingesting even a very small amount of alcohol. Other common triggers are emotional stress, relaxation following stressful times, exposure to heat or cold, glare, hay fever attacks, and occasionally the ingestion of specific foods (eg, eggs, dairy products, chocolate).

There is some evidence that head trauma can precipitate the disorder.[158] Among 180 patients studied by Manzoni et al,[146] previous head injury was reported by 41, with loss of consciousness occurring in 20. This is significantly more frequent than is observed among patients with other types of headaches. Other studies have not found this relationship.

Certain medications can trigger cluster attacks in cluster-prone patients. Sublingual nitroglycerin (1 mg) can initiate an attack.[159] In approximately 70% of cluster patients, an attack can be initiated by subcutaneous histamine.[160]

Diagnostic considerations

The following are the specific IHS criteria that must be fulfilled for the specific diagnosis of cluster headache (IHC 3.1).[3]

1. The patient has experienced at least five attacks fulfilling criteria 2 to 4 below.
2. The pain is severe or very severe unilateral orbital, supraorbital, and/or temporal, lasting 15 to 180 minutes if untreated.
3. The headache is accompanied by at least one of the following characteristics: ipsilateral conjunctival injection and/or lacrimation, ipsilateral nasal congestion and/or rhinorrhea, ipsilateral eyelid edema, ipsilateral forehead and facial sweating, ipsilateral miosis and/or ptosis, a sense of restlessness or agitation.
4. The headache attacks have a frequency ranging from one every other day to eight per day.
5. The headache is not attributed to any other disorder.

Cluster headache can be further subdivided into episodic or chronic variants, according to the timing of the headache periods. When the cluster headache attacks occur in periods lasting 7 days to 1 year, separated by pain-free periods lasting 1 month or longer, they are classified as episodic cluster headache (IHC 3.1.1). When the cluster headache attack periods last between 7 and 365 days and are separated by pain-free remission periods of 1 month or less, they are classified as chronic cluster headache (IHC 3.1.2).

Management

Patient education and trigger avoidance. As with migraine, patients who experience cluster headaches need to understand basic information regarding their pain condition. They need to know that even though the pain is very severe, it is still benign and not an aggressive disease. Probably one of the most important aspects of education is having the patient identify any triggering factors that initiate the attacks. Often patients may have no appreciation for triggers. If the patient can identify a trigger, then proper avoidance can be instituted. Since the attack usually occurs shortly after the trigger, it may be easy for the patient to recognize the trigger.

Since cluster headache is related to the "biologic clock," changes in sleep can affect the attacks. The patient should be encouraged to maintain good sleep hygiene and avoid any afternoon naps. Any change in the sleep cycle, such as vacation schedules, work shift changes, studying habits, or jet lag, can precipitate an attack. Patients who experience long periods of stress, anger, rage, worry, or frustration often experience an attack after the event has passed. Patients should be made aware of these factors and minimize them as much as possible.

Patients should be cautioned about prolonged exposure to volatile substances, such as solvents, gasoline, or oil-based paints, during the cluster periods. Bursts of anger, prolonged anticipatory anxiety, and excessive physical activity should be avoided because cluster attacks are apt to occur during the relaxation period that follows. Prolonged anger, hurt rage, or frustration during a cluster period is often associated with the onset of a new cluster period.

Nonpharmacologic methods. Ekbom[161] found that compression of the superficial temporal artery provided relief for about 40% of his patients, but he also found that this worsened the pain in another 40%. Carotid compression reduced the pain half the time, while worsening the pain 25% of the time. Vigorous physical exertion at the earliest sign of an attack can, in some cases, be remarkably effective in ameliorating or even aborting an attack.[162,163] Ice can also be placed over the painful area. Because attacks come on so quickly, the pain is very severe before any therapy can begin. These therapies are not tremendously effective, but even the smallest reduction in pain is appreciated by the patient.

Pharmacologic methods. As for migraine, pharmacologic management of cluster headache can be divided into two types: medications that are used to abort the headache and medications that are used to prevent attacks.

Since cluster headaches come on so fast, it is difficult to get adequate relief from oral medications. Instead, inhalants can be used. One of the most effective inhalants is 100% oxygen.[164,165] The patient should breathe pure oxygen via a tight-fitting mask at a flow rate of 8 to 10 L/min for 10 to 15 minutes. This therapy can be 80% effective in those patients who find this approach feasible. Since the attacks can occur frequently during the cluster period, oxygen must be made available to the patient in their home or workplace. Oxygen inhalation is especially helpful during nocturnal attacks.

Subcutaneous sumatriptan (Imitrex) is the most effective self-administered medication for the symptomatic relief of cluster headache. In a placebo-controlled study, 6 mg of sumatriptan delivered subcutaneously was significantly more effective than placebo, with 74% of patients having compete relief after 15 minutes compared with 26% of placebo-treated patients.[166] The effectiveness of sumatriptan has been reported to be approximately 8% lower in

patients with chronic cluster headache than in patients with episodic cluster headache.[167]

Sumatriptan nasal spray (20 mg) is less effective than a subcutaneous injection at relieving pain in the great majority of cluster headache sufferers. In an open randomized study comparing the effectiveness and satisfaction of subcutaneous sumatriptan 6 mg versus intranasal sumatriptan 20 mg, 49 of 52 treatments with injection resulted in compete relief of pain within 15 minutes, with a mean time to pain relief of 9.6 minutes. The remaining attacks were reduced by a mean of 87% at 15 minutes. By comparison, only 7 of 52 treatments with nasal spray in the nostril ipsilateral to the pain resulted in complete relief within 15 minutes, with a mean of 13 minutes. No pain relief was obtained in 27 attacks at 15 minutes.[168]

Other inhalants that can be effective in aborting a cluster headache are ergotamine and lidocaine. Ergotamine aerosol at a dosage of 0.36 to 1.08 mg (one to three inhalations) produces peak plasma levels of ergotamine within 5 minutes[169] and is effective in 80% of the patients.[141,170] Kittrelle et al[171] demonstrated that intranasal administration of 1 mL 4% topical lidocaine was effective in terminating attacks in four of five patients. These patients were instructed to lie supine, with their heads extended backward 45 degrees and rotated 30 to 40 degrees toward the side of the headache. One milliliter of lidocaine was slowly dropped into the nostril ipsilateral to the pain while the patient was maintained in that position for several minutes. These investigators believe that the lidocaine reached the sphenopalatine fossa and anesthetized the sphenopalatine ganglion.

Another abortive medication is DHE, which can be given intravenously and usually will abort the headache. The only difficulty with this therapy is that the patient must be in the doctor's office for administration. This limits its use as an abortive medication.

Oral dosages of zolmitriptan have also been used as an abortive medication for cluster headache. A double-blind, controlled trial[172] compared the efficacy of 5 and 10 mg of oral zolmitriptan to placebo for the treatment of acute cluster headache attacks. Significantly more patients reported mild or no pain 30 minutes after treatment with 5 and 10 mg of zolmitriptan (57% and 60%, respectively) than following placebo administration (42%).[172] Although these efficacy rates do not approach those of oxygen or subcutaneous sumatriptan, zolmitriptan is the first orally administered triptan to demonstrate efficacy in the treatment of cluster headache and remains a therapeutic option for patients who cannot tolerate oxygen or subcutaneous sumatriptan.

However, the most appropriate management for cluster headache is to prevent the attacks, especially during the cluster period. Medication should be provided to the patient during the entire cluster period. Once the cluster period has resolved, the medication can be withdrawn. Therapeutically it may be difficult to know exactly when to begin or stop the medications, since the onset of attacks is quick and the duration of cluster period may vary greatly. This often becomes a management problem.

Oral administration of 2 mg of ergotamine tartrate 1 to 2 hours before bedtime can be very effective in preventing nocturnal attacks.[173] However, when a patient is experiencing long periods of cluster attacks, the ergotamine can produce rebound attacks. Therefore, use for a short time is advised. Cluster attacks during the day are best prevented by the prophylactic use of agents such as methysergide, verapamil, lithium, DHE, or prednisone. The use of methysergide, verapamil, and DHE have already been reviewed in the section on migraine. Lithium can be a suitable medication for chronic cluster headache, but care must be taken regarding side effects, and renal and thyroid functions must be regularly monitored. Prednisone has been shown to be 75% effective for the episodic form of cluster headache.[174] The dosage may vary from 10 to 80 mg daily for 7 days, followed by a rapid tapering off over the next 6 days.[30] The paroxysmal pain should cease within hours of the first dose. If it does not, the prednisone should be discontinued. Prolonged or repeated use of prednisone is not advised owing to its general effects on the immune system.

Indomethacin can sometimes be helpful for the prevention of cluster headache.[175] Indomethacin can be given at dosages of 25 to 50 mg three times a day. Stomach irritation is a common side effect that should be monitored. Indomethacin is a very specific drug used in the treatment of paroxysmal hemicrania, a very similar condition to cluster headache that will be discussed in the next section.

Paroxysmal hemicrania (IHC 3.2)

Clinical characteristics

Paroxysmal hemicrania has many clinical characteristics that are similar to cluster headache. Both conditions are characterized by episodes of severe unilateral pain that is consistently reported on the same side. Accompanying the headache are ipsilateral nasal stuffiness and rhinorrhea, along with lacrimation and conjunctival injection. Forehead perspiration may also accompany the severe pain. An aura is rarely present with either cluster or paroxysmal hemicrania. Nocturnal attacks are common with both headaches, and the mean age of onset is between 30 and 34 years.

Because of these similarities, diagnosis can be confusing. Since treatment for these two headaches is different, it is important to focus on the differences. There are five differences that help distinguish paroxysmal hemicrania from cluster headache:

1. While cluster headache is more common in men, paroxysmal hemicrania is five times more common in women than in

men.[176] This statistic is not helpful when establishing a diagnosis for one patient, but it may be considered.

2. Paroxysmal hemicrania attacks occur much more frequently than cluster headache attacks, with a mean of 10.8 attacks during a 42-hour period.[177]

3. Attacks of paroxysmal hemicrania are shorter in duration (mean 13.3 minutes) than cluster headaches (mean 49 minutes).[178]

4. Paroxysmal hemicrania attacks may be "mechanically precipitated," with 10% of the attacks related to flexing or rotating the head.[178] This not common with cluster headache.

5. Another clinical characteristic of paroxysmal hemicrania that differentiates it from cluster headache is prompt, dramatic, and lasting response to indomethacin. This characteristic is almost pathognomonic of the disorder.

The location of the paroxysmal hemicrania headache is usually described as in the temple, forehead, eye, or peri-aural areas, and occasionally in the occiput. The pain can be excruciatingly severe, but there is a continuous fluctuation between severe and moderate attacks. In the worst periods, there may be a continuous sore feeling in the usually painful areas between attacks. The pain usually has a piercing, boring, or claw-like character, but in the initial stages, especially in precipitated attacks, it may be pulsating.

Pathophysiology

The pathophysiology of paroxysmal hemicrania is not well understood. It can probably be viewed as a disorder that is closely related to cluster headache, yet some distinct differences exist. During an attack of paroxysmal hemicrania, there is an increase in the intraocular pressure of the eye on the symptomatic side, along with a rise in the temperature of the cornea. These findings suggest a marked increase in vasodilation within the eye.[179,180] Forehead sweating increases on both sides with paroxysmal hemicrania, yet with cluster headache the sweating is unilateral. This suggests that the pathophysiology may be different.[181]

Abnormalities in the cyclic release of catecholamines and beta-endorphins have been observed.[182,183] Increased levels of CGRP and vasoactive intestinal peptide in the cranial venous blood of the paroxysmal hemicrania sufferer have also been documented. These levels return to normal following treatment with indomethacin.[184]

Paroxysmal hemicrania attacks can be abruptly precipitated by applying pressure to certain particularly sensitive points in the neck or by neck flexion. In only a few seconds, tears appear and the intraocular pressure is increased on the symptomatic side. Obstruction of the flow in the common or internal carotid artery on the symptomatic side does not initiate an attack, nor does rubbing these arteries. The pathway from the neck to the eye would therefore appear to be neurogenic rather than vascular.[185] Although autonomic symptoms predominate during the attacks, they do not seem to cause the pain.[185] The fact that nocturnal attacks are common also suggests a central mechanism or at least a central influence. Perhaps, as with other neurovascular disorders, there is a peripheral mechanism that is influenced by a central dysregulation. The precise mechanism has eluded researchers.

Precipitating factors

As already mentioned, neck movements seem to be a precipitating factor in some patients. At this time, other trigger factors have not been well described. It would not be surprising to learn that common factors that trigger other neurovascular disorders may also trigger paroxysmal hemicrania.

Diagnostic considerations

The following are the specific IHS criteria that must be fulfilled for the specific diagnosis of paroxysmal hemicrania (IHC 3.2).[3]

1. The patient must have experienced at least 20 attacks fulfilling criteria 2 to 4 below.
2. The attacks are characterized by severe unilateral orbital, supraorbital, or temporal pain lasting 2 to 20 minutes.
3. The headache is accompanied by at least one of the following characteristics: ipsilateral conjunctival injection and/or lacrimation, ipsilateral nasal congestion and/or rhinorrhea, ipsilateral eyelid edema, ipsilateral forehead and facial sweating, ipsilateral miosis and/or ptosis.
4. The headache attacks have a frequency of at least five per day for more than half of the time, although periods of lower frequency may occur.
5. Attacks are prevented completely by therapeutic doses of indomethacin.
6. The headache is not attributed to any other disorder.

Paroxysmal hemicrania can be further subdivided into episodic or chronic according to the timing of the headache periods. When the paroxysmal hemicrania attacks occur in periods lasting 7 days to 1 year, separated by pain-free periods lasting 1 month or longer, they are classified as episodic paroxysmal hemicrania (IHC 3.2.1). When the paroxysmal hemicrania attack periods last more than 1 year, without remission or with remission periods lasting less than 1 month, they are classified as chronic paroxysmal hemicrania (IHC 3.2.2).

Management

As mentioned in the diagnosis section, paroxysmal hemicrania can be eliminated by continuous administration of adequate doses of indomethacin.[177,186] The dosage may vary greatly from patient to patient and even from attack to attack in the same individual, depending upon severity. Indomethacin is easily titrated and dosage may vary from 25 to 250 mg/day. Indomethacin is tolerated well, although it may cause dyspepsia. If dyspepsia does occur, a histamine H_2 receptor blocking agent or indomethacin suppositories can be used.

SUNCT (IHC 3.3)

Clinical characteristics

Short-lasting unilateral neuralgiform headaches with conjunctival injection and tearing (SUNCT syndrome) is one of the rarest of the primary headache disorders. The syndrome was first described in 1978 and more fully characterized in 1989 by Sjaastad et al.[187,188] Although the number of documented cases is still small, it appears that there is a male predominance of about 2.25:1.[183,189-191]

SUNCT syndrome is characterized by very brief headache episodes recurring multiple times per day. The age at onset ranges from 23 to 77 years of age (mean 51).[189] The pain is usually maximal in and around the eye and may radiate to the ipsilateral forehead, temple, nose, cheek, and palate.[189] Attacks are typically felt unilaterally; however, in rare cases the pain may be bilateral. The pain is usually burning, stabbing, or electric in nature. Paroxysms begin and end abruptly, reaching maximum intensity within 2 to 3 seconds.[192] Individual headache attacks last between 5 and 250 seconds (mean 49),[189] although attacks lasting 2 hours each have been described.[193] Some patients experience a dull discomfort that persists between acute episodes.[193]

The temporal pattern is also quite variable, with symptomatic periods of pain-free remission occurring in an unpredictable fashion. Symptomatic periods generally last from a few days to several months and occur once or twice a year. Remissions range from 1 week to 7 years but usually are of a few months' duration.[189] During the symptomatic phase, daily attacks recur from 6 to 77 times (mean 28)[192]; however, tremendous variability can occur between patients and even with the same patient. Although attacks occur during the day, night attacks are common.

Acute attacks of headache in SUNCT syndrome are accompanied by a variety of associated symptoms, the most prominent of which are ipsilateral conjunctival injection and lacrimation. Ipsilateral nasal congestion, rhinorrhea, and eyelid edema are less commonly reported. The associated tearing and conjunctival injection usually begin 1 to 2 seconds following the acute episodes of pain and may persist for a few seconds longer than the painful episode.[189]

It has been reported that many patients can precipitate acute attacks by touching certain trigger zones within the territory of V1 to V3.[189] This clinical characteristic separates it from most of the other neurovascular disorders and points to the possibility of neuropathic mechanisms.

Pathophysiology

The pathophysiology of SUNCT is unknown. The clinical characteristics are similar to cluster headache; therefore, similar neurovascular mechanisms are suspected but documentation is scarce at this time. The triggering of painful episodes by light touch to the face has neuralgic similarities (see chapter 17) and therefore a neurologic component is certainly possible. In a few cases, SUNCT seemed to be secondary to a intracranial condition, including homolateral cerebellopontine angle arteriovenous malformation[194,195] and a brain stem cavernous hemangioma.[196]

Precipitating factors

Many patients report that light touch to the face in areas innervated by V1 to V3 can precipitate acute attacks. These areas are called trigger zones and have similarities to neuralgic pain disorders. Precipitants include touching the hair, forehead, face,

nose, and lip on the symptomatic side. Washing, shaving, eating, chewing, toothbrushing, talking, and coughing have also been report to trigger the headache.[189]

Diagnostic considerations

The following are the specific IHS criteria that must be fulfilled for the specific diagnosis of SUNCT (IHC 3.3).[3]

1. The patient must have experienced at least 20 attacks fulfilling criteria 2 to 4 below.
2. Attacks are characterized by unilateral orbital, supraorbital, or temporal stabbing or pulsating pain lasting 5 to 240 seconds.
3. The pain is accompanied by ipsilateral conjunctival injection and lacrimation.
4. The attacks occur with a frequency between 3 and 200 per day.
5. The headache is not attributed to any other disorder.

Management

The SUNCT syndrome has proven to be refractory to a variety of therapeutic approaches. Medications typically employed for the treatment of migraines, cluster, and other short-lived headache syndromes are ineffective, as are anesthetic blockades.[197] Carbamazepine was reported to be of some possible benefit in 5 of 18 patients.[189] Azathioprine, oral sumatriptan, prednisone, valproate, nifedipine, and lamotrigine were mildly efficacious in single reports.[197–200] Verapamil and omeprazole were reported to worsen the condition.[197]

Table 16-4 summarizes the common features of the five major primary headaches that have been reviewed in this chapter.

Other Primary Headaches

The IHS has classified all primary headaches into four categories. The first three

Table 16-4 Common Features Associated with the Major Primary Headaches*

Feature	Migraine headache	Tension-type headache	Cluster headache	Paroxysmal hemicrania	SUNCT
Location of pain	Unilateral	Bilateral	Unilateral, periorbital	Unilateral, orbital, temporal	Unilateral, oribital, temporal
Age at onset	10 to 50 y	Any	> 20 y	6 to 81 y	23 to 77 y
F:M†	F > M	F = M	F < M	F > M	F < M
Pain quality	Throbbing, pulsatile	Pressure, tightening	Stabbing, boring	Stabbing, throbbing	Burning, stabbing, electrical
Pain intensity	Moderate to severe	Moderate	Severe	Severe	Severe
Pain frequency	0/mo to constant	0/mo to constant	0 to 8/d	1 to 40/d	3 to 100/d
Time of day	Any time	Any time	Frequently at night	Any time	Any time
Duration of pain	> 4 h to constant	> 30 min to constant	15 to 180 min (usually > 30 min)	2 to 120 min (mean, 10 to 15 min)	5 to 250 s (mean, 49 s)
Prodromes	Often present	None	None	None	None
Autonomic signs and symptoms	Yes	Rare	Yes	Yes	Yes
Behavior during attack	Rests in quiet, dark room	Activities continue unimpeded	Paces, pounds fist	Paces, rests in quiet, dark room	Paces, pounds fist

*From Silberstein S, Saber J, Freitag F. Migraine: Diagnosis and treatment. In: Silberstein S, Lipton R, Dalessio D (eds). Wolff's Headache and Other Head Pains, ed 7. New York: Oxford University Press, 2001:124.
†F = female; M = male.

categories, and by far the more common headaches, have already been discussed in this chapter: migraine, tension-type headache and cluster and TAC. The IHS recognized the existence of other primary headaches and developed a fourth category simply known as "other primary headaches" (see Table 16-1). Since this chapter is not meant to elaborate on every headache, only a brief description will be given for each of these other primary headaches. The orofacial pain clinician should be aware of their existence so as to be able to include them in a differential diagnosis. The management of these headaches requires more information, and it is suggested that the reader review the IHS Classification publication.[3]

Primary stabbing headache (IHC 4.1) is characterized by transient and localized stabs of pain in the head that occur spontaneously in the absence of organic disease of underlying structures or of the cranial nerves. *Primary cough headache* (IHC 4.2) is precipitated by coughing or straining in the absence of any intracranial disorder. *Primary exertional headache* (IHC 4.3) is precipitated by any form of exercise. Sub-forms such as weightlifters' headache are also recognized. *Primary headache associated with sexual activity* (IHC 4.4) is precipitated by sexual activity, usually starting as a dull, bilateral ache as sexual excitement increases and suddenly becoming intense at orgasm, in the absence of any intracranial disorder. *Hypnic headache* (IHC 4.5) is characterized by attacks of dull headache that always awake the patient from sleep. *Primary thunderclap headache* (IHC 4.6) is characterized by a very intense pain of abrupt onset mimicking that of a ruptured cerebral aneurysm. *Hemicrania continua* (IHC 4.7) is characterized by a persistent strictly unilateral pain that is responsive to indomethacin. *New daily-persistent headache* (NDPH) (IHC 4.8) is characterized by a daily and unremitting pain from a very recent onset (within 3 days at the most). The pain is typically bilateral, pressing, or tightening in quality and mild to moderate in intensity. There may be photophobia, phonophobia, or mild nausea.

Neurovascular Variants

Neurovascular variants are pain disorders that have neurovascular origins, but their clinical presentations are different than those of migraine, tension-type headache, and cluster headache. One of the major differences is in the location. Neurovascular variants can present as a very focal area of pain in the face. When the location of the pain is in the maxilla or mandible, it may be called a lower-face migraine or facial migraine. When this pain is reported near or in the teeth, it presents a particular problem for the dental practitioner. Neurovas-

cular variants may be easily mistaken for neuropathic pain disorders. It is important, therefore, that a thorough history and examination be completed so that these conditions can be differentiated from the episodic neuropathic pains, such as paroxysmal neuralgia, and the constant neuropathic pains, such as neuritis or deafferentation pain (see chapter 17).

Clinical characteristics

The neurovascular pain disorders are of deep somatic rather than neurogenous origin. Neurovascular variants differ from those of neural origin in the following ways:

1. Pain is not limited to the peripheral distribution of a nerve but may spread beyond neurologic boundaries following the vascular arborization.
2. Pain is not precisely controlled by division of the sensory root of a single nerve.
3. Pain is steady, diffuse, aching, and usually throbbing, with milder dull, diffuse, nonpulsatile discomfort bridging the more severe exacerbations. It may last for hours, days, or weeks.
4. Summation effects, such as triggering from slight stimulation, are not observed.
5. The disorder occurs in younger age groups.
6. Attacks of pain are not induced by stimulation of superficial sensory receptors.
7. Vasoconstricting medications usually decrease the intensity of the throbbing component of pain.

Pathophysiology

Little is known regarding the pathophysiology of neurovascular variants. As with other neurovascular disorders, there are likely to be both central and peripheral mechanisms that precipitate the attacks. Perhaps continued research investigations will help the profession better understand these disorders and may even lead to new approaches to classification and management. At this time, this category is used for those disorders that have clinical symptoms that more closely resemble neurovascular disorders than any other pain disorders. This is a very naïve approach to pain classification, but it has some use since their responses to treatment seem to be similar.

Types of neurovascular variants

The location of pain felt with a neurovascular variant varies according to the vascular tissue that is involved. The location of the pain does not affect the quality or characteristics of the pain, but it may greatly influence how the clinician views the condition. If the pain is felt in a tooth, it may become a diagnostic problem for the dental clinician.[201] When the pain is felt in the sinus area, it now becomes a diagnostic problem for the otolaryngologist. Pain felt in the face or cheek may be called *atypical facial pain*,[202] which is a catch-all term for facial pain of unknown etiology. It is the clinician's duty to thoroughly assess the condition before any therapy begins. As one can imagine, this condition can be easily mistreated.

Neurovascular (migrainous) toothache

When a neurovascular variant is felt primarily in a tooth, it is referred to as a *neurovascular toothache* or sometimes a *migrainous toothache*. This type of pain is most commonly felt in the maxillary canine and premolar area (Case 19). The initiating pain is sufficiently similar to true pulpal toothache to convince the patient, and perhaps the dental therapist as well, that a dental cause is present and dental treatment indicated. Unfortunately, such dental treatment may be instituted prior to an accurate diagnosis and followed by still other forms of therapy. For example, such a tooth may be prepared and filled (when minor caries is identified or the tooth has been previously treated), only to be treated endodontically

and finally extracted. Then treatment may begin on adjacent teeth, and sometimes extensive procedures are attempted. Because of the accompanying nasal symptoms, the patient may be treated for sinusitis, then allergic rhinitis, perhaps finally being branded neurotic. As treatment progresses, so does spreading of the complaint. As rapport between patient and doctor breaks down, the patient may blame the initial or subsequent dental treatment for his or her predicament.

The ability of the dental practitioner to recognize and identify this pain condition is extremely important, and only the dental practitioner can do it. Differential diagnostic criteria include the following:

1. The aching tooth is free of reasonable dental cause for the pain.
2. The toothache has a persistent, episodic, recurrent behavior.
3. Analgesic blocking of the tooth proper may stop the pain in some instances and lead the dental clinician to assume that the source is of dental origin. At other times its effect is not precise or conclusive and may even aggravate the pain.
4. Definitive therapy such as endodontic treatment or extraction may give temporary, transitory benefit, only to be followed in due time by recurrence of the complaint.
5. Frequently, there are accompanying ipsilateral autonomic signs involving the eye and nose.
6. With time, the complaint spreads to involve wider areas of the face and neck, even the shoulder. Frequently, occipital muscle effects are observed, with symptoms suggestive of tension-type headache. Very frequently, chewing pains occur due to secondary hyperalgesia or muscle co-contraction of masticatory muscles. Efforts to manage a masticatory muscle disorder may follow.
7. Early in the disorder, the pain complaint may be favorably influenced by carotid

Case 19 — Heterotopic pain felt as a toothache secondary to a neurovascular pain source

Chief Complaint — Maxillary right first premolar toothache.

History

A 46-year-old woman presented with recurrent episodes of mild to severe, variable, intermittent, dull, aching, throbbing pain diffusely located in the maxillary right first premolar tooth, aggravated by tension and fatigue, and accompanied by nasal congestion.

The complaint had been recurrently present for 4 to 5 years, each episode lasting a few days to a week, followed by a remission of several months. The episode seems to spontaneously occur most often at about 5:00 AM, waking her from sleep. The present one began about a month ago. There is mild constant aching in the face and some also in the occipital area, with severe exacerbations described as throbbing toothache lasting up to an hour and occurring once or twice daily, sometimes at night. She has lacrimation and congestion of the nose on the right side that increases when the pain is severe. It was initially treated as sinusitis, then as trigeminal neuralgia, and more recently as allergic rhinitis, all without benefit. Dental treatments have included occlusal adjustments, endodontics, and extraction of the maxillary right second premolar. She has been cleared neurologically. The patient's internist wants the dental pain resolved.

Examination

Intraoral: There is no clinical or radiographic evidence of any dental, oral, or masticatory cause for the complaint. The quality of the previous dental care is excellent. Oral hygiene is good. There is no occlusal instability. Masticatory functioning appears to be normal in all respects.

TMJs: Both joints are structurally and functionally normal.

Muscles: There is no palpable tenderness of any masticatory muscles and no muscular dysfunction. There is vague occipital discomfort that seems to parallel the dental and facial pain.

Cervical: Within normal limits.

Cranial: Within normal limits.

Diagnostic tests: A 50-mg trial dose of oral sumatriptan gave noticeable relief during a spontaneous exacerbation of tooth pain. The occipital discomfort and constant mild aching sensation in the face were not affected.

Impression

There is no dental, oral, or masticatory cause for the complaint. By history, clinical course, present behavioral characteristics, and trial therapy, the entire pain problem suggests a neurovascular pain disorder. The dental, nasal, and ocular symptoms are very likely secondary central excitatory effects of the deep pain that presumably involves the right maxillary artery. Management should be on a medical level by central excitatory effects induced by primary otalgia. Cyclic muscle pain has occurred.

Diagnosis — Toothache secondary to a neurovascular pain disorder.

pressure or administration of oral suma-triptan, which helps identify it as a neu-rovascular pain. This effect diminishes as secondary muscle involvement occurs.

Although a neurovascular variant may fre-quently occur initially as a toothache, it may spread to involve the entire maxilla, side of the face, ear, neck, and shoulder. It is episodic and recurrent. Its throbbing qual-ity and muscular component may simulate both odontogenous and masticatory pains. Its extreme variability and sudden exacerba-tions give it a neuralgic quality that may be mistaken for trigeminal neuralgia (tic douloureux). The acute pains may occur rather regularly at night. As spreading oc-curs, the accompanying autonomic effects, ie, edema of the eyelids and face, lacrima-tion, and nasal congestion, may be con-fused with allergic rhinitis and sinusitis.[202] The component of occipital pain that secondarily refers to the frontal region may induce tension-type headache.

When expressed as a direct central exci-tatory effect, the muscle symptoms almost invariably occur in the masticatory muscles, because these are innervated by the trigem-inal nerve that mediates the pain input. Ac-tual masticatory muscle co-contraction causing true masticatory pain and repre-senting a masticatory muscle disorder can therefore be a direct secondary effect of per-sistent neurovascular pain. When this is true, both the initiating primary neurovas-cular pain and the secondary masticatory pain should be identified, and therapy for both pain problems is required for ade-quate management. This immediately be-comes a multidisciplinary effort. If only the masticatory component is treated, a prompt relapse occurs when active therapy ceases. If only the neurovascular component is treated, the secondary masticatory muscle component remains as a complaint. Proper management depends on diagnostic identi-fication of the dual phenomenon present

and simultaneous therapy administered (Cases 20 and 21).

Neurovascular variants reported as atypical facial pain

When a neurovascular variant is felt in the face or cheek region, it is frequently referred to as *atypical facial pain*. Atypical facial pain is a general term often used to describe fa-cial pain of unknown origin. Although this term is used to describe many different con-ditions, it is included in this section, since neurovascular variants felt in the face are often misunderstood or misdiagnosed. This author believes this term has no real pur-pose since it is not specific for any disorder and therefore useless in leading to a proper management. Often, the use of this term reflects the clinician's inability to properly diagnosis the pain condition.

Diagnostic considerations

The clinician needs to be very familiar with the behavior of facial neurovascular pains. Definite similarities exist between neuro-vascular variants and masticatory muscle pain, since both are representative of deep somatic pain. Both conditions are episodic or recurrent. The pains are steady, not paroxysmal, and have a dull, aching quality. The pains are very poorly localized or frankly diffuse, and both conditions readily induce central excitatory effects. The fol-lowing points should serve as guidelines to help differentiate them.

1. Neurovascular variants usually have a characteristic pulsatile, throbbing quality.
2. Neurovascular variants follow the vascu-lar arborization and therefore violate neuroanatomic boundaries. Frequently the pain is simultaneously felt in the side of the neck, sometimes in the shoulder. Vessel wall edema may occur and is iden-tified as palpable tenderness along the superficial arteries. Occipital muscular discomfort may be present.

Case 20 Cyclic masticatory muscle pain in the masseter secondary to neurovascular pain

Chief Complaint   Left face and ear pain.

History

A 60-year-old man presented with mild to severe, continuous, protracted, steady, dull, aching pain diffusely located in the left auricular and preauricular area, aggravated by mandibular movement, associated with a continuous but quite variable high- and low-intensity throbbing pain in the left maxillary teeth, face, orbit, and neck. When the pain was intense it was accompanied by tearing, swelling, and redness of the left eye, left nasal congestion, and flushing of the left face.

The complaint began about 2 years ago as a recurrent throbbing pain in the left maxillary teeth, several of which were treated dentally without lasting benefit. He was then unsuccessfully treated for sinusitis and allergic rhinitis. About a year ago, the pain became continuous and soon spread to involve the masticatory system. He has been examined medically, neurologically, and otolaryngologically, and the consensus was that he had a temporomandibular disorder. The complaint has remained the same for several months. No medications are presently being taken.

Examination

Intraoral: The teeth and mouth are essentially negative clinically and radiographically. There is pain in the left masseter area with opening beyond 24 mm, with chewing eccentrically, and with clenching the teeth. The mandible deflects to the left after about 24 to 25 mm of opening. The maximum opening is about 30 mm. The occlusal condition appears stable.

TMJs: Both joints are clinically normal except for left side restriction of opening. Radiographically, the left joint is normal structurally and functionally except for evidence of extracapsular restriction of translatory movement with opening.

Muscles: There is palpable tenderness in the left masseter muscle.

Cervical: Within normal limits.

Cranial nerves: Within normal limits.

Diagnostic tests: Analgesic blocking of the left masseter muscle arrested the masticatory component of the complaint but did not affect the diffuse throbbing pain. Administration of 50 mg of sumatriptan reduced the throbbing component when used during a period of high-intensity pain.

Impression

It appears that a neurovascular pain disorder preceded the masticatory complaint and as such represented the primary pain that secondarily induced muscle pain in the left masseter muscle. Cycling has no doubt occurred. The resulting cyclic masticatory muscle pain was induced by nonmasticatory causes.

Diagnosis   Cyclic masticatory muscle pain of the left masseter muscle, secondary to preexisting neurovascular pain.

Case 21 Neurovascular pain disorder mistaken for masticatory pain

Chief Complaint Left occipital and face pain.

History

A 36-year-old woman presented with recurrent episodes of continuous, mild, protracted, steady, dull, aching pain diffusely located in the left occipital and preauricular areas. The pain is aggravated by head movements and hard chewing, punctuated several times daily by spontaneous periods of high-intensity throbbing pain located in the maxillary left teeth and jaw, and associated with ipsilateral lacrimation and nasal congestion, sometimes with noticeable nausea. Each episode lasts several weeks and the episodes are separated by irregular intervals of several months.

The complaint began about 2 years ago and was treated as tension-type headache. When the chewing discomfort occurred, the physician thought it was due to a "TMJ syndrome" and promptly referred the patient for dental treatment. This consisted of refilling several maxillary left teeth and adjustments of the occlusion, all without benefit. At times, the remissions were attributed to medical and/or dental therapy. The present episode had lasted 5 weeks without responding favorably to any treatment. No medications are presently being taken.

Examination

Intraoral: No dental or oral cause for the complaint is found clinically or radiographically. Masticatory function is entirely normal in all respects. No occlusal instability is identified clinically. There is some minor preauricular and temporal discomfort with hard chewing.

TMJs: Both joints are normal clinically and radiographically.

Muscles: There is slight palpable tenderness in the left masseter, temporal, occipital, and trapezius muscles but no dysfunction of any kind.

Cervical: Slight restriction to rotational movement with a soft end feel.

Cranial nerves: Within normal limits.

Diagnostic tests: Sumatriptan (50 mg) was administered several times during the severe episodes. Each time, this arrested the throbbing maxillary component within 30 minutes but had no noticeable effect on the preauricular and occipital discomfort. Nighttime use of amitriptyline seemed to reduce the episodes and intensity of the pain.

Impression

The history, clinical course, and present behavioral characteristics of the pain complaint are highly suggestive of a neurovascular pain disorder accompanied by muscular, cervical, and occipital pain. The left masticatory muscles have become secondarily involved, probably as a central excitatory effect, causing discomfort with hard chewing but no masticatory dysfunction of any kind.

Diagnosis Neurovascular pain disorder with a secondary muscle component mistaken for a masticatory muscle pain disorder.

3. Neurovascular variants vary in intensity from low to high—low enough almost to go unnoticed, followed by a sudden exacerbation of high-intensity pain. This gives it a neuralgic quality, but the pains are not truly paroxysmal, and the intermissions are not completely pain-free. The low-intensity pain is predominantly myalgic and nonpulsatile, whereas the high-intensity exacerbations are usually more characteristically vascular and throbbing. The intense exacerbations may have a temporal regularity unrelated to functioning. These attacks are frequently nocturnal.

4. Neurovascular variants are prone to occur in episodes lasting several weeks and separated by pain-free remissions of several weeks or months. Sometimes they occur in clusters of short, painful episodes followed by long periods of remission. The episodes relate more to emotional stress and fatigue than to functional demands.

5. Neurovascular variants do not cause appreciable dysfunction unless there is a dominant component of secondarily induced muscle co-contraction. Since such effects involve chiefly the masticatory muscles, the symptoms of a masticatory muscle disorder may become evident, and the underlying etiologically important neurovascular pain disorder may go unnoticed. The only indication of its presence may be recurring exacerbations of throbbing pain, a phenomenon wholly inconsistent with true masticatory pain.

6. Neurovascular variants frequently present characteristic autonomic effects, eg, nasal congestion, lacrimation, injection of the conjunctiva, edema of the eyelids and face, on the affected side. These central excitatory effects may be confused with allergic rhinitis and sinusitis clinically. It should be noted, however, that allergic rhinitis is always bilateral.

7. When a neurovascular variant is suspected, the throbbing component (but not the muscular component) may be reduced by applying pressure to the carotid artery manually or by administration of oral sumatriptan.

8. Differentiation between neurovascular variants and true masticatory pain is best made by the accumulation of positive evidence of the presence of neurovascular pain on one hand or of masticatory pain on the other.

9. When the two conditions occur simultaneously, therapeutic trials may be required to confirm the diagnosis.

Neurovascular variants may follow facial trauma, including tooth extraction and other minor oral surgery. As such, they may be confused with other posttraumatic pain problems. Because of the extreme versatility of this type of neurovascular pain and its propensity to simulate other facial pain disorders, especially those involving dental practice, errors in diagnosis may be made. The dental examiner should be constantly alert to these possibilities, because neurovascular pain is very common.

The examiner should have at his or her command sufficient understanding to be able to identify pains of this type. He or she should be especially cautious in advising definitive therapy either of the teeth or the masticatory apparatus until a confirmed diagnosis is established.

Management

Neurovascular variants are managed, in part, according to the clinical characteristics. If the pain is only occasional, abortive medications are used. If the pain is prolonged, preventive medications may be in order. Severe pain is treated more aggressively than mild pain.

When a neurovascular variant has a periodic presentation, 50 to 100 mg of sumatriptan be given orally at the onset of the pain. If relief is achieved, it is quite indicative of a neurovascular origin and therefore can assist in diagnosis. Before any triptan is given, the clinician needs to assess the health of the patient, especially for any cardiovascular disease.

For some patients, analgesic medications such as aspirin, acetaminophen, and NSAIDs (ie, ibuprofen) can be useful in controlling the pain. When these medications are helpful, they should be used because of their low toxicity and side effects. Low dosages of tricyclic antidepressants, such as amitriptyline (25 to 50 mg at bedtime), may be helpful in some neurovascular variants. When the pain condition persists, medications used to manage migraine, such as the triptans or DHE, may be helpful. Preventive medications used for migraine may also be tried (see the section on migraine management).

Vascular Pains of the Mouth and Face

Vascular pains are those pains that originate from the tissues that make up the vessel walls. These pain conditions are far less common than the neurovascular pains discussed in the previous section. Vascular pain originating from inflammation of the vessel wall is referred to as either *arteritis,* in the case of an artery, or *phlebitis,* in the case of a vein. Many different types of vascular conditions can produce head and neck pain. Some of these conditions are arterial hypertension, cerebral venous thrombosis, ischemic stroke, vascular malformation, and intracranial hematoma. Most of these conditions do not refer pain to the orofacial structures and therefore will not be reviewed in this text. There are two vascular pain conditions, however, that can produce pains in the orofacial regions and therefore will be reviewed (Fig 16-4). These conditions are cranial arteritis and carotidynia.

Cranial Arteritis

Clinical characteristics

The term *cranial arteritis* suggests that an artery in the cranial region has become inflamed. The most common artery to be involved is the temporal artery, which is therefore referred to as *temporal arteritis.* Because of its etiology, this condition is also sometimes referred to as *giant cell arteritis* or *polymyalgia rheumatica.* The incidence of temporal arteritis increases greatly after the age of 50. It is rarely seen before this age. It is nine times more frequent in the ninth decade than in the sixth.[204] It appears to be a disease of Caucasians and is rarely seen in Asians[205,206] and African Americans.[207]

Temporal arteritis commonly presents as a severe headache in the temporal region. It is usually unilateral, affecting only one artery, but on occasion can present bilaterally. The pain is often throbbing and boring.[208,209] It may be felt superficially as burning pain with a superimposed lancinating quality. The intensity may range from mild to severe. In half the cases the pain is constant, with the other half intermittent.[210] Palpation of the temporal region will usually find a prominent, tortuous, very tender and enlarged temporal artery.[211] Minor jaw movement will not produce pain; however, with increased use of the jaw, pain will increase significantly (jaw claudication). Blood studies will reveal an elevated erythrocyte sedimentation rate, often greater than 100 mm/h. The disease is confirmed by biopsy of the artery confirming a giant cell arteritis.

Because of the pathophysiology of temporal arteritis, other pains may be present, such as shoulder or hip pain, diplopia, malaise, weakness, weight loss, anorexia, and fever.[212] Complete or partial loss of vision is the most serious consequence of temporal arteritis. This occurs in at least one third of all cases.[213,214] Blindness can occur when the temporal arteritis produces

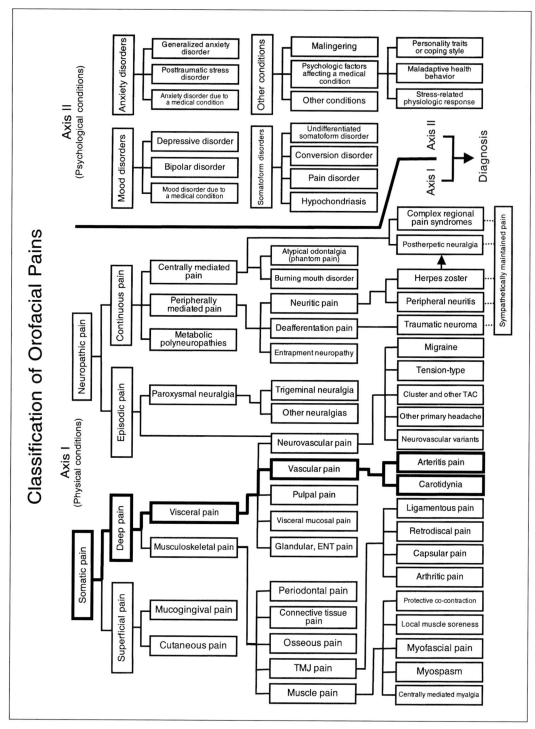

Fig 16-4 Pain classification chart highlighted to show the relationship of vascular pains to other orofacial pain disorders.

a granulomatous inflammation of the posterior ciliary arteries, resulting in an anterior ischemic optic neuropathy.[215,216]

Pathophysiology

The pathophysiology of cranial arteritis is unknown. It is very similar in clinical presentation to polymyalgia rheumatica, which also has an unknown etiology. These disorders may in fact be the same disorder presenting in different regions. These disorders seem to present with a common inflammatory process and the clinical picture may reflect certain host responses to an inciting agent. The inflammatory phase often appears to be self-limiting, but because of the possibility of blindness and stroke, immediate management is essential.

Precipitating factors

At this time there are no known precipitating factors of cranial arteritis. Local provocation of the involved artery will greatly increase the pain, but this does not seem to be the result of anything more than local stimulation.

Diagnostic considerations

According to the IHS classification, cranial arteritis (IHC 6.5.1) is diagnosed by a swollen and tender scalp artery (usually the superficial temporal artery) with an elevated red blood cell sedimentation rate and confirmed by artery biopsy revealing a giant cell arteritis. The diagnosis is also confirmed by disappearance of the headache within 48 hours after the beginning of steroid treatment.

Management

Since cranial arteritis is considered a semiacute inflammatory disease, it demands rapid treatment. Because temporal arteritis can quickly threaten vision, it can be con-

sidered a medical emergency. If symptoms are progressing rapidly, hospitalization may be indicated. The treatment of choice is 40 to 60 mg of prednisone daily.[209,212] This dosage may be rapidly tapered to a maintenance level, depending on the relief of symptoms and the decline in the sedimentation rate toward normal. The duration of treatment is uncertain. It may be necessary to continue corticosteroids for months, although eventually it is possible to discontinue treatment in almost all patients.

Carotidynia

Clinical characteristics

Carotidynia is a pain condition that arises from the cervical carotid artery, resulting in unilateral neck pain that frequently radiates to the ipsilateral face and ear and sometimes to the head. Facial pain is a common primary symptom, and carotid artery tenderness and overlying soft tissue swelling are the major physical findings. There appear to be two forms of this disorder: an acute form and a chronic form. The acute form seems to be the result of a monophasic illness usually lasting for a week or two and tends not to recur. The chronic form is likely to be a neurovascular variant.[217]

Roseman[218] found that carotidynia seems to affect both sexes equally, while Lovshin[219] found women to be affected more frequently than men at a rate of 4:1. Although this condition can present at any age, middle age seems to be the most common. Palpation of the neck reveals tenderness, swelling, and sometimes conspicuous pulsation of the common carotid artery on the affected side.[220] If the thumbs are placed on the common carotid arteries just below the bifurcation and the structures are pressed back against the transverse cervical processes with a rolling movement, severe pain is produced. Pain originating from the carotid artery is often referred to the eye, deep in the malar region, and spreading back to the ear. Pressure on a painful carotid artery will often increase this referred pain pattern.

Pathophysiology

Acute carotidynia appears to be associated with an acute inflammatory response in the carotid artery.[221] The etiology of this inflammation is unknown, but it appears to be self-limiting and usually resolves in 1 to 2 weeks. There is also no evidence that it recurs. The chronic form does recur and can be associated with migraine attacks.

Precipitating factors

There are no known precipitating factors associated with acute carotidynia. Since chronic carotidynia is associated with a neurovascular mechanism, precipitating factors may be similar to those of migraines.

Diagnostic considerations

According to the IHS classification, carotidynia (IHC 6.6.2) is diagnosed by either tenderness, swelling, or increased pulsations overlying the carotid artery, with no other structural findings to explain the pain. The pain is over the affected side of the neck and may project to the ipsilateral side of the head.

Management

Acute carotidynia is a self-limiting disorder, and therefore conservative therapy is all that is indicated. Patient education is helpful, especially in explaining the natural course of the disorder. Mild analgesics may be useful in making the patient more comfortable. If the degree of pain warrants more treatment, 30 mg of prednisone given for 2 days and tapered off over the next 4 days is usually helpful.[222]

For chronic carotidynia, medications used for migraine are usually the treatment of choice.[223,224] Since these pains are neurovascular in origin, migraine therapies are the most appropriate method of intervention.

Differential Diagnosis

Primary deep somatic visceral pain expressed as vascular and neurovascular pain disorders should be distinguished diagnostically from the following conditions:

1. Odontogenous pains
2. Primary musculoskeletal pains, especially myalgia of cervical, occipital, or masticatory origin, and temporomandibular arthralgia
3. Posttraumatic headaches[225]
4. Heterotopic referred pains and secondary hyperalgesias arising from other deep somatic pains
5. Heterotopic projected neuropathic pains
6. Heterotopic pains of central origin
7. Psychologic factors in Axis II

References

1. Wolff HG. Headache and Other Head Pain. New York: Oxford University Press, 1947.
2. Olesen J, Tfelt-Hansen P, Henricksen L, Larsen B. The common migraine attack may not be initiated by cerebral ischaemia. Lancet 1981; 2:438–440.
3. Headache Classification Subcommittee of the International Headache Society. The International Classification of Headache Disorders: 2nd edition. Cephalalgia 2004;24(suppl 1): 9–160.

4. Rasmussen BK, Jensen R, Schroll M, Olesen J. Epidemiology of headache in a general population—A prevalence study. J Clin Epidemiol 1991;44:1174–1157.

5. Hu XH, Markson LE, Lipton RB, Stewart WF, Berger ML. Burden of migraine in the United States: Disability and economic costs. Arch Intern Med 1999;159:813–818.

6. Holmes WF, MacGregor EA, Dodick D. Migraine-related disability: Impact and implications for sufferers' lives and clinical issues. Neurology 2001;56:S13–S9.

7. Walters WE, Silberstein SD, Dalessio DJ. Inheritance and epidemiology of headache. In: Dalessio DJ, Silberstein SD (eds). Wolff's Headache and Other Head Pain, ed 6. New York: Oxford University Press, 1993:42–58.

8. Selby G, Lance JW. Observations on 500 cases of migraine and allied vascular headache. J Neurol Neurosurg Psychiatry 1960;23:23–32.

9. Ely FA. The migraine-epilepsy syndrome. Arch Neurol Psychiatry 1930;24:943–949.

10. Lance JW, Anthony M. Some clinical aspects of migraine. A prospective survey of 500 patients. Arch Neurol 1966;15:356–361.

11. Haan J, Terwindt GM, Ferrari MD. Genetics of migraine. Neurol Clin 1997;15:43–60.

12. Ferrari MD. Migraine. Lancet 1998;351:1043–1051.

13. Dalsgaard-Nielsen T. Migraine and heredity. Acta Neurol Scand 1965;41:287–300.

14. Ziegler DK. Genetics of migraine. In: Rose FC (ed). Handbook of Clinical Neurology. Amsterdam: Elsevier Science, 1986:23–30.

15. Headache Classification Committee of the International Headache Society. Classification and diagnosis criteria for headache disorders, cranial neuralgia, and facial pain. Cephalalgia 1988;8(suppl 7):1–96.

16. Selby G, Lance JW. Observations on 500 cases of migraine and allied vascular headache. J Neurol Neurosurg Psychiatry 1960;23:23–32.

17. Stewart WF, Shechter A, Lipton RB. Migraine heterogeneity. Disability, pain intensity, and attack frequency and duration. Neurology 1994;44:S24–S39.

18. Silberstein SD. Advances in understanding the pathophysiology of headache. Neurology 1992;42(3 suppl 2):6–10.

19. Silberstein SD, Saber JR, Freitag FG. Migraine: Diagnosis and treatment. In: Silberstein S, Lipton R, Dalessio D (eds). Wolff's Headache and Other Head Pains, ed 7. New York: Oxford University Press, 2001:121–237.

20. Blau JN. Migraine prodromes separated from the aura: Complete migraine. Brit Med J 1980;281:658–660.

21. Amery WK, Waelkens J, Vandenbergh V. Migraine warnings. Headache 1986;26:60–66.

22. Russell MB, Rasmussen BK, Fenger K, Olesen J. Migraine without aura and migraine with aura are distinct clinical entities: A study of four hundred and eighty-four male and female migraineurs from the general population. Cephalalgia 1996;16:239–245.

23. Russell MB, Rasmussen BK, Thorvaldsen P, Olesen J. Prevalence and sex-ratio of the subtypes of migraine. Int J Epidemiol 1995;24:612–618.

24. Russell MB, Olesen J. Increased familial risk and evidence of genetic factor in migraine. BMJ 1995;311:541–544.

25. Russell MB, Olesen J. A nosographic analysis of the migraine aura in a general population. Brain 1996;119(Pt 2):355–361.

26. Drummond PD. A quantitative assessment of photophobia in migraine and tension headache. Headache 1986;26:465–469.

27. Drummond PD. Scalp tenderness and sensitivity to pain in migraine and tension headache. Headache 1987;27:45–50.

28. Kuritzky A, Ziegler KE, Hassanein R. Vertigo, motion sickness and migraine. Headache 1981;21:227–231.

29. Olesen JA. Some clinical features of the acute migraine attack. An analysis of 750 patients. Headache 1978;18:268–271.

30. Raskin NH. Headache. New York: Churchill Livingstone, 1988.

31. Blau JN. Resolution of migraine attacks: Sleep and the recovery phase. J Neurosurg Psychiatry 1982;47:223–226.

32. Coffey RJ, Rhoton AL. Pain-sensitive cranial structures. In: Dalessio DJ, Silberstein SD (eds). Wolff's Headache and Other Head Pain, ed 6. New York: Oxford University Press, 1993:19–41.

33. Hannington-Kiff JG. Pain Relief. Philadelphia: Lippincott, 1974.

34. Ferrari MD. Systemic biochemistry. In: Olesen J, Tfelt-Hansen P, Welch KM (eds). The Headaches. New York: Raven Press, 1993:179–183.

35. Dvilansky A, Rishpon S, Nathan I, Zolotow Z, Korczyn AD. Release of platelet 5-hydroxytryptamine by plasma taken from patients during and between migraine attacks. Pain 1976;2:315–318.

36. Anthony M, Hinterberger H, Lance JW. Plasma serotonin in migraine and stress. Arch Neurol 1967;16:544–552.

37. Moss RA, Lombardo TW, Cooley JE, et al. Effects of sleep duration on classic migraine and depression headache pain: Case reports. J Craniomandib Pract 1987;5:88–94.

38. Govitrapong P, Limthavon C, Srikiatkhachorn A. 5-HT$_2$ serotonin receptor on blood platelet of migraine patients. Headache 1992;32:480–484.

39. Moskowitz MA. Brain mechanisms in vascular headache. Neurol Clin 1990;8:801–815.

40. Krabbe AA, Olesen J. Headache provocation by continuous intravenous infusion of histamine: Clinical results and receptor mechanisms. Pain 1980;8:253–259.

41. Clifford T, Lauritzen M, Bakke M, Olesen J, Moller E. Electromyography of pericranial muscles during treatment of spontaneous common migraine attacks. Pain 1982;14:137–147.

42. Bakke M, Tfelt-Hansen P, Olesen J, Moller E. Action of some pericranial muscles during provoked attacks of common migraine. Pain 1982;14:121–135.

43. Moss RA. Oral behavioral patterns in common migraine. J Craniomandib Pract 1987;5:197–202.

44. Moss RA. A structural imbalance/muscular hyperactivity interactional theory of common migraine pain. J Craniomandib Pract 1988;6:87–89.

45. Lapeer GL. Reduction of the painful sequelae of migraine headache by use of occlusal diagnostic splint: An hypothesis. J Craniomandib Pract 1988;6:83–86.

46. Olesen J. Clinical and pathophysiological observations in migraine and tension-type headache explained by integration of vascular, supraspinal and myofascial inputs. Pain 1991;46:125–132.

47. Solomon GD. Therapeutic advances in migraine. J Clin Pharmacol 1993;33:200–209.

48. Peroutka S. Developments in 5-hydroxytriptamine receptor pharmacology in migraine. Neurol Clin 1990;8:829–839.

49. Buzzi MG, Moskowitz MA. The antimigraine drug, sumitriptan specifically blocks neurogenic plasma extravasation from blood vessels in dura mater. Br J Pharmacol 1990;99:202–206.

50. Hartman BK, Swanson LW, Raichle ME, Preskorn SH, Clark HB. Central adrenergic regulation of cerebral microvascular pemeability and blook flow, anatomic and physiologic evidence. Adv Exp Med Biol 1980;131:113–126.

51. Olesen J, Larsen B, Lauritzen M. Focal hyperemia followed by spreading oligemia and impaired activation of rCBF in classical migraine. Ann Neurol 1981;9:344–352.

52. Friberg L, Olsen TS, Roland PE, Lassen NA. Focal ischaemia caused by instability of cerebrovascular tone during attacks of hemiplegic migraine. A regional cerebral blood flow study. Brain 1987;110:917–934.

53. Laeo AAP. Spreading depression of activity in the cerebral cortex. J Neurophysiol 1944;7:359–390.

54. Adams RW, Lambert GA, Lance JW. Stimulation of brainstem nuclei in the cat: Effect on neuronal activity in the primary visual cortex of relevance to cerebral blood flow and migraine. Cephalalgia 1989;9:107–118.

55. Lance JW. The pathophysiology of migraine. In: Dalessio DJ, Silberstein SD (eds). Wolff's Headache and Other Head Pain, ed 6. New York: Oxford University Press, 1993:59–95.

56. Raskin NH. Chemical headaches. Annu Rev Med 1981;32:63–71.

57. Schaumberg HH, Buckley CE, Gerstl R, Mashman JH. Monosoduim L-glutamate: Its pharmacology and role in the Chinese restaurant syndrome. Science 1969;163:826–828.

58. Littlewood JT, Glover V, Davies PTG, Sandler M, Davies PT, Rose FC. Red wine as a cause of migraine. Lancet 1988;1:558–559.

59. Silberstein SD, Saper JR. Migraine: Diagnosis and treatment. In: Dalessio DJ, Silberstein SD (eds). Wolff's Headache and Other Head Pain, ed 6. New York: Oxford University Press, 1993:96–170.

60. Van den Bergh V, Amery WK, Waelkens J. Trigger factors in migraine: A study conducted by the Belgian migraine society. Headache 1987;27:191–196.

61. Epstein MT, Hockaday JM, Hockaday TDR. Migraine and reproductive hormones throughout the menstrual cycle. Lancet 1975;1:543–548.

62. Ratinahirana H, Darbois Y, Bousser MG. Migraine and pregnancy: A prospective study in 703 women after delivery. Neurology 1990;40:437–441.

63. Lance JW. Mechanisms and Management of Headache. Boston: Butterworth, 1982:16–21.

64. Saper JR. Headache Disorders: Current Concepts and Treatment Strategies. Boston, MA: Wright PSG, 1983.

65. Oleson J, Tfelt-Hansen P, Welch KM. The Headaches. Philadelphia: Lippincott, Williams and Wilkins, 1999.

66. Silberstein SD, Lipton RB, Dalessio DJ. Wolff's Headache and Other Head Pain, ed 7. New York: Oxford University Press, 2001.

67. Larsson B, Melin L. Follow-up on behavioral treatment of recurrent headache in adolescents. Headache 1989;29:249–253.

68. Blanchard EB, Appelbaum KA, Radnitz CL, et al. A placebo-controlled evaluation of abbreviated progressive muscle relaxation and relaxation combined with cognitive therapy in the treatment of tension headache. J Consult Clin Psychol 1990;58:210–215.

69. Vasudeva S, Claggett AL, Tietjen GE, McGrady AV. Biofeedback-assisted relaxation in migraine headache: Relationship to cerebral blood flow velocity in the middle cerebral artery. Headache 2003;43:245–250.

70. Richter IL, McGrath PJ, Humphreys PJ, Goodman JT, Firestone P, Keene D. Cognitive and relaxation treatment of paediatric migraine. Pain 1986;25:195–203.

71. Andrasik F. Psychological and behavioral aspects of chronic headache. Neurol Clin 1990; 8:961–976.

72. Baumann RJ. Behavioral treatment of migraine in children and adolescents. Paediatr Drugs 2002;4:555–561.

73. Miller FG. Treatment of acute migraine. Lancet 2002;359:802.

74. Martins IP, Parreira E. Behavioral response to headache: A comparison between migraine and tension-type headache. Headache 2001;41: 546–553.

75. Dodick DW. Acute and prophylactic management of migraine. Clin Cornerstone 2001;4: 36–52.

76. Blumenthal HJ, Weisz MA, Kelly KM, Mayer RL, Blonsky J. Treatment of primary headache in the emergency department. Headache 2003; 43:1026–1031.

77. Bigal ME, Tepper SJ. Ergotamine and dihydroergotamine: A review. Curr Pain Headache Rep 2003;7:55–62.

78. Saddah H. Abortive headache therapy in the office with intravenous dihydroergotamine plus prochlorperazine. Headache 1992;23:143–146.

79. Mondell B, Giuliano R. A prospective evaluation of intramuscular dihydroergotamine for the control of acute migraine in the office setting; Preliminary findings. Headache 1992;32: 251–252.

80. Freitag FG, Diamond M, Urban G, Diamond S. Subcutaneous dihydroergotamine in the acute treatment of menstrual migraine. Headache 1992;32:252–253.

81. Treves TA, Kuritzky A, Hering R, Korczyn AD. Dihydroergotamine nasal spray in the treatment of acute migrane. Headache 1998;38: 614–617.

82. Cady R, Wendt J, Lirchner J, Sargent J, Rothrock J, Skaggs H. Treatment of acute migraine with subcutanous sumatriptan. JAMA 1991;265:2831–2835.

83. Goadsby P, Zagami A, Donnan G, et al. Oral sumatriptan in acute migraine. Lancet 1991; 338:782–783.

84. Group FS. A placebo-controlled study of intranasal sumatriptan for the acute treatment of migraine. Eur Neurol 1991;31:332–338.

85. Peroutka S. 5-Hydroxytryptamine receptor subtypes. Ann Rev Neurosci 1988;11:45–60.

86. Silberstein SD, Goadsby PJ. Migraine: Preventive treatment. Cephalalgia 2002;22:491–512.

87. Rahimtoola H, Buurma H, Tijssen CC, Leufkens HG, Egberts AC. Migraine prophylactic medication usage patterns in The Netherlands. Cephalalgia 2003;23:293–301.

88. Diener H. Pharmacological approaches to migraine. J Neural Transm Suppl 2003:35–63.

89. Andersson K, Vinge E. Beta-adrenoceptor blockers and calcium antagonists in the prophylaxis and tratment of migraine. Drugs 1990;39: 355–373.

90. Diamond S, Medina JL. Double blind study of propranolol for migraine prophylaxis. Headache 1976;16:24–27.

91. Adelman JU, Adelman RD. Current options for the prevention and treatment of migraine. Clin Ther 2001;23:772–788; discussion 771.

92. Silberstein SD. Methysergide. Cephalalgia 1998; 18:421–435.

93. Rasmussen BK, Jensen R, Olesen J. A population-based analysis of the criteria of the International Headache Society. Cephalalgia 1991;11: 129–134.

94. Iversen HK, Langemark M, Andersson PG, Hansen PE, Olesen J. Clinical characteristics of migraine and tension-type headache in relation to new and old diagnostic criteria. Headache 1990;30:514–519.

95. Rasmussen BK, Jensen R, Schroll M, Olesen J. Epidemiology of headache in a general population—A prevalence study. J Clin Epidemiol 1991;44:1147–1157.

96. Friedman AP, Von Storch TJC, Merritt HH. Migraine and tension headaches. A clinical study: 2000 cases. Neurology 1954;4:773–788.

97. Pikoff H. Is the muscular model of headache viable? A review of conflicting data. Headache 1984;24:186–198.

98. Feuerstien M, Bush C, Corpisiero P. Stress and chronic headache: A psychophysiological analysis of mechanisms. J Psychosom Res 1982;26: 176–182.

99. Schoenen J, Gerard P, De Pasqua V, Juprelle M. EMG activity in pericranial muscles during postural variation and mental activity in healthy volunteers and patients with chronic tension-type headaches. Headache 1991;31: 321–324.

100. Schoenen J. Neurophysiology: Tension-type headache, cluster headache and miscellaneous headaches. In: Olesen J, Tfelt-Hansen P, Welch KMA (eds). The Headache. New York: Raven Press, 1993:463–470.

101. Blanchard EB, Kirsch CA, Appelbaum KA, Jaccard J. The role of psychopathology in chronic headache: Cause and effect. Headache 1989; 29:295–301.

102. Schulman B. Psychiatric management of the headache patient. In: Diamond S, Dalessio DJ (eds). The Practicing Physician's Approach to Headache. Baltimore: Williams & Wilkins, 1992: 217–223.

103. Holte KA, Vasseljen O, Westgaard RH. Exploring perceived tension as a response to psychosocial work stress. Scand J Work Environ Health 2003;29:124–133.

104. Bertolotti G, Vidotto G, Sanavio E, Frediani F. Psychological and emotional aspects and pain. Neurol Sci 2003;24(suppl 2):S71–S5.

105. Olesen J, Schoenen J. Synthesis: Tension-type headache, cluster headache and miscellaneous headaches. In: Olesen J, Tfelt-Hansen P, Welch KMA (eds). The Headaches. New York: Raven Press, 1993:493–496.

106. Bovim G. Cervicogenic headache, migraine, and tension-type headache. Pressure-pain threshold measurements. Pain 1992;51:169–173.

107. Andrasik F, Passchier J. Psychological aspects: Tension type-headache, cluster headache and miscellaneous headaches. In: Olesen J, Tfelt-Hansen P, Welch KMA (eds). The Headaches. New York: Raven Press, 1993:489–492.

108. Spierings EL, Ranke AH, Honkoop PC. Precipitating and aggravating factors of migraine versus tension-type headache. Headache 2001;41: 554–558.

109. Jensen R, Paiva T. Episodic tension-type headache. In: Olesen J, Tfelt-Hansen P, Welch KMA (eds). The Headaches. New York: Raven Press, 1993:497–502.

110. Blau JN. Sleep deprivation headache. Cephalalgia 1990;10:157–160.

111. Sahots PK, Dexter JD. Sleep and the headache syndromes: A clinical review. Headache 1990; 30:80–84.

112. Rasmussen BK. Migraine and tension-type headache in a general population: Precipitating factors, female hormones, sleep pattern and relation of lifestyle. Pain 1993;53:65–72.

113. Solomon S, Lipton RB, Newman LC. Clinical features of chronic daily headache. Headache 1992;23:325–329.

114. Spierings EL, Schroevers M, Honkoop PC, Sorbi M. Presentation of chronic daily headache: A clinical study. Headache 1998;38: 191–196.

115. Baumgartner CP, Wessely P, Bingol C, Maly J, Holzner F. Long term prognosis of analgesic withdrawal in patients with drug induced headaches. Headache 1989;29:510–514.

116. Mathew NT, Reuveni U, Perez F. Transformed or evolutive migraine. Headache 1987;27: 102–106.

117. Diener HC, Tfelt-Hansen P. Headache associated with chronic use of substances. In: Olesen J, Tfelt-Hansen P, Welch KMA (eds). The Headaches. New York: Raven Press, 1993:721–727.

118. Warner JS. Frequent migraine and migraine status without tension-type headaches: An unusual presentation of rebound headaches. Cephalalgia 2003;23:309–313.

119. Jensen R, Olesen J. Oromandibular dysfunction, tension type-headache, cluster headache and miscellaneous headaches. In: Olesen J, Tfelt-Hansen P, Welch KMA (eds). The Headaches. New York: Raven Press, 1993:479–482.

120. Forssell H, Kangasniemi P. Mandibular dysfunction in patients with muscle contraction headache. Proc Finnish Dent Soc 1984;80: 211–216.

121. Gelb H, Tarte J. A two year clinical dental evaluation of 200 cases of chronic headache: The craniocervical-mandibular syndrome. J Am Dent Assoc 1975;91:1230–1236.

122. Heloe B, Heloe LA, Heiberg A. Relationship between sociomedical factors and TMJ symptoms in Norwegians with myofascial pain-dysfunction syndrome. Community Dent Oral Epidemiol 1977;5:207–212.

123. Jensen R, Rasmussen BK, Pedersen B, Olsen J. Muscle tenderness and pressure-pain thresholds in headache. A population study. Pain 1993;52: 193–199.

124. Mongini F, Ciccone G, Ibertis F, Negro C. Personality characteristics and accompanying symptoms in temporomandibular joint dysfunction, headache, and facial pain. J Orofac Pain 2000;14:52–58.

125. Magnusson T, Enbom L. Signs and symptoms of mandibular dysfunction after introduction of experimental balancing side interferences. Acta Odontol Scand 1984;42:129–135.

126. Mathew NT, Reuveni U, Perez F. Transformed or evolutive migraine. Headache 1987;27:102–106.

127. Saper JR. Ergotamine dependency—A review. Headache 1987;27:435–438.

128. Andrasik F, Gerber WD. Relation, biofeedback and stress-coping therapies. In: Olesen J, Tfelt-Hansen P, Welch KMA (eds). The Headaches. New York: Raven Press, 1993:833–842.

129. Okeson JP. Treatment of masticatory muscle disorders. In: Management of Temporomandibular Disorders and Occlusion. St Louis: Mosby-Year Book, 2003:413–435.

130. Ondo W, Vuong K, Derman H. Botulinum toxin A for chronic daily headache: A randomized, placebo-controlled, parallel design study. Cephalalgia 2004;24:60–65.

131. Blumenfeld A. Botulinum toxin type A as an effective prophylactic treatment in primary headache disorders. Headache 2003;43:853–860.

132. Dodick DW. Botulinum neurotoxin for the treatment of migraine and other primary headache disorders: From bench to bedside. Headache 2003;43(suppl 1):S25–S33.

133. von Lindern JJ, Niederhagen B, Berge S, Appel T. Type A botulinum toxin in the treatment of chronic facial pain associated with masticatory hyperactivity. J Oral Maxillofac Surg 2003;61:774–778.

134. Loder E, Biondi D. Use of botulinum toxins for chronic headaches: A focused review. Clin J Pain 2002;18:S169–S176.

135. Behmand RA, Tucker T, Guyuron B. Single-site botulinum toxin type a injection for elimination of migraine trigger points. Headache 2003;43:1085–1089.

136. Winner P. Botulinum toxins in the treatment of migraine and tension-type headaches. Phys Med Rehabil Clin N Am 2003;14:885–899.

137. Binder WJ, Brin MF, Blitzer A, Pogoda JM. Botulinum toxin type A (BOTOX) for treatment of migraine. Dis Mon 2002;48:323–335.

138. Mathew NT, Kaup AO. The use of botulinum toxin type A in headache treatment. Curr Treat Options Neurol 2002;4:365–373.

139. Wheeler AH. Botulinum toxin A, adjunctive therapy for refractory headaches associated with pericranial muscle tension. Headache 1998;38:468–471.

140. Sheean G. Botulinum toxin for the treatment of musculoskeletal pain and spasm. Curr Pain Headache Rep 2002;6:460–469.

141. Kudrow L. Cluster Headache: Mechanisms and Management. New York: Oxford University Press, 1980:53–70.

142. Andersson PG. Migraine in patients with cluster headache. Cephalalgia 1985;5:11–16.

143. Kudrow L, Kudrow DB. Inheritance of cluster headache and its possible link to migraine. Headache 1994;34:400–407.

144. Russell MB. Genetic epidemiology of migraine and cluster headache. Cephalalgia 1997;17:683–701.

145. Russell D. Cluster headache: Severity and temporal profile of attacks and patient activity prior to and during attacks. Cephalalgia 1981;1:209–219.

146. Manzoni GC, Terzano MG, Bono G, Micieli G, Martucci N, Nappi G. Cluster headache—Clinical findings in 180 patients. Cephalalgia 1983;3:21–30.

147. Lance JW, Anthony M. Migrainous neuralgia or cluster headache? J Neurol Sci 1971;13:401–414.

148. Horton BT, MacLean AR, Craig WM. A new syndrome of vascular headache: Results of treatment with histamine: Preliminary report. Mayo Clin Proc 1939;14:257–260.

149. Ekbom K, Greitz T. Carotid angiography in cluster headache. Acta Radiol (Stockh) 1970;10:177–186.

150. Aebelholt-Krabbe A, Henriksen L, Olesen J. Tomographic determination of cerebral blood flow during attacks of cluster headache. Cephalalgia 1984;4:17–23.

151. Salvesen R, Bogucki A, Wysocka-Bakaowska MM, Antonaci F, Fredriksen TA, Sjaastad O. Cluster headache pathogenesis: A pupillometric study. Cephalalgia 1987;7:273–284.

152. Boccuni M, Morace G, Pietrini U, Porciani MC, Fanciullacci M, Sicuteri F. Coexistence of pupillary and heart sympathergic asymmetries in cluster headache. Cephalalgia 1984;4:9–15.

153. Anthony M, Lance JW. Histaminic and serotonin in cluster headache. Arch Neurol 1971;25:225–231.

154. Dimitriadou V, Henry P, Brochet B, Mathiau P, Aubineau P. Cluster headache: Ultrastructural evidence for mast cell degranulation and interaction with nerve fibers in the human temporal artery. Cephalalgia 1990;10:221–228.

155. Moore-Ede MC, Czeisler CA, Richardson GS. Circadian timekeeping in health and disease. N Engl J Med 1983;309:469–479.

156. Sadun AA, Schaechter JD, Smith LEH. A retinohypothalamic pathway in man: Light mediation of circadian rhythms. Brain Res 1984;302:371–377.

157. Raskin NH. Cluster headache. In: Headache. New York: Churchhill Livingstone, 1988: 236–240.

158. Turkewitz LJ, Wirth O, Dawson GA, Casaly JS. Cluster headache following head injury: A case report and review of the literature. Headache 1992;32:504–506.

159. Ekbom K. Nitroglycerin as a provocative agent in cluster headache. Arch Neurol 1968;19: 487–493.

160. Horton BT. Histamine cephalgia. Md State Med J 1961;10:92–98.

161. Ekbom K. Some observations on pain in cluster headache. Headache 1975;14:219–225.

162. Atkinson R. Physical fitness and headache. Headache 1977;17:189–195.

163. Ekbom K, Lindahl J. Effect of induced rise in blood pressure on pain in cluster headache. Acta Neurol Scand 1970;46:585–600.

164. Kudrow L. Response of cluster headache attacks to oxygen inhalation. Headache 1981;21: 1–4.

165. Fogan L. Treatment of cluster headache. A double-blind comparison of oxygen vs. air inhalation. Arch Neurol 1985;42:362–363.

166. Ekbom K. Treatment of cluster headache: Clinical trials, design and results. Cephalalgia 1995;15(suppl 15):33–36.

167. Gobel H, Lindner V, Heinze A, Ribbat M, Deuschl G. Acute therapy for cluster headache with sumatriptan: Findings of a one-year long-term study. Neurology 1998;51:908–911.

168. Hardebo JE, Dahlof C. Sumatriptan nasal spray (20 mg/dose) in the acute treatment of cluster headache. Cephalalgia 1998;18:487–489.

169. Ekbom K, Krabbe AA, Paalzow G, Paalzow L, Tfelt-Hansen P, Waldenlind E. Optimal routes of administration of ergotamine tartrate in cluster headache patients. A pharmacokinetic study. Cephalalgia 1983;3:15–20.

170. Speed WG. Ergotamine tartrate inhalation: A new approach to the management of recurrent vascular headaches. Am J Med Sci 1960;240: 327–331.

171. Kittrelle JP, Grouse DS, Seybold ME. Cluster headache: Local anesthetic abortive agents. Arch Neurol 1985;42:496–498.

172. Bahra A, Gawel MJ, Hardebo JE, Millson D, Breen SA, Goadsby PJ. Oral zolmitriptan is effective in the acute treatment of cluster headache. Neurology 2000;54:1832–1839.

173. Kudrow L, McGinty DJ, Phillips ER. Sleep apnea in cluster headache. Cephalalgia 1984;4: 33–38.

174. Kudrow L. Comparative results of prednisone, methysergide, and lithium therapy in cluster headache. In: Greene R (ed). Current Concepts in Migraine Research. New York: Raven Press, 1978:159–163.

175. Goadsby PJ, Lipton RB. A review of paroxysmal hemicranias, SUNCT syndrome and other short-lasting headaches with autonomic feature, including new cases. Brain 1997;120: 193–209.

176. Raskin NH. The indomethacin responsive syndromes. In: Headache. New York: Churchill Livingstone, 1988:255–268.

177. Sjaastad O, Dale I. Evidence for a new (?) clinical headache entity: "Chronic paroxysmal hemicrania." Acta Neurol Scand 1976;54:140–149.

178. Russel D. Chronic paroxysmal hemicrania: Severity, duration and time of occurrence of attacks. Cephalalgia 1984;4:53–56.

179. Horven I, Sjaastad O. Cluster headache syndrome and migraine, ophthalmological support for a two-entity therory. Acta Ophthalmol (Copenh) 1977;55:35–50.

180. Horven I, Russel D, Sjaastad O. Ocular blood flow changes in cluster headache and chronic paroxysmal hemicrania. Headache 1989;29: 373–376.

181. Sjaastad O. Chronic paroxysmal hemicrania. In: Vinken PJ, Bruyn GW, Klawans HI (eds). Headache, vol 48, Handbook of Clinical Neurology. Amsterdam: Elsevier, 1986:257–266.

182. Micieli G, Cavallini A, Facchinetti F, Sances G, Nappi G. Chronic paroxysmal hemicrania: A chronobiological study (case report). Cephalalgia 1989;9:281–286.

183. Goadsby PJ, Lipton RB. A review of paroxysmal hemicranias, SUNCT syndrome and other short-lasting headaches with autonomic feature, including new cases. Brain 1997;120(Pt 1):193–209.

184. Goadsby PJ, Edvinsson L. Neuropeptide changes in a case of chronic paroxysmal hemicrania— Evidence for trigemino-parasympathetic activation. Cephalalgia 1996;16:448–450.

185. Sjaastad O. Chronic paroxsymal hemicrania and similar headaches. In: Dalessio DJ, Silberstein SD (eds). Wolff's Headache and Other Head Pain, ed 6. New York: Oxford University Press, 1993:198–202.

186. Delcanho RE, Graff-Radford SB. Chronic paroxysmal hemicrania presenting as toothache. J Orofac Pain 1993;7:300–306.

187. Sjaastad O, Saunte C, Salvesen R, et al. Short-lasting unilateral neuralgiform headache attacks with conjunctival injection, tearing, sweating, and rhinorrhea. Cephalalgia 1989;9: 147–156.

188. Sjaastad O, Kruszewski P. Trigeminal neuralgia and SUNCT syndrome: Similarities and differences in the clinical pictures. An overview. Funct Neurol 1992;7:103–107.

189. Pareja JA, Sjaastad O. SUNCT syndrome. A clinical review. Headache 1997;37:195–202.

190. Pareja JA, Pareja J, Palomo T, Caballero V, Pamo M. SUNCT syndrome: Repetitive and overlapping attacks. Headache 1994;34:114–116.

191. Pareja JA, Sjaastad O. SUNCT syndrome in the female. Headache 1994;34:217–220.

192. Pareja JA, Shen JM, Kruszewski P, Caballero V, Pamo M, Sjaastad O. SUNCT syndrome: Duration, frequency, and temporal distribution of attacks. Headache 1996;36:161–165.

193. Pareja JA, Joubert J, Sjaastad O. SUNCT syndrome. Atypical temporal patterns. Headache 1996;36:108–110.

194. Bussone G, Leone M, Dalla Volta G, Strada L, Gasparotti R, Di Monda V. Short-lasting unilateral neuralgiform headache attacks with tearing and conjunctival injection: The first "symptomatic" case? Cephalalgia 1991;11: 123–127.

195. Morales F, Mostacero E, Marta J, Sanchez S. Vascular malformation of the cerebellopontine angle associated with "SUNCT" syndrome. Cephalalgia 1994;14:301–302.

196. De Benedittis G. SUNCT syndrome associated with cavernous angioma of the brain stem. Cephalalgia 1996;16:503–506.

197. Pareja JA, Kruszewski P, Sjaastad O. SUNCT syndrome: Trials of drugs and anesthetic blockades. Headache 1995;35:138–142.

198. Hannerz J, Greitz D, Hansson P, Ericson K. SUNCT may be another manifestation of orbital venous vasculitis. Headache 1992;32: 384–389.

199. Ghose RR. SUNCT syndrome. Med J Aust 1995;162:667–668.

200. D'Andrea G, Granella F, Cadaldini M. Possible usefulness of lamotrigine in the treatment of SUNCT syndrome. Neurology 1999;53:1609.

201. Penarrocha M, Bandres A, Penarrocha MA, Bagan JV. Relationship between oral surgical and endodontic procedures and episodic cluster headache. Oral Surg Oral Med Oral Pathol Oral Radiol Endod 2001;92:499–502.

202. McArdle MJ. Atypical facial neuralgia. In: Hassler R, Walker AE (eds). Trigeminal Neuralgia. Stuttgart: Thieme, 1970:35–42.

203. Campbell JK. Cluster headache. J Craniomandib Disord Facial Oral Pain 1987;1:27–33.

204. Bengtsson BA, Malmvall BE. Giant cell arteritis. Acta Medica Scand 1982;658:1–102.

205. Kobayashi S, Yano T, Matsumoto Y, et al. Clinical and epidemiologic analysis of giant cell (temporal) arteritis from a nationwide survey in 1998 in Japan: The first government-supported nationwide survey. Arthritis Rheum 2003;49: 594–598.

206. Cullen JF, Chan CM, Chuah KL. Giant cell arteritis (temporal arteritis, cranial arteritis) and a case from Singapore. Singapore Med J 2003; 44:306–308.

207. Liang GC, Simkin PA, Hunder GG, Wilske KR, Healey LA. Familial aggregation of polymyalgia rheumatica and giant cell arteritis. Arthritis Rheum 1974;17:19–24.

208. Scheitler LE, Balciunas BA. Carotidynia. J Oral Maxillofac Surg 1982;40:121–122.

209. Redillas C, Solomon S. Recent advances in temporal arteritis. Curr Pain Headache Rep 2003;7: 297–302.

210. Solomon S, Cappa KG. The headache of temporal arteritis. J Am Geriatr Soc 1987;35:163–165.

211. Dalessio D. Evaluation of the patient with chronic facial pain. Am Fam Physician 1977;16: 84–92.

212. Dalessio DJ, Williams GW. Giant cell arteritis and polymyalgia rheumatica. In: Dalessio DJ, Silberstein SD (eds). Wolff's Headache and Other Head Pain, ed 6. New York: Oxford University Press, 1993:262–275.

213. Powers WH, Britton BH. Nonotogenic otalgia: Diagnosis and treatment. Am J Otol 1980;2: 97–104.

214. Acetta D, Kelly JP, Tubbs RR. An elderly black woman with a painful swollen face. Ann Allergy 1985;55:819–823.

215. Wall M, Corbett JJ. Arteritis. In: Olesen J, Tfelt-Hansen P, Welch KMA (eds). The Headaches. New York: Raven Press, 1993:653–662.

216. Liozon E, Loustaud-Ratti V, Ly K, et al. Visual prognosis in extremely old patients with temporal (giant cell) arteritis. J Am Geriatr Soc 2003;51:722–723.
217. Murray TJ. Carotidynia: A cause of neck and face pain. Can Med Assoc J 1979;120:441–443.
218. Roseman DM. Carotidynia. A distinct syndrome. Arch Otolaryngol 1967;85:81–84.
219. Lovshin L. Carotidynia. Headache 1977;17:192–195.
220. Troiano MF, Gaston GW. Carotid system arteritis: An overlooked and misdiagnosed syndrome. J Am Dent Assoc 1975;91:589–593.
221. Upton PD, Smith JG, Charnock DR. Histologic confirmation of carotidynia. Otolaryngol Head Neck Surg 2003;129:443–444.
222. Bank H. Idiopathic carotiditis. Lancet 1978;1:726.
223. Valle N, Gonzalez-Mandly A, Oterino A, Pascual J. A case of carotidynia with response to almotriptan. Cephalalgia 2003;23:155–156.
224. White JR, Bell WL. Dysphonia associated with carotidynia and migraine responding to dihydroergotamine. Headache 2003;43:69–71.
225. Campbell JK. Posttraumatic headaches. J Craniomandib Disord Facial Oral Pain 1987;1:75–77.

Neuropathic Pains

Unlike superficial and deep somatic pain, neuropathic pain has its etiology in the neural tissue itself and not in the structures that it innervates. Neuropathic pain has been defined by the International Association for the Study of Pain as pain "initiated or caused by a primary lesion or dysfunction in the nervous system."[1] Whereas somatic pains are predominantly a warning system that noxious stimulation (ie, tissue injury) is present, neuropathic pain represents either a structural or functional abnormality in the peripheral or central nervous system (CNS). There are a variety of etiologies that can lead to neuropathic pain. Some of these are infections, trauma, metabolic abnormalities, chemotherapy, surgery, radiation, neurotoxins, nerve compression, inflammation, and tumor infiltration. Neuropathic pains are not rare. It is estimated that in the United States approximately 3.8 million individuals have neuropathic pain (this includes neuropathic back pain).[2] Neuropathic pains pose a real problem for the clinician, because at this time management is very difficult and therefore they often present as a chronic pain condition.

In recent years there has been great progress toward understanding the etiology of neuropathic pain; however, much is still unknown. It is apparent that some neuropathic pains have a strong peripheral component, while others seem to have a significant central component. Even within one specific neuropathic pain disorder, there are often both peripheral and central mechanisms. A widely accepted classification for neuropathic pain does not exist at this time. The classification used in this text is based on both the etiology of the condition and the location of the neuropathic mechanism that appears to be responsible for the pain experience. Some neuropathic pains present as episodic, and some are more continuous. In instances when there appears to be a strong peripheral component, the category of *peripherally mediated neuropathic pain* will be used. When central mechanisms seem to predominate, the category of *centrally mediated neuropathic pain* will be used. In still other instances there appears to be a systemic disorder underlying the pain condition, in which case the category will be *metabolic polyneuro-*

pathies. The rationale for this classification is to help the clinician group neuropathic pain conditions into categories with similar mechanisms so that common treatment strategies can be used. In some instances, neuropathic mechanisms are relatively simple and uncomplicated, allowing treatment strategies to work well. Unfortunately, some continuous neuropathic pain disorders are very complicated, with both peripheral and central factors contributing to the pain condition. When this occurs, the classification is less useful. This is a reflection of the many unknowns associated with neuropathic pain. Perhaps a more useful classification will develop as our understanding of neuropathic pain mechanism becomes more complete.

Behavior of Neuropathic Pains

Neuropathic pain presents with some clinical characteristics that can help differentiate it from other pain conditions. Boureau et al[3] provided evidence that six sensory adjectives were significantly more frequently chosen by patients with neuropathic pain. These six adjectives were electric shock, burning, cold, pricking, tingling, and itching. Of these, electric shock, burning, and tingling where the most common (53%, 54%, and 48%, respectively).

Neuropathic pains can be divided into two broad categories according to their clinical characteristics: those that are episodic and those that are continuous. These categories are diagnostically helpful and will therefore be used in this text. *Episodic neuropathic pains* are pains of neurogenous source that have periods of complete remission between episodes. The episodes may be frequent or separated by long periods of time. Episodic neuropathic pains are nor-

mally triggered by some event or stimulus but can be spontaneous. There are two categories of episodic neuropathic pains: *neurovascular pains* and *neuralgic pains*. Neurovascular pains have been discussed in the previous chapter. They are considered in this chapter because their etiology is tied to a neurovascular mechanism that triggers the cascade of events already presented in chapter 16. They will not be discussed further in this chapter.

The second type of episodic neuropathic pain is that associated with neuralgia. Neuralgic pain is characterized by sudden volleys of electrical-like pain. This paroxysmal pain is quite characteristic of the neuralgias, assisting greatly in diagnosis.

Continuous neuropathic pains present with periods of high and low intensity but no periods of total remission. They may be felt as dull aching or sharp and burning. They are often provoked or aggravated by relatively normal sensory stimuli. These clinical characteristics make it difficult to differentiate them from other pain conditions. The key identifying factor is the lack of any somatic source for the pain. Continuous neuropathic pains are divided into three categories: peripherally mediated neuropathic pain, centrally mediated neuropathic pain, and metabolic polyneuropathies. Each type of neuropathic pain will now be discussed along with the subcategories.

Episodic Neuropathic Pains: Paroxysmal Neuralgias

Since the neurovascular pains have already been discussed in chapter 16, this discussion of episodic neuropathic pains will discuss only those pains of the neuralgic variety, ie, paroxysmal neuralgia.

Clinical Characteristics

Paroxysmal neuralgia (Fig 17-1) is characterized by sudden bursts of electric-like pain that projects heterotopically along the course of a nerve. The pains are bright and stimulating. They are usually described as burning, hot, or shocking and can be accurately located by the patient. There is typically a peripheral site on the face that, when lightly touched, triggers the paroxysmal pain. The relationship between the initiating stimulus or trigger and location of the pain is anatomically related. The relationship between the initiating stimulus and intensity of the pain, however, is inaccurate in that the pains are extremely intense compared with the degree of stimulation. In fact, the pains are often triggered by normal daily activities, and frequently the patient will refrain from actions that excite the pains. Such activities as eating, talking, washing the face, and shaving may become too painful to bear. The impulses from surface stimulation or movement received by the sensory receptors of the nerve are painless until they summate to the threshold level; then they burst through as excruciating pain. There may be delays of up to half a minute between stimulation and pain response. Frequently after a period of severe pain, there may be an interval during which pain cannot be induced, a so-called refractory period.

There are no central excitatory effects, no referred pains or secondary hyperalgesias, no autonomic effects, and no secondary muscle effects. There are usually no sensory changes or muscle effects, other than the hard contractions induced by the paroxysms of pain and some residual muscular soreness incidental to such contractions. Both the pain and the triggering are promptly arrested by analgesic blocking of the sensory pathways that conduct impulses from the peripheral receptors of the affected nerve. If such impulses arise in the oral mucosa, application of a topical anes-

thetic at that site likewise may arrest the pain and triggering.[4]

Most neuralgias occur after the age of 50. The typical pains last only seconds, but on occasion they may last up to 20 or 30 seconds. The pains are unilateral and felt in the precise distribution of the involved nerve. They present as rapidly repeated volleys or jabs separated by pain-free intermissions. This feature is characteristic; however, not all neuralgias present with a completely pain-free intermittent behavior. In addition to the paroxysms, some patients with true neuralgia may have a mild, steady, background aching sensation that usually is bearable.[5]

In summary, paroxysmal neuralgias are characterized by the following features[6-8]:

1. Severe paroxysmal pain
2. Unilateral location
3. Initiation of the pain by minor superficial stimulation in the peripheral distribution of sensory fibers of the same nerve that is affected

Types of cranial neuralgias

Although the clinical characteristics of most cranial neuralgias are similar, the location is dependent upon the nerve that is affected. This section will review the unique features and locations of the following cranial neuralgias: trigeminal neuralgia, glossopharyngeal neuralgia, geniculate neuralgia, superior laryngeal neuralgia, and occipital neuralgia.

Trigeminal neuralgia

Trigeminal neuralgia[7,9-16] sometimes called *tic douloureux,* has been known for centuries and is one of the most painful afflictions of humanity. Hundreds of years ago trigeminal neuralgia was thought to be caused by evil sprits and/or mental disorders. More recently, has it been recognized as a true neuropathy. It occurs predominantly during middle and old age, with the incidence

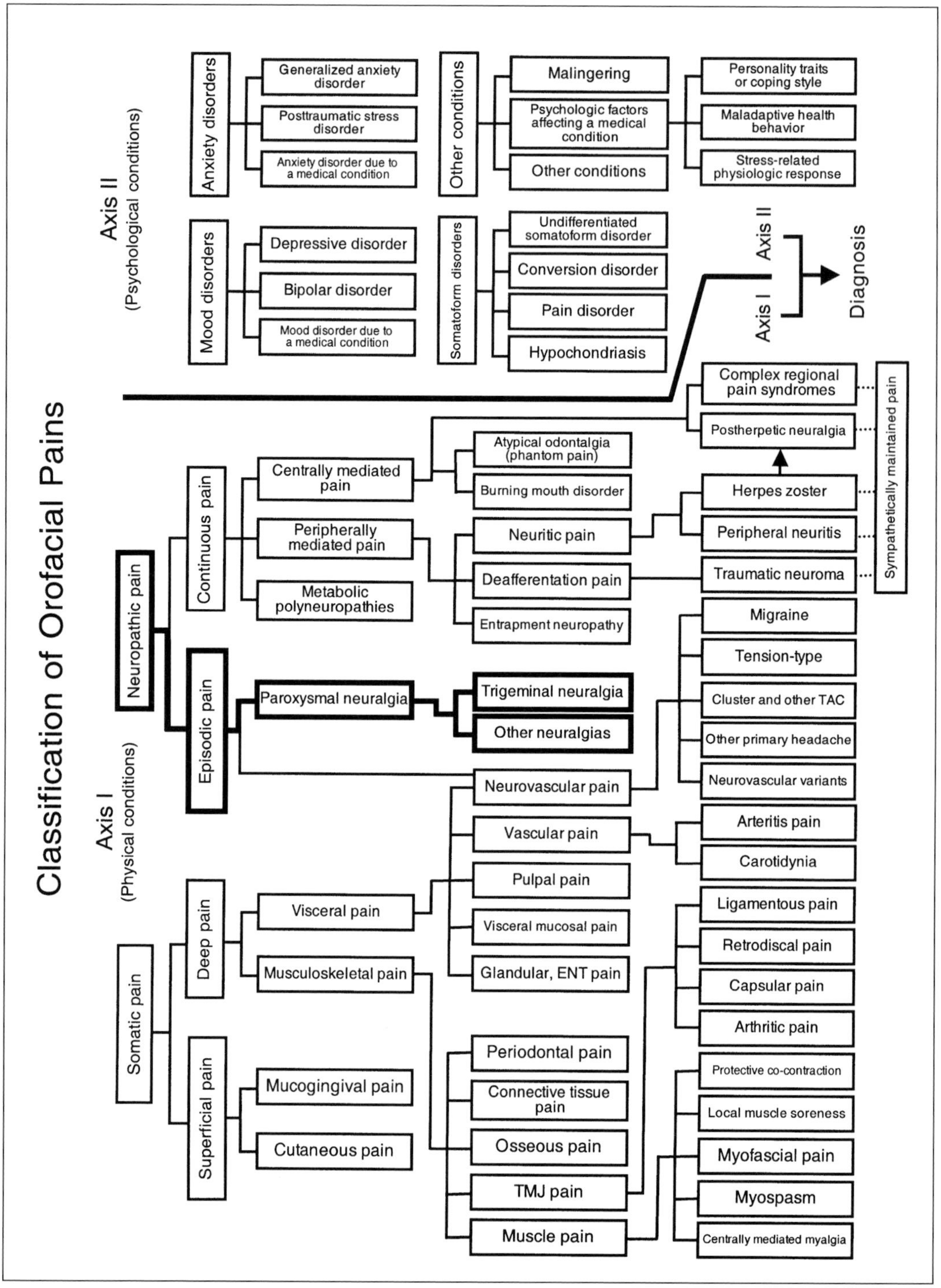

Fig 17-1 Pain classification chart highlighted to show the relationship of paroxysmal neuralgia pains to other orofacial pain disorders.

increasing with age. It occurs more frequently in women. A single nerve branch may be affected without involving other branches, the entire division, or other divisions of the nerve. The pains and triggering occur in the receptor area of the affected nerve so precisely that analgesic blocking to interrupt the passage of impulses from the superficial peripheral receptors accurately arrests both pain and triggering. This effect is diagnostic. Yet the peripheral receptors are not hyperalgesic. The stimulus for pain is the normal sensation induced by surface stimulation due to such factors as movement, contact, and thermal change, which gives the paroxysms a spontaneous character. Triggering may occur from a light touch or movement of the same receptor areas.

The pain usually is unilateral and remains in the anatomic distribution of the affected nerve, regardless of intermissions or remissions. Sometimes it may slowly spread to involve more extensive portions of the nerve, even sometimes affecting all divisions of the nerve simultaneously. There have been reports of pain occurring bilaterally but not at the same time. Rapid spreading, bilateral involvement or simultaneous involvement with other nerve trunks should suggest a systemic involvement, such as multiple sclerosis or expanding cranial tumor (to be discussed under pathophysiology). Examples of simultaneous involvement with other major nerve trunks are *tic convulsive*,[15,17,18] which afflicts both the fifth and seventh cranial nerves, and occurrence of symptoms in both the trigeminal and glossopharyngeal areas, a condition that is not rare (to be discussed).

Usually, the longer the condition lasts, the more typical it becomes. Sometimes incipient trigeminal neuralgia has rather atypical features and is difficult to diagnose accurately. Occasionally only the auriculotemporal branch may be involved. The pains and triggering are located in the auricle as well as in the temple region. This entity may be confused with geniculate and glossopharyngeal neuralgias (to be discussed). Analgesic blocking clearly differentiates them (Case 22).

Since triggering may relate to facial and tongue movements incidental to chewing and swallowing, trigeminal neuralgia must be differentiated from masticatory pain that has the clinical characteristics of deep somatic rather than neuropathic pain. Masticatory pain is induced by jaw movements, and it may be intense, but true triggering by a light superficial touch and slight movement does not occur. Masticatory pain is not arrested by a conventional mandibular local anesthetic block, because the nerves mediating the pain from the joint or the masticatory muscles are not anesthetized (Case 23).

Neuropathies such as trigeminal neuralgia can cause tooth pains of nondental origin that at times may be difficult to identify properly. In the past it has not been unusual to examine a patient with obvious trigeminal neuralgia who had lost some or all of the teeth up to the midline on the side of pain. Such cases bear witness that true neuralgia of the maxillary or mandibular divisions of the trigeminal nerve causes pain that may be felt as a toothache of sufficient intensity to induce the patient to demand removal of the painful tooth (Case 24). The clinician needs to be aware that the following characteristics of true neuralgia contribute to the misdiagnosis of a nonodontogenic toothache (see chapter 11):

1. Stimulation of a tooth by percussion or other means may trigger the neuralgia paroxysm, or a spontaneous paroxysm may be felt in the tooth. This is because the teeth are part of the sensory receptor system of the affected nerve trunk.

2. The pain is immediately and completely arrested by analgesic blocking of the tooth that hurts, which leads the dental practitioner and patient to believe that the "proper offending tooth" has been identified.

Case 22   Paroxysmal neuralgia of the auriculotemporal nerve

Chief Complaint   Sharp, burning pain in the left temple.

History

A 75-year-old woman presented with recurrent episodes of mild to severe, sharp, steady, bright, burning pain localized in the left auricular, periauricular, and temporal areas, aggravated by jaw movements as well as by superficial touch and movement of the painful structures. Exacerbations were nearly paroxysmal.

The complaint had been recurrent for several years in irregular episodes of several weeks or months, separated by pain-free remissions of several months' duration. The discomfort was of low intensity except when stimulated by opening, chewing, or touching the left ear, periauricular structures, and temple. Such stimulation caused a sudden volley of paroxysmal pain. She had been treated with vitamins, including B_{12}, with iron, and with liver extract. She had been cleared medically for sinusitis, allergies, nutritional deficiency, anemia, and diabetes. Her complaint was presumed to be of masticatory origin. Her dentist had adjusted the occlusion, altered her partial dentures, and extracted several teeth without benefit. He referred the patient for a TMD examination. The present episode began 6 months ago.

Examination

Intraoral: There is no dental or oral cause for the complaint. The masticatory system functions normally and no pain results from any mandibular movement except when the speed and amplitude causes movement of the temporal and auricular structures.

TMJs: Both joints are structurally and functionally normal.

Muscles: There is no palpable tenderness in any masticatory muscle and no muscular dysfunction of any kind.

Cervical: Within normal limits.

Cranial nerves: Mild hyperesthesia, especially following an episode of pain. All other functions are normal.

Diagnostic tests: Intraoral analgesic blocking of the left inferior alveolar nerve did not affect the pain. Blocking of the left auriculotemporal nerve where it crosses the zygomatic arch anterior to the tragus promptly and completely arrested all pain and triggering for the duration of anesthesia.

Impression

There is no dental, oral, or masticatory cause for the pain complaint. The history, clinical course, behavioral characteristics, and effect of analgesic blocking are indicative of neuropathic pain involving the auriculotemporal branches of the left trigeminal nerve. The complaint probably should be classified clinically as trigeminal neuralgia with some atypical clinical features.

Diagnosis   Auriculotemporal paroxysmal neuralgia mistaken for masticatory pain.

Case 23 Paroxysmal neuralgia of the maxillary branch of the trigeminal nerve

Chief Complaint   Severe left face pain.

History

A 63-year-old woman presented with recurrent episodes of frequent, intermittent, short paroxysms of severe bright burning pain located in the left face, upper lip, nose, and lower eyelid, occurring both spontaneously and triggered by light touch to the upper lip and nose and by movement of the face and jaw, especially opening widely, chewing food, and touching the palate with the tongue.

The complaint began about 2 years ago. It was diagnosed as a left TMJ pain and treated by injections with corticosteroids. During the pain-free remissions, it was thought that the injections had been beneficial. The present episode began about 2 months ago and continued despite joint therapy. Another dentist gave the patient muscle relaxants without benefit. Her physician thought the complaint consisted largely of "nerves" and prescribed phenothiazine therapy. Since the complaint persisted, she was referred for a TMD examination.

Examination

Intraoral: The mouth is completely edentulous and the patient is wearing artificial dentures that appear to be satisfactory. There is no hyperemia or palpable tenderness. Masticatory function is entirely normal in all respects. The severe face pain is triggered by light touch, face and lip movement, and extended mandibular movements. Episodes are accompanied by contraction of the facial muscles. The pain continues even when the mandible is stabilized by biting against a bite block.

TMJs: Both joints are structurally and functionally normal.

Muscles: There is no palpable tenderness in any masticatory muscle and no muscular dysfunction.

Cervical: Within normal limits.

Cranial nerves: Within normal limits.

Diagnostic tests: Analgesic blocking of the left infraorbital and anterior palatine nerves promptly and completely arrested both the pain and the triggering for the duration of anesthesia.

Impression

By the history, clinical course, behavioral characteristics, and effect of analgesic blocking, it is concluded that no masticatory pain is present. Rather, the complaint is that of neuropathic origin, likely trigeminal neuralgia of the maxillary division of the left trigeminal nerve.

Diagnosis   Trigeminal neuralgia (tic douloureux) mistaken for masticatory pain.

Case 24   Paroxysmal neuralgia of the mandibular branch of the trigeminal nerve

Chief Complaint   Severe left mandibular toothache.

History

A 65-year-old woman presented with severe, intermittent, momentary paroxysms of bright, burning pain localized to the mandibular left teeth, jaw, tongue, and lower lip. The paroxysms sometimes occurred so frequently as to cause nearly continuous pain for up to 5 minutes. The pain was spontaneous and triggered by light touch and movement of the lower lip, and sometimes the tongue as well. The pains were accompanied by muscular contractions of the face that left minor discomfort between attacks. Otherwise, the intermissions were entirely pain-free.

The pains began about 3 weeks ago and increased slightly in frequency and severity. She had on average about five severe paroxysms daily, none at night. She promptly went to her dentist because of the dental pain, but when he was unable to decide which tooth was responsible for the pain, he referred her for a more complete diagnostic evaluation. No medications are presently in use, since analgesics seem to do no good.

Examination

Intraoral: There is no clinical or radiographic evidence that the pain originates from the teeth or mouth. All the teeth are asymptomatic and there is no evidence of any occlusal problems. The pain may sometimes be triggered by very light touch or minor movement of the lower lip. Manual palpation, pressure, and gross movement do nothing.

    TMJs: Both joints are clinically within normal limits.

    Muscles: There is no palpable tenderness in any masticatory muscle and no discernible muscular dysfunction.

    Cervical: Within normal limits.

    Cranial nerves: Although light touch seems to initiate the pain, there is no hyperesthesia, hyperalgesia, or paresthesia.

Diagnostic tests: Analgesic blocking of the left mandibular nerve promptly and completely arrested all pain and triggering for the duration of anesthesia. Trial therapy with 300 mg of oxcarbazepine twice a day reduced the pain to limits readily controllable with simple analgesics in about 3 days.

Impression

No dental, oral, or masticatory cause is present for the pain complaint. The behavioral characteristics and results of trial therapy are indicative of typical paroxysmal neuralgia of the mandibular division of the left trigeminal nerve.

Diagnosis   Trigeminal neuralgia with referring pain to the teeth and other orofacial structures.

3. Extraction of the tooth, or for that matter any surgery or even the analgesic block itself, may interrupt the neuralgic paroxysms for days or weeks, thereby convincing both patient and clinician that the offending cause has been found and removed.

These characteristics of the usual behavior of neuralgia should be well known to the dental practitioner so that he or she may guard against being deceived by them and be able to convince the patient that such dental treatment is unnecessary and futile.

There is still another clinical presentation of trigeminal neuralgia that can lead to an incorrect diagnosis. This condition is called *pre–trigeminal neuralgia*.[19,20] Fromm et al[19] described 18 patients who originally presented with a toothache or sinusitis-like pain that lasted up to several hours. This pain did not have a paroxysmal characteristic but was instead constant during the painful episode. Sometimes this pain was triggered by jaw movements or by drinking hot or cold liquids and presented more as a musculoskeletal pain disorder. Typical trigeminal neuralgia symptoms developed a few days to 12 years later, and in all cases affected the same division of the trigeminal nerve. Six additional patients experiencing what appeared to be pre–trigeminal neuralgia became pain-free when taking carbamazepine or baclofen. These early symptoms are considered the prodrome of trigeminal neuralgia; thus the term *pre–trigeminal neuralgia*. Recognition of pre–trigeminal neuralgia is often difficult, since the symptoms are not that of trigeminal neuralgia. Typically the clinician will begin treating what he or she believes is a musculoskeletal pain disorder (ie, a temporomandibular disorder) or a toothache with no success, and only later—when the symptoms change to the more classic presentation of trigeminal neuralgia—will the correct diagnosis be made and proper treatment rendered. As a general rule, whenever treatment fails to re-solve the disorder, the clinician should always consider the possibility of a misdiagnosis. The clinician should re-evaluate the clinical signs and symptoms and think of other possible diagnoses. Failure of treatment does not always mean the treatment was not done well. Once again, the clinician should always consider reversible treatments before any irreversible therapies are begun.

Glossopharyngeal neuralgia

Glossopharyngeal neuralgia, or ninth cranial nerve neuralgia,[4,6,11,21–23] is characterized by severe pain in the region of the tonsil and ear. Its clinical features are similar to those of trigeminal neuralgia, but the pain is initiated by yawning and swallowing or contact of food with the tonsillar region. Since the pain relates to jaw use, it may easily be confused with pain emanating from the temporomandibular joint (TMJ) or masticatory muscles (Case 25). Patients suffering with glossopharyngeal neuralgia will often refrain from any food or drink, which quickly compromises their health. The pain of glossopharyngeal neuralgia can be provoked by touching the lateral aspect of the throat. A second episode cannot be immediately provoked because of the refractory period associated with paroxysmal neuralgias.

Glossopharyngeal neuralgia can occur in conjunction with trigeminal neuralgia. Unless they are separate entities, a neurologic search should be made to determine whether a common lesion is responsible.

Sometimes the pain is felt deeply in the ear only, and when this occurs, it is usually designated as *tympanic plexus neuralgia*. The ear pain may be excruciating. Such neuralgia may be indistinguishable from geniculate neuralgia when that disorder occurs only in the ear. Precise differentiation may at times require surgical exposure of these nerves under local anesthesia and direct stimulation to determine which nerve is involved.[6,23]

Case 25   Paroxysmal neuralgia of the glossopharyngeal nerve

Chief Complaint   Severe throat, ear, and tongue pain.

History

A 61-year-old woman presented with recurrent episodes of mild to severe, intermittent, short paroxysms of bright, burning pain located in the right ear, postmandibular area, throat, and tongue, occurring both spontaneously and triggered by jaw movements, talking, and swallowing.

The complaint began 5 years ago as sharp pains in the right ear, throat, and tongue induced by jaw use. Her ear, nose, and throat (ENT) physician found no ear cause and thought it was neuralgia. Her neurologist thought the pain was TMJ arthralgia, so her dentist remade her dentures to "correct the bite." Soon a pain-free remission occurred and lasted 3 years with only minor breakthrough. Two years ago, it recurred as before. The neurologist treated with vitamin B$_{12}$, nicotinamide, alcohol injection of the right mandibular nerve, corticosteroids, and various injections. An oral surgeon was then consulted. He did several TMJ injections, used ethyl chloride spray, performed physical therapy, and finally did a right condylectomy. After 3 months another remission of 7 months occurred, after which the present episode began. Another oral surgeon again blocked the right mandibular nerve with alcohol, then referred her for a TMD exam.

Examination

Intraoral: The mouth has been edentulous for 8 years with satisfactory dentures. There is no oral cause for the pain. She has right TMJ hypomobility and localized tenderness, presumably a result of the surgery. This is not her chief complaint. There is mandibular anesthesia from the alcohol blocks. All other functions are normal.

TMJs: Radiographically, a surgical defect in the right condyle is seen and there is condylar fixation due presumably to cicatrization. Left joint is normal. There is palpable tenderness over the right condyle.

Muscles: There is palpable tenderness over the masseter muscle, presumably secondary to the arthralgia.

Cervical: Within normal limits.

Cranial nerves: Within normal limits.

Diagnostic tests: Neurologic consultation was requested to differentiate between very likely paroxysmal neuralgia and TMJ arthralgia, which was presumed to reflect only the surgical interference, numerous injections, and cicatrization. The neurologist's diagnosis, based chiefly on topical anesthesia of the throat, was glossopharyngeal neuralgia. Complete relief followed ninth nerve rhizotomy.

Impression

No doubt the recurrent glossopharyngeal neuralgia was the chief complaint during the 5 years. Unfortunately, triggering from jaw movements misled all concerned and was diagnosed repeatedly as masticatory pain. Only after the failure of TMJ therapy was neuropathic pain considered. Then it was diagnosed as trigeminal instead of glossopharyngeal.

Diagnosis   Trigeminal neuralgia with referring pain to the teeth and other orofacial structures.

Glossopharyngeal neuralgia may be accompanied by vagal symptoms, and the examiner should be watchful for such signs. Syncope, arrhythmia, and even cardiac arrest may accompany the paroxysms of glossopharyngeal neuralgia.[23]

Clinical differentiation of glossopharyngeal neuralgia from masticatory pain may be made by the following criteria:

1. Masticatory pain has the clinical features of deep somatic pain, whereas glossopharyngeal neuralgia is neuropathic.
2. Masticatory pain is arrested or decreased by immobilization of the mandible with a bite block. This does not prevent triggering of neuralgia by tongue movement and swallowing.
3. Masticatory pain is not arrested by application of a topical anesthetic to the pharyngeal mucosa, but glossopharyngeal neuralgia can be if the trigger area is anesthetized.

Glossopharyngeal neuralgia has pain characteristics similar to those of trigeminal neuralgia, but the location of the initiating stimulus for both spontaneous and triggered pain is different. This distinction can be made by immobilizing the mandible and face by having the patient bite on a bite block, which minimizes stimulation of the trigeminal structures, and by noting whether pain still occurs from tongue movement and swallowing. A more positive means of distinguishing between the two neuralgias is by application of a topical anesthetic to the pharyngeal mucosa. This arrests glossopharyngeal neuralgia triggering, but it does not affect that of trigeminal neuralgia.

At this time it is unknown whether glossopharyngeal neuralgia ever initially presents with pre–glossopharyngeal neuralgia symptoms, like pre–trigeminal neuralgia. Although this may occur, the incidence of glossopharyngeal neuralgia is so low that no data have ever been published. We may learn that all of the neuralgias mentioned in this section can initially present with different clinical symptoms, making the early diagnosis very difficult.

Nervus intermedius neuralgia

The sensory component of the facial nerve that innervates the external auditory meatus, parts of the pinna of the ear, and a small zone of skin beneath and behind the lobe of the ear is called the nerve intermedius. When a paroxysmal neuralgia affects this nerve it is called *nervus intermedius neuralgia*.[4,6,11,13,23] This condition is also referred to as *geniculate* or *seventh nerve neuralgia*. The pain is felt in the tympanic membrane, walls of the auditory canal, the external auditory meatus, and the external structures of the ear. On occasions the pain may be felt in the palate, tongue, and even deeply in the facial musculature. When the triggering is caused by touching the ear, topical anesthesia of the external auditory canal may arrest it.

In the neuralgic process, one part of the afferent distribution may be involved without implication of the whole nerve, and the site of pain varies accordingly. Since fibers of the facial nerve innervate the anterior two thirds of the tongue and part of the soft palate, the actual propensity for numerous sites of pain and triggering is great indeed.

The pains, although typical of neuralgic pains, are not especially dramatic, and the diagnosis may not be evident. Neurosurgical exposure of the cerebellopontine angle under local anesthesia makes possible the accurate identification of the affected nerve prior to sectioning. The nervus intermedius can be isolated so that no facial paralysis results from rhizotomy to control nervus intermedius neuralgia.

Nervus intermedius neuralgia may sometimes be clinically confused with a migraine variant. The following guidelines may be helpful in differentiating these conditions:

1. Neurovascular pain has characteristics of deep somatic pain, usually with a component of throbbing. The pain distribution often follows the vascular arborization. Neuralgia is neuropathic and has a precise, though widespread, distribution that makes anatomic sense to a knowledgeable examiner.
2. Neurovascular pain is often accompanied by central excitatory effects not evident with neuralgia.
3. If a surgical approach is contemplated and positive identification of the affected nerve is required, this can be done by a neurosurgical suboccipital exposure under local anesthesia for direct stimulation of the nervus intermedius.[6,23]

This condition may be associated with a herpes zoster infection of the geniculate ganglion, which will be reviewed under the category of neuritis.

Superior laryngeal neuralgia
The superior laryngeal nerve is a branch of the vagus and innervates the cricothyroid muscle of the larynx, which stretches, tenses, and adducts the vocal cord. Paralysis of this nerve causes hoarseness and fatigued voice, with altered pitch. The clinical characteristics of superior laryngeal neuralgia are periodic, unilateral submandibular pain radiating through the ear, eye, or shoulder. It is sometimes difficult to differentiate this condition from glossopharyngeal neuralgia. The pain is paroxysmal, lasting momentarily, and may be provoked by swallowing, straining the voice, turning the head, coughing, sneezing, yawning, or blowing the nose. The patient may report an irresistible urge to swallow. A trigger is frequently located just superior and lateral to the thyroid cartilage.[24]

Occipital neuralgia
The greater occipital nerve is a continuation of the dorsal ramus of the second cervical nerve. It moves superiorly between the sternocleidomastoid and trapezius muscles to innervate the posterior scalp. Compression of this nerve induces paresthesia or dysesthesia in the back of the head. True occipital neuralgia is rare, but when present, the paroxysmal pains are felt in the posterior occipital region radiating up the back of the head. The pain may also be felt in the cervical region.

Most pain and tenderness felt in the posterior occipital region is not neuralgic pain but instead musculoskeletal. Many of these conditions are secondary to trauma (eg, a cervical strain). When evaluating the cervical region, the clinician needs to be constantly aware of the difference in clinical characteristics of neuropathic pains and musculoskeletal pains.

Pathophysiology of neuralgic pain

Until recently, the mechanism of neuralgic pain was not known. Kerr and Miller[25,26] have shown that significant pathologic change occurs in the myelin sheath of fibers in the ganglion, dorsal root, or both. This change, recognizable by both light and electron microscopy, consists of disintegration of the myelin sheath—ie, demyelination. There is some evidence that demyelination results from a progressive degenerative process.[9] Demyelination affects the fibers in such a way as to permit ephaptic exchange of neural signals at the site of neuropathy.

There are likely to be several reasons for demyelination of the nerve fiber. It may be associated with a structural abnormality, whereby an adjacent structure applies constant force to the nerve root.[27] In the case of trigeminal neuralgia, the nerve root can be affected in the posterior fossa as it exits the pons before reaching the gasserian ganglion. One source of such compression is an aberrant loop of the superior cerebellar artery that lies on the nerve root and produces a significant microvascular compression.[21,28,29] This compression is thought to cause the demyelination of the nerve.

Other sources of compression that need to be considered are space-occupying lesions in this region of the brain, the most frequent of which is a cerebellopontine angle tumor.[30-32] Posterior fossa tumors or basilar artery aneurysms are also possible sources, along with a meningioma of Meckel's cavity or an epidermoid cyst. It is established that malignant tumors that initiate pain are extramedullary.[6,15] Destructive lesions of the nerve located within the brain tissue from the entrance of the trigeminal nerve into the pons throughout the numerous sensory circuits to the cortex do not cause neuralgia.[33]

Demyelination of the trigeminal nerve may result from a systemic condition, such as multiple sclerosis.[6,10,11,15,34] Approximately 1 out of every 100 multiple sclerosis patients suffer from trigeminal neuralgia. Multiple sclerosis may present with pain as the initial symptom that, once established, may continue throughout the course of the disease. Occasionally, the pain may be paroxysmal trigeminal pain associated with trigeminal neuralgia. At autopsy, sclerotic plaques have been found at the root entrance zone of the trigeminal nerve when trigeminal neuralgia had been present. Such plaques in the descending root and sensory nucleus have been observed without associated paroxysmal pains.

When trigeminal neuralgia occurs in a patient with known multiple sclerosis, several features can help determine the etiology. If it is the initiating symptom, the patient's age may be important, since multiple sclerosis is most likely to develop between the ages of 20 and 40. Neuralgia from this cause may be bilateral, which is rare with other causes of trigeminal neuralgia.

In a series of papers Rappaport, Devor, and associates[7,8,35] proposed a hypothesis for the mechanism of trigeminal neuralgia, and any neuralgia, for that matter. They suggested that the compression and demyelination of the nerve root cause ectopic firing of a focal group of trigeminal ganglion neurons. This causes this same cluster of neurons to become hyperexcitable. When this activity is supplemented by activity evoked from a peripheral trigger, especially light touch, the aggregate focus activity produces a chain reaction spread of activity to passive neighboring cells in the ganglion. After a brief period of autonomous firing, activity is quenched, and a refractory period is initiated by an intrinsic suppressive (hyperpolarizing) process engaged as a result of the rapid firing. Since the primary abnormality resides in the trigeminal ganglion and nerve root, normal sensation is present in the periphery between periods of ectopic paroxysmal discharges.

The International Headache Society[36] (IHS) has classified trigeminal neuralgia (IHC 13.1) into two categories according to etiology. Trigeminal neuralgia associated with a vascular compression of the nerve root is considered *classical trigeminal neuralgia* (IHC 13.1.1). When the trigeminal neuralgia is caused by a demonstrable structural lesion other than a vessel, the term is *symptomatic trigeminal neuralgia* (IHC 13.1.2).

Precipitating factors

As just discussed, precipitating factors of neuralgic pains are often a relatively innocuous peripheral stimulation. A light touch to the face or facial movement associated with smiling or swallowing may be enough to evoke the pain. The location of the trigger shows no evidence of tissue abnormality, which is diagnostic of the disorder. The patient will go to great effort not to stimulate the trigger area. Local and sometimes topical anesthetic in the location of the trigger area will temporary stop the pain episodes.

Diagnostic considerations

Symptomatic neuralgias

About 2% of the paroxysmal neuralgias of the orofacial region result from pathologic lesions. Although such symptomatic neuralgias are encountered only rarely, they must be considered in the diagnosis of neuropathic pains about the face and mouth. Symptomatic neuralgias usually present certain clinical features that indicate the presence of some pathologic lesion. When one or more of the following features are observed by the clinician, referral for a neurologic consultation is indicated:

1. Atypical manifestations, such as prolonged or nearly continuous paroxysms of pain
2. Definite bridging of paroxysms with a more continuous aching or burning pain
3. Bilateral neuralgic pains
4. Neuralgic involvement of two or more cranial nerves simultaneously
5. Neuralgia accompanied by other sensory manifestations such as hypoesthesia, paresthesia, dysesthesia, or anesthesia
6. Neuralgia accompanied by muscular weakness or paralysis or by unusual autonomic signs
7. Rapid or significant change in behavior of the symptom complex
8. Failure of the complaint to respond to reasonable therapy
9. Typical paroxysmal neuralgia in young persons

Neuralgia Versus Masticatory Pain

Neuropathic pains in the orofacial region that are influenced by jaw movement may be mistaken for masticatory pain. It is necessary that they be clearly differentiated. The examiner can distinguish between paroxysmal neuralgic pains of all types and true masticatory pain by observing the following points:

1. Neuralgia is a precisely localized, bright, stimulating, burning pain occurring in spontaneous or triggered paroxysms induced by normal functioning, light touch, superficial stimulation, or movement, with the pain being wholly disproportionate to the stimulus and exhibiting characteristics of temporal and spatial summation. Masticatory pain, in contrast, is a poorly localized, dull, depressing, aching pain, sometimes punctuated by sharper lancinating pain or having a minor burning component. It is more consistently related to functional demands and is not so clearly intermittent or triggered by insignificant stimulation. The pain is more proportional to the stimulus and does not exhibit characteristics of summation.
2. Neuralgia is not accompanied by dysfunction, other than muscular contractions with severe paroxysms or the inhibitory influence of fear of the pain. Masticatory pain is usually related to symptoms of masticatory dysfunction and commonly induces secondary referred pains and cyclic muscle pain.
3. Neuralgia is promptly and completely arrested by interrupting the input from the sensory receptors of the affected nerve. This can be done by analgesic blocking. Mucosal triggering can be arrested by application of a topical anesthetic. Masticatory pain is arrested by analgesic blocking of the source only, which is either the TMJ or the masticatory muscles.
4. To differentiate glossopharyngeal neuralgia from masticatory pain, both of which are stimulated by mastication, it is useful to insert a small bite block between the teeth to restrain movements of the masticatory muscles and joints. With the mandible thus stabilized, if throat stimulation and tongue movements continue to trigger the pain, it is probably of glossopharyngeal origin. Analgesic blocking of the joint, masticatory muscles, or both does not arrest glossopharyngeal pain, but topical anesthesia of the throat does.
5. The best differentiation between masticatory pain and the paroxysmal neuralgias is done by identification of positive

evidence of masticatory pain, via completion of an adequate examination and application of trial palliative therapy to arrive at a confirmed working diagnosis.

The IHS has published criteria[36] and a classification number for each neuralgia mentioned in this section. To assist in diagnosis and for consistency between medical professions, the classification is listed in Table 17-1.

Management

There are several approaches to the management of paroxysmal neuralgias. Since trigeminal neuralgia is the most common neuralgia, it will be highlighted in this section. Similar approaches are indicated for the other neuralgias.

Treatment considerations should begin with knowledge of the etiology. When a systemic condition such as multiple sclerosis is responsible, treatment is directed toward the disease itself. Likewise, if a space-occupying lesion is found in the posterior fossa, it needs to be appropriately managed. The remaining treatments can be divided into to two categories: pharmacologic and neurosurgical.

Pharmacologic management

The most effective drug used to treat trigeminal neuralgia is carbamazepine (Tegretol).[37,38] In fact this drug is so effective that when it is tried and it effectively eliminates the symptoms, it confirms the diagnosis of trigeminal neuralgia. Carbamazepine is an anticonvulsant medication that enhances inactivation of voltage-gated sodium channels by reducing high-frequency repetitive firing of the action potential.[39,40] This mechanism of action is believed to result from a shift in sodium channels to an inactive state, from which recovery is delayed, and is likely to be responsible for the reduction of spontaneous activity in experimental neuromas.[41] Carba-

Table 17-1 The IHS Classification of Headaches for Cranial Neuralgias and Central Causes of Facial Pain[36]

13.1 Trigeminal neuralgia
    13.1.1 Classical trigeminal neuralgia
    13.1.2 Symptomatic trigeminal neuralgia
13.2 Glossopharyngeal neuralgia
    13.2.1 Classical glossopharyngeal neuralgia
    13.2.2 Symptomatic glossopharyngeal neuralgia
13.3 Nervus intermedius neuralgia
13.4 Superior laryngeal neuralgia
13.5 Nasociliary neuralgia
13.6 Supraorbital neuralgia
13.7 Other terminal branch neuralgias
13.8 Occipital neuralgia

Used with permission.

mazepine has been shown to depress the posttetanic potentiation at the spinal cord level in animals and significantly inhibit polysynaptic reflex activity in the spinal cord.[42] Unfortunately, this medication does not address the etiology of the neuralgia and therefore may need to be taken long-term. Although it is very effective, long-term use is not without medical complications. Initial side effects may include ataxia, drowsiness, and fatigue. Idiosyncratic side effects include leukopenia, agranulocytosis, and aplastic anemia. It is therefore advisable to obtain pretreatment baseline values of blood and platelets and to repeat these tests at regular intervals (eg, monthly) during treatment. The medication should be begun slowly and titrated to the minimal dosage that is needed to eliminate the paroxysms.

More recently, oxcarbazepine (Trileptal) has been introduced. Oxcarbazepine is a keto-analog of carbamazepine, which is metabolized via oxidative pathways.[38,43,44] Cytosolic enzymes reduce oxcarbazepine to the monohydroxyl derivative, which is responsible for most of its pharmacologic effect. As a result, the active metabolite of carbamazepine that contributes to its adverse side effects is not produced. Oxcarbazepine shares the effects of carbamazepine on voltage-dependent sodium channels and inhibition of release of excitatory neurotransmitters. In a recent study, administration of oxcarbazepine led to inhibition of high-frequency firing of cutaneous afferent fibers following repetitive stimulation, without affecting impulse conduction.[45] Because of its reduced side effects, oxcarbazepine has become the drug of choice for trigeminal neuralgia, with carbamazepine being used only if it fails.

Another drug that has proven to be very helpful with neuralgic pain is gabapentin (Neurontin).[46] Gabapentin is an anticonvulsive medication that has become popular with clinicians because of its relatively low side-effect profile. The mechanism of action responsible for the antineuralgic properties of gabapentin is still being evaluated. Data from animal models of pain have shown that the efficacy of gabapentin is not mediated by binding to gamma-aminobutyric acid (GABA), opioid, dopamine, serotonin, or neurokinin-1 receptors.[47] Gabapentin was found to increase the CNS concentration of GABA and may enhance the release of nonvesicular GABA.[48] Although the maximum dosage suggested for seizures is 1,800 mg per day, pain clinicians have found that higher levels can and may be used for neuropathic pains.[49] The greatest side effect is drowsiness, and therefore this medication should be slowly titrated to a therapeutic dose.

Topiramate (Topamax) is another anticonvulsant medication that may be helpful in reducing the symptoms of trigeminal neuralgia. Topiramate is a sulfonamide derivative with multiple mechanisms of action.

Although topiramate was initially believed to strongly modulate voltage-sensitive sodium channels, recent data have shown that at therapeutically relevant concentrations, topiramate limited sustained repetitive discharges to a variable extent in cultured mouse spinal neurons, causing an effect in about one third of neurons and only intermittent limitation of sustained repetitive firing in another third.[50] It may also enhance the ability of GABA.[51] Possible adverse effects of topiramate include somnolence, fatigue, anxiety, memory or concentration difficulties, and kidney stones. The clinician should avoid abrupt withdrawal of this medication.

Still another drug that can be helpful is baclofen (Lioresal).[52,53] Baclofen depresses excitatory synaptic transmission in the spinal trigeminal nucleus. It has been shown to increase the latency of response and decrease the number of spikes in trigeminal nucleus neurons elicited by maxillary nerve stimulation.[54] Although baclofen is not as effective as carbamazepine, it is associated with fewer side effects, especially those associated with blood disorders. However, patients may report significant drowsiness, weakness, nausea, and vomiting.

Another medication sometimes used to treat trigeminal neuralgia is lamotrigine (Lamictal).[55] Lamotrigine is a phenothiazine derivative, which is not structurally related to other anticonvulsive drugs. It acts by stabilizing the slow inactivated conformation of sodium channels and inhibiting repetitive firing of action potentials under conditions of sustained neuronal depolarization.[56] Lamotrigine may also inhibit the release of excitatory neurotransmitters.[57] Adverse effects such as dizziness, somnolence, nausea, and diplopia are similar to those of the other anticonvulsants. The greatest concern with this drug is the hypersensitivity rash that may develop and progress to Stevens-Johnson syndrome. In case of rash, the medication should be immediately reduced but not immediately discontinued. This medication needs to be tapered down gradually over at least 2 weeks.

When trigeminal neuralgia presents with mild symptoms, less aggressive medication such as the tricyclic antidepressants can be used (eg, amitriptyline, desipramine). Clonazepam, a benzodiazepine, has also shown some value with trigeminal neuralgia and may be a reasonable choice when symptoms are mild.

Since the medications used to treat paroxysmal neuralgias may have significant medical side effects, the clinician needs to be well versed in managing these complications. An appropriate plan for the long-term management of the patient's medical condition needs to be considered.

Neurosurgical management

Since trigeminal neuralgia is such a painful and debilitating condition, patients have been willing to submit to variety of surgical procedures in the hope of eliminating their pain. Unfortunately, between 25% and 50% of the patients treated pharmacologically will report an unsatisfactory result.[11] Before a neurosurgical procedure is attempted, the patient must be completely and clearly informed of the nature of the operation, the procedures to be undertaken, possible side effects, costs, morbidity, and mortality.

In early years, aggressive ablative procedures were attempted. Peripheral neurosurgical procedures such as peripheral neurectomy[58,59] and neurolytic block[60-62] are now less enthusiastically undertaken because of a better understanding of the problems that attend deafferentation of peripheral nerves. The benefit of such procedures must be weighed against the possibility of dysesthesia and the continued pain of anesthesia dolorosa (to be discussed). Although such procedures can provide pain relief, the benefit is often not lasting.

Another temporary alternative to invasive neurosurgery for trigeminal neuralgia is radiofrequency thermolysis of the peripheral nerve.[63,64] Although pain thresholds and pain tolerance are significantly raised, it is said that the sensory threshold to tactile-discriminative stimuli is not permanently altered. This suggests that the method is somewhat selective for small myelinated and unmyelinated fibers.[65] These procedures may be more useful than a more aggressive neurosurgical approach to the problem, particularly in medically compromised patients.

Today, there are two types of neurosurgical procedures that are commonly used for trigeminal neuralgia: rhizotomy and microvascular decompression. *Rhizotomy* is a neurosurgical procedure by which selected nerve fibers near or within the gasserian ganglion are either traumatized or destroyed. This is accomplished by placing a needle guided by radiographic fluoroscopy into the foramen ovale of the sedated patient. After careful manipulation and solicitation of feedback from the patient, the selected nerve fibers involved in the pain condition are located. At that time the selected nerve fibers are destroyed by either radiofrequency thermocoagulation (called radiofrequency rhizotomy[34,63,64]) or by depositing a toxic substance such as glycerol (called glycerol rhizotomy[66]). A third type of rhizotomy can be used that merely traumatizes the nerves fibers by inflating a tiny balloon in the area of the involved nerve fibers (called percutaneous microcompression[67,68]). This procedure appears to be effective without risking neural destruction.

Rhizotomy procedures can generally be accomplished on an outpatient basis and therefore do not incur any major hospital expenses. Although the effectiveness of the procedure is good, there may be a return of symptoms in 1 to 2 years. Complications of these procedures are loss of facial sensation and occasionally masseter muscle weakness. The most significant complication is corneal anesthesia, which may eventually lead to blindness.

An alternative to rhizotomy is *microvascular decompression* of the trigeminal ganglion and dorsal root. This was first described in 1952 by Taarnhoj[69] in Denmark and by Love[70] in the United States. More recently Janetta[71] refined and popularized this operation. This procedure involves a craniotomy in which the posterior fossa is opened and explored.[72] The cortex is carefully lifted, exposing the root entry zone of the trigeminal nerve. The offending vessel or lesion that is producing the compression on the nerve root is located. The superior cerebellar artery is the most common offending vessel. When this is the case, the vessel is carefully dissected from the trigeminal nerve and a sponge is placed between the structures. Remarkable relief immediately follows this procedure.[73-75]

Although this neurosurgical procedure appears to have great long-term success, it is considered major surgery. Patient selection is therefore extremely important. Relatively young, healthy patients are obviously the best candidates. The neurosurgeon must select the appropriate patients for this procedure.

Continuous Neuropathic Pains

Continuous neuropathic pains are pain disorders that have their origin in neural structures and are expressed as constant, ongoing, and unremitting pain. They will often have high and low intensity but no periods of total remission. Continuous neuropathic pains can be subdivided into three types: peripherally mediated neuropathic pain, centrally mediated neuropathic pain, and metabolic polyneuropathies. There appear to be some common mechanisms involved in continuous neuropathic pains, and these mechanisms will be discussed here before the specific subcategories are reviewed in more detail later in the chapter.

Mechanisms of Continuous Neuropathic Pains

The neurophysiologic mechanisms that lead to continuous neuropathic pains are very complex and certainly not completely understood at this time. Evidence suggests that there are both peripheral and central mechanisms that may contribute at different levels, explaining the variety of clinical presentations of continuous neuropathic pains. It is well established that the release of inflammatory mediators following a nerve injury results in the altered expression and distribution of sodium channels at the level of the injured nociceptors and their associated dorsal root ganglia. In addition to sodium channels, novel ion channels can be expressed in the regenerating axons, including adrenergic receptors[76] and calcium channels.[77] This results in a lowering of the nociceptor depolarization threshold and in ectopic discharges, a phenomenon known as *peripheral sensitization*.[78,79]

This peripheral sensitization leads to an ongoing barrage of deep pain nociceptive input, which causes the release of tachykinins such as substance P and neurokinin A centrally. These neuropeptides bind with neurokinin receptors in the second-order neurons (ie, wide dynamic range [WDR]) and trigger the release of intracellular calcium, facilitating the up-regulation of the N-methyl-D-aspartate (NMDA) receptors.[80-84] In turn, excitatory amino acids such as aspartate and glutamate[85,86] are released into the synapse between the primary and secondary neuron. These excitatory amino acids result in a further influx of calcium into the cell. This intracellular calcium results in a cascade of enzymatic activity and genetic effects that have long-term consequences, such as a lowering the threshold of spinal tract neurons. The lowering of the threshold results in what is known as *central sensitization* (see chapter 4). When this becomes a prolonged condition, there can be an induction of early gene expression that causes the release of the proto-oncogenes c-fos and c-jun.[87] The release of these substances by the cell alters mRNA, which in turn can changes the type and number of receptors that are formed on the cell membrane. As the number and type of receptors change, so also does the cell's function. This condition, called *neuroplasticity,* has been discussed in chapter 4. In addition to these cellular changes, resprouting and reorganization of these spinal tract neurons can also occur, especially when there has been peripheral nerve injury. Although neuroplasticity has an important function in many brain activities (eg, learned motor function, memory), it does not seem to play a positive role in prolonged, ongoing nociception. In fact, it may lead to the changes associated with chronic continuous neuropathic pain disorders.

As the spinal tract neurons become more sensitized, additional primary afferent input is enhanced and/or misinterpreted (Figs 17-2a and 17-2b). With time, the original source of peripheral nociception can resolve, but if the second-order neuron maintains its sensitization, pain is still felt (Fig 17-2c). Once a second-order neuron has become sensitized, even normally nonnoxious A-beta input, such as light touch, can be perceived as painful. This condition is called *allodynia* (Fig 17-2d).

Another feature of central sensitization involves the other afferent neurons that converge on the sensitized secondary neuron. This condition is characterized by spreading or a widening of the receptive field. Clinically this presents as a neuropathic condition that is far greater in area than the original location.

Once neuroplasticity has occurred, the original source of pain can resolve, leaving a neuropathic pain disorder that seems to have no apparent clinical source (see Fig 17-2c). This can be extremely frustrating to the clinician who does not appreciate this condition. All of the pain disorders reviewed in this section produce continuous pain and therefore may be the result of neuroplasticity. This central sensitization only complicates the condition and explains why local treatment often fails to relieve the pain.

Since continuous neuropathic pains can have both peripheral and central mechanisms, they may present with a variety of symptoms, according to the predominant mechanism. Rowbotham et al[88] proposed a mechanism-based approach to neuropathic pain. They suggested that there were three types of continuous neuropathic conditions. The first group is made up of patients with prominent allodynia and minimal sensory deficits. In these patients, such as those with the intense pain of acute herpes zoster, there is an intense state of central sensitization that is maintained by abnormal activity in primary afferent nociceptors. These patients respond to treatment with local anesthetics that attenuate the abnormal activity in the peripheral nociceptors. The second group includes those patients with spontaneous pain, little or no allodynia, and marked sensory deficits in the areas of greatest pain. The contribution of primary afferent nociceptors to pain in these patients appears to be minimal, which suggests that their spontaneous pain is caused by a different mechanism, perhaps central hyperactivity resulting from deafferentation. The third group includes those patients with both sensory deficits and allodynia, a pattern of signs and symptoms that may be explained by yet another mechanism. Perhaps these patients are experiencing deafferentation pain accompanied by central reorganization involving sprouting of large myelinated fibers into the substantia gelatinosa, where contact is made onto neurons that were formally innervated by nociceptors.[89]

Understanding this mechanism of neuropathic pain introduces some very interesting clinical implications. If a constant barrage of nociceptive input carried by the C fiber can sensitize the second-order neu-

Fig 17-2 Continuous neuropathic pain may develop with a sensory barrage of afferent input in the central nervous system.

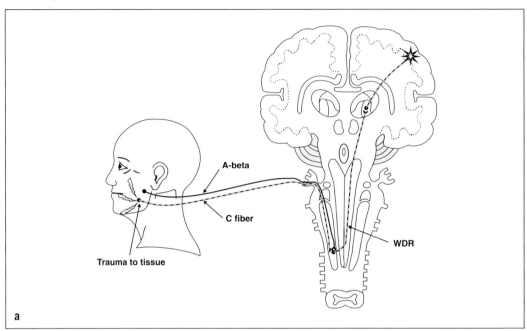

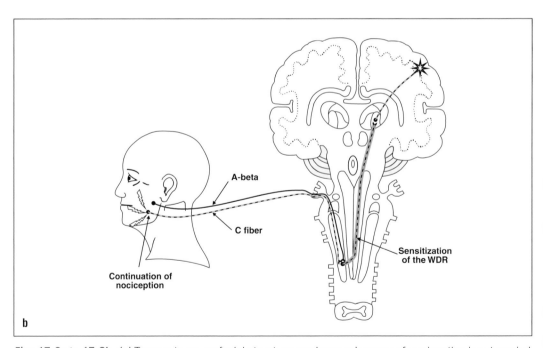

Figs 17-2a to 17-2b *(a)* Trauma to an orofacial structure produces a barrage of nociceptive input carried by the primary afferent neuron (C fiber) to the second-order neuron (WDR neuron). The WDR neuron then carries the input to the thalamus, which sends it on to the cortex for interruption (pain). *(b)* If the sensory input is great or persistent, the second-order neuron may become sensitized, lowering its action potential threshold. This is known as *neuroplasticity*.

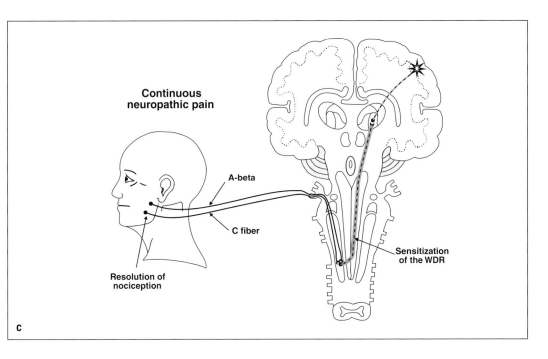

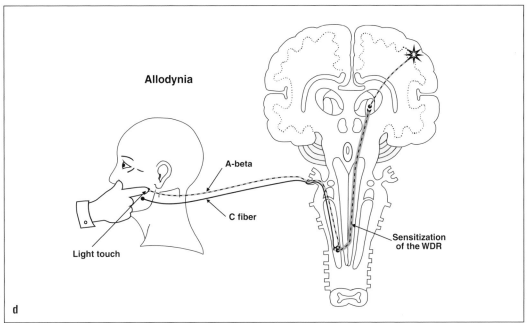

Figs 17-2c to 17-2d *(c)* If the WDR neuron remains sensitized, the original nociceptive input may stop, but pain may still be perceived by the cortex as a result of the altered plasticity of the WDR. *(d)* Even light touch, which only activates the normally nonnociceptive A-beta afferent fibers, can elicit a pain response (known as *allodynia*).

ron, then it would make clinical sense that if known tissue damage were planned, blocking nociceptive input to the second-order neuron would lessen the likelihood of central sensitization. An example of known trauma is surgery. With most dental procedures, local anesthesia is performed before tissue damage is begun. In this instance the C fibers are blocked before there is any chance of nociception reaching the second-order neuron. When this is done, the chance of any central sensitization occurring is minimal. If, on the other hand, a patient receives a surgical procedure under general anesthesia, a different condition exists. General anesthesia blocks neural impulses from reaching the cortex at the level of the brainstem or higher. Surgery under general anesthesia would allow nociceptive input to reach the dorsal horn; therefore, sensitization could still occur. This is likely demonstrated by studies that report that patients who received local anesthesia prior to surgery have less postoperative pain than those who receive general anesthesia without local tissue blockade.[90–93] Preemptive analgesia may an important consideration in the prevention of some neuropathic pains. This same management consideration may be equally important in managing any acute musculoskeletal pain disorder.[94]

Peripherally Mediated Neuropathic Pains

The category of peripherally mediated pain is made up of a group of neuropathic disorders that have their etiology within the peripheral nerve itself and not in the CNS (Fig 17-3). There are three subcategories according to etiology: Neuritic pain associated with infection or inflammation; deafferentation pain associated with nerve injury; and entrapment neuropathies associated with pressure or impingement on a nerve. Each subcategory is discussed below.

Neuritic pain

Neuritic pain,[11,95–97] sometimes referred to as *neuritic neuralgia,* occurs as the result of alteration of the afferent fibers in a nerve trunk. It is felt as projected heterotopic pain in the peripheral distribution of the affected nerve. Presumed to be inflammatory as the result of traumatic, bacterial, viral, or toxic causes, the process alters the fibers that mediate pricking and burning pain, elevating the threshold for pricking pain but lowering it for burning pain.[11] This gives the pain a characteristic burning quality along with the other characteristics of neuropathic pain, such as a bright, stimulating, precisely localizable pain that is accurately related in location to the site of inflammation as far as the anatomic distribution of those fibers is concerned. It is inaccurately related, however, to the intensity of the stimulus. In fact, the pain persists regardless of added stimulation, only increasing when stimulated. No secondary excitatory effects are seen. Although it is variable in degree, neuritic pain has a strange constancy that relates to the incidence and resolution of the inflammatory process. Its temporal behavior is less dramatic than that of other neuropathic pains.

The clinical symptoms of neuritis relate to which fibers are affected and to what degree. This gives neuritis important identifying characteristics. Neuritis may also present with other sensory effects, such as hyperesthesia, hypoesthesia, paresthesia, dysesthesia, and anesthesia. If motor efferent fibers are present in the nerve trunk and are also affected, then muscular signs such as muscular tics, weakness, or paralysis become evident. If autonomic fibers are present, various autonomic effects become clinically evident. The symptom complex therefore depends on the types of fibers affected, the degree of change, the peripheral distribution of the affected fibers, and the state of the inflammatory process. A knowledgeable examiner can utilize these clinical

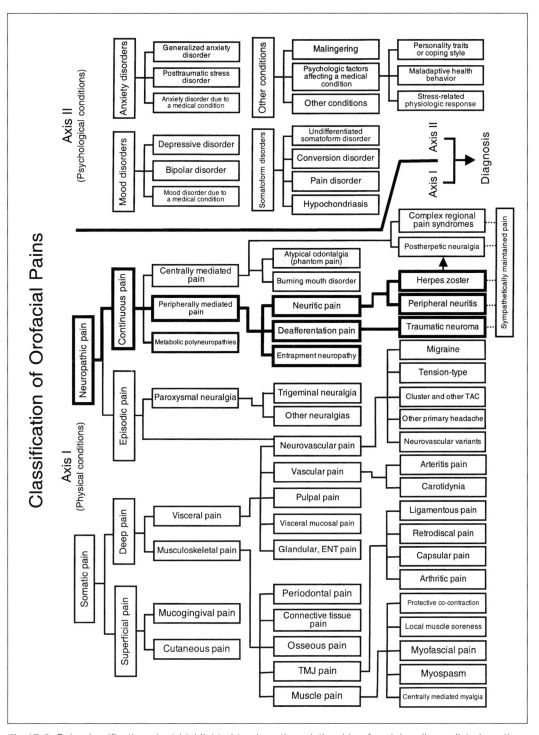

Fig 17-3 Pain classification chart highlighted to show the relationship of peripherally mediated continuous neuropathic pain to other orofacial pain disorders.

symptoms to locate the site of inflammation. When the inflammatory process occurs within a bony canal, compression effects from the inflammatory exudate may occur. The relationship between the clinical symptoms and inflammatory process is strictly anatomic. The effects are the direct result of peripheral fiber involvement and do not represent central excitatory phenomena.

Neuritic pains of the mouth and face may be classified as peripheral neuritis or herpes zoster. In some patients, after an initial herpes zoster infection, a chronic continuous neuropathic pain condition may develop called postherpetic neuralgia, which will also be reviewed in a later section.

Peripheral neuritis

Clinical characteristics. Peripheral neuritis is a pain condition that relates to the entire peripheral nerve trunk, not just nerve endings and terminal branches. Sensory, motor, and autonomic symptoms may be present, depending on the fiber content of the affected nerve. Peripheral neuritic pain has a persistent, unremitting, burning quality that is fairly characteristic of neuritic pain.

Trigeminal peripheral neuritis most frequently involves branches of alveolar nerves. More centrally located inflammatory lesions may induce pain that is more widely located peripherally. With the mandibular division, it may be accompanied by weakness or paralysis of masticatory muscles. Some salivary gland and taste effects may occur, depending on the location of the inflammation. Auriculotemporal neuritis deserves special attention, since it can be mistaken for masticatory pain such as TMJ pain.

Toothache and other pains felt in and around the teeth, periodontal structures, and oral mucogingival tissues may be the result of neuritis. The pain is a direct neurologic manifestation of a nerve trunk, and the symptoms relate to the types of nerve fibers thus inflamed and to the precise anatomic distribution of those fibers. Referred pains and other central excitatory effects do not occur. Therefore a direct organic relationship exists between the toothache and its neuritic cause, and the symptoms presented identify this relationship. For example, if dental pain is the only symptom, the location of the neuritis should be sought in the terminal dental branches of the maxillary or mandibular nerves (ie, the superior alveolar plexus above and the inferior alveolar nerve below). If the neuritis is more centrally located, sensory symptoms in other areas would be expected, along with muscular and autonomic signs when such fibers are present in the nerve trunk at the site of inflammation.

A toothache from neuritic cause would be expressed as discomfort that differs considerably from a typical odontogenous toothache (see chapter 11). Perhaps more important is that neuritis almost invariably causes sensory symptoms other than hyperalgesia, especially paresthesia or anesthesia. Such symptoms occur in the peripheral distribution of the affected nerve, so that other teeth may feel strange or "dead" and may thus respond to electric pulp testing. Either pain, dysesthesia, paresthesia, or anesthesia may occur in the superficial soft tissues supplied by the affected nerve. This would include not only the cutaneous distribution of the infraorbital and mental nerves above and below, respectively, but also the areas of mucogingiva supplied by the affected nerves. A good understanding of the local neuroanatomy therefore is essential for the diagnosis of neuritic symptoms.

Pathophysiology. The assumed cause of peripheral neuritis is an inflammatory process along the course of a nerve trunk secondary to traumatic, bacterial, viral, or toxic causes. The inflammation process alters the fibers that mediate pricking and burning pain and elevates the threshold for pricking pain but lowers it for burning pain.[11] The cause of a neuritic toothache arising from the dental branches of the maxillary and mandibular nerves should be well understood. Neuritis of the superior dental plexus occurs most frequently as a result of contiguous inflammation in the maxillary sinus. The dental nerves frequently lie just below the lining mucosa or are separated by very thin osseous structures. They are vulnerable to involvement by direct extension. It should be noted that this is not a tooth-root relationship but a neural relationship. When antral disease causes inflammation of the dental nerve plexus, a neuritic toothache may occur in any maxillary tooth on that side. The symptoms may be pain, hypoesthesia, paresthesia, and/or anesthesia of a tooth, several teeth, mucogingiva, or the cutaneous area supplied by the infraorbital nerve. When anterior teeth are thus affected, and they frequently are, especially when the antral symptoms are silent because of the relative insensibility of the antral mucosa, a very real diagnostic problem confronts the dental clinician. Many teeth so affected have been treated endodontically and even extracted, only to find continuance of the pain. For example, such an endodontically treated tooth may not only continue to ache, but the pain may actually be excited by electric stimulation—a condition that is anatomically impossible when the pain arises from pulpal sources. Therefore, a diffuse maxillary toothache occurring as a direct result of maxillary sinusitis may be neuritic if its behavior follows the rules that apply to neuritis. This should be well understood by all dental practitioners and otolaryngologists (Case 26).

A neuritic toothache arising from inflammation of the inferior dental nerve occurs most frequently from contiguous inflammation in the mandibular canal, usually from trauma or infection. The most common source is surgery involving deeply embedded mandibular third molars. However, spreading of dental sepsis to the mandibular canal is also a cause of this condition (Fig 17-4). Sometimes such neuritic pain involves all mandibular teeth to the midline. Frequently, paresthesia or anesthesia of the lower lip is encountered. Paresthesia sensed as tightness of dental contacts, and various "dead" feelings may be described. Mucogingival pain and sensations of swelling in the peripheral distribution of the inferior alveolar nerve are common. All such mandibular toothache complaints that are a result of inferior alveolar neuritis follow the rules that apply to neuritis (Case 27).

Facial nerve neuritis (also called *Bell's palsy*) results from inflammation of the facial nerve. The location is usually but not necessarily within the facial canal. Although some deeply situated neuritic pain, along with a persistent burning pain of the auricular area is noticeable, the predominant effects are weakness or paralysis of facial muscles, because efferent fibers to the muscles of facial expression are numerically greater. Other sensory effects, autonomic effects, and taste aberrations also may be recognized.

One possible etiology for facial nerve neuritis is a herpes simplex virus infection.[98] It is thought that the virus may be dormant in the geniculate ganglion; with activation, the nerve becomes inflamed.[99] Another possible etiology of facial nerve neuritis is Lyme disease.[100,101] When Lyme disease is suspected, therapy needs to be directed toward this disease.

Compression effects arising from angioneurotic edema within the facial canal can also cause facial paralysis that may be indistinguishable from true facial neuritis. Clinically, it may be assumed that sudden painless and otherwise nonsymptomatic facial paralysis of a transitory type that accompanies other allergic manifestations results from angioneurotic edema rather than facial neuritis.

Glossopharyngeal neuritis is characterized by neuritic pain in the throat and the postmandibular and auricular areas. The pain may be aggravated by throat and mandibu-

Case 26 Peripheral neuritis secondary to maxillary sinusitis, expressed as toothache

Chief Complaint   Maxillary right toothache.

History

A 65-year-old woman presented with mild to severe, variable but protracted, continuous, steady, bright, burning pain located in the maxillary right teeth and gingiva, accompanied by some sensations of hyperesthesia and paresthesia. The pain was located in the maxillary right canine and incisor region, where the teeth had recently been extracted.

The complaint began 3 months ago as intermittent, burning pain in the maxillary anterior teeth, which were treated endodontically without benefit. After about 30 days, she had some burning pain and sensations of swelling of the right labial and buccal maxillary mucogingival tissues. This had persisted as a variable tingling and numb sensation. About 6 weeks ago, the dental pain became severe and more constant. A few days previously the maxillary right canine and lateral incisor were extracted in a futile attempt to control the patient's pain.

Examination

Intraoral: The maxillary right canine area shows evidence of recent operation for removal of the canine and incisor teeth. No surgical complications are evident. The remaining maxillary right teeth appear to be normal clinically and radiographically, except for decreased response to pulp testing of the maxillary right first and second premolars.

TMJs: Entirely negative.

Muscles: Entirely negative.

Cervical: Within normal limits.

Cranial nerves: Sensory alterations in the region of the extraction sites, especially to light touch. Hyperesthesia and paresthesia are present in this region.

Diagnostic tests: Local anesthetic infiltration of the extraction region failed to arrest the pain. Right second division analgesic block nearly completely arrested the pain for the duration of anesthesia.

Impression

The persistent, bright, burning pain accompanied by other definite sensations, especially in the absence of central excitatory effects such as referred pain and secondary muscle symptoms, is highly suggestive of neuropathic pain rather than true odontalgia. A presumptive diagnosis, therefore, is superior alveolar neuritis, probably secondary to a previous maxillary sinus infection. Subsequent consultation with an otolaryngologist confirmed the diagnosis.

Diagnosis   Superior alveolar neuritis due to maxillary sinusitis, felt as neuritic toothache.

Fig 17-4 Radiograph of a mandibular third molar showing extensive radiolucency indicative of an interradicular abscess that communicated with the mandibular canal. The patient's clinical symptoms were those of localized periodontal odontogenous pain in third molar region, accompanied by neuritic pain in other mandibular teeth, with paresthesia and hypoesthesia of the structures supplied by the mental nerve.

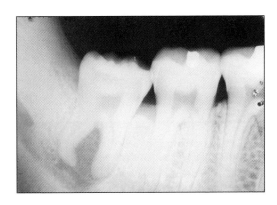

lar movement and therefore may be mistaken for masticatory pain. Traumatic involvement of a prominent styloid process may cause glossopharyngeal neuritis that may be confused with masticatory pain because of its relationship with mandibular functioning (Case 28). Styloid process pain usually can be identified by manual palpation through the tonsillar fossa, with pressure being directed laterally toward the styloid process. Elongation of the styloid process and/or calcification of the stylohyoid ligament is commonly known as Eagle syndrome.[102] The symptoms are those of glossopharyngeal neuritis and sometimes of carotidynia.

Tools-Hunt syndrome is a rare and relatively poorly understood disorder that is thought to arise from inflammation of the third, fourth, or sixth cranial nerve. It can originally present as intermittent pain in the region of the orbit, but when progressive, it leads to constant pain. It often leads to paralysis of one or more of the third, fourth, or sixth cranial nerves, leading to the inability to move the eye.

Precipitating factors. Often neuritis begins in association with local trauma or inflammation. Once present, the pain is constant, burning, and located in the distribution of the involved nerve. Since the pain is constant, there are no precipitating factors.

The pain, however, is usually accentuated by local stimulation of the involved area.

Diagnostic considerations. Analgesic blocking peripheral to the site of neuropathy may reduce discomfort by shutting off the input of noxious impulses received by the sensory receptors, but it does not arrest the ongoing burning pain that characterizes neuritis. Analgesic blocking central to the site of neuropathy arrests the neuritic pain.

Since peripheral neuritis can present as toothache, the clinician needs to be aware of the proper differential diagnosis. The following characteristics are associated with neuritic toothache and therefore can be helpful in differentiating it from odontalgic toothache:

1. The pain is less variable, more persistent, less likely to be accompanied by central excitatory effects, and has more of a burning quality than true odontogenous pain.
2. The pain is likely to be accompanied by other sensory effects such as hypoesthesia, dysesthesia, paresthesia, or anesthesia in other teeth or in the superficial mucogingival and cutaneous tissues innervated by fibers of the affected nerve.
3. More centrally located inflammation involving a nerve trunk may cause motor or autonomic symptoms if efferent so-

Case 27 — Neuritic pain of the inferior alveolar nerve, expressed as a mandibular toothache

Chief Complaint   Burning pain in the mandibular left teeth.

History

A 45-year-old woman presented with mild, continuous but variable, protracted, steady, bright, burning pain located in the mandibular left teeth, accompanied by some paresthesia described as a tingling sensation. The discomfort increased with firm biting pressure on the teeth and when she was tired and nervous.

The complaint began about 4 months ago following the extraction of the mandibular left third molar about 2 months before. The immediate postoperative pain was intense for several days. This was followed by a period of numbness that lasted several weeks and then subsided. As the numbness decreased, the present mild burning pain was felt in several mandibular left teeth, especially the second molar. The "toothache" has been more annoying than actually painful. It worried her and made her nervous. During the last few weeks the complaint seemed to be decreasing gradually. The medical history is negative for cause. No medications are presently being taken.

Examination

Intraoral: The mandibular left teeth are clinically and radiographically free of obvious cause for the complaint. The mandibular left alveolus appears to be healing satisfactorily. The root apex of the extracted tooth appears to have been in close proximity to the mandibular canal. There is no palpable tenderness. All teeth respond within normal limits to pulp testing.

   TMJs: Within normal limits.

   Muscles: Within normal limits.

   Cervical: Within normal limits.

   Cranial nerves: Sensory alterations in the region of the extraction sites, especially to light touch. Hyperesthesia and paresthesia are present in this region.

Impression

The descriptive behavior of the complaint from its inception is highly suggestive of neuropathic pain of neuritic type rather than any form of true odontogenous pain. It appears that the inflammatory process incidental to the surgery and the healing process enveloped the mandibular neurovascular bundle, causing first severe pain, then anesthesia, and subsequently a peripheral neuritis. The dental pain and tingling sensation seem to be subsiding as the inflammatory process resolves naturally.

Diagnosis   Neuritic toothache due to postoperative neuritis of the left inferior alveolar nerve.

Case 28 — Neuritis of the glossopharyngeal nerve due to a fractured styloid process, mistaken for masticatory pain

Chief Complaint Burning pain in the mandibular left teeth.

History

A 44-year-old woman presented with mild, continuous, variable, protracted, steady, bright, aching, stinging, and burning pain located in the left ear and throat, which was aggravated by chewing, talking and swallowing and was accompanied by rawness of the throat and a sensation of "wetness" in the left ear.

The complaint began about 30 days ago following a severe blow to the left face. That evening she had pain in the left ear and postmandibular area that increased with opening the mouth. Her ENT physician found no aural cause for the complaint and advised a corticosteroid injection of the left TMJ. The patient's internist suggested a dental examination before the steroid injection was performed. Her dentist found no dental or oral cause for the pain. A panoramic radiographic revealed the left styloid process to be very long, with an obvious fracture in its midbody.

Examination

Intraoral: No dental or oral source of pain.

TMJs: Both joints are structurally and functionally normal.

Muscles: There is no palpable tenderness in any masticatory muscle and no muscular dysfunction of any kind.

Cervical: Cervical muscle palpation is negative, but palpation of the sternocleidomastoid muscle increases the pain. Swallowing also increases the pain.

Cranial nerves: Within normal limits.

Diagnostic tests: Application of topical anesthetic to the throat did not arrest the pain. Analgesic blocking of the left mandibular nerve intraorally and of the left TMJ proper extraorally did not arrest the pain.

Impression

The only masticatory relationship is extensive mandibular movement that stretches the stylomandibular ligament. The behavioral characteristics are highly suggestive of neuropathic pain involving the left glossopharyngeal nerve. Radiographic evidence of fracture of the left styloid process suggests a possible etiology of a glossopharyngeal neuritis induced by trauma. Eagle syndrome is ruled out due to the constancy of the pain and neuropathic quality of the pain.

Diagnosis Glossopharyngeal neuritis mistaken for masticatory pain.

matic and visceral fibers are present in the nerve trunk at the site of inflammation.

4. Electric pulp testing may give results indicative of the varied sensory responses characteristic of neuritis.

5. Neuritis of the superior dental plexus may be confirmed by evidence of maxillary sinus disease. A radiographic of the maxillary sinus, in particular a computerized tomographic (CT) scan, can provide evidence of maxillary sinusitis.

Management. The management of peripheral neuritis begins with an understanding of the etiology of the inflammation. When a bacterial source is suspected, antibiotics are indicated. Other treatments needed to eliminate the infection should be undertaken. When a viral infection is suspected, antiviral medications such as acyclovir can be helpful.

When no obvious infection exists, administration of steroids should be considered.[103,104] Steroids can reduce swelling of the nerve tissue, which may be extremely important when neuritis affects a nerve that exits a cranial foramen. It is thought that this swelling is responsible for the paralysis seen in Bell's palsy and Tools-Hunt syndrome. Early treatment with steroids in these conditions may spare the patient permanent paralysis.

Herpes zoster

Clinical characteristics. Herpes zoster is an acute neuritis of viral source that presents with severe pain in the exact distribution of the involved nerve. The viral infection often causes production of tiny vesicles in the peripheral distribution of the nerve. These vesicles usually present 4 to 5 days after the onset of the pain and typically burst open to produce surface lesions. Herpes zoster most commonly occurs in the thoracic nerves innervating the trunk and is called *shingles.* The most typical areas of involvement in the head and neck are in the distribution of the ophthalmic division of the trigeminal nerve and the occipitocervical junction. Most attacks are unilateral.

Pathophysiology. Acute herpes zoster[6,9,11] is a self-limiting viral infection of the ganglion, sensory root, or medullary tract of a nerve. The cause of the infection is the varicella zoster virus, or chickenpox.[105] It is unlike the virus of herpes simplex. The heterotopic neuritic pain and herpetic eruptions are located superficially in the exact anatomic peripheral distribution of the affected nerve. Strong evidence supports the hypothesis that herpes zoster occurs as the result of reactivation of the virus after having remained inactive and latent since the initial varicella infection.[106] Ordinarily, one attack renders the subject immune. Sometimes, however, recurrences do occur. It may persist in chronic form as postherpetic neuralgia, especially in the elderly. Although most patients recover within 6 weeks, immunocompromised patients may develop serious infections that can become life-threatening.[107,108]

Trigeminal herpes zoster may involve any of the divisions but most frequently involves the ophthalmic. The maxillary and mandibular divisions may be affected individually, in conjunction with each other, or with the ophthalmic. The cutaneous and mucosal eruptions are located in the superficial peripheral sensory distribution of the particular nerve affected, and the pain is felt in exactly the same area (Fig 17-5). Intraoral lesions may be the only eruptions, and therefore the condition may be confused with aphthous stomatitis or herpes simplex. The diagnostic clue that the condition is herpes zoster is the anatomic location of the lesions, which is identical to that of the peripheral superficial distribution of the sensory nerve mediating the pain. Herpes zoster pain is not arrested by the application of a topical anesthetic or by regional block anesthesia. Sometimes it may occur before or after the appearance of the mucosal or cu-

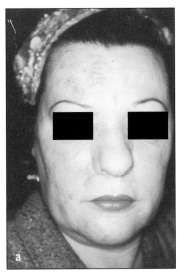
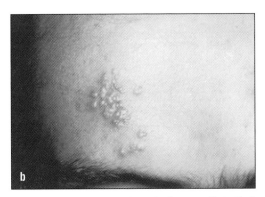

Fig 17-5 *(a)* Herpes zoster involving all divisions of the right trigeminal nerve. Note that cutaneous herpetic lesions are confined to the peripheral distribution of the nerve on the right side of the patient's face. *(b)* Herpes zoster involving only the ophthalmic division of the right trigeminal nerve (*b* is courtesy of Dr Donald E. Falace, Lexington, Kentucky).

taneous lesions and occasionally without superficial lesions (Case 29).

Ramsay Hunt syndrome is herpes zoster of the nervus intermedius, the sensory component of the facial nerve. This rare syndrome causes neuritic pain and superficial herpetic lesions in the external ear, auditory canal, and mastoid area, and sometimes on the tympanic membrane. Intraorally, the heterotopic pain and herpetic lesions affect the fauces, soft palate, and anterior part of the tongue.[6] Herpes zoster does not display muscular symptoms.

Geniculate herpes involves the viral infection of the facial nerve and geniculate ganglion.[109,110] The pain is often felt deep in the ear and is referred to the retro-orbital, posterior nasal, malar, and palatal regions of the face. There may also be a loss of taste. Vesicles may appear on the face and also in the external auditory canal.

Precipitating factors. There are no other precipitating factors other then the viral infection itself. Once the pain is present, any sensory stimulation such as light touch exacerbates the pain. Even clothing that touches the involved area is not tolerated.

Diagnostic considerations. Herpes zoster may be difficult to diagnosis in the very early stage, when pain is the only symptom. Once the vesicles appear, the diagnosis becomes more obvious. Laboratory examination of spinal fluid shows elevated protein levels and pleocytosis.

Case 29 Herpes zoster involving the mandibular nerve, expressed intraorally

Chief Complaint   Left mandibular pain.

History

A 66-year-old woman presented with moderately severe, steady, bright, burning pain located in the left mandible from the mental foramen to the ear and in the lower lip and labial gingiva from the mental foramen to the mandibular symphysis.

The pain began without apparent cause about 4 to 5 days ago and has continued as a protracted complaint ever since. She had a similar but milder attack about 10 months ago. It lasted 5 to 6 weeks and finally disappeared without therapy. Her dentist checked her dentures and prescribed a muscle relaxant, without benefit. There appears to be no history of prior illness, infection, trauma, or allergy. Simple analgesics are presently being used with very little help.

Examination

Intraoral: The mouth is edentulous and the dentures appear to be satisfactory. No hyperemia or ulceration is seen. The tissues around the mental foramen and the entire lower lip are hyperalgesic.

   TMJs: Negative.

   Muscles: Negative.

   Cervical: Within normal limits.

   Cranial nerves: Tissues innervated by the mandibular branch of the left trigeminal nerve were very hyperalgesic and hyperesthetic. All other sensory and motor functions were within normal limits.

Diagnostic tests: Local anesthetic mandibular block caused a mild burning sensation in the left lower lip prior to anesthesia. A few hours later, the patient noticed some superficial swelling of the lower lip. This was followed by some vesiculation of the inner mucosa of the lip. About two days later, herpetic-type ulceration became evident located precisely in the peripheral distribution of the left mental nerve.

Impression

This complaint presents the features of neuritic pain of herpetic origin, probably recurrent.

Diagnosis   Herpes zoster involving the mandibular division of the left trigeminal nerve.

Management. Since herpes zoster is usually a self-limiting disease, treatment is normally directed toward making the patient comfortable during the painful stage. Unfortunately, this is not always easy with neuritic pain. Education and reassurance are important. Mild analgesics may be useful, while topical anesthetics do not usually provide much help. The most serious complication of herpes zoster is another continuous neuropathic pain condition called *postherpetic neuralgia.* Postherpetic neuralgia is an intractable condition that is maintained by CNS changes and is therefore included later in this chapter under the category of centrally mediated neuropathic pains. The severity of the pain and inflammation associated with herpes zoster are well established risk factors for postherpetic neuralgia.[111] Therefore, if the pain and inflammation are severe they should be aggressively managed by appropriate analgesics and anti-inflammatory medications. It is thought that this early management might reduce the likelihood of the development of a chronic pain condition.

Deafferentation pain

Deafferentation means that there is a loss of normal afferent input to the CNS (Fig 17-6). Earlier it was felt that if a painful condition could not be managed, simply cutting the nerve was a reasonable treatment. Although this assumption seemed logical at first, we have now learned that deafferentation can itself produce pain. Deafferentation can result from physical, chemical, or thermal trauma to the nerve.

Deafferentation symptoms in the orofacial region are commonplace. Only a few such conditions, however, elicit pain. The most frequent complaint is anesthesia and paresthesia following injury of the mandibular nerve that is incidental to the removal of teeth. Despite considerable regeneration, some sensory abnormality may persist.

However, since they are nonpainful, such conditions are beyond the scope of this text.

Deafferentation of nerve fibers can occur in the peripheral tissues as well as centrally. The most common painful deafferentation disorder of the mouth and face that occurs in the peripheral tissues is a traumatic neuroma.

Traumatic neuroma

Clinical characteristics. Crushing and lacerating injuries of the mouth and face, as well as surgery and denervation procedures, interrupt the flow of normal afferent impulses in sensory neurons. Damage to peripheral nerves can cause changes not only in the central terminals but also in other peripheral and central cells that are functionally related. Such deafferentation therefore may initiate a variety of symptoms, including pain. Such pains arise within the nervous system itself and are not significantly influenced by the subject's activities, nor are they effectively controlled by measures that reduce peripheral nociceptive stimulation. Some deafferentation symptoms may remain, even when considerable regeneration takes place. Thus, sensory symptoms including anesthesia, hypoesthesia, paresthesia, dysesthesia, hyperesthesia, hyperalgesia, and spontaneous pain may be felt in the region innervated by an injured nerve. These strange sensations may be felt in an area larger than that subserved by the injured nerve, because deafferentation causes an enlargement of the receptive field. Such symptoms may persist indefinitely. Deafferentation symptoms may follow such simple surgical procedures as tooth extraction and pulp extirpation[112] (Case 30).

Persistent conditions about the mouth and face that follow as complications of trauma or surgery are usually divided into two categories: *(1)* hyperalgesia, in which dysesthesia and pain predominate; and *(2)* anesthesia dolorosa, in which a denervated area continues to hurt even though it is anesthetic.

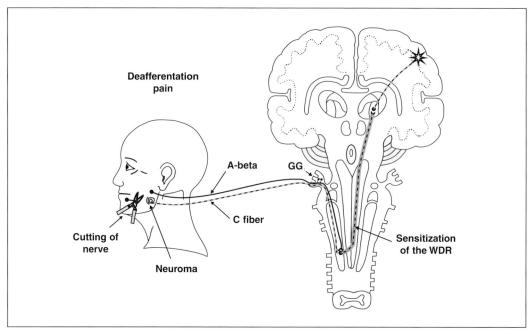

Fig 17-6 Deafferentation pain. When a peripheral nerve is damaged or cut, there is a loss of afferent input to the CNS. The cut neuron sprouts in an attempt to reinnervate the area. If the neurolemma sheath is damaged or displaced, a neuroma may form. The newly developed neural tissue is sensitized to norepinephrine, resulting in spontaneous ectopic nociceptive impulses. The cell bodies of the deafferented neurons in the gasserian ganglion (GG) can also produce ectopic nociceptive impulses. These impulses excite the second-order neuron (drawn here as the WDR neuron), which carries the impulse onto the higher centers for interpretation, often felt as pain. As this afferent barrage continuous, the WDR neuron can become sensitized (neuroplasticity), producing a continuous neuropathic pain felt in an anesthetic tissue area.

It has been demonstrated that deeply located, permanent, degenerative change may take place in the afferent neurons following peripheral nerve trauma.[113] It is now recognized that varying degrees of anesthesia, paresthesia, dysesthesia, and hyperalgesia characterize deafferentation, and it is only when regeneration is sufficient and orderly that the return of normal sensibility effectively masks otherwise abnormal sensations. A relative deficiency in the regeneration mechanism leaves a residue of altered sensations that may range from numbness to severe pain.

Perhaps the most frequent of such disorders is the familiar paresthesia that may follow the surgical removal of impacted mandibular third molars. Either the inferior alveolar or the lingual nerve may be involved. But posttraumatic hyperalgesia may develop and persist following the extraction of teeth and other minor surgical procedures, including gingivectomy and endodontic therapy. Major surgical intervention and maxillofacial trauma present more serious hazards.

Posttraumatic trigeminal neuralgia presents features that identify it as neuropathic. It combines the characteristics of both painful neuritis and paroxysmal neuralgia, so that the examiner may be unable to clearly call it one or the other. The disor-

Case 30   Deafferentation pain expressed as toothache

Chief Complaint   Left mandibular toothache.

History

A 42-year-old woman presented with mild, continuous, protracted, steady, bright, burning pain located in the left mandibular teeth and accompanied by paresthesia. The patient described a sensation of "high teeth" and "gingival swelling."

The complaint began 5 years ago following the surgical removal of an impacted mandibular left third molar. After a few months, dental pain began in the mandibular left first molar, which was extracted and replaced with a fixed prosthesis that felt "too high" in spite of repeated occlusal adjustment and finally was remade. A year later, the mandibular left second molar was treated endodontically because of pain along with the mandibular left first and second premolars later. The fixed partial denture was replaced after the second premolar and first molar were extracted with a removable partial denture that could not be tolerated because of pain. Then some diffuse temporal muscle discomfort began, which led the periodontist to fabricate a stabilization appliance, which did not help. Presently the patient has an excellent prosthesis but she cannot wear it because of pain and a sensation of gingival swelling. It feels no better when she leaves it out.

Examination

Intraoral: The missing mandibular left teeth were replaced with an excellent removable partial denture, which she does not wear. No dental cause is evident either clinically or radiographically. There is a spot that is acutely tender to finger pressure located in the mucosal scar residual to the surgery for removal of the mandibular left third molar.

TMJs: The joints were clinically and radiographically normal.

Muscles: There was minor tenderness in the left temporal muscle area, which was interpreted to be a secondary response to the chronic pain condition. Analgesic blocking of that muscle arrested the muscle pain only.

Cervical: Within normal limits.

Cranial nerves: Hyperalgesia, paresthesia, and dysesthesia are noted at the gingival tissue over the former extraction sites.

Diagnostic tests: Injection of a local anesthetic into the mucosal scar immediately gave considerable relief of pain and, therefore, it was presumed to represent a painful neuroma. Excision, however, gave only transitory relief, and after a few weeks all pain returned.

Impression

The behavioral characteristics of this pain problem suggest a posttraumatic peripheral neuritis that has resulted in a centrally mediated pain condition. There is no evidence that the pain originates from dental, oral, or masticatory causes.

Diagnosis   Deafferentation toothache caused by a previous nerve injury.

der has the persistent, unremitting though variable, bright, burning pain that suggests painful neuritis, and it may be accompanied by other sensory, motor, and/or autonomic effects that characterize a neuritic manifestation. These effects are anatomically direct and do not behave as central excitatory effects. This basic background neuritic pain is interrupted by paroxysms of neuralgic pain. The term *atypical trigeminal neuralgia* has been used to designate this syndrome.

Deafferentation may induce complete anesthesia of the area innervated by the severed or damaged nerve. This may be accompanied by paresthesia. If the abnormal sensation becomes unpleasant, dysesthesia complicates the symptom picture. Hyperesthesia also may occur, or hyperalgesia and spontaneous pain. When pain occurs in an anesthetic area, the condition is termed *anesthesia dolorosa*.[114] Such pain may follow trauma or surgery involving facial structures. It is also one of the hazards of rhizotomy for the control of facial pain. Anesthesia dolorosa is a chronic, intractable pain syndrome that may persist indefinitely. It is a hazard of peripheral neurectomy and neurolytic alcohol or glycerol blocks for the control of trigeminal neuralgia. Sometimes the deafferentation syndrome plagues the patient more than the condition for which treatment was instituted.

Pathophysiology. Traumatic neuralgia is the result of an injury to a nerve that causes either partial or complete deafferentation. If the injury is minor, the nerve tissue may gradually repair, resulting in a return of normal neural function. When injury is significant, total repair may not be possible. Injuries that result in significant crushing of the nerve or complete severing and nerve displacement are especially difficult to heal. A cut nerve will sprout a new nerve ending. If the neurolemma sheath is present, the nerve sprout is directed by the sheath to the peripheral distribution of the nerve, and reinnervation can occur with time. If the nerve sheath has been damaged or displaced, the sprouting neurons will likely growth haphazardly into a small growth called a *neuroma*. Traumatic neuromas are not true neoplasms. Rather, they consist of a random overgrowth of intertwined extraneural and intraneural tissues and Schwann cells that develops as part of the regeneration process after a nerve is cut. This disorganized mass of young nerve sprouts is extremely sensitive to norepinephrine, which is released by the sympathetic fibers in the area. The result is an ectopic firing of the neurons that make up the neuroma, creating a source of nociceptive input carried centrally to the second-order neuron. This condition seems to be further aggravated by ectopic impulses that seem to be generated by the cell bodies of these injured neurons found in the dorsal (gasserian) ganglion[115] (Fig 17-7). Traumatic neuromas can therefore produce spontaneous pain. Other factors that can aggravate or extenuate the pain are pressure, impingement, or stretching.

Large traumatic neuromas are not reported in the oral structures, presumably because of the size of the nerve trunks that may be sectioned. Many sensory nerves are situated within bony canals, where they are protected from injury, and if sectioning should occur and a neuroma develops, it is unlikely that pain would occur because the overlying osseous tissue provides protection. Following fracture of facial bones and deep lacerations, one should be alert to the inherent possibility of neuroma formation as a cause of posttraumatic pain. The oral surgeon especially should know the characteristic features of this source of neuropathic pain.

Of considerable importance is the formation of minute neuromas in scar tissue, because these may be a cause of painful scars.[13] Microscopic examination of painful scar tissue excised from the mouth is not remarkable, and the pathologist should not expect to find typical end-bulb neuromas.

Fig 17-7 A panoramic radiograph of a gunshot injury to the right angle of the mandible. One month following this injury, the patient began complaining of constant burning pain in the region of the injury. Mechanical allodynia is present, even though the patient reports the area as "numb." This condition reflects a deafferentation pain disorder secondary to a traumatic neuroma.

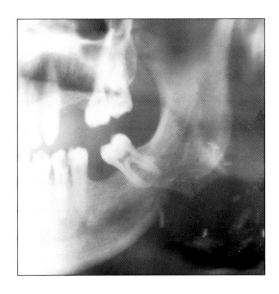

Usually, considerable fibrous tissue is seen with small nerve fibers that appear thicker than normal and nodular and terminate in small whorls. The time lapse between wound healing and the development of a painful scar varies considerably. Once a painful neuroma becomes clinically evident, the complaint will continue until the mass is surgically excised.

Precipitating factors. The most important precipitating factor associated with traumatic neuralgia is a significant history of trauma (see Fig 17-7). Most patients have no difficulty relating the onset of their pain disorder to a traumatic event. Other precipitating factors may be locally associated with provocation of the injured tissue or neuroma by touch, pressure, or any form of local irritation.

Diagnostic considerations. Traumatic neuromas are characterized by continuous neuropathic pain associated with prior trauma. Mucogingival scars following minor oral surgical procedures such as extraction of teeth and alveoloplasty can elicit typical neuropathic pain. This type of mucogingival scar reveals increased pain when finger pressure is applied over the area or when compressed by a denture base. Such minute painful spots can easily be overlooked by the examiner (Case 31).

The following features of mucogingival scars with neuroma formation are diagnostic:

1. History of prior surgery or lacerating injury at the site of pain
2. Usually no visible or palpable mass
3. No complaint of pain except when the site is aggravated by pressure or stretching
4. Decisive arresting of pain for the duration of anesthesia by injection of a drop of anesthetic at the pain site

Traumatic neuromas may form in TMJ adhesions and contractures that result from an operation or lacerating trauma (Case 32). Pain from this source must be differentiated from arthralgia arising from inflammatory conditions of the joint. Such pains also may be confused with neuralgic pains of the trigeminal and glossopharyngeal nerves. True paroxysms of the spontaneous type do not occur, and triggering from slight stimulation of the peripheral sensory receptors does not take place.

Case 31 — Traumatic neuroma pain located in edentulous mucogingival tissue (postsurgical)

Chief Complaint   Constant denture ridge pain.

History

A 65-year-old woman presented with mild to severe, bright, steady, burning pain induced momentarily by denture or finger pressure at a point in the maxillary right edentulous ridge area about halfway between the crest of the ridge and the mucobuccal fold. The pain was proportionate to the pressure. There was no spontaneous or triggered pain. Location was precise and the pain predictable.

Complaint began about 30 years ago following the extraction of the anterior maxillary teeth and had remained the same ever since. Many doctors had been consulted and therapy of different types unsuccessfully tried, including all types of topical applications, systemic medications, denture adjustments, and surgical smoothing of the underlying alveolar bone. No medications are presently being taken.

Examination

Intraoral: The mouth is edentulous with no evidence of hyperemia, ulceration, or palpable tenderness other than precisely at the site in question. That site appears normal radiographically and there is no abnormal prominence of the bone beneath. Pain is readily elicited when this site is pressed with the finger.

TMJs: Within normal limits.

Muscles: Within normal limits.

Cervical: Within normal limits.

Cranial nerves: Extreme hyperalgesia and hyperesthesia in the central area of pain. All other sensory and motor functions are normal.

Diagnostic tests: Application of a topical anesthetic to the painful site did not prevent pain when pressed. Injection of a drop of local anesthetic directly into the painful site immediately arrested all pain from pressure for the duration of anesthesia.

Impression

The complaint is typical of that elicited by pressing upon a painful neuroma located in the mucoperiosteum. Full-thickness excision of the painful site was done and the pathologic diagnosis obtained by biopsy of the excised tissue was "neuromatous formation, benign, involving skeletal muscle tissue." The pain did not return following excision.

Diagnosis   Painful traumatic neuroma (deafferentation pain) located in the mucoperiosteum of an edentulous maxillary right alveolar ridge.

Case 32 Traumatic neuroma pain in the TMJ as a result of trauma

Chief Complaint Sharp momentary left TMJ pain.

History

A 27-year-old man presented with mild to severe, momentary, intermittent, steady, bright, burning pain located in the left TMJ area, induced by mandibular movements, and accompanied by some restriction of jaw movements.

The complaint began about 6 months ago and had remained much the same ever since. Some 12 months prior, the patient sustained bilateral mandibular condylar fractures in an automobile accident. Reduction was closed via maxillomandibular fixation for 6 weeks. When fixation was released, his opening was said to have been about 15 mm. This increased to about 32 mm during the ensuing year with little or no change since. Although he had some restriction of mandibular movements and definite malocclusion, his chief complaint during the last 6 months was the acute burning pain that occurred almost every time he tried to open the mouth to chew. Presently, he is wearing an occlusal appliance that seems to have improved his occlusion, but it has not altered the sharp pains.

Examination

Intraoral: There is malocclusion, which seems to have been very well corrected with an occlusal appliance. All mandibular movements are restricted, with lateral and protrusive movements less than 2 mm. He has some mild, dull, constant discomfort in the left masseter and joint area, but this does not seem to constitute his chief complaint. There is sharp, burning pain when he opens 32 mm and with extended protrusive and lateral excursions. This pain does not occur in the occlusal position, with eccentric biting, or with actual chewing.

TMJs: Both joints show evidence of malposition, presumed to be a result of the trauma and cicatrization. The condyles are radiographically normal in appearance.

Muscles: There is palpable tenderness in the left masseter muscle.

Cervical: Within normal limits.

Cranial nerves: Within normal limits.

Diagnostic tests:: Analgesic blocking of the left masseter muscle reduced the discomfort only partially. Trial therapy consisting of one corticosteroid injection into the left TMJ did nothing to reduce the pain complaint.

Impression

Since the sharp, burning pain does not originate from the muscles or inflamed adhesions, and since the behavioral characteristics are those of neuropathic pain, it is presumed that the pain arises from a painful neuroma formation associated with the cicatrization sequential to trauma. Surgical management is suggested.

Diagnosis Painful neuroma formation in scar tissue of the left TMJ secondary to trauma.

The following diagnostic features are common with traumatic neuromas in TMJ adhesions and help differentiate them from inflammatory arthralgia:

1. Prior history of surgery or lacerating trauma
2. Clinical characteristics of neuropathic rather than deep somatic pain
3. Evidence that adhesions restrain joint movements
4. No complaint of pain except at the moment that the adhesion is stretched

Management. In some cases of traumatic injury, microsurgical repair of injured peripheral sensory nerves of the face has been accomplished successfully. Trauma-induced paresthesia and lacerated nerves offer opportunities for oral surgery of this type. Regeneration of afferent fibers may be sufficient to restore useful sensation.[116] Surgical decompression and other microneurosurgical techniques may be helpful in the treatment of mandibular nerve paresthesia and neuritis resulting from surgical trauma to the inferior alveolar nerve or to accidental involvement of the nerve canal during endodontic procedures.[117-124]

A relatively conservative approach to the treatment of traumatic neuralgia is the application of topical medications to the painful area. In some instances topical application of local anesthetic can assist in reducing the ongoing nociceptive input and improve the condition. Any decrease in nociceptive input lessens the barrage of afferent input that may be responsible for the neuroplasticity. Capsaicin (Zostrix) can also be used to desensitize the primary afferent neurons. Capsaicin is the active ingredient in hot chili peppers and has been shown to stimulate the primary afferent neuron to release substance P into the synapse at the second-order neuron.[125] Capsaicin seems to affects unmyelinated fibers without inducing degeneration.[126] The enzyme fluoride-resistant acid phosphatase

disappears from central terminals within a few days, and substance P and cholecystokinin are depleted in the region of spinal cord terminals within 2 weeks.[127] Capsaicin reduces nociceptive, heat, and nonnociceptive warm responses. However, it does not alter responses to touch, vibration, cold, or nonnociceptive pressure.[128] Fitzgerald[129] has reviewed the limitations of assumptions that should be drawn from the local and neonatal use of capsaicin to simulate the effects of mechanical deafferentation.

At first, application of capsaicin causes an increase in pain. It has been found, however, that repeated applications of capsaicin can deplete the primary afferent neurons of substance P, decreasing their influence on the second-order neuron. It is thought that this shutdown of the primary afferents may provide an opportunity for the desensitization of the second order neuron. The capsaicin should be applied five times a day to the affected area for the first week and three times a day for the next 3 weeks. If this treatment is too painful for the patient, the cream can be mixed with 5% lidocaine ointment.

In some instances, a low dosage of tricyclic antidepressant (amitriptyline, 25 to 50 mg daily) may help reduce the pain experienced with traumatic neuralgia, but this rarely totally controls the condition. Gabapentin (Neurontin) has also demonstrated usefulness in managing the pain associated with traumatic neuroma.[130] New medications are being developed at this time to block the NMDA receptor, which will hopefully help manage this and other neuropathic pain conditions.

Although a traumatic neuroma has its source in the peripheral tissues, the loss of afferent input also affects the central processing of input into the higher centers. Therefore, deafferentation pains often have both peripheral and central mechanisms. With this in mind, medications used for centrally mediated neuropathic pain disorders can also be helpful. A description of these medications will be discussed in the section on centrally mediated neuropathic pains.

Entrapment neuropathy

Entrapment neuropathies refer to those disorders caused by circumstances that lead to application of pressure to a nerve, nerve root, or ganglion and the resulting neurologic symptoms. These conditions are quite common in the spine as nerve roots exit the spine to innervate the somatic tissues. Entrapment neuropathies are far less common in the face, because the trigeminal nerve root and ganglion are contained within the cranium and well protected from mechanical manipulation. Once the branches of trigeminal nerve exit the foramen, they are still relatively protected from being entrapped by adjacent structures. However, some entrapment neuropathies can occur and for thoroughness, this neuropathic condition has been included in this chapter.

Clinical characteristics

Entrapment neuropathies are characterized by symptoms that are felt in the peripheral distribution of the nerve that is affected. These symptoms can be anesthesia, hypoesthesia, paresthesia, dysesthesia, hyperesthesia, hyperalgesia, and/or pain. When pain is felt, it is by definition a projected pain (see chapter 4). If the mandibular branch is involved, the symptoms may be felt in the mandibular teeth, gingival tissue, tongue, and/or lip. These symptoms may also be felt in the TMJ, which can be a diagnostic problem.

Pathophysiology

A common cause of an entrapment neuropathy in the trigeminal region is a tumor in the masticatory structures. A tumor or cyst in the mandible may expand, applying pressure to the mandibular nerve trapped in the mandibular canal. If the pressure on the nerve is prolonged, it may result in a demyelination of the nerve. As with other demyelination disorders the affected nerve can become sensitized, thresholds are lowered, spontaneous ectopic firing can occur, and symptoms are felt at the location of the entrapment as well as radiating out to the peripheral distribution of the nerve. It is also likely that nociception is initiated by the nervi nervorum, which innervates the nerve fiber itself (see chapter 2).

In some instances the entrapment may be associated with musculoskeletal structures such as tendons or ligaments. When this occurs, the entrapment symptoms may come and go depending on changes in muscle activity. For example, if the buccal nerve passes through the masseter muscle, prolonged contraction of this muscle could affect nerve function. In this instance a patient with sleep-related bruxing may awaken with a numb face secondary to an entrapped buccal nerve.

Precipitating factors

The key to understanding the precipitating factor associated with an entrapment neuropathy is recognizing the source of entrapment. Successful management is therefore dependent upon the removal of the source of entrapment. In the case of a muscle entrapment, the precipitating factor is the function of the involved muscle. The history is usually the key in appreciating this relationship.

Diagnostic considerations

When a tumor or cyst is suspected, proper imaging should be ordered to investigate the area of concern. This may include standard radiographs, CT scans, and/or soft tissue imaging such as magnetic resonance. In cases of soft tissue or muscle entrapment, standard nerve conduction testing may help reveal the presence and sometimes the location of nerve entrapment.

Management

Successful management of an entrapment neuropathy is directed toward the removal of the source of entrapment. In the case of a tumor or cyst, surgical removal is normally indicated and will hopefully eliminate the entrapment symptoms. When muscle entrapment is suspected, therapy is directed toward reduction of muscle activity. In the case of buccal nerve entrapment increased by bruxism, an occlusal appliance for nighttime use may be helpful.

In some instances the neuropathic symptoms may persist even after the cause of the entrapment has been eliminated. When this occurs it is likely that neuroplastic changes have occurred that are now independent of the original entrapment. When this occurs, the pain symptoms should be managed in the same manner used for other continuous neuropathic pain disorders.

Centrally Mediated Neuropathic Pains

The subcategory of centrally mediated pain is designated to include those continuous neuropathic pain disorders that have a significant central component contributing to the condition (Fig 17-8). There are five neuropathic conditions included in this subcategory: atypical odontalgia (phantom pain), burning mouth disorders (BMDs), postherpetic neuralgia, complex regional pain syndromes (CRPS), and sympathetically maintained pains (SMPs). Each condition will be discussed in this section.

Atypical odontalgia (phantom pain)

Phantom pain is well recognized in the neurologic literature. It is most commonly associated with the loss of a limb and therefore called phantom limb pain. Phantom limb pain is not an uncommon finding in individuals who have lost an arm or leg. Dental clinicians, however, are less familiar with this condition, yet it can certainly present as an orofacial pain disorder. When it

does, the dental practitioner can become confused and often offer treatment that is ineffective and inappropriate. This is especially true when the phantom pain presents as a toothache. In the dental literature, phantom pain felt in a tooth has been called *atypical odontalgia.*

Atypical odontalgia is probably one of the most frustrating conditions that plague the dental practitioner. By definition atypical odontalgia means "toothache of unknown cause."[131] This condition has also been referred to as phantom tooth pain.[132,133] Most patients who suffer with atypical odontalgia will have had multiple dental procedures completed before the diagnosis is established. These unnecessary procedures are performed because the patient is often totally convinced that the pain is coming from a tooth. When the treatment fails, the patient will often encourage or sometimes even demand that the dental clinician continue with additional therapy. The dentist will often closely evaluate the last treatment and critically look for reasons to explain the failure. For example, if the last treatment was an endodontic procedure, the dental clinician may closely evaluate the radiograph and find that the fill was not perfect. In such cases the root canal procedures may be repeated, or perhaps even an apicoectomy may be attempted. When this treatment fails, the frustration increases for both the patient and the clinician. Often the patient will eventually demand the extraction of the painful tooth, only to learn that this does not stop the pain. Acknowledgment of the existence of this condition is the first step in diagnosis.

Although phantom pains may be felt in different structures of the face and oral structures, this text will highlight phantom pains as they are felt in the teeth, since this is common and a condition every dental practitioner must be able to recognize and manage.

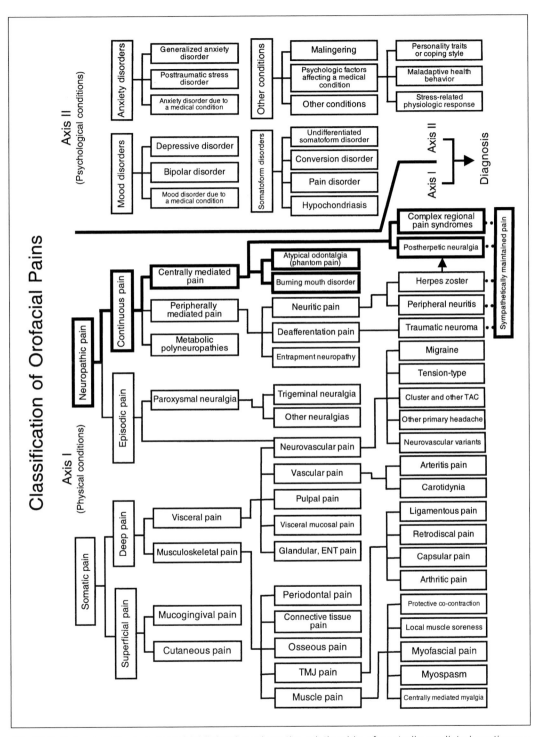

Fig 17-8 Pain classification chart highlighted to show the relationship of centrally mediated continuous neuropathic pains to other orofacial pain disorders.

Clinical characteristics

Atypical odontalgia is felt as a toothache and often without other symptoms. The patient can usually locate the exact tooth that is responsible, or at least felt to be responsible, for the pain. The pain is felt as dull, aching, and persistent. Often the toothache has been present for months or even years, with no significant change in clinical characteristics. It may increase and decrease in intensity but rarely resolves. The most common areas affected are the maxillary premolar or molar regions. It appears to occur more frequently in women in their fourth or fifth decade of life. There is no explanation for this prevalence. Although the pain is felt in the tooth or alveolar process, there is no local pathology present to explain the pain. Local provocation of the tooth or surrounding tissues does not alter the pain.

Pathophysiology

In past years there has been some controversy regarding the etiology of atypical odontalgia. Earlier, this condition was thought to be associated with a vascular pain condition.[134,135] Later, a neurovascular etiology was suggested.[136] However, the clinical characteristics of the condition do not meet the criteria for either vascular or neurovascular origin. For example, the pain is continuous, which is unlike vascular and or neurovascular pain. Also, the pain does not respond to vascular or neurovascular therapies.

Another theory suggested was that atypical odontalgia has a psychogenic etiology.[134,137,138] This theory was proposed when it was observed that many patients with atypical odontalgia also had psychopathologic disorders. For example, in one study[139] depression was found to be present in 42% of the patients with atypical odontalgia. In this study, however, it was pointed out that this percentage was very similar to the percentage of patients found with depression in any medical population seeking treatment for pain conditions.[140] A question must then be asked: Did the depression cause the pain condition or did the pain condition cause the depression? The general opinion at this time is that more evidence exists to suggest that the presence of chronic pain is likely to be associated with the development of depression.[141] This relationship, however, is not a simple one. There is little doubt in this author's mind that psychologic factors likely contribute to the pain of atypical odontalgia. As previously discussed, all pain is influenced by Axis II factors. Since atypical odontalgia is a chronic pain condition, Axis II factors can become a significant portion of the condition. On the other hand, little evidence exists to support the concept that this condition is caused by psychologic factors.

The clinical characteristic of this pain disorder more closely places it in the category of deafferentation pain with a strong central component. As with other deafferentation pains, the pain is constant, sometimes even described as burning or pressing. It does not present with periods of remission. Often a history of trauma or deafferentation is present. The clinician should remember that removal of pulpal tissue or extraction of teeth represent deafferentation procedures.

Precipitating factors

Some patients with atypical odontalgia will report that the onset was associated with prolonged pain felt in the region of the pain, for example, an endodontic procedure that was accompanied by persistent pain. Perhaps this pain experience, in combination with the deafferentation associated with pulp removal, resulted in the condition. There are, however, many patients who report no past or present trauma associated with the onset of the pain. At this time there is no explanation for this condition.

Diagnostic considerations

It is extremely important to differentiate atypical odontalgia from toothache of pulpal source. The following characteristics are common to atypical odontalgia and not pulpal toothache:

1. Constant pain is present in the tooth, with no obvious source of local pathology.
2. Local provocation of the tooth does not relate consistently to the pain. Hot, cold, or loading stimulation does not reliably affect the pain.
3. The toothache is unchanging over weeks or months. Pulpal pain tends to worsen or improve with time.
4. Repeated dental therapies fail to resolve the pain.
5. Response to local anesthesia is equivocal.

A condition that may lead to diagnostic confusion is that atypical odontalgia may be associated with neurogenic inflammation leading to secondary hyperalgesia. Since the pain is felt in the tooth, the neurogenic inflammation may present as secondary hyperalgesia in the periodontal ligament. The clinical presentation is an increased response to local provocation of the tooth. This can often lead the clinician to assume that the etiology is pulpal. The clinician must always be suspicious of atypical odontalgia, especially when a local cause is not obvious.

Management

As with many continuous neuropathic pains, management of atypical odontalgia can be difficult. Most of the success comes from addressing the central mechanisms that seem to dominate the condition. There is some evidence that tricyclic antidepressants may be of some benefit.[134,135,138,139] It is likely that this effect is not related to the management of depression but instead to the analgesic effects of relatively low dosages of the tricyclic antidepressants. These medications inhibit the reuptake of serotonin and norepinephrine, thus increasing the effectiveness of the descending inhibitory system. Dosages ranging from 25 to 100 mg seem to be adequate for pain relief; however, total elimination of pain is rare.

Another drug that that may be helpful is gabapentin (Neurontin).[46] Gabapentin may be slowly titrated until pain is reduced or to a maximum dosage of 3,600 mg.[49] Gabapentin is an anticonvulsant medication originally developed for seizures but has found a place in the management of neuropathic pains. The greatest side effect is drowsiness, which is why it should be slowly titrated to a therapeutic dose.

There may also be some use of the topical application of capsaicin to the site of the painful tooth.[125] As previously discussed, application of capsaicin to the painful tissue appears to deplete the C fiber of substance P, thus reducing its ability to further stimulate the second-order neuron.[142,143] Capsaicin ointment should be applied to the area four times a day for 4 weeks.[142] If this treatment is too painful, the capsaicin ointment can be mixed with a topical anesthetic.

At this time there is no suitable medication that reliably reduces the pain of atypical odontalgia. The future holds promise that new medications will better address this pain condition.

BMDs

BMDs (sometimes referred to as *burning mouth syndromes*) are painful oral conditions featuring burning sensations of the tongue, lips, and mucosal regions of the mouth. The etiology of BMDs is poorly understood and is likely related to a variety of conditions, some local and some systemic. Local conditions that lead to burning of the oral tissues were discussed in chapter 10. Once local factors have been eliminated as a cause, the more central factors need to be considered. The most common central mechanism that likely explains burning mouth disorders is a centrally mediated continuous neuropathic pain. For that reason, BMDs are placed in this category of neuropathic pains.

Clinical characteristics

BMDs are characterized by unexplained, usually persistent, burning sensations of the oral soft tissues. Symptoms range in intensity from mild to severe, with most patients experiencing moderate levels of pain that appear on awakening or later in the day.[144-146] The tongue is the most frequently affected area, particularly in the anterior one third of the dorsal surface. The next most common areas affected are the lips, with the palate, gingiva, and oropharynx affected less often. Although patients experience a distinct burning sensation, clinical examination often reveals few clinical abnormalities. As a result most patients consult several health care provides in an attempt to find relief.[147]

Approximately 1% to 3% of adult populations in developed countries are affected with BMDs.[148-150] There is a predilection for women at a 6:1 ratio, mostly of the peri- or postmenopausal age.[145,148-150] At least 50% of BMD patients also report oral dryness and taste abnormalities (dysgeusia).[145,146,148,151,152]

Pathophysiology

BMDs can be a symptom of several different conditions, and therefore the specific condition needs to be identified so that treatment can be properly selected. Some of these conditions have their origin in the surface of the tissue that is burning, such as candidiasis[151,153,154] (see chapter 10). Lichen planus and geographic tongue can also cause burning mouth pain,[146,155,156] Some BMDs are caused by systemic conditions such as diabetes mellitus[149,157-159]; nutritional deficiencies[149,160-163] (eg, iron, folate, or vitamin B_{12}); and disturbances in salivary flow.[145,146,152,164-166] Sometimes decreased

salivary flow may be a result of xerostomic medications, such as an angiotensin-converting enzyme (ACE) inhibitor.[167-169] The exact mechanisms by which these conditions cause the burning symptoms are unknown. Perhaps some of these mechanisms are similar to the polyneuropathies that will be discussed later in this chapter. One might assume that a common mechanism of all these conditions is an association with an alteration of basic neural function—common to this class of continuous neuropathic pains.

A common belief is that BMDs occur in patients with high levels of psychosocial issues. Some of the psychometric evaluations mentioned earlier in the in text (see chapter 8) can be used to help identify the presence of any significant emotional or psychologic distress (eg, the Symptom Checklist-90[170] or the Multidimensional Pain Inventory[171]). However, a recent study[172] suggests that most patients who suffer from BMDs do not have psychologic disturbances.

Precipitating factors

The precipitating factors responsible for a BMD relate to the onset of the condition that is found to be responsible. Therefore, a thorough history that identifies not only the underlying condition but also the temporal association of this condition with the beginning of the burning symptoms is critical. The history taken from a BMD patient needs to include the medical history for underlying diseases, including dry mouth. Sometimes trauma to the oral mucosa can precipitate a BMD. This may include dental treatment, spicy foods, or a local burn from hot food.[146,156,173] It is therefore important that the clinician investigate these circumstances in the history.

Diagnostic considerations

Each of the known conditions that can lead to BMDs needs to be systematically ruled out so that treatment can be appropriately selected. This is accomplished by thorough history taking, clinical examination, and appropriate laboratory tests. When a positive finding identifies an underlying cause, treatment is directed as such. However, in a significant number of BMD patients the history, examination, and laboratory test findings are not conclusive. In this population, psychometric evaluations may have greater significance.

When dry mouth is suspected, baseline measures of salivary flow should be performed. To be of value, collection of saliva must be performed precisely. Salivary rates can be measured by having the patient collect whole saliva into a container by drooling or by expectorating two to three times every minute for at least 5 minutes. Resting flow rates in healthy individuals are between 0.3 and 0.4 mL/min. Stimulated flow rates range from 0.75 to 2 mL/min.[174] When hyposalivation is present, medication side effects and Sjögren syndrome need to be ruled out.

Management

The management of a BMD is complicated by the fact that so many etiologies exist. This is not a single symptom related to a single condition. Therefore the clinician must perform the proper workup to know what treatment will be effective. When systemic disorders such as diabetes mellitus and nutritional deficiency are suspected, these individuals should be referred for proper medical care. When candidiasis is suspected and verified by a positive culture, antifungal medications are prescribed. When hyposalivation is present and medication use and Sjögren syndrome have been ruled out, attempts should be made to increase moisture in the mouth. This may be accomplished by salivary substitutes (eg, Moi-Stir, Xerolube, Orex) used throughout the day or medications (sialogogues) that stimulate increased saliva flow. A few examples of sialogogues that may help are 5 mg of pilocarpine hydrochloride three times a

day, 25 mg of urecholine three times a day, or 30 mg of cevimeline three times a day.

When the local and systemic conditions have been ruled out, basic management of BMDs falls into the category of a centrally mediated continuous neuropathic pain. It has been demonstrated that clonazepam (Klonopin) can be helpful in reducing the symptoms of BMD.[146,175] When clonazepam is used it should be initially tried at the lowest dose (0.25 mg per day) and slowly titrated higher (0.25 mg per week) as needed for pain relief (maximum of 3 mg per day). Alternatively, chlordiazepoxide may be prescribed.[155]

As with other continuous neuropathic pains, A low dosage of tricyclic antidepressants may help reduce the pain experienced associated with BMDs. In this instance amitriptyline is usually avoided because of its anticholinergic effects (dry mouth). The tricyclic of choice is desipramine (Norpramin), beginning with 25 mg at bedtime and escalating by 25 mg weekly up to 100 mg per day or until symptoms resolve. Gabapentin (Neurontin) may also be helpful and should be attempted.[155] If these fail, other anticonvulsants can be tried.

Postherpetic neuralgia

Clinical characteristics

In some instances acute herpes zoster persists, resulting in a condition known as *postherpetic neuralgia*. This rarely occurs prior to 40 years of age. The incidence of postherpetic neuralgia is about 10% at the age of 40 and increases dramatically with age, reaching an incidence of about 75% at the age of 90.[176] Postherpetic neuralgia occurs as an intractable, chronic, burning pain. The heterotopic pain of postherpetic neuralgia is felt superficially in the area affected by the acute attack. If it lasts longer than a year, it is likely to persist indefinitely and be resistant to all therapies. The pain is usually accompanied by other sensory symptoms, such as dysesthesia, hypoesthesia, and hyperesthesia in the cutaneous distribution of the affected nerve. The syndrome may display episodes of exacerbated symptoms. Occasionally, spontaneous pain reduction occurs. Usually the pain remains moderate in intensity, but the constancy and intractability may render it intolerable.

Pathophysiology

Like herpes zoster, postherpetic neuralgia is caused by the varicella zoster virus. It occurs in patients who have been exposed to herpes zoster and the virus lies dormant in the nerve ganglion cell bodies. In approximately 10% of the patients infected, the virus will become active and produce postherpetic neuralgia.[177] Sixty percent of those affected are over the age of 45 years.

It is thought that one reason for the extreme difficulty in managing this syndrome, even by trigeminal deinnervation, is because the virus involves central pathways in the brainstem and cerebral hemispheres.[178] It is thought that the virus destroys the large inhibitory fibers, opening the spinal gate, allowing smaller fibers to predominate the input.[179] This increases the C-fiber nociceptive input. It is for this reason that postherpetic neuralgia is considered to belong to the category of centrally mediated neuropathic pain.

Precipitating factors

Postherpetic neuralgia is caused by the reactivation of the herpesvirus that lies dormant in the nerve ganglion. The precipitating factors that may reactivate the virus are not completely known. Some possible factors that have been suggested are re-exposure to the virus, stress and fatigue, immunosuppression, and Hodgkin disease.

Diagnostic considerations

A prior infection with the varicella zoster virus is required, but this may not always be a significant finding in the history. If the patient had experienced an episode of herpes zoster, the history will likely reveal this finding. However, even a childhood infection of chickenpox can leave the dormant virus.

Management

The management of postherpetic neuralgia is very difficult. Analgesics can be given, but they provide little relief. Amitriptyline[180–182] can be helpful in enhancing the descending inhibitory system so that central pain modulation can be most effective. Gabapentin (Neurontin) has demonstrated usefulness in reducing the pain of postherpetic neuralgia.[183–185] Its mechanism of action is not well understood, but because it has a low side-effect profile it has become a popular choice for management of postherpetic neuralgia.

The topical application of capsaicin cream (0.025% or 0.075%) can also be helpful in reducing the pain.[177] There is a report that topical ketamine may be useful.[186] Sometimes antineuralgic agents and even repeated intravenous infusions of procaine or lidocaine may be helpful.[180] Suzuki et al[187] reported the use of cryocautery of sensitized skin areas in refractory postherpetic neuralgia. The success rate was reported to be good. Spinal trigeminal nucleotomy has been used to control the pain of postherpetic neuralgia, painful dysesthesia, and some deafferentation disorders, with variable levels of success.[188–190]

CRPS

Complex regional pain syndromes[191,192] is a term that has been proposed to replace the terms *causalgia* and *reflex sympathetic dystrophy* (RSD) (to be discussed later in this chapter). It represents a group of clinical symptoms that are associated with a neuropathic pain condition related to nerve injury. It is primarily described in terms of a limb injury, but may have some implications for orofacial pain. Since the medical literature describes this continuous neuropathic condition as it relates to limb injury and pain, it will be described in these terms in this section. Although some of the common clinical signs of CRPS are found in the face, many are not. Therefore some clinicians question the existence of CRPS in the orofacial structures.

Clinical characteristics
Spontaneous burning pain felt in the distal part of the affected extremity is a common clinical symptom. The pain is disproportionate in intensity to the inciting event. Stimulus-evoked pains are a striking clinical feature, along with mechanical and thermal allodynia and/or hyperalgesia. Typically, pain is elicited by movements and pressure to joints that may not even be directly affected by the inciting lesion. There are normally autonomic abnormalities including swelling, and changes in sweating and blood flow to the skin. There may also be temperature changes in the affected limb. In the acute phase of CRPS, the limb is normally warmer than the contralateral limb. As the condition becomes more chronic, the limb becomes colder than the contralateral limb. There may be weakness of all muscles of the affected distal extremity and there may be trophic changes such as thin glossy skin, increased or decreased hair growth, and fibrosis.

Because of the chronicity and intensity of the pain experienced in CRPS, patients often exhibit significant amounts of psychologic distress. Many patients become overwhelmed by the pain and associated symptoms. Without adequate psychosocial support, the patients may develop maladaptive coping skills. These observations in connection with normal neurophysiologic test results in CRPS led to the hypothesis that CRPS is primarily a psychogenic disorder.[193,194] However, well-designed studies and comprehensive review of the available literature have suggested that psychologic symptoms are the result and not the cause of CRPS.[195–198]

Pathophysiology
The pathophysiology of CRPS is not fully known, but evidence from human experimentation and animal studies provides some insight. Certainly the clinical presentation of skin blood flow, temperature, and sweating suggests a sympathetic component of what might be considered a broader autonomic dysfunction. Under normal conditions, sympathetic activity does not interact with the nociceptive neurons in the periphery.[199] However, in CRPS (as well as with other sympathetically maintained pains) sympathetic neurons seem to affect the peripheral nociceptors, causing increased firing and thus increased nociceptive input. The exact mechanism of this "peripheral generator" is not known, but certainly the increased number of adrenergic receptors that appear associated with the injured nerve plays an important part. These receptors are then excited by the norepinephrine released by the sympathetic fibers.

There is increasing evidence that a localized neurogenic inflammation might be involved in the generation of acute edema, vasodilation and increased sweating.[200] The CNS is likely to play a significant role in the pathophysiology of CRPS, as noted by the extreme allodynia. There may even be a centrally mediated impulse abnormality in the motoneuron pool.[201] Although the precise mechanisms of CRPS are unclear, there are certainly both peripheral and central components that combine to form this very painful, disabling neuropathic condition.

Precipitating factors
The single common precipitating factor in CRPS is trauma associated with nerve injury. The traumatic event may be very minor or massive. In fact the amount of trauma helps determine the type of CRPS (discussed below). Another clinical feature of CRPS is that the pain does not begin immediately following the nerve injury, but is delayed by some time.

Diagnostic considerations

The International Association for the Study of Pain defines CRPS using the following clinical criteria[191]:

1. The syndrome usually, but not always, develops in the wake of an initiating noxious event (optional criterion).
2. There is continuing pain and allodynia and/or hyperalgesia, disproportionate to the initiating event; this precipitating event at times can appear trivial and heal quickly (mandatory criteria).
3. The pain becomes associated at some point in time with changes in skin blood flow, edema, and/or abnormal sweating in the region of the pain (mandatory criterion).
4. There is no evidence of another condition that could account for the pain and dysfunction (mandatory criterion).

According to the type of nerve injury, CRPS is further divided into two subcategories: CRPS I and CRPS II. In CRPS I the injury to the nerve is very minor and often not even associated with trauma that concerns the patient. For example, CRPS I may develop following a minor sprain, soft tissue trauma, frostbite, or skin lesions. A bone fracture or surgery can initiate the conditions. An important feature of CRPS I is that the severity of the symptoms is disproportionate to the trauma that caused the condition. CRPS I has replaced the term *reflex sympathetic dystrophy.*

In the case of CRPS II there has been a major injury to a relatively large peripheral nerve. CRPS II is often associated with major tissue injuries such as the crushing of a limb or amputation. CRPS II has replaced the term *causalgia.*

Management

Since the precise etiology of CRPS is unknown and likely to be multifactorial, the treatment remains quite elusive. It should be remembered that most of the evidence of CRPS is reported as it relates to injury in limbs. Although some CRPS-like symptoms are common to continuous neuropathic pain in the orofacial structures, many of these symptoms, such as trophic skin changes, significant swelling, and sweating are rarely seen in the face. CRPS is therefore not a condition that most dental practitioners will primarily treat. In fact CRPS requires a multidisciplinary approach, including neurologists, anesthesiologists, orthopedic specialists, physiotherapists, and psychologists.

Literature review outcome studies that investigate the management of CRPS are discouraging, finding little consistent information regarding pharmacologic agents and other methods of treatment. Certainly analgesics are important, along with the tricyclic antidepressants. GABA agonists such as baclofen, valproic acid, and benzodiazepines have been used with moderate effects. As with other neuropathic pain disorders, gabapentin has shown some promise. Transdermal application of the alpha-2 adrenoceptor agonist clonidine,[202,203] which is thought to prevent the release of catecholamines by a presynaptic action, may be helpful.

The key for the dental clinician is that CRPS is not a primary problem of the orofacial structures. It is useful for the dentist to know about this pain condition, but treatment should not be primarily managed out of a dental office. For additional information on CRPS, the reader should review more extensive texts dedicated to this subject.

SMP

Clinical characteristics

It has been recognized for a number of years that some pain conditions can be maintained by activity of the sympathetic nervous system. These pain conditions are therefore referred to as *sympathetically maintained pain.* These pains are often characterized by constant burning sensations that are frequently associated with a prior history of tissue damage. There are several different terms that have been used to describe pain conditions that involve the sympathetic nervous system. One of the original terms is *causalgia*. Causalgia was first reported in 1872 by Mitchell[204,205] as a condition associated with nerve damage to limbs of injured soldiers during the American Civil War. Causalgia was described as a painful burning condition usually felt in a limb that had received the trauma. The pain may appear immediately or be delayed for weeks or months. More recently, causalgia has been defined as burning pain, allodynia, and hyperpathia, usually in the hand or foot after partial injury of a nerve or one of its major branches.[206] Causalgia has been generally replaced by the term CRPS II.

Another term used to describe a pain condition associated with the sympathetic nervous system is *reflex sympathetic dystrophy*.[207,208] RSD is described as continuous pain in a portion of an extremity after trauma that does not involve a major nerve and is associated with sympathetic hyperactivity.[117] RSD has been generally replaced by the term CRPS I.

In 1986, Roberts[209] proposed a hypothesis that attempted to explain the mechanism behind pain conditions that were influenced by sympathetic activity. He coined the term *sympathetically maintained pain*. According to Roberts, SMP is characterized by a history of past physical trauma in the painful area, continuous burning pain, mechanical hyperalgesia and allodynia. Also included in his description was the relief of pain following a sympathetic blockade. If a patient has all of the symptoms but does not respond to a sympathetic block, the pain is called *sympathetically independent pain* (SIP).

Sympathetically maintained pains are characterized by pain in an area that is associated with prior trauma. The pain may not begin immediately following the trauma but in fact may present itself several weeks or months later. SMP is typically a constant, diffuse, intense, burning sensation, not necessarily confined to the sensory distribution of the injured nerve. The skin is usually sensitive and excruciatingly painful, even to innocuous stimulation such as touch, air drafts, thermal changes, vibration, noise, or emotional stress. Autonomic symptoms can be seen as changes in cutaneous temperature, color, texture, and perspiration but are rare in the orofacial structures.

Over time it has been appreciated that sympathetic activity can influence several of the continuous neuropathic pain conditions. Therefore, in the pain classification, a dotted line connects SMP to the subcategories of continuous neuropathic pain, both peripherally and centrally meditated. This is to acknowledge that any of these conditions may be influenced and/or maintained by even normal sympathetic activity (Fig 17-9).

Pathophysiology

SMP seems to begin with trauma to peripheral tissues and/or peripheral nerves. The primary afferent neuron carries the nociceptive input into the dorsal horn and synapses with the second-order neuron (Fig 17-10a). With time, this input can centrally sensitize the second-order neuron (ie, WDR neuron) as discussed in an earlier section. As the WDR neuron becomes sensitized, even normal mechanical input from the A-beta fibers can produce a nociceptive response (allodynia)[210] (Fig 17-10b). It appears that changes may occur at the original site of tissue damage that maintain activity of the primary afferents to continue the sensitization of the second-order neuron[211] (a peripheral generator). It is thought that following the trauma, alpha-1 adrenoreceptors are expressed on the primary afferent nociceptors and that these receptors are activated by norepinephrine released by the sympathetic efferents in the area[212,213]

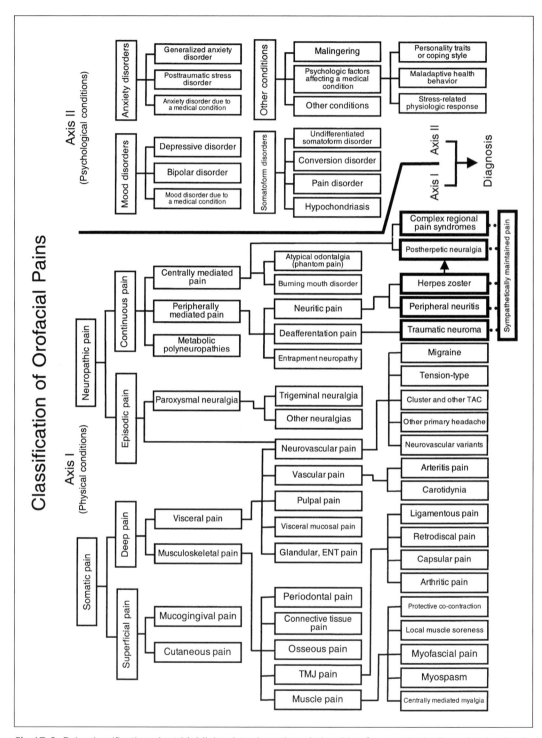

Fig 17-9 Pain classification chart highlighted to show the relationship of sympathetically maintained pain and the other continuous neuropathic pain conditions.

(Fig 17-10c). It is interesting to note that injection of norepinephrine in normal patients does not elicit a pain response. However, injection of norepinephrine in the area of a neuroma results in a marked increase in pain.[214] This suggests that SMPs do not arise from too much norepinephrine but rather from the presence of adrenergic receptors in the area of the tissue injury that are coupled to nociceptors. Therefore, even normal activity of the postganglionic sympathetic neurons is adequate to fire these altered primary afferents. Since normal activity of the sympathetics can activate the primary afferents, nociceptive input becomes constant, which further enhances the central sensitization of the second-order neuron. A self-maintaining loop is established, which is known as SMP.

Further contributing to this pain condition is the evidence that sympathetic activity may directly affect the second-order neurons in the dorsal horn and nucleus caudalis, contributing to the neuroplasticity and sensitization.[215] The findings that sympathetic activity can influence painful conditions both centrally and peripherally add to the understanding of many painful conditions and will hopefully lead to more effective therapies.

Precipitating factors

As already stated, trauma to peripheral tissues seems to be a precipitating factor in SMP. Fortunately, not all trauma results in this pain condition. At this time we do not know what unique characteristics are present to initiate this condition. In some instances, the trauma may be minor and not even associated with the condition. This is further complicated by the fact that SMP may not present immediately.

Since this condition is maintained and enhanced by sympathetic activity, it is not surprising to find that any condition that increases the sympathetic system will likely increase the pain experience. Increased levels of emotional stress and even visual or auditory stimuli can markedly increase the pain intensity.

Diagnostic considerations

SMPs are best diagnosed by the pain characteristics and clinical presentation. Confirmation of SMP is achieved by regional blockade of the sympathetic nerve input to the painful region. In the case of the orofacial structures, this is accomplished with a stellate ganglion block. Anesthetic blocking of the stellate ganglion should immediately reduce or eliminate the pain condition.

Although rare, SMP may cause a toothache of nondental origin. Toothache from this cause has descriptive characteristics that differ from those of true pulpal pain. The pain is described as a persistent, unremitting, only slightly variable, burning sensation in and around the tooth. It is characterized by a neuritic quality and is not characteristic of an odontogenous toothache (Case 33).

SMPs may be confused with masticatory pain (Case 34). They may be differentiated from masticatory pain by the following criteria:

1. The underlying ongoing, persistent, constant, diffusely located, burning sensation does not suggest masticatory pain, which is characterized by variability linked to functional demands and by an aching quality, the source of which can be clinically identified by manual palpation and analgesic blocking.
2. SMP can be differentially diagnosed by a stellate ganglion block.
3. As with all differential diagnosis, true masticatory pain should be identified by positive evidence, as obtained by a satisfactory and exacting examination by the examiner.

Management

Managing SMPs is no easy task. Much confusion still exists regarding etiology and pathophysiology, and without this knowl-

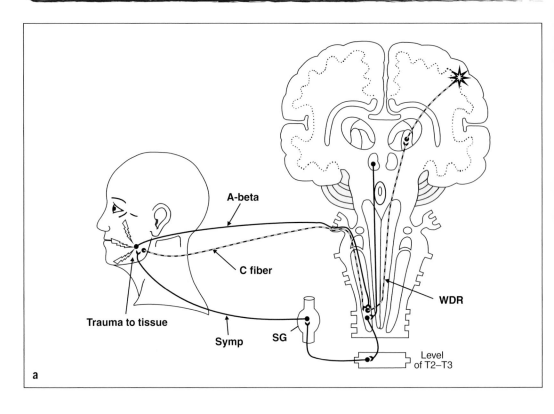

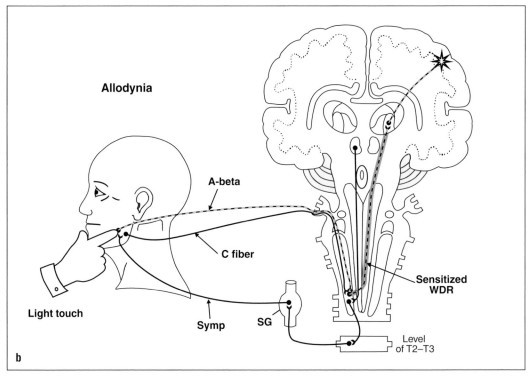

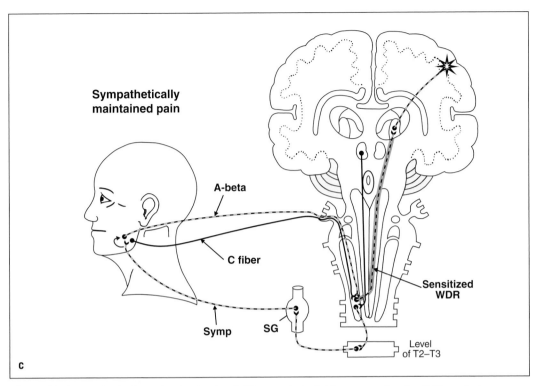

Sympathetically maintained pain

A-beta

C fiber

Symp   SG

Sensitized WDR

Level of T2–T3

c

Fig 17-10 Sympathetically maintained pain. *(a)* Trauma to facial tissues excites the C fibers that carry nociceptive impulses to the second-order neuron (WDR), which then relays the impulse to the higher centers, resulting in pain. Note that the sympathetic fibers (Symp) have been included in this diagram. The sympathetic fibers descend from the hypothalamus to the dorsal horn in the region of T2 and T3, where they exit the spinal column to enter the sympathetic chain. From there they ascend to the stellate ganglion (SG) and exit to innervate the facial tissues. *(b)* The afferent sensory input can lead to a sensitization of the WDR neuron (neuroplasticity), so that light touch (A-beta fiber stimulation) will produce pain (allodynia). *(c)* Release of norepinephrine by the sympathetic fibers in the area of the peripheral injury can excite the A-beta fibers, resulting in continued input to the sensitized second-order neuron. This establishes a self-maintaining loop known as sympathetically maintained pain.

edge, treatment is quite lacking. It is believed that the earlier the condition is treated, the better the results. This is likely due to the reduced sensitization or neuroplasticity of the central neurons. Medications such as clonidine have been suggested[213,216] as a topical agent that may reduce the sympathetic activity in the region of the peripheral generator. Clonidine is an alpha-2 agonist that suppresses norepinephrine release. Clonidine has also been used orally. Although it does provide some reduction in sympathetic activity, as demonstrated by decreased vasoconstrictor ice response, its actual reduction of pain may not be much better than that of placebo.[217]

Case 33 Sympathetically maintained pain felt in a tooth

Chief Complaint Right mandibular toothache.

History

A 45-year-old woman presented with mild to severe, variable but continuous, steady, dull, burning pain diffusely located in the mandibular right teeth and edentulous area, described as persistent toothache in the remaining teeth as well as phantom toothache in the mandibular right teeth and edentulous area.

The complaint began following an automobile accident in which the patient sustained injuries to the back and head. A neurologic examination at the time indicated a cerebral concussion and fracture of T-11, plus complaints that included transient leg numbness, headaches, facial paresthesias, and visual disturbance, although there were no abnormal sensory or motor nerve findings. All the cranial nerves were said to be intact.

After the accident, the patient felt toothache in the mandibular right first and second molars; after 2 weeks these were extracted without benefit. Two months later, the mandibular right second premolar was also extracted, but the complaint continued as before. Percodan is used to control the pain.

Examination

Intraoral: Recent extraction of the mandibular teeth is evident. Healing appears to be normal. The remaining teeth and mouth are clinically and radiographically negative for cause of the pain.

TMJs: Clinically normal.

Muscles: No tenderness or dysfunction noted.

Cervical: Marked pain to palpation of cervical muscles and right trapezius. Restriction to head rotation and bending.

Cranial nerves: Marked dysesthesia, hyperalgesia, and allodynia noted directly over the edentulous area. All other sensory and motor functions within normal limits.

Diagnostic tests: Analgesic blocking of the right mandibular and maxillary teeth did not arrest the pain, although satisfactory anesthesia was promptly obtained. The patient was referred to an anesthesiologist for consultation and diagnostic analgesic blocking of the right stellate ganglion. This block arrested the mandibular pains.

Impression

There does not appear to be any dental, oral, or masticatory cause for the complaint. The toothache and other pains appear to be mediated by afferent sympathetic fibers from the head. The stimulus appears to arise central to the level of intraoral analgesic blocking of the mandibular nerve. The neuritic-like pain appears to be part of a posttraumatic condition.

Diagnosis Sympathetically maintained pain referred as a toothache.

Case 34 Deafferentation pain, maintained by sympathetic activity

Chief Complaint
Left face and jaw pain.

History

A 41-year-old woman presented with mild, continuous, protracted, steady, dull, burning pain diffusely located in the left jaw and face and aggravated by peripheral stimulation of the entire painful area as well as by masticatory movements.

The complaint began about 6 months ago as pain following the extraction of several mandibular left posterior teeth. Initially, it was treated as an acute alveolitis, but the pain persisted after healing occurred. Soon it was felt as earache. The patient's ENT physician found the ear to be normal and advised that the dentist "adjust her bite." Her dentist replaced the missing teeth, without benefit. As the pain spread to the masseter, temporal, and orbital areas, the dentist adjusted the occlusion several times, prescribed ibuprofen and muscle relaxants, remade the partial denture, tried an anterior repositioning appliance, and injected corticosteroid into the left joint. When the complaint persisted, the patient was referred for a TMD evaluation. Presently, she is only taking the ibuprofen.

Examination

Intraoral: The teeth and mouth are clinically and radiographically negative for cause of pain. The left mandibular edentulous area is hypersensitive to touch. There is subjective increase in discomfort with all mandibular movements, but there is no identifiable masticatory dysfunction of any kind. The auricular, masseter, temporal, and orbital areas all seem to be hyperalgesic to touch.

TMJs: Both joints are clinically and radiographically normal.

Muscles: There is vague subjective discomfort in the masseter and temporal muscles with manual palpation but no muscular dysfunction of any kind.

Cervical: Within normal limits.

Cranial nerves: Marked dysesthesia, hyperalgesia, and allodynia noted directly over the edentulous area. All other sensory and motor functions within normal limits.

Diagnostic tests: Analgesic blocking of the left masseter and temporal muscles, followed by blocking of the left TMJ proper, did not arrest the complaint. Consultation with an anesthesiologist was requested for the purpose of making an analgesic block of the left stellate ganglion. This block arrested all left orofacial pain and two subsequent similar blocks repeated at weekly intervals eliminated the complaint without relapse.

Impression

The history, clinical course, and present behavioral characteristics suggested an autonomic involvement. This presumptive diagnosis was confirmed by analgesic blocking of the stellate ganglion.

Diagnosis
Deafferentation pain felt in the teeth and maintained by sympathetic activity.

Alpha-1 and alpha-2 agonists, such as phentolamine, have also been suggested to decrease the sympathetic activity and reduce the pain.[218] These medications are infused intravenously and therefore must be administered under proper supervision. Sometimes repeated infusions may gradually reduce the pain condition and therefore become of therapeutic benefit. For those patients who experienced a significant reduction of pain during a diagnostic stellate ganglion block, repeated blocks may also result in gradual pain reduction. These blocks can be repeated weekly until the pain is eliminated or until no more reduction is achieved.

Since SMPs are very difficult to manage, they are often best treated by a trained chronic pain specialist such as an appropriately trained anesthesiologist. It is most important for the clinician to recognize this type of pain condition, so that inappropriate treatments are avoided and the patient can be quickly managed by appropriately trained personnel. Remember, the sooner appropriate therapy is introduced, the more successful the results.

Metabolic Polyneuropathies

Clinical characteristics

The orofacial pain clinician needs to be aware that certain metabolic disorders can lead to neuropathies that may present as facial pain (Fig 17-11). In the medical arena, sensory complaints in the area of the mandible and mouth often escape notice or remain undiagnosed. This attests to the importance role of the dental practitioner in appreciating the etiologic connection between the metabolic condition and the neuropathic orofacial pain. Some of the more common disorders that can lead to metabolic polyneuropathies are diabetes, hypothyroidism, alcoholism, malnutrition,

and vitamin deficiencies. In most of these disorders the pain associated with the metabolic polyneuropathies is not found in the orofacial structures, but instead in other regions, especially the limbs. Although orofacial pain is rare, one must appreciate the possibilities when establishing the diagnosis so that proper therapy can be initiated. This section is added to this orofacial pain text for completeness and is not meant to provide detailed information regarding any of these disorders. For a more thorough review, other medical texts should be consulted.

Probably the most common metabolic polyneuropathy is associated with diabetes. One study found a prevalence of neuropathy in a diabetic population of 48%,[219] with the frequency increasing with age and the length of time the patient experienced the disease. Of these neuropathies however, orofacial pain was relatively rare. Fraser et al[220] reported that the median, ulnar, and lateral popliteal nerves were most commonly affected and cranial neuropathy was relatively uncommon. According to Irkec et al,[221] the incidence of cranial nerve involvement ranges anywhere from 3% to 14%.

Hypothyroid neuropathy is actually quite common, appearing in 71.8 % of patients with this disorder.[222] The most common type of hypothyroid neuropathy is a focal nerve involvement, such as median neuropathy at the wrist or ulnar neuropathy at the elbow. A common presentation of hypothyroid neuropathy is paresthesia of the distal extremities, especially the hands. Once again, this type of neuropathy is not often seen in the cranial nerves.

There appears to be a relationship between alcoholism and metabolic polyneuropathies, but the exact nature is uncertain. Scientists do not know whether alcoholism causes neuropathies directly or by way of malnutrition. Patients will divert money to buying alcohol and replace the protein in their diet with simple carbohydrates. This imbalance has been postulated to increase

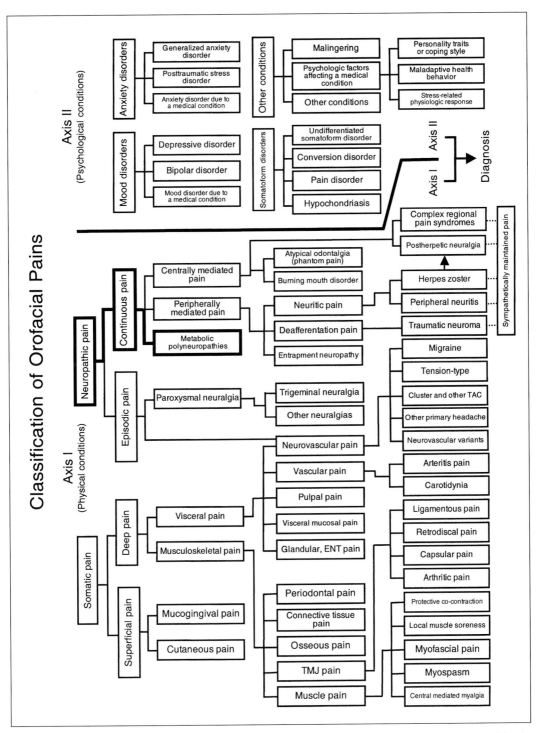

Fig 17-11 Pain classification chart highlighted to show the relationship of metabolic polyneuropathies to other orofacial pain disorders.

the load on the vitamin B_1 (thiamine) enzymatic system, thus increasing the requirement for vitamin B_1 in the diet.[222]

Pathophysiology

It is uncertain as to how these various metabolic disorders cause polyneuropathies. Perhaps each disorder affects the peripheral nerves differently, or there may be common peripheral and central mechanisms. Chronic hyperglycemia appears to be the main risk factor for diabetic polyneuropathies. It has been suggested that hyperglycemia causes damage to microvessels, leading to ischemia that eventually causes nerve injury.[219] Diabetes also causes changes in lipids, alcohol sugars, and myo-inositol that may also relate to the neuropathy.[223,224] Perhaps similar conditions are present with hypothyroidism, alcoholism, and vitamin deficiencies.

Precipitating factors

In each of the metabolic polyneuropathies, the specific underlining metabolic condition is responsible for the symptoms. Therefore the clinician needs to be cognizant of the orofacial pain patient's overall health and any systemic conditions so that these possibilities are not overlooked. A thorough history should uncover the likelihood of these disorders and when suspicion is raised, proper tests should be ordered (see chapter 8).

Diagnostic considerations

The diagnosis of a metabolic polyneuropathy begins with identifying the specific laboratory test used to confirm the presence of the metabolic condition in question. Once the disorder is confirmed, the patient should be referred to the appropriate medical specialist for a comprehensive workup and treatment plan.

Some authors have found that electrophysiologic testing may be helpful. Irkec et

al[221] reported that 70% of diabetics with confirmed polyneuropathies outside the facial also have prolonged facial nerve distal latencies. These distal latencies, as well as the amplitudes of muscle response to facial nerve stimulation, showed a statistically significant difference from controls.

Using electromyographic recording of the trigeminal reflexes and motor responses, Cruccu et al[225] looked at trigeminal nerve dysfunction in 50 patients with peripheral neuropathies. Trigeminal reflex recordings (early and late blink reflex after supraorbital stimulation, early and late masseter inhibitory reflex after mental stimulation, and jaw jerk) disclosed abnormalities caused by sensory trigeminal neuropathy in 13 out of 23 patients with severe diabetic polyneuropathy, and in none of 12 patients with mild diabetic polyneuropathy. Six patients had abnormal motor responses in facial or masseter muscles. The response affected most frequently was the masseter early inhibitory reflex (also called first silent period) after mental nerve stimulation, with its latency being strongly delayed. They concluded that peripheral polyneuropathies often cause subclinical damage to the trigeminal nerve, especially to its mandibular branch. They suggested that the nerve fibers running along the alveolar-mandibular pathway are exposed to more damage because of their cramped anatomic route in the mandibular canal and below the internal pterygoid muscle and fascia. The use of electrophysiologic data in identifying metabolic polyneuropathies has been suggested for diabetes and hypothyroidism, but the data are still very subjective and these are not considered standard diagnostic procedures.[222]

Management

Since the underling etiology of the metabolic polyneuropathy is the metabolic disorder, the primary treatment should be directed toward this condition. This is rarely within the practice of the orofacial pain practitioner. Therefore when this condition is identified, the patient should be immediately referred to the appropriate medical specialist to manage the systemic condition. The medical specialist should then develop the appropriate treatment plan and be in charge of carrying it out. The orofacial pain practitioner may supplement treatment for the neuropathy if it is agreed upon in advance by the medical specialist. It is important that both practitioners coordinate their roles in managing the patient's condition. It should be remembered that treatment of the neuropathic pain without managing the overall metabolic condition is counterproductive and may lead to worsening of the patient's pain and health.

The literature on managing metabolic neuropathies is directed more at management of the disease than the actual neuropathic condition. It is reasonable to believe that this pain condition will respond similar to other continuous neuropathic pain disorders, and therefore certain medications can be used in conjunction with the therapy provided by the medical specialist for the systemic disorder. A relatively conservative approach is the application of topical medications to the painful area. In some instances, topical application of local anesthetic can assist in reducing the ongoing nociceptive input and improve the condition. Any decrease in nociceptive input lessens the barrage of afferent input that may be responsible for the neuroplasticity. Capsaicin (Zostrix) can also be used to desensitize the primary afferent neurons.[125]

As with other continuous neuropathic pains, low dosage of tricyclic antidepressants (amitriptyline, 25 to 50 mg daily) may help reduce the pain experienced associated with metabolic polyneuropathies. Gabapentin (Neurontin) may also be helpful and should be attempted. If these fail, other anticonvulsants should be tried.

Summary

At this time, the management of neuropathic pains is both an exciting and frustrating area of study. The excitement stems from the recent significant research investigations into this most complex type of pain. Each day, new research provides a clearer understanding of the mechanisms responsible for this source of chronic suffering. The frustration felt by the clinician, however, stems from the present inability to effectively manage the neuropathic pain. Each day, new mechanisms, neurotransmitters, and receptor sites are being uncovered. However, additional research is required to discover a safe and effective manner to interrupt these pain processes. The development of effective treatment follows the understanding of etiology. The delay, however, is very frustrating to the suffering patient and the concerned clinician. Presently researchers are working on both peripheral and central methods of interrupting this type of pain. The author believes the profession is on the verge of making a major impact on this common source of chronic pain and suffering.

References

1. Merskey H. Clarifying definition of neuropathic pain. Pain 2002;96:408–409.
2. Bennett G. Neuropathic pain: An overview. In: Borsook D (ed). Molecular Neurobiology of Pain. Seattle, WA: IASP Press, 1997:109–113.
3. Boureau F, Doubrere JF, Luu M. Study of verbal description in neuropathic pain. Pain 1990; 42:145–152.
4. Walker AE. The differential diagnosis of trigeminal neuralgia. In: Hassler R, Walker AE (eds). Trigeminal Neuralgia. Stuttgart: Thieme, 1970:30–34.

5. McArdle MJ. Atypical facial neuralgia. In: Hassler R, Walker AE (eds). Trigeminal Neuralgia. Stuttgart: Thieme, 1970:35–42.

6. Stookey B, Ransohoff J. Trigeminal Neuralgia. Springfield, IL: Thomas, 1959:85–111.

7. Rappaport ZH, Devor M. Trigeminal neuralgia: The role of self-sustaining discharge in the trigeminal ganglion. Pain 1994;56:127–138.

8. Devor M, Amir R, Rappaport ZH. Pathophysiology of trigeminal neuralgia: The ignition hypothesis. Clin J Pain 2002;18:4–13.

9. Kerr FWL. Evidence for a peripheral etiology of trigeminal neuralgia. J Neurosurg 1967;(suppl 26):168–174.

10. Jensen TS, Rasmussen P, Reske-Nielsen E. Association of trigeminal neuralgia with multiple sclerosis: Clinical and pathological features. Acta Neurol Scand 1982;65:182–189.

11. Dalessio DJ. The major neuralgias, postinfectious neuritis, and atypical facial pain. In: Dalessio DJ, Silberstein SD. Wolff's Headache and Other Head Pain, ed 6. New York: Oxford University Press, 1993:345–364.

12. Finneson BE. Diagnosis and Management of Pain Syndromes. Philadelphia: Saunders, 1969.

13. Rovit RL, Murali R, Jannetta PJ. Trigeminal Neuralgia. Baltimore: Williams & Wilkins, 1990:1–77.

14. Earl C. Disorders of cranial nerves V, VII, IX, and XII. In: Asbury AK, Mackhann GM, McDonald WI (eds). Diseases of the Nervous System, Clinical Neurobiology. Philadelphia: Saunders, 1986:577–579.

15. Gardner WJ. Trigeminal neuralgia. In: Hassler R, Walker AE (eds). Trigeminal Neuralgia. Stuttgart: Thieme, 1970:162–165.

16. Love S, Coakham HB. Trigeminal neuralgia: Pathology and pathogenesis. Brain 2001;124:2347–2360.

17. Pyen JS, Whang K, Hu C, et al. Tic convulsif caused by cerebellopontine angle schwannoma. Yonsei Med J 2001;42:255–257.

18. Iwasaki K, Kondo A, Otsuka S, Hasegawa K, Ohbayashi T. Painful tic convulsif caused by a brain tumor: Case report and review of the literature. Neurosurgery 1992;30:916–919.

19. Fromm GH, Graff-Radford SB, Terrence CF, Sweet WH. Pre-trigeminal neuralgia. Neurology 1990;40:1493–1495.

20. Juniper RP, Glynn CJ. Association between paroxysmal trigeminal neuralgia and atypical facial pain. Br J Oral Maxillofac Surg 1999;37:444–447.

21. Stevens JC. Cranial neuralgias. J Craniomandib Disord Facial Oral Pain 1987;1:51–53.

22. Gorlin RJ, Pindborg JJ. Syndromes of the Head and Neck. New York: McGraw-Hill, 1964:201–203.

23. Walker AE. Neuralgia of the glossopharyngeal, vagus, and intermedius nerves. In: Knighton RS, Dumke PR (eds). Pain. Boston: Little, Brown, 1966:421–429.

24. Saper JR, Silberstein SD, Gordon CD, Hamel RL. Handbook of Headache Management. Baltimore: Williams & Wilkins, 1993:128–129.

25. Kerr FWL, Miller RH. The pathology of trigeminal neuralgia: Electron microscopic studies. Arch Neurol 1966;15:308–319.

26. Kerr FWL. Fine structure and functional characteristics of the primary trigeminal neuron. In: Hassler R, Walker AE (eds). Trigeminal Neuralgia. Stuttgart: Thieme, 1970:11–21.

27. De Ridder D, Moller A, Verlooy J, Cornelissen M, De Ridder L. Is the root entry/exit zone important in microvascular compression syndromes? Neurosurgery 2002;51:427–433; discussion 433–434.

28. Dandy WE. Concerning the cause of trigeminal neuralgia. Am J Surg 1934;24:447–455.

29. Jannetta PJ. Neurocompression in cranial nerve and systemic disease. Ann Surg 1980;192:518–525.

30. Youmans JR. Neurological Surgery. Philadelphia: Saunders, 1973:2959–3003.

31. Kobata H, Kondo A, Iwasaki K. Cerebellopontine angle epidermoids presenting with cranial nerve hyperactive dysfunction: Pathogenesis and long-term surgical results in 30 patients. Neurosurgery 2002;50:276–285; discussion 285–286.

32. Revuelta R, Soto-Hernandez JL, Vales LO, Gonzalez RH. Cerebellopontine angle cysticercus and concurrent vascular compression in a case of trigeminal neuralgia. Clin Neurol Neurosurg 2003;106:19–22.

33. Kaemmerer EF. A review of the etiologic factors in trigeminal neuralgia. In: Hassler R, Walker AE (eds). Trigeminal Neuralgia. Stuttgart: Thieme, 1970:175–179.

34. Sweet WH, Wepsic JG. Controlled thermocoagulation of trigeminal ganglion and rootlets for differential destruction of pain fibers: I. Trigeminal neuralgia. J Neurosurg 1974;39:143–156.

35. Devor M, Govrin-Lippmann R, Rappaport ZH. Mechanism of trigeminal neuralgia: An ultrastructural analysis of trigeminal root specimens obtained during microvascular decompression surgery. J Neurosurg 2002;96:532–543.

36. Headache Classification Committee of the International Headache Society. The International Classification of Headache Disorders: 2nd edition. Cephalalgia 2004;24(suppl 1):9–160.

37. Tremont-Lukats IW, Megeff C, Backonja MM. Anticonvulsants for neuropathic pain syndromes: Mechanisms of action and place in therapy. Drugs 2000;60:1029–1052.

38. Carrazana E, Mikoshiba I. Rationale and evidence for the use of oxcarbazepine in neuropathic pain. J Pain Symptom Manage 2003;25: S31–S35.

39. Backonja MM. Use of anticonvulsants for treatment of neuropathic pain. Neurology 2002;59: S14–S17.

40. Macdonald RL, Kelly KM. Antiepileptic drug mechanisms of action. Epilepsia 1995;36(suppl 2):S2–S12.

41. Burchiel KJ. Carbamazepine inhibits spontaneous activity in experimental neuromas. Exp Neurol 1988;102:249–253.

42. Fromm GH. Pharmacological consideration of anticonvulsants. Headache 1969;9:35–41.

43. Beydoun A, Kutluay E. Oxcarbazepine. Expert Opin Pharmacother 2002;3:59–71.

44. Zakrzewska JM, Patsalos PN. Long-term cohort study comparing medical (oxcarbazepine) and surgical management of intractable trigeminal neuralgia. Pain 2002;95:259–266.

45. Ichikawa K, Koyama N, Kiguchi S, Kojima M, Yokota T. Inhibitory effect of oxcarbazepine on high-frequency firing in peripheral nerve fibers. Eur J Pharmacol 2001;420:119–122.

46. Backonja MM. Anticonvulsants (antineuropathics) for neuropathic pain syndromes. Clin J Pain 2000;16:S67–S72.

47. Taylor CP, Gee NS, Su TZ, et al. A summary of mechanistic hypotheses of gabapentin pharmacology. Epilepsy Res 1998;29:233–249.

48. Petroff OA, Rothman DL, Behar KL, Lamoureux D, Mattson RH. The effect of gabapentin on brain gamma-aminobutyric acid in patients with epilepsy. Ann Neurol 1996;39:95–99.

49. Cheshire WP Jr. Defining the role for gabapentin in the treatment of trigeminal neuralgia: A retrospective study. J Pain 2002;3:137–142.

50. McLean MJ, Bukhari AA, Wamil AW. Effects of topiramate on sodium-dependent action-potential firing by mouse spinal cord neurons in cell culture. Epilepsia 2000;41(suppl 1): S21–S24.

51. Schneiderman JH. Topiramate: Pharmacokinetics and pharmacodynamics. Can J Neurol Sci 1998;25:S3–S5.

52. Sindrup SH, Jensen TS. Pharmacotherapy of trigeminal neuralgia. Clin J Pain 2002;18: 22–27.

53. Terrence CF, Fromm GH, Tenicela R. Baclofen as an analgesic in chronic peripheral nerve disease. Eur Neurol 1985;24:380–385.

54. Fromm GH, Terrence CF, Maroon JC. Trigeminal neuralgia. Current concepts regarding etiology and pathogenesis. Arch Neurol 1984;41: 1204–1207.

55. Solaro C, Messmer Uccelli M, Uccelli A, Leandri M, Mancardi GL. Low-dose gabapentin combined with either lamotrigine or carbamazepine can be useful therapies for trigeminal neuralgia in multiple sclerosis. Eur Neurol 2000;44: 45–48.

56. Xie X, Lancaster B, Peakman T, Garthwaite J. Interaction of the antiepileptic drug lamotrigine with recombinant rat brain type IIA Na+ channels and with native Na+ channels in rat hippocampal neurones. Pflugers Arch 1995; 430:437–446.

57. Teoh H, Fowler LJ, Bowery NG. Effect of lamotrigine on the electrically-evoked release of endogenous amino acids from slices of dorsal horn of the rat spinal cord. Neuropharmacology 1995;34:1273–1278.

58. Ziccardi VB, Janosky JE, Patterson GT, Jannetta PJ. Peripheral trigeminal nerve surgery for patients with atypical facial pain. J Craniomaxillofac Surg 1994;22:355–360.

59. Freemont AJ, Millac P. The place of peripheral neurectomy in the management of trigeminal neuralgia. Postgrad Med J 1981;57:75–76.

60. Wilkinson HA. Trigeminal nerve peripheral branch phenol/glycerol injections for tic douloureux. J Neurosurg 1999;90:828–832.

61. Goto F, Ishizaki K, Yoshikawa D, Obata H, Arii H, Terada M. The long lasting effects of peripheral nerve blocks for trigeminal neuralgia using high concentration of tetracaine dissolved in bupivacaine. Pain 1999;79:101–103.

62. Wood KM. The use of phenol as a neurolytic agent: A review. Pain 1978;5:205–229.

63. Silverberg GD, Britt RH. Percutaneous radiofrequency rhizotomy in the treatment of trigeminal neuralgia. West J Med 1978;129:97–100.

64. Sengupta RP, Stunden RJ. Radiofrequency thermocoagulation of Gasserian ganglion and its rootlets for trigeminal neuralgia. Br Med J 1977;1:142–143.

65. Gregg JM, Banerjoe T, Ghia JN, Campbell R. Radiofrequency thermoneurolysis of peripheral nerves for control of trigeminal neuralgia. Pain 1978;5:231–243.

66. Young RF. Glycerol rhizolysis for treatment of trigeminal neuralgia. J Neurosurg 1988;69:39–45.

67. Meglio M, Cioni B. Percutaneous procedures for trigeminal neuralgia: Microcompression versus radiofrequency thermocoaulation. Pain 1989;38:9–16.

68. Natarajan M. Percutaneous trigeminal ganglion balloon compression: Experience in 40 patients. Neurol India 2000;48:330–332.

69. Taarnhoj P. Decompression of the trigeminal root as treatment in trigeminal neuralgia: Preliminary communication. J Neurosurg 1952;9:288–298.

70. Love JG. Decompression of the gasserian ganglion and posterior root; a new treatment for trigeminal neuralgia; preliminary report. Mayo Clin Proc 1952;27:257–258.

71. Janetta PJ. Treatment of trigeminal neuralgia by suboccipital and transtentorial cranial operations. Clin Neurosurg 1977;24:538–549.

72. Hitotsumatsu T, Matsushima T, Inoue T. Microvascular decompression for treatment of trigeminal neuralgia, hemifacial spasm, and glossopharyngeal neuralgia: Three surgical approach variations: Technical note. Neurosurgery 2003;53:1436–1441; discussion 1442–1443.

73. Kalkanis SN, Eskandar EN, Carter BS, Barker FG 2nd. Microvascular decompression surgery in the United States, 1996 to 2000: Mortality rates, morbidity rates, and the effects of hospital and surgeon volumes. Neurosurgery 2003;52:1251–1261; discussion 1261–1262.

74. Bederson JB, Wilson CB. Evaluation of microvascular decompression and partial sensory rhizotomy in 252 cases of trigeminal neuralgia. J Neurosurg 1989;71:359–367.

75. Ishikawa M, Nishi S, Aoki T, et al. Operative findings in cases of trigeminal neuralgia without vascular compression: Proposal of a different mechanism. J Clin Neurosci 2002;9:200–204.

76. Sato J, Perl ER. Adrenergic excitation of cutaneous pain receptors induced by peripheral nerve injury. Science 1991;251:1608–1610.

77. Xie YK, Xiao WH, Li HQ. The relationship between new ion channels and ectopic discharges from a region of nerve injury. Sci China B 1993;36:68–74.

78. Devor M. Neuropathic pain and injured nerve: Peripheral mechanisms. Br Med Bull 1991;47:619–630.

79. Devor M, Govrin-Lippmann R, Angelides K. Na+ channel immunolocalization in peripheral mammalian axons and changes following nerve injury and neuroma formation. J Neurosci 1993;13:1976–1992.

80. Dubner R, Hylden JLK, Nahin RL, Traub RJ. Neuronal plasticity in the superficial dorsal horn following peripheral tissue inflammation and nerve injury. In: Cervero F, Bennett GJ, Headley PM (eds). Processing of Sensory Information in the Superficial Dorsal Horn of the Spinal Cord. New York: Plenum, 1989:429–442.

81. Torebjork HE, Lundeberg L, LaMotte RH. Central changes in processing of mechanoreceptive input in capsaicin-induced secondary hyperalgesia in humans. J Physiol 1992;448:765–780.

82. Ren K, Dubner R. Central nervous system plasticity and persistent pain. J Orofac Pain 1999;13:155–163; discussion 164–171.

83. Yu XM, Sessle BJ, Haas DA, Izzo A, Vernon H, Hu JW. Involvement of NMDA receptor mechanisms in jaw electromyographic activity and plasma extravasation induced by inflammatory irritant application to temporomandibular joint region of rats. Pain 1996;68:169–178.

84. Cairns BE, Sessle BJ, Hu JW. Temporomandibular-evoked jaw muscle reflex: Role of brain stem NMDA and non-NMDA receptors. Neuroreport 2001;12:1875–1878.

85. Coderre TJ, Katx J, Vaccarino AL, Melzack R. Contribution of central neuroplasticity to pathological pain: Review of clinical and experimental evidence. Pain 1993;52:259–285.

86. Woolf CJ, Thompson WN. The induction and maintenance of central sensitization is dependent on N-methyl-D-aspartic acid receptor activation; Implications for the treatment of post-injury pain hypersensitivity states. Pain 1991;44:293–300.

87. Abbadie C, Besson JM, Calvino B. c-Fos expression in the spinal cord and pain-related symptoms induced by chronic arthritis in the rat are prevented by pretreatment with Freund adjuvant. J Neurosci 1994;14:5865–5871.

88. Rowbotham M, Petersen K, Fields HL. Is postherpetic neuralgia more than one disorder? Pain Forum 1998;7:231–237.

89. Woolf CJ, Shortland P, Coggeshall RE. Peripheral nerve injury triggers central sprouting of myelinated afferents. Nature 1992;355:75–78.

90. Ejlersen E, Anderson HB, Eliasen K, Mogensen T. A comparison between preincisional and postincisional lidocaine infiltration and postoperative pain. Anesth Analg 1992;74:495–498.

91. Jebeles JA, Reilly JS, Gutierrez JF, Bradley EL Jr, Kissin I. The effect of pre-incisional infiltration of tonsils with bupivacaine on the pain following tonsillectomy under general anesthesia. Pain 1991;47:305–308.

92. McQuay HJ, Carroll D, Moore RA. Postoperative orthopedic pain: The effects of opiate premedication and local anesthetic blocks. Pain 1988;33:291–295.

93. Ringrose NH, Cross MJ. Femoral nerve block in knee joint surgery. Am J Sports Med 1984;12:398–402.

94. Linton SJ, Hellsing AL, Andersson D. A controlled study of the effects of an early intervention on acute musculoskeletal pain problems. Pain 1993;54:353–359.

95. Wolff HG, Wolf S. Pain. Springfield, IL: Thomas, 1958.

96. Agnew DC. Painful neurological disorders. In: Aronoff GM (ed). Evaluation and Treatment of Chronic Pain. Baltimore: Urban & Schwarzenberg, 1985:65–67.

97. LaBanc JP, Epker BN. Serious inferior alveolar nerve dysesthesia after endodontic procedure: Report of three cases. J Am Dent Assoc 1984;108:605–607.

98. Hadar T, Tovi F, Sidi J, Sarov B, Sarov I. Specific IgG and IgA antibodies to herpes simplex virus and varicella zoster virus in acute peripheral facial palsy patients. J Med Virol 1983;12:237–245.

99. Burgess RC, Michaels L, Bale JF Jr, Smith RJ. Polymerase chain reaction amplification of herpes simplex viral DNA from the geniculate ganglion of a patient with Bell's palsy. Ann Otol Rhinol Laryngol 1994;103:775–779.

100. Pachner AR, Steere AC. The triad of neurologic manifestations of Lyme disease: Meningitis, cranial neuritis, and radiculoneuritis. Neurology 1985;35:47–53.

101. Clark JR, Carlson RD, Sasaki CT, Pachner AR, Steere AC. Facial paralysis in Lyme disease. Laryngoscope 1985;95:1341–1345.

102. Eagle WW. Elongated styloid process: Further observations and a new syndrome. Arch Otolaryngol Head Neck Surg 1948;47:630–640.

103. Lagalla G, Logullo F, Di Bella P, Provinciali L, Ceravolo MG. Influence of early high-dose steroid treatment on Bell's palsy evolution. Neurol Sci 2002;23:107–112.

104. Austin JR, Peskind SP, Austin SG, Rice DH. Idiopathic facial nerve paralysis: A randomized double blind controlled study of placebo versus prednisone. Laryngoscope 1993;103:1326–1333.

105. Mitchell BM, Bloom DC, Cohrs RJ, Gilden DH, Kennedy PG. Herpes simplex virus-1 and varicella-zoster virus latency in ganglia. J Neurovirol 2003;9:194–204.

106. Straus SE, Reinhold W, Smith HA, et al. Endonuclease analysis of viral DNA from varicella and subsequent zoster infections in the same patient. N Engl J Med 1984;311:1362–1364.

107. Shepp DH, Dandliker PS, Meyers JD. Treatment of varicella-zoster virus infection in severely immunocompromised patients. N Engl J Med 1986;314:208–212.

108. Johnson RW. Herpes zoster in the immunocompetent patient: Management of post-herpetic neuralgia. Herpes 2003;10:38–45.

109. Wakisaka H, Kobayashi N, Mominoki K, et al. Herpes simplex virus in the vestibular ganglion and the geniculate ganglion—Role of loose myelin. J Neurocytol 2001;30:685–693.

110. Carreno M, Ona M, Melon S, Llorente JL, Diaz JJ, Suarez C. Amplification of herpes simplex virus type 1 DNA in human geniculate ganglia from formalin-fixed, nonembedded temporal bones. Otolaryngol Head Neck Surg 2000;123:508–511.

111. Opstelten W, van Wijck AJ, Stolker RJ. Interventions to prevent postherpetic neuralgia: Cutaneous and percutaneous techniques. Pain 2004;107:202–206.

112. Gobel S, Binck JM. Degenerative changes in primary trigeminal axons and in neurons in nucleus caudalis following tooth pulp extirpation in the cat. Brain Res 1977;132:347–354.

113. Gregg JM. Posttraumatic pain: Experimental trigeminal neuropathy. J Oral Surg 1971;29:260–267.

114. Wall PD, Scadding JW, Tomkiewicz MM. The production and prevention of experimental anesthesia dolorosa. Pain 1979;6:175–182.

115. Wall PD, Devor M. Sensory afferent impulses originate from dorsal root ganglia as well as from the periphery in normal and nerve injured rats. Pain 1983;17:321–339.

116. Mozsary PG, Middleton RA. Microsurgical reconstruction of the infraorbital nerves. J Oral Maxillofac Surg 1983;41:697–700.

117. Merrill RG. Oral neurosurgical procedures for nerve injuries. In: Walker RV (ed). Oral Surgery. London: Livingstone, 1970:131–140.

118. LaBanc JP, Epker BN. Serious inferior alveolar dysesthesia after endodontic procedure: Report of three cases. J Am Dent Assoc 1984;108:605–607.

119. Wessberg GA, Wolford LM, Epker BN. Experiences with microsurgical reconstruction of the inferior alveolar nerve. J Oral Maxillofac Surg 1982;40:651–655.

120. Mozsary PG, Syers CS. Microsurgical correction of the injured inferior alveolar nerve. J Oral Maxillofac Surg 1985;43:353–358.

121. Noma H, Kakizawa T, Yamane G, Sasaki K. Repair of the mandibular nerve by autogenous grafting after partial resection of the mandible. J Oral Maxillofac Surg 1986;44:31–36.

122. Kaban LB, Upton J. Cross mental nerve graft for restoration of lip sensation after inferior alveolar nerve damage: Report of case. J Oral Maxillofac Surg 1986;44:649–651.

123. LaBanc JP, Epker BN, Jones DL, Milam S. Nerve sharing by an interpositional sural nerve graft between the great auricular and inferior alveolar nerve to restore lower lip sensation. J Oral Maxillofac Surg 1987;45:621–627.

124. Mozsary PG, Middleton RA. Microsurgical reconstruction of the lingual nerve. J Oral Maxillofac Surg 1984;42:415–420.

125. Epstein JB, Marcoe JH. Topical application of capsaicin for treatment of oral neuropathic pain and trigeminal neuralgia. Oral Surg Oral Med Oral Pathol 1994;77:135–140.

126. Nagy JI, Hunt SP, Iversen LL. Effects of capsaicin on dorsal root afferents. In: Bonica JJ, Lindblom U, Iggo A (eds). Proceedings of the Third World Congress on Pain, vol 5, Advances in Pain Research and Therapy. New York: Raven Press, 1983:77–82.

127. Ainsworth A, Hall P, Wall PD. Effects of capsaicin applied locally to adult peripheral nerves: II. Anatomy and enzyme and peptide chemistry of peripheral nerve and spinal cord. Pain 1981;11:379–388.

128. Buck SH, Miller MS, Burks TF. Specific sensory deficits in adult guinea pigs induced by the putative substance P neurotoxin, capsaicin, and its active analogs [abstract]. Pain 1981;11(suppl 1):134.

129. Fitzgerald M. Capsaicin and sensory neurons: A review. Pain 1983;15:109–130.

130. Rozen TD. Relief of anesthesia dolorosa with gabapentin. Headache 1999;39:761–762.

131. Rees RT, Harris M. Atypical odontalgia: Differential diagnosis and treatment. Br J Oral Surg 1978;16:212–218.

132. Marbach J, Hulbrock J, Hohnn C, Segal AG. Incidence of phantom tooth pain: An atypical facial neuralgia. Oral Surg Oral Med Oral Pathol 1982;53:190–193.

133. Marbach JJ. Phantom tooth pain. J Endod 1978;4:362–371.

134. Rees RT, Harris M. Atypical odontalgia. Br J Oral Surg 1979;16:212–218.

135. Brooke RI. Atypical odontalgia. J Oral Surg 1980;49:196–199.

136. Moskowitz MA. The neurobiology of vascular head pain. Ann Neurol 1984;16:157–168.

137. Lascelles RG. Atypical facial pain and depression. Br J Psychiatry 1966;112:651–659.

138. Kreisberg MK. Atypical odontalgia: Differential diagnosis and treatment. J Am Dent Assoc 1982;104:852–854.

139. Graff-Radford SB, Solberg WK. Atypical odontalgia. J Craniomandib Disord Facial Oral Pain 1992;6:260–266.

140. Smith DP, Pilling LF, Pearson JS, Rushton JG, Goldstein NP, Gibilisco JA. A psychiatric study of atypical facial pain. Can Med Assoc J 1969;11:286–291.

141. Magni G, Moresch C, Rigatti-Luchini S, Merskey H. Prospective study on the relationship between depressive symptoms and chronic musculoskeletal pain. Pain 1994;56:289–297.

142. Rumsfield JA, West DP. Topical capsaicin in dermatologic and peripheral pain disorders. Ann Pharmacother 1991;25:381–387.

143. Bernstein JE, Bickers DR, Dahl MV, Roshal JY. Treatment of chronic postherpetic neuralgia with topical capsaicin. J Am Acad Dermatol 1987;17:93–96.

144. Rhodus NL, Carlson CR, Miller CS. Burning mouth (syndrome) disorder. Quintessence Int 2003;34:587–593.

145. Grushka M. Clinical features of burning mouth syndrome. Oral Surg Oral Med Oral Pathol 1987;63:30–36.

146. Danhauer SC, Miller CS, Rhodus NL, Carlson CR. Impact of criteria-based diagnosis of burning mouth syndrome on treatment outcome. J Orofac Pain 2002;16:305–311.

147. Hampf G. Dilemma in treatment of patients suffering from orofacial dysaesthesia. Int J Oral Maxillofac Surg 1987;16:397–401.

148. Bergdahl M, Bergdahl J. Burning mouth syndrome: Prevalence and associated factors. J Oral Pathol Med 1999;28:350–354.

149. Basker RM, Sturdee DW, Davenport JC. Patients with burning mouths. A clinical investigation of causative factors, including the climacteric and diabetes. Br Dent J 1978;145:9–16.

150. Ship JA, Grushka M, Lipton JA, Mott AE, Sessle BJ, Dionne RA. Burning mouth syndrome: An update. J Am Dent Assoc 1995;126:842–853.

151. Gorsky M, Silverman S Jr, Chinn H. Burning mouth syndrome: A review of 98 cases. J Oral Med 1987;42:7–9.

152. Maresky LS, van der Bijl P, Gird I. Burning mouth syndrome. Evaluation of multiple variables among 85 patients. Oral Surg Oral Med Oral Pathol 1993;75:303–307.

153. Zegarelli DJ. Burning mouth: An analysis of 57 patients. Oral Surg Oral Med Oral Pathol 1984;58:34–38.

154. Samaranayake LP, Lamb AB, Lamey PJ, Mac-Farlane TW. Oral carriage of Candida species and coliforms in patients with burning mouth syndrome. J Oral Pathol Med 1989;18:233–235.

155. Gorsky M, Silverman S Jr, Chinn H. Clinical characteristics and management outcome in the burning mouth syndrome. An open study of 130 patients. Oral Surg Oral Med Oral Pathol 1991;72:192–195.

156. Grushka M, Epstein JB, Gorsky M. Burning mouth syndrome. Am Fam Physician 2002;65:615–620.

157. Lamey PJ, Lamb AB. Prospective study of aetiological factors in burning mouth syndrome. Br Med J (Clin Res Ed) 1988;296:1243–1246.

158. Hatch CL. Glossodynia as an oral manifestation of diabetes mellitus. Ear Nose Throat J 1989;68:782–785.

159. Silverman S Jr. Oral changes in metabolic diseases. Postgrad Med 1971;49:106–110.

160. Brooke RI, Seganski DP. Etiology and investigation of the sore mouth. Dent J 1977;43:504–506.

161. Main DM, Basker RM. Patients complaining of a burning mouth. Further experience in clinical assessment and management. Br Dent J 1983;154:206–211.

162. Lamey PJ, Hammond A, Allam BF, McIntosh WB. Vitamin status of patients with burning mouth syndrome and the response to replacement therapy. Br Dent J 1986;160:81–84.

163. Lamey PJ, Lewis MA. Oral medicine in practice: Burning mouth syndrome. Br Dent J 1989;167:197–200.

164. Rhodus NL, Liljemark W, Bloomquist C, Bereuter J. Candida albicans levels in patients with Sjögren's syndrome before and after long-term use of pilocarpine hydrochloride: A pilot study. Quintessence Int 1998;29:705–710.

165. Glick D, Ben-Aryeh H, Gutman D, Szargel R. Relation between idiopathic glossodynia and salivary flow rate and content. Int J Oral Surg 1976;5:161–165.

166. Rhodus NL. Xerostomia and glossodynia in patients with autoimmune disorders. Ear Nose Throat J 1989;68:791–794.

167. Brown RS, Krakow AM, Douglas T, Choksi SK. "Scalded mouth syndrome" caused by angiotensin converting enzyme inhibitors: Two case reports. Oral Surg Oral Med Oral Pathol Oral Radiol Endod 1997;83:665–667.

168. Savino LB, Haushalter NM. Lisinopril-induced "scalded mouth syndrome." Ann Pharmacother 1992;26:1381–1382.

169. Glass BJ. Drug-induced xerostomia as a cause of glossodynia. Ear Nose Throat J 1989;68:776, 779–781.

170. Derogatis LR. SCL-90-R: Administration, Scoring and Procedures Manual-II for the Revised Version. Towson, MD: Clinical Psychometric Research, 1977.

171. Turk DC, Rudy TE. Toward a comprehensive assessment of chronic pain patients: A multiaxial approach. Behav Res Ther 1987;25:237–249.

172. Carlson CR, Miller CS, Reid KI. Psychosocial profiles of patients with burning mouth syndrome. J Orofac Pain 2000;14:59–64.

173. McCabe JF, Basker RM. Tissue sensitivity to acrylic resin. A method of measuring the residual monomer content and its clinical application. Br Dent J 1976;140:347–350.

174. Sreebny LM, Yu A, Green A, Valdini A. Xerostomia in diabetes mellitus. Diabetes Care 1992;15:900–904.

175. Grushka M, Epstein J, Mott A. An open-label, dose escalation pilot study of the effect of clonazepam in burning mouth syndrome. Oral Surg Oral Med Oral Pathol Oral Radiol Endod 1998;86:557–561.

176. De Marages JH, Rierlord BP. The outcome of patients with herpes zoster. Arch Dermatol 1957;75:193–196.

177. Watson CP, Evans RJ, Watt VR. Post-herpetic neuralgia and topical capsaicin. Pain 1988;3:333–340.

178. Sweet WH. Trigeminal neuralgia. In: Alling CC, Mahan PE (eds). Facial Pain. Philadelphia: Lea & Febiger, 1977:71–93.

179. Watson C, Morshead C, Van der Kooy D, Deck J, Evans RJ. Post-herpetic neuralgia: Postmortem analysis of a case. Pain 1988;34:129–138.

180. Watson CPN, Evans RJ. Post-herpetic neuralgia: A review. Arch Neurol 1986;43:836–840.

181. Dworkin RH, Schmader KE. Treatment and prevention of postherpetic neuralgia. Clin Infect Dis 2003;36:877–882.

182. Fox CH. Tricyclics and opioids effective for treatment of postherpetic neuralgia. J Fam Pract 2003;52:517–518.

183. Singh D, Kennedy DH. The use of gabapentin for the treatment of postherpetic neuralgia. Clin Ther 2003;25:852–889.

184. Stacey BR, Glanzman RL. Use of gabapentin for postherpetic neuralgia: Results of two randomized, placebo-controlled studies. Clin Ther 2003;25:2597–2608.

185. Curran MP, Wagstaff AJ. Gabapentin: In postherpetic neuralgia. CNS Drugs 2003;17:975–982.

186. Quan D, Wellish M, Gilden DH. Topical ketamine treatment of postherpetic neuralgia. Neurology 2003;60:1391–1392.

187. Suzuki H, Ogawa S, Nakagawa H, et al. Cryocautery of sensitized skin areas for the relief of pain due to postherpetic neuralgia. Pain 1980; 9:355–362.

188. Kunc Z. Vertical trigeminal partial nucleotomy. In: Bonica JJ, Liebeskind JC, Albe-Fessard DG (eds). Proceedings of the Second World Congress on Pain, vol 3, Advances in Pain Research and Therapy. New York: Raven Press, 1979: 325–330.

189. Schvarez JR. Stereotactic spinal trigeminal nucleotomy for dysesthetic facial pain. In: Bonica JJ, Liebeskind JC, Albe-Fessard DG (eds). Proceedings of the Second World Congress on Pain, vol 3, Advances in Pain Research and Therapy. New York: Raven Press, 1979:331–336.

190. Tasker RR. Surgical approaches to the primary afferent and the spinal cord. In: Fields HL, Dubner R, Cervero F (eds). Proceedings of the Fourth World Congress on Pain: Seattle, vol 9, Advances in Pain Research and Therapy. New York: Raven Press, 1985:799–824.

191. Merskey H, Bogduk N. Classification of Chronic Pain: Descriptions of Chronic Pain Syndromes and Definition of Terms, ed 2. Seattle: IASP Press, 1994.

192. Wasner G, Backonja MM, Baron R. Traumatic neuralgias: Complex regional pain syndromes (reflex sympathetic dystrophy and causalgia): Clinical characteristics, pathophysiological mechanisms and therapy. Neurol Clin 1998; 16:851–868.

193. Ochoa JL. Truths, errors, and lies around "reflex sympathetic dystrophy" and "complex regional pain syndrome." J Neurol 1999;246: 875–879.

194. Verdugo RJ, Ochoa JL. Abnormal movements in complex regional pain syndrome: Assessment of their nature. Muscle Nerve 2000;23:198–205.

195. Ciccone DS, Bandilla EB, Wu W. Psychological dysfunction in patients with reflex sympathetic dystrophy. Pain 1997;71:323–333.

196. Van Houdenhove B, Vasquez G, Onghena P, et al. Etiopathogenesis of reflex sympathetic dystrophy: A review and biopsychosocial hypothesis. Clin J Pain 1992;8:300–306.

197. van der Laan L, van Spaendonck K, Horstink MW, Goris RJ. The Symptom Checklist-90 Revised questionnaire: No psychological profiles in complex regional pain syndrome-dystonia. J Pain Symptom Manage 1999;17:357–362.

198. Geertzen JH, de Bruijn-Kofman AT, de Bruijn HP, van de Wiel HB, Dijkstra PU. Stressful life events and psychological dysfunction in Complex Regional Pain Syndrome type I. Clin J Pain 1998;14:143–147.

199. Baron R, Wasner G, Borgstedt R, et al. Effect of sympathetic activity on capsaicin-evoked pain, hyperalgesia, and vasodilatation. Neurology 1999;52:923–932.

200. Oyen WJ, Arntz IE, Claessens RM, Van der Meer JW, Corstens FH, Goris RJ. Reflex sympathetic dystrophy of the hand: An excessive inflammatory response? Pain 1993;55:151–157.

201. Wasner G, Schattschneider J, Binder A, Baron R. Complex regional pain syndrome—Diagnosis, mechanisms, CNS involvement and therapy. Spinal Cord 2003;41:61–75.

202. Davis KD, Treede RD, Raja SN, Meyer RA, Campbell JN. Topical application of clonidine relieves hyperalgesia in patients with sympathetically maintained pain. Pain 1991;47: 309–317.

203. Byas-Smith MG, Max MB, Muir J, Kingman A. Transdermal clonidine compared to placebo in painful diabetic neuropathy using a two-stage 'enriched enrollment' design. Pain 1995;60: 267–274.

204. Mitchell SW. Injuries of Nerves and Their Consequences. Philadelphia: Lippincott, 1872.

205. Livingston WK. Silas Weir Mitchell and his work on causalgia. In: Knighton RS, Dumke PR (eds). Pain. Boston: Little, Brown, 1966:561–572.

206. International Association for the Study of Pain, Subcommittee on Taxonomy. Classification of chronic pain. Descriptions of chronic pain syndromes and definitions of pain terms. Pain 1986;(suppl 3):S1–S226.

207. Bonica JJ. The Management of Pain. Philadelphia: Lea & Febiger, 1953:230–243.

208. Bonica JJ. Management of intractable pain. In: Way EL (ed). New Concepts in Pain. Philadelphia: Davis, 1967:155–167.

209. Roberts WJ. A hypothesis on the physiological basis for causalgia and related pains. Pain 1986; 24:297–311.

210. Campbell JN, Raja SN, Meyer RA, Mackinnon SE. Myelinated afferents signal the hyperalgesia associated with nerve injury. Pain 1988;32: 89–94.

211. Gracely RH, Lynch SA, Bennett GJ. Painful neuropathy: Altered central processing maintained dynamically by peripheral input. Pain 1992; 51:175–194.

212. Campbell JN, Meyer RA, Raja SN. Is nociceptor activation by alpha-1 adrenoreceptors the culprit in sympathetically maintained pain? Am Pain Soc J 1992;1:3–11.

213. Raja SN, Davis KD, Campbell JN. The adrenergic pharmacology of sympathetically maintained pain. J Reconstr Microsurg 1992;8: 63–69.

214. Choi B, Rowbotham MC. Effect of adrenergic receptor activation on post-herpetic neuralgia pain and sensory disturbances. Pain 1997;69: 55–63.

215. Gillette RG, Kramis RC, Roberts WJ. Sympathetic activation of cat spinal neurons responsive to noxious stimulation of deep tissues in the low back. Pain 1994;56:31–42.

216. Davis KD, Campbell JN, Raja SN, Treede RD, Lin C, Meyer RA. Topical application of an alpha-2 adrenergic agonist relieves hyperalgesia in sympathetically maintained pain [abstract]. Pain 1990;(suppl 5):S421.

217. Glynn C, Jones P. An investigation of the role of clonidine in the treatment of reflex sympathetic dystrophy. In: Stanton-Hicks M, Jänig W, Boas RA (eds). Reflex Sympathetic Dystrophy. Boston: Kluwer, 1990:187–196.

218. Raja SN, Treede RD, Davis KD, Cambell JN. Systemic alpha-adrenergic blockade with phentolamine: A diagnostic test for sympthetically maintained pain. Anesthesiology 1991;74: 691–698.

219. Dyck PJ, Davies JL, Wilson DM, Service FJ, Melton LJ 3rd, O'Brien PC. Risk factors for severity of diabetic polyneuropathy: Intensive longitudinal assessment of the Rochester Diabetic Neuropathy Study cohort. Diabetes Care 1999;22:1479–1486.

220. Fraser DM, Campbell IW, Ewing DJ, Clarke BF. Mononeuropathy in diabetes mellitus. Diabetes 1979;28:96–101.

221. Irkec C, Nazliel B, Yetkin I, Kocer B. Facial nerve conduction in diabetic neuropathy. Acta Neurol Belg 2001;101:177–179.

222. Beghi E, Delodovici ML, Bogliun G, et al. Hypothyroidism and polyneuropathy. J Neurol Neurosurg Psychiatry 1989;52:1420–1423.

223. Dyck PJ, Kratz KM, Karnes JL, et al. The prevalence by staged severity of various types of diabetic neuropathy, retinopathy, and nephropathy in a population-based cohort: The Rochester Diabetic Neuropathy Study. Neurology 1993;43:817–824.

224. Dyck PJ, Zimmerman BR, Vilen TH, et al. Nerve glucose, fructose, sorbitol, myo-inositol, and fiber degeneration and regeneration in diabetic neuropathy. N Engl J Med 1988;319:542–548.

225. Cruccu G, Agostino R, Inghilleri M, Innocenti P, Romaniello A, Manfredi M. Mandibular nerve involvement in diabetic polyneuropathy and chronic inflammatory demyelinating polyneuropathy. Muscle Nerve 1998;21:1673–1679.

Psychologic Factors and Orofacial Pain: Axis II

In recent years, the advancement of medical science has been phenomenal. We know more today about disease processes then ever before. As we study a disease and begin to understand the mechanisms responsible for its development, we learn ways of interrupting its progression, thereby terminating the disease. This new knowledge has certainly improved the health and well-being of the human race. This processing of information, however, can pose some interesting conflicts in the understanding and management of pain.

Most of the medical community has a belief that every disease has a physical condition associated with it. Once the physical condition that is responsible for the disease is found, it can be corrected and the disease is terminated. This mechanistic model of disease makes complete sense for some diseases, such as pulpitis. When a caries lesion nears the dental pulp, the pulpal tissues become inflamed and painful symptoms begin. If the caries lesion is removed and the pulpal tissue recovers, the symptoms resolve. The successful management of this type of pulpal disease occurs every day in

the practice of dentistry. If removal of the caries lesion does not resolve the pain symptoms, it is assumed that the pulpal tissues are necrotic and a new therapy (endodontics) is performed. When this disease process is present, the removal of the pulp eliminates the painful symptoms. These clinical findings reinforce the physical cause-and-effect (mechanistic) approach to treating pulpal pain. Since pulpal pain fits this model so well, it perfectly supports the mechanistic approach to disease.

Taking this example one step further, however, helps demonstrate the limitations of the mechanistic model of disease. Assume that after the endodontic procedure was completed on the tooth, the pain continued. The mechanistic approach would suggest that the endodontic therapy has failed, even though no clinical evidence of failure exists, and the tooth would logically be extracted. Unfortunately, after extraction of the tooth, the pain continues. Since there is no longer evidence of disease, the mechanistic approach to the disease fails to explain the pain. It is at this time the clinician will often blame the pain on some psychologic factor. Since the condition is now psychologic, the clinician who is not trained in the management of psychologic issues will likely feel inadequate and without any treatment strategies. A common occurrence at this time is for the clinician to brand the patient as neurotic. This type of thinking greatly limits the clinician's ability to manage pain.

Every clinician who manages pain needs to appreciate that no pain is without some influence of psychologic factors. As nociception enters the brainstem, it ascends to the higher centers for interpretation and evaluation. As it reaches the thalamus, the nociceptive input is influenced by neural interaction between the limbic structures, the cortex, and the hypothalamus. It is at this level that the nociceptive input is given meaning. The limbic structures add instincts, drives, and emotions to the input. The cortex adds the influence of prior experiences and present environmental conditions to the input. The hypothalamus prepares the body to react to the input through responses of the autonomic nervous system (eg, blood pressure, heart rate, vigilance). It is this unique response at the thalamic level that makes the experience of pain so individual and personal. It is at this level that one can begin to understand why the experience of pain is dependent upon the attention drawn to the injury and the consequence of the injury (see chapter 1).

As discussed in chapter 1, nociception is merely the mechanism by which noxious information is carried into the central nervous system (CNS). Pain is an unpleasant sensation perceived in the cortex, usually as a result of incoming nociceptive input. The presence or absence of nociceptive input, however, does not always relate closely to pain. The term *suffering* refers to still another phenomenon. Suffering refers to how the human reacts to the perception of pain. It is at this level that the complex interaction of the cortex, thalamus, hypothalamus, and limbic structures becomes evi-

dent. Suffering, therefore, may not be proportionally related to nociception or pain. Patients experiencing little pain may suffer greatly, while others with significant pain may suffer less. *Pain behavior* is something different still. Pain behavior refers to the individual's audible and visible actions that communicate his suffering to others. Pain behavior is sometimes the only observed evidence the clinician receives regarding the pain experience. This behavior is as individual as people themselves.

When one appreciates the complexity of the pain experience, it becomes evident that the mechanistic model of disease is inadequate in the management of pain conditions. A more suitable model is the *biopsychosocial model* of disease (Fig 18-1). The "bio" represents the nociceptive input arising from the somatic tissues and the "psychosocial" component represents the influence of the interaction between the thalamus, cortex, and limbic structures. It is interesting to note that the neurotransmission of impulses between all these higher centers is responsible for what we call the *psychologic aspects of pain*. In fact, like all neural functions, psychologic factors and moods are based on neurotransmitter activity. Although some clinicians cling to the notion that psychologic activity somehow operates independently of somatic structures, there is a preponderance of evidence that points to an organic neural basis for all such activity. Receptors, neurons, synapses, electric charges, and neurochemicals are the structural elements that underlie all functional activities, psychologic as well as physiologic. Neurochemistry seems to be the key to such mechanisms. As mentioned in chapter 5, psychology could be construed as actually neurology that is not yet fully understood. No doubt, as these mechanisms are better understood, we shall know a great deal more about suffering and pain behavior.

It is with this appreciation of pain that a dual-axis classification of orofacial pain has

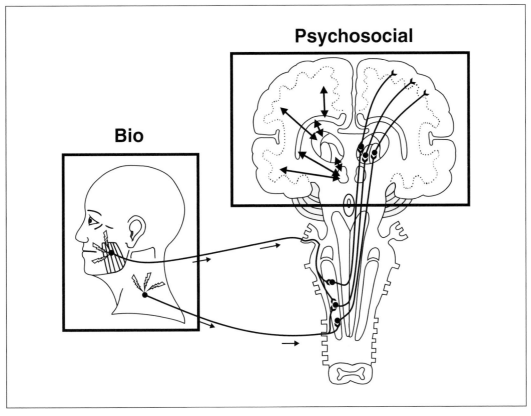

Psychosocial

Bio

Fig 18-1 A graphic depiction of the biopsychosocial model of disease. Nociceptive input arises from the masseter and the trapezius muscles. This input represents the "bio" portion of model. Once the nociceptive input enters the CNS and ascends to the higher centers, the interaction of the thalamus, limbic structures, hypothalamus, and cortex interrupts the input and labels it as painful or not. This higher center interaction represents the "psychosocial" portion of the model. Both areas are likely to be of equal importance in the pain experience.

been developed for this text. Axis I represents those conditions that have a physical basis, while Axis II represents those conditions with a psychosocial basis. A detailed review of Axis I conditions was presented in chapters 9 through 17. The clinician must appreciate that each Axis I diagnosis is likely to be influenced by the presence of an Axis II diagnosis. For complete patient management, the presence and influence of each axis must be accessed for proper diagnosis. In some pain conditions, treatment of only the Axis I factors will fail to manage the patient's complaints. Unfortunately, this concept is foreign to many health professionals.

Acute Pain Versus Chronic Pain and the Biopsychosocial Model

As discussed in chapter 5, acute pains are of short duration and are often closely related to somatic tissue changes, such as those produced by trauma or disease. *Chronic pain* refers to pains of long duration, and these pains take on a different therapeutic meaning. Most clinicians use the term to describe any pain that has lasted longer than 6 months, regardless of its origin. Although this is the classic definition, perhaps a better concept of chronic pain would be pains that last longer than normal healing time. It is expected that tissue damage will produce nociception and pain, but when healing is complete, pain should subside. If pain continues after normal healing time, the origin of the pain is in doubt. One reason for continued pain is the influence of the Axis II psychologic factors. As pain becomes protracted, a shift in the origin of the pain can be expected from primary somatosensory input to the affective, cognitive, and behavioral inputs of pain. As the duration of pain input continues, the level of suffering increases, even when the intensity of somatosensory input remains the same (Fig 18-2). In fact, chronic pain can be sustained at high level of discomfort, even though the intensity of the somatosensory input may decrease or disappear altogether. As pain becomes chronic, management options shift from local to systemic modalities. Pain that could initially be managed on a purely Axis I level may require extensive and coordinated interdisciplinary therapy to be effective.

When considering the effects of acute and chronic pains within the biopsychosocial model, one realizes that early in the pain experience the somatosensory input (bio) often has the greatest influence on the pain experience. As pain becomes protracted, the influence from the higher centers (psychosocial) will likely become predominant. As already stated, this has therapeutic significance.

Psychologic intensification of pain is a normal modulating effect peculiar to humans and has to do with their evaluation of the consequences attending the experience. All pains are subject to some degree of intensification. It is only when psychogenic factors (Axis II) dominate the complaint that it becomes a significant therapeutic consideration. Since duration increases pain intensification, a component of Axis II factors become an ingredient in the development of chronicity.

Another element that appears to be important in the development of chronic pain is the continuity of nociceptive input. Intermittency lessens the likelihood of the development of pain chronicity, as is seen in such conditions as trigeminal neuralgia and migraine. Even though they persist and recur indefinitely, such disorders usually do not change appreciably in their response to therapy and therefore are not likely maintained by Axis II factors. Pain disorders that have a constant input, even if it is of variable high and low intensity, are more likely to develop symptoms of chronicity. A combination of duration and continuity of nociceptive input predisposes a patient to pain chronicity.

In the past, the term *atypical facial pain* was used to categorize a group of patients who had chronic facial pain of unknown etiology. In a study of 34 cases of chronic atypical facial pain, Mock et al[1] reported that all of the patients displayed nonanatomic distribution with no identifiable organic or physiologic cause and complained of symptoms that were not compatible with any known neurologic syndrome. Of the 34 patients, 76.5% were women. More than 50% had undergone some dental treatment for the pain that made it worse rather than

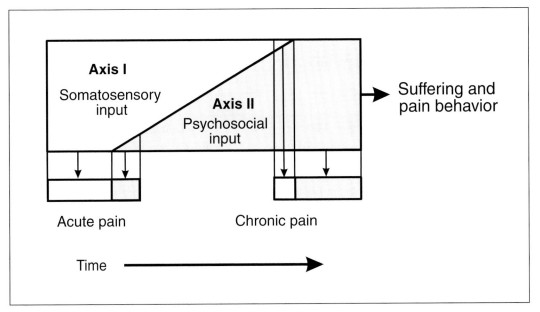

Fig 18-2 Axis I input represents the somatosensory (bio) input that contributes to the patient's pain and suffering. Axis II represents the psychosocial input that contributes to pain and suffering. Both Axis I and Axis II factors must be considered when evaluating a patient's pain and suffering. Early in the pain experience, Axis I input often dominates the degree of pain and suffering. As the condition becomes chronic, Axis II factors often become the dominant input. An understanding of this relationship is important in therapy.

better. Some 38% reported a sensory complaint such as anesthesia, paresthesia, or hyperesthesia; 55% had headaches; and 73% had associated depression, anxiety, or a highly stressed state. Of course these findings would be expected by definition in a population of patients classified as having atypical facial pain. It would appear that this general classification should diminish as the profession becomes more knowledgeable of orofacial pain mechanisms. For this reason, the term *atypical facial pain* will not be used in this text.

It is important to note that pain experienced in the orofacial structures may be significantly related to Axis II factors. In a review[2] of 430 patients with psychogenic regional pain, the head and heart regions were the most frequent sites of pain. In a study of 40,000 patients with orofacial pain,[3] 2% to 5% had no organic disease or

had exaggerated responses to minimal pathologic conditions. It was noted that depressive illness occurred especially with glossodynia, glossopyrosis, recalcitrant masticatory pain, and atypical facial pain. In one clinic that treated chronic pain patients of all types,[4] 40% complained of chronic craniofacial and neck pains. In these patients, there were few or no signs of Axis I pathosis, or it was not consistent with the degree of discomfort. The characteristics that these patients displayed included the following:

1. A high level of stress expressed as anxiety and depression
2. A marked tendency toward tolerance, dependence, and addiction, not only to medications but also to surgery and treatments of all kinds

3. A marked dependency on family, friends, and doctors
4. Evidence of loss of self-esteem, impotence, apathy, regressive attitude, and withdrawal behavior
5. Hostility

Moulton[5] identified two types of patients with chronic pain: *(1)* people who were overtly dependent on someone who was either inadequate, overdominant, or unapproachable and thus became angry and hostile; and *(2)* unusually competent people who were obsessive and domineering and therefore became hostile secretly. The author warned that local treatment in patients with chronic pain may serve to focus their attention on the area treated, with the result that they would continue to seek relief on a purely peripheral level thereafter.

Beck et al[6] associated depression with glossodynia, myofascial pain, and atypical facial pains. They listed the symptoms of mild depression as disappointment, lack of self-confidence, and feelings of inadequacy; a desire to be alone and inactive; undue concern for physical appearance; decreased mental and physical alertness; and loss of weight and disturbed sleep. They listed the symptoms of severe and potentially suicidal depression as apathy, self-hate, despondency, immobility, poor posture, decreased muscle tone, insomnia, and fatigue.

Fordyce[7] pointed out that pain behavior, which consists of audible and visible communications that imply suffering, is subject to the influence of conditioning or "learning." Examples of such conditioning are *(1)* the effect of imitating the behavior of others who suffer (social modeling); *(2)* the reinforcement of the "reality" of pain by medications prescribed to be used as needed, as well as by the attention received from others because of suffering; and *(3)* the indirect reinforcement of pain by avoidance of obligations, commitments, or duties to escape or minimize pain. Pain behavior that is contingent upon expectancy or secondary gain

may be reinforced by cues in the environment that suffering may be imminent when actually no noxious stimulation is ever sensed. It may be necessary only to anticipate that pain may occur for overt pain behavior to be displayed.

Sternbach[8] observed that subjective improvement in a patient's pain condition follows behavioral improvement. This suggests that pain responses change if the state of mind changes. Thus, if the pain behavior of chronic pain patients is acquired or learned, it may be unlearned by proper techniques. Chronic pain is modifiable through coping strategies.

Roberts[9] attempted to control chronic pain by focusing on the patient's behavior and not on the source of nociception nor on an attempt to change an alleged emotional state. His objective was to rehabilitate the patient rather than to alleviate the pain. He believed that it is better to teach the patient to live a normal life, even though pain may still be present. In chronic pain disorders, treatment measures that are aimed only to alleviate pain tend to reinforce the "pain concept" that the patient holds.

It should be noted that in patients with chronic pain, the endorphin system does not offer protection of any importance.[10] Perhaps the experience of chronic pain depletes the CNS of these pain modulators. Although the action of tricyclic antidepressants in normal subjects has no greater effect on the pain threshold than does placebo,[11] in depressed individuals the analgesic effect parallels the antidepressant action.[12]

Symptoms of Chronicity

It is important that chronicity be identified as early as possible. Even though pains that are truly intermittent are often of greater intensity, they are less prone to be associated with the symptoms of chronicity, such as depressive illness. The relief between attacks seems to prevent physical and emotional deterioration. Thus, with paroxysmal neuralgia and neurovascular pain disorders, chronicity seldom becomes a problem. However, the persistence of continuous neuropathic pains, such as deafferentation pain or neuritis, or continuous masticatory pains should lead the examiner to identify evidence of chronicity as early as possible. Guidelines based on units of time are not dependable, because chronicity is extremely variable. Rather, identification of chronicity depends on such factors as the following:

1. Constancy and continuity of peripheral input
2. Evidence of increased suffering in spite of otherwise effective peripheral therapeutic efforts
3. Persistence or prompt relapse of symptoms in spite of different methods of therapy used by different clinicians
4. Increasing anxiety on the patient's part
5. Patient's obsessive concern with his suffering expressed by relief-seeking efforts of all types
6. Progressive depression and withdrawal behavior
7. Physical and emotional deterioration

The Psychologic Significance of Orofacial Pains

All pains carry with them certain importance and meaning. As already mentioned, the attention drawn to the injury and the consequence of the injury directly determine the degree of suffering experienced by the patient. This concept is extremely important when addressing facial pain. The clinician should never forget the significant psychologic meaning of pain in this portion of the body. The face and mouth are the primary structures needed for survival. Without these, the individual will not be able to take in food. These structures are basic to life itself. Damage or significant loss of function is a significant threat to the individual.

The orofacial structures are also basic to communication. In our social environment, where communication is so vital, dysfunction of these structures threatens meaningful existence. These structures provide the means by which we relate to others our feelings, goals, opinions, and aspirations. They are a source of gratification and satisfaction physically, emotionally, spiritually, and sexually. When these structures are threatened by pain or dysfunction, the quality of life can greatly diminish.

Not only do the mouth and face have unusual emotional significance for the individual, but they also relate to concepts of body image, in that the individual interprets a damaged face as a damaged self. Distortion of body image results in anxiety that is frequently expressed as pain.[13] This is likely to have an important bearing on the severity and duration of chronic post-traumatic pain syndromes of the maxillofacial region. This trauma may be not only that of actual tissue damage to the face, but also that of emotional trauma such as that associated with physical or sexual abuse.[14–20]

It is wise for the clinician to always be mindful of the unique emotional significance of the orofacial structures. The clinician should always approach the patient with care and respect, never too quickly or abruptly. The successful clinician learns the appropriate examination and management style that gains the confidence of the patient.

Axis II: Classification of Mental Disorders

Understanding the complex neurologic interaction between the thalamus, cortex, hypothalamus, and limbic structures is indeed a difficult task. Dysfunction of this neural interaction results in what are referred to as *mental disorders*. The study of mental disorders encompasses an enormous body of information. The main purpose of this text is to provide information to the clinician regarding orofacial pain disorders. Although the Axis II conditions described as mental disorders are enormously important, they cannot be reviewed completely in this text. This author has therefore limited the discussion in this chapter to a few of the more important mental disorders that may involve orofacial pain conditions. For a thorough discussion of mental disorders, a review of the *Diagnostic and Statistical Manual of Mental Disorders* (DSM-IV), published by the American Psychiatric Association,[21] is recommended.

There are four general categories of mental disorders that will be reviewed in this chapter. The description of each disorder will be in accord with the DSM-IV[21] publication. The categories that will be discussed are mood disorders, anxiety disorders, somatoform disorders, and a broad category that includes other conditions that may be a focus of clinical attention. Each of these categories will be divided into important subcategories and will be discussed strictly for the purpose of identification and not treatment. It is important for the dental clinician and physician to recognize these conditions so that optimum therapy is provided by appropriate health care personnel.

Mood Disorders

Mood disorders are mental disorders that are characterized by disturbances in the patient's mood. Mood disorders are divided into three categories: depressive disorders, bipolar disorders, and mood disorders resulting from a medical condition (Fig 18-3).

Depressive disorders

A depressed mood is characterized by markedly diminished interest or pleasure in all, or almost all, activities most of the day, nearly every day. The depressed mood is described subjectively by the patient as an overwhelming feeling of sadness or emptiness. There is often uncontrolled crying and a common complaint of fatigue or loss of energy nearly every day. Depressive disorders often result in either an increase or decrease in appetite, leading to a change of more than 5% of body weight in a month. There is usually a diminished ability to think or concentrate, with much indecision. Insomnia or hypersomnia usually accompany depressive disorders. Depressive disorders may range in severity from minor to major. In major depressive disorders, recurrent thoughts of death or considerations of suicide are common. When severe depression is suspected, it is important for the clinician to question the patient regarding his or her thoughts regarding suicide. If considerable risk is present, the patient should not be released without proper evaluation.

Bipolar disorders

Bipolar disorders are characterized by depressive periods followed or preceded by an opposite mood swing, called a manic

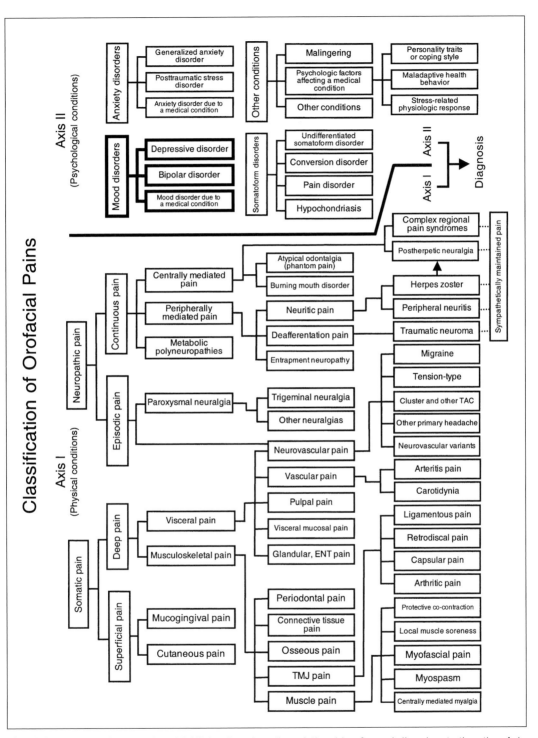

Fig 18-3 Pain classification chart highlighted to show the relationship of mood disorders to the other Axis I and Axis II conditions.

episode. A common term for this disorder is *manic-depressive illness*. The manic episode is characterized a distinct period of an abnormally and persistently elevated, expansive, or irritable mood. The mood often includes an inflated self-esteem or grandiosity, decreased need for sleep, rapid speech, flight of ideas, distractibility, and an increased involvement in goal-directed activities. The expansive quality of the mood is characterized by unceasing and indiscriminate enthusiasm for interpersonal, sexual, or occupational interactions. For example, the person may spontaneously start extensive conversations with strangers in public places. Although the mood may initially have an infectious quality for the uninvolved observer, it is recognized as excessive by those who know the person well. Sometimes the mood becomes irritable rather than elevated or expanded.

A bipolar disorder is characterized by alternating manic and depressive periods. Specific subdivisions are identified according to the frequency and severity of the mood changes.[21]

Mood Disorders Resulting from a Medical Condition

This category of mood disorders is extremely important when considering orofacial pain disorders. Many studies have investigated the common occurrence of depression and chronic pain disorders.[22-25] Although some have concluded that depression can lead to chronic pain,[26] the more convincing evidence suggests that chronic pain can lead to depression.[27] This category of mood disorders is reserved for those patients who experience a prominent and persistent disturbance in mood that is a direct physiologic consequence of a general medical condition. The mood may be depressive or bipolar or any other mood disorder. The physical condition may be a chronic pain disorder or any other medical condition. For example, the condition may be listed as a "depressive disorder due to chronic osteoarthritis of the temporomandibular joint." The common occurrence of both Axis I and Axis II conditions challenges the clinician to astutely evaluate each patient so as to maximize therapeutic results.

Anxiety Disorders

Anxiety disorders are characterized by an unusual increase in anxiety and worry that last longer than a normal or appropriate period of time. Three categories of anxiety disorders will be discussed in this text: generalized anxiety disorders, posttraumatic stress disorders, and anxiety disorders resulting from a medical condition (Fig 18-4).

Generalized anxiety disorders

Generalized anxiety disorders are characterized by excessive anxiety and worry that occurs for a majority of days for at least 6 months. The person reveals an intensity, duration, and frequency of the anxiety and worry that is far out of proportion to the actual likelihood or impact of the feared event. The increase in apprehension and expectation is associated with certain events or activities. These events may be related to work, school, or home functions. The person will often find it difficult to control the worry and be restless or "keyed up." The person will often have difficulty concentrating and the mind may suddenly go blank. Generalized anxiety disorders create irritability, muscle tension, and poor-quality sleep. The sleep disturbance is often characterized by either difficulty falling asleep or staying asleep. The anxiety, worry, or physical symptoms will cause clinically significant distress or impairment in social, occupational, or other important areas of functioning.

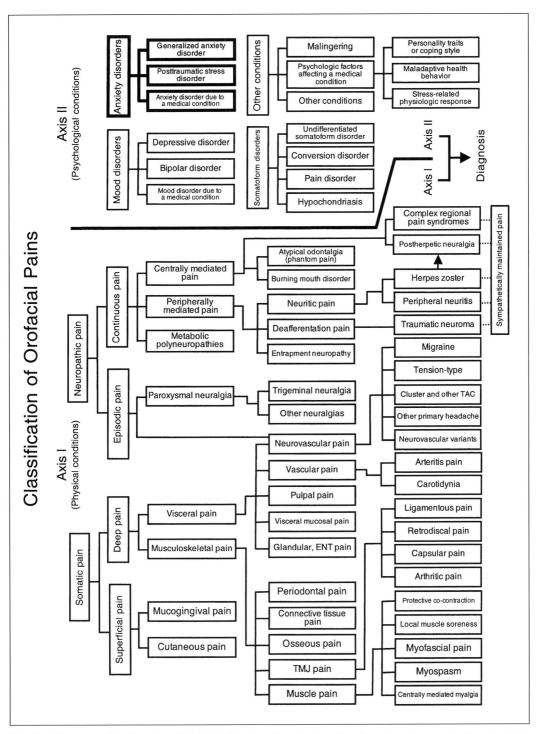

Fig 18-4 Pain classification chart highlighted to show the relationship of anxiety disorders to the other Axis I and Axis II conditions.

Posttraumatic stress disorders

A posttraumatic stress disorder is a type of anxiety disorder that can develop following an individual's exposure to an extremely traumatic stressor. The stressor may be associated with a direct personal experience that threatened death or serious injury or threatened one's physical integrity. It may result from witnessing an event that involves death, injury, or threat to the physical integrity of another person. It may even result from learning about an unexpected or violent death, serious harm, or threat of death or injury experienced by a family member or other close associate. The person's response to the event involves intense fear, helplessness, or horror. The person experiencing a posttraumatic stress disorder will often report persistent re-experiencing of the traumatic event and avoid any stimuli associated with the trauma. The person will reveal a numbing of general responsiveness, yet also show persistent symptoms of increased arousal.

The traumatic event may be re-experienced in various ways. Commonly the person has recurrent and intrusive recollections of the event or recurrent, distressing dreams during which the event is replayed. In rare instances, the person may experience dissociative states that last from a few seconds to several hours, even days. During this time, the components of the event are relived and the person may behave as though experiencing the event at that moment. Often, intense psychologic distress or physiologic reactivity occurs when the person is exposed to triggering events that resemble or symbolize an aspect of the traumatic event. A well-known example is the combat veteran who overresponds to a loud sound, such as the backfiring of an automobile. Another example is the woman who had been previously assaulted reliving the same fear when approaching her car in a dark parking lot.

It should always be remembered that the traumatic event does not have to appear traumatic to the clinician to be significant. It must only be traumatic to the patient. This is an important concept to remember when taking a history from the patient. The clinician should not place his or her own values on the patient.

Posttraumatic stress disorders are likely to represent a generalized up-regulation of the autonomic nervous system. As discussed in earlier chapters, stressful events are countered by the fight-or-flight reaction. This response is controlled by the autonomic nervous system. In the presence of a sudden environmental challenge, the sympathetic nervous system increases heart rate, blood pressure, and breathing rate while pooling blood to vital organs. This is a normal response to the challenge. When the challenge is eliminated or resolves, the system should return to normal levels of function. In posttraumatic stress disorders, the events are so traumatically imprinted in the person's mind that the autonomic nervous system remains up-regulated as if needed to counter an ongoing challenge. This state of hypervigilance can be seen as irritability, difficulty falling asleep or staying asleep, difficulty concentrating, or an exaggerated startle response.

Often this autonomic up-regulation or hypervigilance can lead to subtle changes in peripheral functions. For some patients, these persistent changes may present as pain in structures that are free of obvious pathology. Physical or sexual abuse, especially involving the face, may be a common source of unexplained chronic orofacial pain.[14-20,28] Patients with histories of physical or sexual abuse often experience posttraumatic stress disorders related to these prior traumatic events. This concept of sympathetic up-regulation is important and will be discussed further in the section on therapy.

Anxiety disorders resulting from a medical condition

Anyone with a significant medical condition will likely experience some degree of apprehension or anxiety. This is certainly a normal finding. Some patients, however, may reveal that the anxiety produced by the presence of the physical condition is far greater than normal, and in fact may actually impair social, occupational, or other important areas of functioning. When this occurs, it represents an anxiety disorder that is due to a general medical condition. Symptoms may include prominent generalized anxiety symptoms, panic attacks, or obsessions or compulsions.

There must be evidence from the history, physical examination, or laboratory findings that the disturbance is the direct physiologic consequence of a general medical condition. The anxiety disorder should not be better explained by some other mental disorder but should in fact be related to the physical condition. The relationship between the physical condition and the anxiety disorder may be supported by a temporal association. In other word, there should be an association between the onset, exacerbation, and remission of the general medical condition and the symptoms of anxiety.

Somatoform Disorders

Somatoform disorders represent a group of mental disorders in which physical symptoms are present that suggest a general medical condition, and yet there are insufficient positive physical signs to support the diagnosis of a physical condition; hence the term *somatoform*. The term *somatization disorder* refers very specifically to a person who is older than 30 years, has had symptoms extending for years, and complains of a combination of pain and gastrointestinal, sexual, and pseudoneurologic symptoms.[21]

Since the inclusionary criteria for this category are large, it is not commonly seen in chronic orofacial pain patients and therefore will not be elaborated in this section. Instead, four more common categories seen in orofacial pain patients will be discussed. They are: undifferentiated somatoform disorders, conversion disorders, somatoform pain disorders, and hypochondriasis (Fig 18-5).

Undifferentiated somatoform disorders

The clinical features of an undifferentiated somatoform disorder are one or more physical complaints that persist for 6 months or longer. The most frequent complaints are chronic fatigue, loss of appetite, or gastrointestinal or genitourinary symptoms. Of course, pain can also be present, but it is not the major complaint in this category. The symptoms cannot be fully explained by any known general medical condition or the direct effects of a substance. The physical complaints or resultant impairment are grossly in excess of what would be expected from the history, physical examination, or laboratory findings. This category is used when the symptoms do not fully meet all the criteria used for somatization disorders.

Conversion disorders

Conversion disorders are those mental disorders characterized by the presence of symptoms or deficits affecting voluntary motor or sensory function that suggest a neurologic or other general medical condition. Psychologic factors are judged to be associated with the symptom or deficit, a judgment based on the observation that the initiation or exacerbation of the symptom or deficit is preceded by conflicts or other stressors.

Conversion disorders are related to voluntary motor or sensory functioning and are thus referred to as pseudoneurologic. Motor symptoms or deficits include im-

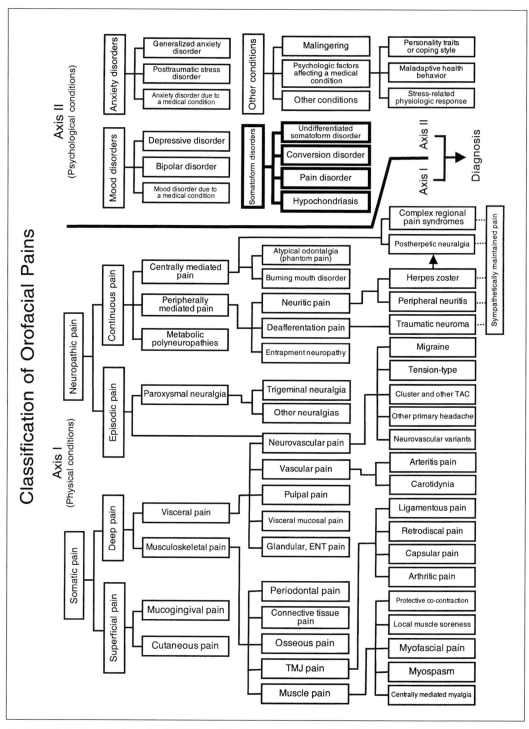

Fig 18-5 Pain classification chart highlighted to show the relationship of somatoform disorders to the other Axis I and Axis II conditions.

paired coordination or balance, paralysis or localized weakness, aphonia, difficulty swallowing or a sensation of a lump in the throat, and urinary retention. Sensory symptoms or deficits include loss of touch or pain sensation, double vision, blindness, deafness, and hallucinations.

The diagnosis of a conversion disorder can only be made after careful examination has ruled out a neurologic or general medical etiology. Because of the physical symptoms, this may be a very difficult task, taking considerable time. Conversion symptoms are often inconsistent and the astute clinician may be able to diagnosis the condition by careful observation. For example, when paralysis is the symptom, small movements of the involved limb may be noticed when dressing or during other activities.

Conversion disorders may also be related to secondary gains, and when so, the clinician needs to be aware of this. If a conversion disorder results in a paralyzed leg, work becomes impossible. The condition may in fact become the escape from work and the circumstances or stressors that are actually responsible for the disorder. The condition, therefore, becomes the treatment that eliminates the etiology. Although this may sound very logical, the clinician should not assume that the patient is actually thinking in this manner on a conscious level. In fact, most conversion disorders are not intentionally produced, and therefore the patient is as baffled as the doctor.

Somatoform pain disorders

The essential feature of a somatoform pain disorder is pain. Therefore, this disorder is an important condition to recognize in the orofacial pain patient. In a somatoform pain disorder, pain is the predominant focus of the clinical presentation and is of sufficient severity to warrant clinical attention. The pain is in one or more anatomic sites and causes the person significant distress or impairment in social, occupational, or other important areas of functioning. There is no obvious pathology present to explain the pain; however, the patient is not intentionally producing the pain (as with a factitious disorder or malingering). Psychologic factors are judged to have an important role in the onset, severity, exacerbation, or maintenance of the pain.

Somatoform pain disorders can certainly pose a significant diagnostic problem for the clinician evaluating orofacial pain complaints. One might be suspicious of this condition if the pain is not associated with any local somatic tissue changes. This statement, however, is very naive when one thinks of the numerous pain disorders that have been described in this text that are not associated with any obvious source of pathology. For example, most neuropathic pains have no local tissue changes that explain their presence. The clinician must therefore always be mindful of somatoform pain disorders, so that an improper diagnosis does not lead to mistreatment. When a patient complains of orofacial pain, always consider all possibilities (Case 35).

Hypochondriasis

Hypochondriasis is a somatoform disorder in which the person is preoccupied with the fears of having, or the idea that one has, a serious disease based on a misinterpretation of one or more bodily signs or symptoms. A thorough medical evaluation does not identify a general medical condition that fully accounts for the person's concerns about disease or for the physical signs or symptoms. The fear or idea of having a disease persists, despite medical reassurance that nothing is present. The preoccupation in hypochondriasis may be with bodily functions, with minor physical abnormalities, or with vague and ambiguous physical sensations. The concern may involve several body systems, at different times or simultaneously. Repeated physical examinations, diagnostic tests, and reassurance from the

Case 35	Clinical presentation of a somatoform pain disorder with some possibility of a posttraumatic stress disorder

Chief Complaint   Bilateral TMJ and tooth pain.

History

A 28-year-old woman presented with protracted, continuous, mild, steady, dull, aching pain diffusely located in and around the TMJs and teeth bilaterally. It was described as an itchy uncomfortable sensation punctuated occasionally by lancinating pains through the face. These pains did not seem to relate to masticatory function. Discomfort was worse in early mornings and was accompanied by a "bad taste" in the mouth.

It began 9 to 10 months earlier following her third marriage and at first seemed to involve only the teeth. She wanted them removed but her dentist found no valid reason. Then it spread to involve the entire masticatory system including the teeth, joints, muscles, lips, tongue, and floor of the mouth bilaterally. She was diagnosed by her regular dentist as having a masticatory muscle pain disorder and was referred for confirmation and therapy.

Due to the vagueness of the complaint, a psychologic survey was done, revealing an emotional overlay that needed further exploration.

Examination

Intraoral: Negative for any cause of the pain.

   TMJs: Clinical and radiographically normal.

   Muscles: Some muscle tenderness but not increased with any jaw use.

   Cervical: Within normal limits; however, the patient reports pain originating from her neck. No evidence of any pain source.

   Cranial nerves: Within normal limits.

Diagnostic tests: Further psychologic investigation revealed a traumatic childhood and a sexually traumatic first marriage, which ended in divorce. A second marriage was short lived. She then isolated herself from male companions for some time. A third marriage, 11 months ago, seems to have reactivated her old feelings due to what she describes as a very aggressive husband. She seeks ways to avoid sexual relations with him.

Impression

The face pain problem may be related to either a somatoform pain disorder or a posttraumatic stress disorder.

Diagnosis   An Axis II mental disorder, clinically manifesting as a masticatory muscle pain disorder.

physician do little to allay the concern about bodily disease or affliction. An individual with hypochondriasis may become alarmed by reading or hearing about disease; knowing someone who becomes sick; or from observations, sensations, or occurrences within their own body. The concern about the feared illness often becomes a central feature of the individual's self-image, a topic of social discourse, and a response to life stresses.

Other Conditions That May Be a Focus of Clinical Attention

When developing the DSM-IV,[21] the American Psychiatric Association felt it important to include a category recognizing the presence of conditions that do not fully meet the specific criteria for a given mental disorder but in fact may be a contributing influence to the patient's symptoms. This category is described as "other conditions that may be a focus of clinical attention." There are numerous possibilities in this category, but this text will only review a few. Fig 18-6 reveals a category of "other conditions" to acknowledge all the other possibilities. There are two categories that should be mentioned in this section: malingering and psychologic factors affecting a medical condition.

Malingering

Malingering is a mental disorder that is characterized by an individual's intentional production of false or grossly exaggerated physical or psychologic symptoms, motivated by external incentives such as avoiding work, military duty, or social encounters. The malingering patient may use the symptoms to obtain drugs or financial compensation, such as in a medicolegal issue.

Malingering should be suspected when there is a marked discrepancy between the person's claimed stress or disability and the objective clinical findings, or if the person is not cooperative during the diagnostic evaluation. Persons who do not comply with suggested therapies should also be suspected of malingering, especially if no logical explanation is given. Of course, ongoing medicolegal issues may also raise suspicion.

Psychologic Factors Affecting a Medical Condition

This category of mental disorders is characterized by the presence of one or more specific psychologic or behavioral factors that adversely affect a general medical condition. These factors may affect the medical condition either by affecting its course, by interfering with the treatment, or by constituting an additional health risk for the individual. There are several psychologic factors that may affect a medical condition, but only three will be reviewed in this text. They are: personality traits or coping style, maladaptive health behavior, and stress-related physiologic responses.

Personality traits or coping style
An individual's personality traits or a maladaptive coping style can sometimes influence the course of treatment of a general medical condition. Some of these traits may actually contribute to the medical condition, such as a type A personality that reveals hostile behavior and continuous pressures affecting coronary artery disease. In some instances, problematic personality traits can interfere with the working relationship of the health care providers, resulting in adverse consequences in treatment.

Maladaptive health behavior
Maladaptive health behaviors can greatly affect the outcome of a general medical condition. For example, a sedentary lifestyle, overeating, excessive alcohol, and drug abuse can greatly affect the medical condition. Behaviors, such as unsafe sexual prac-

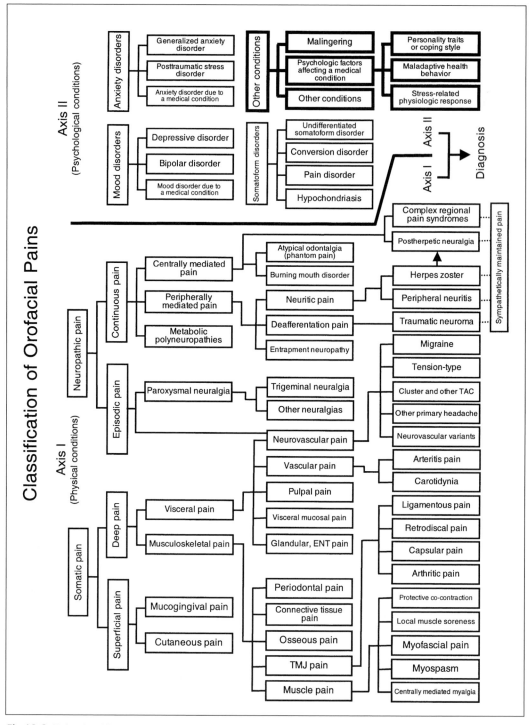

Fig 18-6 Pain classification chart highlighted to show the relationship of the other mental conditions to the other Axis I and Axis II conditions.

tices, also influence medical conditions. These maladaptive health behaviors need to be evaluated and appropriately addressed when treating the general medical condition.

Stress-related physiologic response

Sometimes stress-related physiologic responses can affect the outcome of a general medical condition. This may be seen in an individual who, when emotionally stressed, experiences chest pains. As previously discussed, an up-regulation of the autonomic nervous system may be responsible, in part, for maintaining some chronic pain conditions. For these patients, treatment to decrease the responsiveness of the autonomic nervous system is appropriate.

Other conditions

This category of mental disorders is listed in the orofacial pain classification merely to remind the reader that the mental disorders that have been reviewed in this text are only a few of the many mental disorders that may be present in the orofacial pain patient. The clinician should be mindful of the possible presence of other disorders such as attention disorders, cognitive disorders, substance-related disorders, psychotic disorders, factitious disorders, eating disorders, sleep disorders, adjustment disorders, and personality disorders. These disorders are best diagnosed and managed by appropriate trained health professionals.

General Therapeutic Considerations

The treatment of chronic orofacial pain is no easy task. Not only is the clinician required to have a sound understanding of the physiology of the somatic and neurogenous structures, but he or she also must demonstrate a significant understanding of the Axis II conditions. Most clinical training programs orient their teachings to one or the other but not to both. Only recently have programs been developed that emphasis the significance and interaction of both Axis I and Axis II factors. Since it is difficult to master all aspects of pain, a multidisciplinary approach works best in most settings. In a temporomandibular disorders (TMD) management setting, the minimum support needed is a dental clinician, a clinical psychologist, and a physical therapist. As the practice expands to include all of orofacial pain, it should also expand to include the appropriate medical personnel to manage the pain conditions. These personnel may include an internist, a neurologist, an otolaryngologist, a rheumatologist, a physiatrist, a psychiatrist, and a pain management specialist. On occasion the group may need the expertise of a radiologist, a neurosurgeon, or even a pediatrician. This type of interaction may be necessary to manage complex pain conditions.

Although it is difficult for one clinician to manage all pain conditions, each clinician should be aware of certain basic principles in pain management. These principles are based on the understanding of the pain mechanisms that have been presented in this text. Remember, pain is the result of modulated nociception on its way to the cortex. If this modulation can be favorably influenced, the pain experience can be lessened. As mentioned in chapter 1, the amount of suffering that an individual experiences is not dependent upon tissue damage but instead on the amount of attention drawn to the injury and the consequence of the injury. The clinician should always be mindful of the factors that tend to increase the pain experience. Examples of such factors are attention, expectancy, anxiety, fear, and anger. Factors that tend to lessen the pain experience are confidence, self-efficacy, assurance, distraction, relaxation, and positive emotion. The caring therapist will recognize these influencing factors and encourage the patient's behavior to shift away from the exciting factors to more of the inhibitory factors. In many instances, this becomes more the art of pain management than the science.

All pain management should begin with educating the patient to his or her pain condition. The following suggestions will emphasize the inhibitory pain-modulating factors:

Provide a Definitive Diagnosis

Whenever possible, the patient should be given a definitive diagnosis of the pain condition. There is nothing more unsettling to the patient than fear of the unknown. Patients who are not given a diagnosis will often feel that their condition is unknown and unique only to them. Some patients may feel that their problem is so unique that no one has ever even seen it before. These feelings will promote fear and anxiety, which in turn will likely increase the pain experience.

Provide Assurance

Most orofacial pain conditions are not the result of a life-threatening disease. Once it has been determined that the condition is not life-threatening, the patient should be assured of his or her safety. Certainly the fear of losing one's life increases anxiety and attention and perhaps even produces anger. When explaining the significance of the disease, care should be taken not to downplay the significance of the pain. The clinician should carefully report that the condition is not life-threatening but at the same time show concern for the manner in

which the pain is influencing the quality of the patient's life. This reassurance is the foundation of a positive doctor/patient relationship that may greatly influence the success of future treatment.

Explain the Condition in Appropriate Terms

Each patient should be adequately informed regarding the etiology and treatment indicated for his or her pain condition. Often this information provides the patient with an understanding that not only decreases the excitatory pain–influencing factors but may also help him or her manage the condition. The clinician should present information regarding the pain condition in a manner that can be understood by the patient. The patient should be given time to ask the clinician questions to assure maximum understanding. Once the diagnosis is established, too often the clinician will want to move directly into therapy and overlook this important communication. Patient education is extremely important for maximum therapeutic success.

Do Not Deny the Patient's Pain

Too often in the past when the clinician could not find somatic evidence to explain the pain, the patient was thought to have a psychologic problem. Since the clinician assumed the problem was only in the mind, the pain was not real but instead merely fabricated. One of the purposes of this text is to emphasize that all pains are not somatic, and therefore the origin may not be obvious upon examination. Only in very rare instances is pain fabricated. The clinician should always assume that the patient's pain complaints are real and respect his or her report. Absolutely no benefit can be achieved by initially denying the patient's pain or by claiming that it cannot exist. These claims will only create a poor doctor/patient relationship, lessening the likelihood of treatment success.

Provide Realistic Expectations

Unfortunately, not all pain conditions can be completely resolved. Pain that has its origin in diseased structures that cannot be healed will likely continue, even in the presence of the best medical therapy. There are certain neuropathic pain conditions that are also resistant to therapy. It is important that patients be informed of the likely outcome of their disorder. Many disorders have a natural course that represents a specific time frame, with an increase in pain and then resolution. When these conditions exist, the patient should be informed of the normal time required for healing and the likely outcome. The patient's treatment expectations should be realistic, so as to minimize disappointment. Many patients believe the clinician has all the treatments needed to resolve the pain. When this is not true, the patient needs to appreciate this fact earlier in therapy.

The management of a pain disorder should always begin with conservative therapy. Aggressive treatments should generally be reserved for later considerations. Appropriate pain medications should be used for the condition being treated. With our improved understanding of central sensitization, acute pains should be adequately controlled to minimize the afferent barrage to the second-order neuron. This should be accomplished by proper preemptive analgesia with local anesthesia as well as oral medications.[29]

The Concept of Physical Self-Regulation

An important part of pain management is providing therapies in which the patient can actively participate. A condition that enhances the pain experience is the feeling of helplessness. When a patient can actively participate in his or her treatment, a feeling of control develops. This control helps down-regulate the pain experience. There are multiple strategies that can help the patient gain some control of the certainly physiologic processes thereby reducing the pain. Collectively they are called *physical self-regulation* (PSR). When a patient successfully accomplishes these strategies, he or she gains some control of the pain, which ultimately decreases the pain experience.

One area that can significantly influence many pain conditions is control of autonomic nervous system activity. As mentioned in many sections of this text, the autonomic nervous system often plays an important role in pain. This is especially true in certain musculoskeletal disorders and in the sympathetically maintained pain conditions. Increased levels of environmental challenges or emotional stress increase sympathetic nervous system activity. Although this increased activity is certainly appropriate for acute stressors, chronic maintenance of this up-regulation is not appropriate. However, many patients with chronic pain do just that. These patients are found to maintain a rather rapid rate of breathing from the chest instead of from the diaphragm. Their hand and feet temperatures are colder than normal and their heart rates will increase more rapidly in the presence of stressors.[30] This represents a state of hypervigilance, which increases the pain experience. This is precisely what appears to be present in many posttraumatic stress disorders.

A reasonable treatment approach in the management of chronic TMD and orofacial pains is to develop interventions that address the specific characteristics commonly found in chronic TMD patients. In our research laboratory at the University of Kentucky, we have developed a program of research[31,32] that suggests that patients with chronic muscle-related orofacial pains are distinguished by five characteristics. First, these individuals report significant pain intensity when compared to other pain patients, and they are also more sensitive to painful stimuli in the trigeminal region. This sensitivity to painful stimuli is consistent with research findings in other orofacial pain settings.[33,34] Second, these patients display significant levels of fatigue that impairs normal functioning. This fatigue may be closely related to the third important characteristic, depression, which is common among these patients. Our data, however, further suggest that a significant component of the fatigue is not linked to depression itself. A fourth characteristic of these patients is that breathing patterns are disrupted, so that end-tidal carbon dioxide levels are lower in these patients than in comparable controls. This finding suggests that altered breathing patterns may be contributing to the overall feeling of "physical dysregulation" reported by these patients. Finally, pain patients report significant sleep disturbances involving either sleep-onset difficulties or disruptive awakenings. These five characteristics represent a constellation of symptoms indicative of "autonomic dysregulation" and provide direction for the application of specific intervention strategies to address the underlying physiologic disturbances that may be contributing to the maintenance of the pain disorder.

The following is a treatment approach for chronic orofacial pains that is based on the interpretations of our research findings developed by Drs Peter Bertrand and

Charles Carlson in 1993. This treatment focuses on four areas: *(1)* addressing the pain and fatigue as physiologic disturbances in need of correction, *(2)* managing autonomic dysregulation, *(3)* altering dysfunctional breathing patterns, and *(4)* improving sleep. Since this approach involves entrainment of specific skills to alter physiologic parameters, the approach has been called physical self-regulation (PSR) training. A training manual for PSR was developed by Drs Carlson and Bertrand in 1995 to codify and standardize the procedures.[35] In 2001, Bertrand and Carlson conducted a randomized, controlled clinical trial of the PSR approach in a clinical sample of orofacial pain patients at the National Naval Dental Center in Bethesda, Maryland.[36] The clinical trial included randomization of 44 patients with an average age of 34.6 years and with pain lasting for 52 months into either a group receiving PSR or a group receiving standard dental care (SDC) that included a stabilization appliance. Both treatments resulted in significant decreases in pain intensity and life interference from the pains 6 weeks after treatment was initiated. At 6 months' follow-up, however, the PSR group reported less pain than the SDC group. Comfortable and maximum mouth opening improved for both groups initially as well. At the 6-month follow-up, the PSR group had greater comfortable and maximum mouth opening than did the SDC group. These results provide support for the use and continued evaluation of the PSR approach for managing orofacial pains.

The PSR approach consists of eight areas of education and training.

1. First, patients are provided with an explanation of their condition and given an opportunity to develop personal ownership of the problem.
2. Second, the patients are given instructions regarding the rest positions for structures in the orofacial region[37] and the importance of diminishing muscle

activation by recognizing whether head and neck muscle responses are relevant for specific tasks.

3. Third, specific skills are provided for improving awareness of postural positioning, especially of the head and neck regions. This is termed "proprioceptive re-education," and the rationale for this is further elaborated by Carlson et al.[36]

4. Fourth, a skill for relaxing upper back tension is also imparted to patients through an exercise involving gentle movement of the rhomboid muscle groups.

5. Fifth, a brief progressive relaxation procedure involving the positioning of body structures is given to patients, along with instructions to take at least two periods during daily activities to deeply relax muscle and reduce tension.

6. Sixth, the relaxation training is followed by specific diaphragmatic breathing entrainment instructions so that patients regularly take time to breathe with the diaphragm at a slow, relaxed pace when the body's major skeletal muscles are not being employed in response to stimuli.

7. Seventh, patients are given instructions for beginning sleep in a relaxed position, along with other sleep hygiene recommendations.

8. Finally, patients are provided with instructions on the role of fluid intake, nutrition, and exercise for the restoration of normal functioning.

The entire PSR program is presented within a framework that focuses on understanding pain as a physiologic disturbance that is best managed by addressing those disturbances through rest, nutrition, tissue repair, behavioral regulation of autonomic functioning, and appropriate activity. The PSR approach focuses on limiting any activity that increases the sense of discomfort or pain to promote return of pain-free function.

Our clinical experience in working with PSR over the past 10 years suggests it is a valuable treatment for a variety of orofacial pain conditions. Although it was initially designed predominantly for masticatory muscle pain disorders, we have found it also helpful in managing many intracapsular disorders. PSR assists in managing intracapsular disorder by enabling recognition of inappropriate muscle activity that can lead to co-contraction and inhibition of efficient synovial fluid diffusion into previously overloaded joints. By reducing muscle loading, PSR helps re-establish normal function with pain-free range of motion. In fact, PSR is helpful in most orofacial pain conditions because it enables the patient to gain control of many physiologic functions and reverse the "dysregulation" of their physiologic systems. For those interested in adding this approach to their clinical practices, a more detailed description of the PSR approach can be obtained elsewhere.[35,36] While more clinical trials are needed to further evaluate the PSR approach, our current data, both from controlled scientific study and clinical practice, indicate that patients can receive substantial benefit from PSR training.

A Closing Note

Perhaps the most important concepts for the clinician to remember when managing pain are: Listen carefully, consider all possibilities, cure if you can, manage if you cannot, but always console.

References

1. Mock D, Frydman W, Gorden AS. Atypical facial pain: A retrospective study. Oral Surg Oral Med Oral Pathol 1985;59:472–474.
2. Walters A. The psychogenic regional pain syndrome and its diagnosis. In: Knighton RS, Dumke PR (eds). Pain. Boston: Little, Brown, 1966:439–456.
3. Gerschman J, Burrows G, Reade P. Chronic orofacial pain. In: Bonica JJ, Liebeskind JC, Albe-Fessard DG (eds). Proceedings of the Second World Congress on Pain, vol 3, Advances in Pain Research and Therapy. New York: Raven Press, 1979:317–323.
4. Donaldson D, Kroening R. Recognition and treatment of patients with chronic orofacial pain. J Am Dent Assoc 1979;99:961–966.
5. Moulton RE. Psychiatric considerations in maxillofacial pain. J Am Dent Assoc 1955;51:408–414.
6. Beck FM, Kaul TJ, Weaver JM. Recognition and management of the depressed dental patient. J Am Dent Assoc 1979;99:967–971.
7. Fordyce WE. Behavior conditioning concepts in chronic pain. In: Bonica JJ, Lindblom U, Iggo A (eds). Proceedings of the Third World Congress on Pain, vol 5, Advances in Pain Research and Therapy. New York: Raven Press, 1983:781–788.
8. Sternbach RA. Fundamentals of psychological methods in chronic pain. In: Bonica JJ, Lindblom U, Iggo A (eds). Proceedings of the Third World Congress on Pain, vol 5, Advances in Pain Research and Therapy. New York: Raven Press, 1983:777–780.
9. Roberts AH. Contingency management methods in the treatment of chronic pain. In: Bonica JJ, Lindblom U, Iggo A (eds). Proceedings of the Third World Congress on Pain, vol 5, Advances in Pain Research and Therapy. New York: Raven Press, 1983:789–794.
10. Lindblom U, Tegner R. Are the endorphins active in chronic pain states? Narcotic antagonism in chronic pain patients. Pain 1979;7:65–68.
11. Chapman CR, Butler SH. Effects of doxepin on perception of laboratory induced pain in man. Pain 1978;5:253–262.
12. Ward NG, Bloom VL, Frieder RO. The effectiveness of tricyclic antidepressants in the treatment of coexisting pain and depression. Pain 1979;7:331–341.
13. Pilling LF. Psychosomatic aspects of facial pain. In: Alling CC, Mahan PE (eds). Facial Pain, ed 2. Philadelphia: Lea & Febiger, 1977:213–226.
14. Wurtele SK, Kaplan GM, Keairnes M. Childhood sexual abuse among chronic pain patients. Clin J Pain 1990;6:110–113.
15. Haber JD, Roos C. Effects of spouse abuse and/or sexual abuse in the development and maintenance of chronic pain in women. In: Fields HL, Dubner R, Cervero F (eds). Proceedings of the Fourth World Congress on Pain: Seattle, vol 9, Advances in Pain Research and Therapy. New York: Raven Press, 1985:889–895.
16. Domino JV, Haber JD. Prior physical and sexual abuse in women with chronic headaches: Clinical correlates. Headache 1988;27:310–314.
17. Curran SL, Sherman JJ, Cunningham LL, Okeson JP, Reid KI, Carlson CR. Physical and sexual abuse among orofacial pain patients: Linkages with pain and psychologic distress. J Orofac Pain 1995;9:340–346.
18. Fillingim RB, Maixner W, Sigurdsson A, Kincaid S. Sexual and physical abuse history in subjects with temporomandibular disorders: Relationship to clinical variables, pain sensitivity, and psychologic factors. J Orofac Pain 1997;11:48–57.
19. Fillingim RB, Wilkinson CS, Powell T. Self-reported abuse history and pain complaints among young adults. Clin J Pain 1999;15:85–91.
20. Finestone HM, Stenn P, Davies F, Stalker C, Fry R, Koumanis J. Chronic pain and health care utilization in women with a history of childhood sexual abuse. Child Abuse Negl 2000;24:547–556.
21. Diagnostic and Statistical Manual of Mental Disorders (DSM-IV). Washington, DC: American Psychiatric Association, 1994.
22. Leino P, Magni G. Depressive and distress symptoms as predictors of low back pain, shoulder pain, and other musculoskeletal morbidity. Pain 1993;53:89–94.
23. Magni G. On the relationship between chronic pain and depression when there is no organic lesion. Pain 1987;31:1–21.
24. Magni G, Caldieron C, Rigatti-Luchini S, Merskey H. Chronic musculoskeletal pain and depressive symptoms in the general population. An analysis of the 1st National Health and Nutrition Examination Survey data. Pain 1990;43:299–307.

25. Magni G, Marchetti M, Moreschi C, Merskey H, Luchini SR. Chronic musculoskeletal pain and depressive symptoms in the National Health and Nutrition Examination. I. Epidemiologic follow-up study. Pain 1993;53:163–168.

26. Carroll LJ, Cassidy JD, Cote P. Depression as a risk factor for onset of an episode of troublesome neck and low back pain. Pain 2004;107:134–139.

27. Magni G, Moreschi C, Rigatti-Luchini S, Merskey H. Prospective study on the relationship between depressive symptons and chronic musculoskeletal pain. Pain 1994;54:289–297.

28. Green CR, Flowe Valencia H, Rosenblum L, Tait AR. Do physical and sexual abuse differentially affect chronic pain states in women? J Pain Symptom Manage 1999;18:420–426.

29. Yaksh TL, Abram SE. Preemptive analgesia: A popular misnomer, but a clinically relevant truth? Am Pain Soc J 1993;2:116–121.

30. Carlson CR, Okeson JP, Falace DA, Nitz AJ, Curran SL, Anderson DT. A comparison of psychological and physiological functioning between patients with masticatory muscle pain and controls. J Orofac Pain 1993;7:15–22.

31. Curran SL, Carlson CR, Okeson JP. Emotional and physiologic responses to laboratory challenges: Patients with temporomandibular disorders versus matched control subjects. J Orofac Pain 1996;10:141–150.

32. Carlson CR, Reid KI, Curran SL, et al. Psychological and physiological parameters of masticatory muscle pain. Pain 1998;76:297–307.

33. Maixner W, Fillingim R, Booker D, Sigurdsson A. Sensitivity of patients with painful temporomandibular disorders to experimentally evoked pain. Pain 1995;63:341–351.

34. Svensson P, Arendt-Nielsen L, Nielsen H, Larsen JK. Effect of chronic and experimental jaw muscle pain on pain-pressure thresholds and stimulus-response curves. J Orofac Pain 1995;9:347–356.

35. Carlson CR, Bertrand P. Self-Regulation Training Manual. Lexington, KY: University Press, 1995.

36. Carlson C, Bertrand P, Ehrlich A, Maxwell A, Burton RG. Physical self-regulation training for the management of temporomandibular disorders. J Orofac Pain 2001;15:47–55.

37. Carlson CR, Sherman JJ, Studts JL, Bertrand PM. The effects of tongue position on mandibular muscle activity. J Orofac Pain 1997;11:291–297.

Terminology

Terms that constitute the language of pain should be defined precisely enough to prevent ambiguity and misunderstandings. Many of the definitions listed below are based on terminology proposed by the Subcommittee on Taxonomy of the International Association for the Study of Pain.[1-4] Some are from a standard medical dictionary.[5] A few are specially defined to express a precise meaning by the author. The reader is urged to become familiar with these definitions.

Algogenic Causing pain.

Allodynia Pain resulting from a stimulus that does not normally provoke pain. *(Note: This condition is seen in patients when touch, light pressure, or moderate cold or warmth evoke pain when applied to apparently normal skin.)*

Analgesia Absence of pain in response to stimulation that would normally be painful.

Anesthesia Absence of all sensation.

Anesthesia dolorosa Pain in an area or region that is anesthetic.

Antidromic Conducting impulses in a direction opposite to the normal.

Arthralgia Pain that is felt in joint structures *(Note: If the site of pain represents the source, the arthralgia would be arthrogenous; otherwise, it would be heterotopic.)*

Arthrogenous pain Pain originating from joint structures.

Causalgia A syndrome of sustained burning pain, allodynia, and hyperpathia resulting from a traumatic nerve lesion, often combined with vasomotor and sudomotor dysfunction and later trophic changes. *(Note: Causalgia and the changes listed above are closely associated with complex regional pain syndrome [CRPS].)*

Central pain Pain initiated or caused by a primary lesion or dysfunction in the central nervous system.

Deafferentation The partial or total loss of afferent neural activity to a particular body region through removal of part of the neural pathway.

Denervation Resection or removal of the nerves to an organ or part of the body.

Dysesthesia An unpleasant abnormal sensation, whether spontaneous or evoked. *(Note: Paresthesia is an abnormal sensation whether unpleasant or not. Paresthesia includes dysesthesia, but not vice versa.)*

Heterotopic pain A general term to designate pain that is felt in an area other than its true site of origin. *(Note: Peripheral heterotopic pain may be felt as projected pain, referred pain, or secondary hyperalgesia.)*

Hypalgesia Diminished sensitivity to stimulation-evoked pain.

Hyperalgesia An increased response to a stimulus that is normally painful. *(Note: Primary hyperalgesia is stimulation-evoked primary pain resulting from a lowered local pain threshold. Secondary hyperalgesia is stimulation-evoked pain that occurs without appreciable change in the local pain threshold. Secondary hyperalgesia has a central component.)*

Hyperesthesia Increased sensitivity to stimulation, excluding the special senses. *(Note: When the sensation is painful, the terms allodynia and hyperalgesia are appropriate.)*

Hyperpathia A painful syndrome characterized by an abnormally painful reaction to a stimulus, especially a repetitive stimulus, as well as an increased threshold. *(Note: This may occur with allodynia, hyperesthesia, hyperalgesia, or dysesthesia.)*

Hypoesthesia Diminished sensitivity to stimulation. *(Note: When the sensation is painful, the terms hypalgesia and analgesia are appropriate.)*

Inflammatory pain Pain that emanates from tissue that is inflamed.

Musculoskeletal pain Deep somatic pain that originates in skeletal muscles, fascial sheaths, and tendons (myogenous pain); in bones and periosteum (osseous pain); in joints, joint capsules, and ligaments (arthralgic pain); and in soft connective tissues (soft connective tissue pain).

Myalgia Pain that is felt in muscle tissue. *(Note: If the site of pain represents its source, the myalgia would be myogenous; otherwise, it would be heterotopic.)*

Myofascial trigger point A hyperirritable spot, usually within a taut band of skeletal muscle or in the muscle fascia, that is painful on compression and that can give rise to characteristic referred pain, tenderness (secondary hyperalgesia), and autonomic phenomena.[6]

Neuralgia Neuropathic pain felt in the distribution of a nerve or nerves. *(Note: Paroxysmal neuralgia consists of sudden bursts of burning pain.)*

Neuropathic pain Pain initiated or caused by a primary lesion or dysfunction in the nervous system.

Neuropathy A disturbance of function or pathologic change in a nerve. If it occurs in one nerve, it is termed mononeuropathy; if it occurs in several nerves, it is called mononeuropathy multiplex; if it is diffuse and bilateral, the term polyneuropathy should be used.

Neuroplasticity The dynamic ability of the central nervous system to alter the processing of impulses in response to continued input and/or other factors.

Nociception The mechanism that provides for the reception and conversion of noxious or potentially noxious stimuli into neural impulses and the transmission of such impulses by A-delta and C fibers to the central nervous system, where they are modulated and acted on.

Nociceptive pathway An afferent neural pathway that mediates pain impulses.

Nociceptor A receptor that is preferentially sensitive to a noxious stimulus or to a stimulus that would become noxious if prolonged.

Noxious stimulus A stimulus that is damaging to normal tissues.

Odontalgia Pain that is felt in a tooth. *(Note: If the tooth is the source of the pain, the odontalgia would be odontogenous; if not, it would be heterotopic.)*

Odontogenous pain Deep somatic pain that originates in dental pulps, periodontal ligaments, or both.

Orthodromic Conducting impulses in the normal direction.

Pain An unpleasant sensory and emotional experience associated with actual or potential tissue damage, or described in terms of such damage.

Pain behavior The subject's audible and visible actions that communicate his or her suffering to other.

Pain threshold The least experience of pain that a subject can recognize.

Pain tolerance level The greatest level of pain that a subject is prepared to tolerate.

Paresthesia An abnormal sensation, whether spontaneous or evoked. *(Note: If an abnormal sensation is unpleasant, the term dysesthesia is appropriate.)*

Peripheral neurogenic pain Pain initiated or caused by a primary lesion or dysfunction or transitory perturbation in the peripheral nervous system.

Peripheral neuropathic pain Pain initiated or caused by a primary lesion or dysfunction in the peripheral nervous system.

Periodontal pain Odontogenous pain that emanates from the periodontal ligaments.

Primary pain Pain that identifies the true source of nociceptive input.

Projected pain Heterotopic pain that is felt in the anatomic peripheral distribution of the same nerve that mediates the primary pain.

Pulpal pain Odontogenous pain that emanates from the dental pulps.

Referred pain Heterotopic pain that is felt in an area that is innervated by a nerve different from the one that mediates the primary pain. *(Note: Referred pain implies that it occurs without provocation at the site of pain.)*

Reflex sympathetic dystrophy A syndrome of unremitting, burning pain as the result of deafferentation.

Secondary hyperalgesia Heterotopic pain that is evoked by stimulation at the site of pain.

Secondary pain Heterotopic pain that is induced by deep somatic pain as a central excitatory effect.

Site of pain The anatomic site where pain is felt.

Somatic pain Pain originating in any body structure other than neurogenous structures.

Source of pain The origin of the nociceptive process that is causing the pain experience.

Suffering The emotional response to pain and other factors that reflect the subject's anticipated impending and future threat to his or her well-being. It is influenced by factors that may or may not relate to the initiating pain experience.

Sympathetically maintained pain Pain sustained through activity of the sympathetic nervous system.

Symptoms The objective and subjective evidence of change in structure or function that is indicative of abnormality, dysfunction, or disease.

Vascular pain A type of deep somatic pain of visceral origin that emanates from the afferent nerves that innervate blood vessels. *(Note: Inflammatory vascular pain should be designated as vasculitis.)*

Visceral pain Deep somatic pain that originates in visceral structures such as mucosal linings, walls of hollow viscera, parenchyma of organs, glands, dental pulps, and vascular structures.

References

1. Merskey H. Pain terms: A list with definitions and notes on usage. Pain 1979;6:249–252.
2. Merskey H. Pain terms: A supplementary note. Pain 1982;14:205–206.
3. Merskey H, Bogduk N, IASP Task Force on Taxonomy (eds). Classification of Chronic Pain, ed 2. Seattle: IASP Press, 1994:209–214.
4. Merskey H. Pain specialists and pain terms. Pain 1996;64:205.
5. Anderson DM. Dorland's Illustrated Medical Dictionary, ed 26. Philadelphia: Saunders, 1994:1252.
6. Travell JG, Simons DG. Myofascial Pain and Dysfunction. Baltimore: Williams & Wilkins, 1983.

Index

Page numbers followed by "f" denote figures; those followed by "t" denote tables.

A

A fibers, 19
Abducent nerve
  anatomy of, 36f, 38
  evaluation of, 57f, 156
Accessory nerve
  anatomy of, 36f, 39
  evaluation of, 158
Accommodation reflex, 156, 157f
Acetaminophen, 201
Acetylcholine, 49
Acoustic nerve
  anatomy of, 36f
  evaluation of, 158
Action potential, nerve, 45–46
Acupuncture
  description of, 85–86
  transcutaneous electrical nerve stimulation
    vs., 86
Acute cellulitis, 385
Acute dental alveolitis. *See* Dry-socket pain.
Acute malocclusion, 295
Acute necrotizing ulcerative gingivitis, 247,
  250f
Acute pain
  biopsychosocial model of, 522
  characteristics of, 108, 197
  chronic pain vs., 522
  definition of, 101
  diagnosis of, 177
  physiology of, 85
Acute pulpal pain, 263–264, 265f
Acute retrodiscitis, 348–349
Acyclovir, 210

Addiction, 202
A-delta fibers, 81, 120
Adjuvant analgesics, 203
Afferent neuron, 11, 15, 69, 71–74
A-fiber mechano/heat-sensitive nociceptors,
  17–18
Aggravating factors, 149–150
Allergic responses, 247
Alleviating factors, 149–150
Allodynia, 73, 467, 469f
Amitriptyline, 207
Amygdala, 26
Analgesic agents
  narcotic, 201–203
  nonnarcotic, 201
  temporomandibular joint pains treated with,
    369–370
Analgesic blocking, for pain diagnosis
    confirmation
  dental pain, 274, 277
  equipment for, 182–183
  indications for, 182
  injections
    description of, 183–184
    intra-articular, 191
    intracapsular, 190–191, 191f
    muscle, 184–186, 185f
    nerve block, 186, 188–190, 189f–190f
  local anesthetic used in, 183
  myotoxicity caused by, 183
  rules for, 183
Analgesic system, 82
Anesthesia dolorosa, 117–118, 484
Anesthetic agents
  injectable, 203–206
  topical, 203, 204f

Anterior mandibular positioning appliance, 370–372
Anterior open bite, 353, 354f
Anterolateral spinothalamic tract, 21
Antianxiety agents, 208
Anticonvulsive agents, 210
Antidepressants, 207–208
Antidromic, 63
Antihistamine agents, 210
Anti-inflammatory agents, 206–207
Antimicrobial agents, 209–210
Antiviral agents, 210
Anxiety disorders
  classification of, 529f
  description of, 139
  generalized anxiety disorder, 528
  posttraumatic stress disorder, 530, 543
Aqueduct of Sylvius, 28
Arachidonic acid, 53, 63
Arteritis
  cranial, 437, 439
  definition of, 437
Arthralgia
  characteristics of, 329
  masticatory, 329, 330f
  nonmasticatory origin of, 364
  pain caused by, 335
  temporomandibular joint
    as capsular pain, 351
    description of, 346
    hyperuricemia as cause of, 359
    inflammatory, 363
    inflammatory fibrous ankylosis, 361
    intermittent, 363
    malignant tumors, 362
Arthritis
  osteoarthritis, 329, 353–355, 354f, 357f, 358
  rheumatoid, 353, 354f
  signs and symptoms of, 356
  traumatic, 353, 356
Articular disc, 331, 332f
Aspartate, 50
Aspirin, 199
Association tracts, 25
Atypical facial pain, 431, 433–435, 522–523
Atypical odontalgia, 282–283, 490, 492–493
Aura, migraine with
  description of, 405–406
  diagnosis of, 413–414
Auricular pain, 397, 399
Auriculotemporal nerve block, 186, 188, 189f
Autonomic nerves, 37f

Autonomic nervous system
  definition of, 10, 31
  evaluation of, 159
  functions of, 31, 34
  pain management and, 539
  parasympathetic division of, 33f, 33–34
  sympathetic division of, 31–33, 32f
Axis I
  characteristics of, 523
  description of, 129–138, 133t, 178f, 521
  schematic diagram of, 178f, 244f, 260f, 288f, 330f, 382f, 402f
Axis II
  characteristics of, 523
  description of, 129, 133t, 138–139, 521
  mental disorders. *See* Mental disorders.
  schematic diagram of, 178f, 244f, 260f, 288f, 330f, 382f, 402f
Axolemma, 14
Axon, 14f, 14–15, 45
Axon transport system, 56, 110
Axoplasm, 14

B

Baclofen, 464
Balance, 161
Basal ganglia, 26
Behavior
  learned, 228
  pain-related, 8–9, 141–142, 220, 520, 524
Behavioral modification training, 220–226
Beta-adrenergic blocking agents, 209
Beta-endorphin, 51
Biofeedback, 222–223
Biopsychosocial model, 98–99, 100f, 520
Bipolar disorder, 526, 528
Botulinum toxin A, 318, 420
Bradykinin, 51–53, 63
Brain, 9–10
Brain tumors, 119–120
Brainstem
  anatomy of, 22, 23f, 27–28
  arousal level of, 95–96
Bruxing, 316
Bulboreticular formation area, 59
Burning mouth disorders, 253–255, 493–495

C

C fibers, 19–20, 63, 81
Cafergot, 415
Calcitonin gene-related peptide, 64, 407
Calcium channel blockers, 415–416

Calcium channels, 48
Capsaicin, 488, 496
Capsular fibrosis, 350, 352
Capsular pain, of temporomandibular joint
  capsulitis, 350
  causes of, 350
  fibrosis, 350, 352
  synovitis, 350
Capsulitis, 350
Carbamazepine, 210, 463
Cardiac toothache, 279–281
Carotidynia, 364, 439–440
Causalgia, 119, 498–499. *See also* Complex
    regional pain syndrome.
Cellulitis, 385
Central nervous system
  brainstem, 22, 23f
  cerebellum, 23
  cerebrum. *See* Cerebrum.
  description of, 10, 15
  diencephalon, 24–25
  muscle pain affected by, 294
Central pain, 67
Central sensitization, 68–76, 466–467
Centrally mediated myalgia
  characteristics of, 112, 291, 311, 313
  management of, 321–322, 323f
Cerebellopontine angle tumors, 119
Cerebellum, 23
Cerebrospinal fluid, 27f, 27–28
Cerebrum
  basal ganglia, 26
  cerebral cortex, 25–26
  description of, 22, 25
  limbic structures, 26–27
Cervical evaluation, 160–161, 161f
Cervical spinal nerves, 38–39
C-fiber mechano/heat-sensitive nociceptors,
    17–18
c-fos, 68
Chemical synapse, 46
Chief complaint, 145–150
Chondromalacia, 345
Chronic mandibular hypomobilities, 360
Chronic myalgia disorders, 294
Chronic pain
  acute pain vs., 522
  biopsychosocial model of, 522
  considerations related to, 226–228
  definition of, 522
  depression and, 228
  description of, 101, 108, 197

diagnosis of, 177
management of, 522
neuroplasticity and, 120–121
nociceptive input, 522
treatment of, 537–539
Chronic pulpal pain, 265–266, 266f
Chronicity, 524–525
Cingulate gyrus, 26–27
c-jun, 68
Class II malocclusions, 347
Clinical examination
  autonomic functioning, 159
  balance, 161
  cervical evaluation, 160–161, 161f
  coordination, 161
  cranial nerve evaluation, 153, 156–158
  ears, 160
  eyes, 160
  imaging, 174
  laboratory tests, 174, 176
  location of pain determined by, 152–153
  masticatory evaluation. *See* Masticatory
      evaluation.
  muscles. *See* Muscle examination.
  psychologic assessment, 176–177
  summary of, 156t
  superficial reflexes, 159
  vital signs, 153
Clinical pain, 3–4, 108
Clonazepam, 208, 495
Clonidine, 503
Cluster headache
  autonomic features of, 421–422
  characteristics of, 421–422, 429t
  description of, 421
  diagnosis of, 423
  duration of, 422
  epidemiology of, 421–422
  ergotamine for, 424–425
  indomethacin for, 425
  lidocaine for, 424
  management of, 423–425
  pathophysiology of, 422
  periodicity of, 422
  precipitating factors, 422–423
  sumatriptan for, 424
  trauma and, 422–423
  zolmitriptan for, 425
Co-contraction
  muscle, 74, 112
  myofascial pain and, 297

protective
  characteristics of, 291–293
  management of, 315–316
Commissural tracts, 25
Complex regional pain syndrome, 138, 496–498
Concomitant symptoms, 148
Conditioning, 96, 524
Condyle-disc complex, 331, 333–334, 334f
Consultations
  history taking regarding, 150
  medical, 176
  pain diagnosis confirmation by, 192
Continuous neuropathic pain, 116–119, 138,
    179, 179f
Continuous neuropathic toothache, 282
Convergence, 65
Conversion disorder, 151, 531, 533
Coolant therapy, 368
Coordination, 161
Coping strategies, 220
Corneal reflex, 159
Cortex
  afferent impulse transmission to, 56–59
  anatomy of, 9–10
Corticosteroids, 206–207
Counseling, 218–220
Counterirritation, 212
Cranial arteritis, 437, 439
Cranial nerves. See also specific nerve.
  anatomy of, 36f, 38–39
  evaluation of, 153, 156–158
Cranial neuralgias
  classification of, 463t
  description of, 451
  glossopharyngeal neuralgia, 457–459
  nervus intermedius neuralgia, 459–460
  pathophysiology of, 460–461
  trigeminal neuralgia
    characteristics of, 114–115, 115f, 281, 451,
      453
    classification of, 461
    posttraumatic, 482, 484
    pre-, 457
    triggers of, 453
Crepitation, 170
Cutaneous pain
  behavior of, 243
  differential diagnosis, 255–256
  of face, 245
Cutaneous stimulation, 212–214, 213f
Cyclic muscle pain, 293–294, 363, 434
Cyclobenzaprine, 321, 324

Cyclooxygenase, 53, 63, 201, 370

D

Deafferentation pain
  description of, 117–118, 255–256, 481
  pathophysiology of, 482f
  toothache, 282
  traumatic neuroma, 481–489
Decubitus ulcers, 247, 248f
Deep heat therapy, 216
Deep massage, 217
Deep somatic pain
  cervical causes of, 308
  characteristics of, 109, 112–114, 135–137,
    180–181
  diagnosis of, 180–181, 363
  differential diagnosis, 385–386
  primary, 387
  treatment of, 386
Deep tendon reflexes, 306
Deflection of mandibular opening, 168, 169f
Degenerative joint disease. See Osteoarthritis.
Dendrites, 14, 14f, 45
Dental pain
  behavior of, 261–262
  central inhibition deficiency as cause of, 272
  classification of, 260f
  myofascial trigger points and, 273–274
  periodontal origin of, 269–272
  prevalence of, 259
  pulpal pain. See Pulpal pain.
  referred, 272
  secondary effects of, 272–273
  stimulus of, 262
  tender teeth, 273
Dental practitioner, 4–5
Dentin sensitivity, 261
Depolarization, 45
Depression, 202, 228, 524, 526
Dermatomes, 70f–71f, 71
Descending inhibitory system, 82–85, 83f, 228
Desipramine, 495
Deviation of mandibular opening, 168, 169f
Diabetes mellitus, 506
Diagnosis
  confirmation of
    analgesic blocking for. See Diagnostic
      analgesic blocking.
    consultation for, 192
    diagnostic drugs for, 192
    trial therapy for, 192
  definitive, 218

description of, 129
difficulties associated with, 141–142
evaluation of pain condition, 142
history taking for. *See* History taking.
objective of, 141
pain category determined, 177–182
preliminary interview for, 142–144
steps involved in, 142
Diagnostic analgesic blocking
  for dental pain, 274, 277
  equipment for, 182–183
  indications for, 182
  injections
    description of, 183–184
    intra-articular, 191
    intracapsular, 190–191, 191f
    muscle, 184–186, 185f
    nerve block, 186, 188–190, 189f–190f
  local anesthetic used in, 183
  myotoxicity caused by, 183
  rules for, 183
Diencephalon, 24–25
Dietary changes, 211–212
Diffuse noxious inhibitory control, 82, 110
Diffuse pain, 148
Diffusion, 52
Dihydroergotamine, 415, 424
Disc derangement, 338–343
Divergence, 65
Dopamine, 50
Dry mouth syndrome. *See* Xerostomia.
Dry-socket pain, 383–384
Dynamic nerve terminal, 46–47
Dynorphin, 82

E

Eagle syndrome, 364
Ear evaluation, 160
Ear pain, 397, 399
Earache, 314, 399
Efferent neurons, 74–75
EGS, 216
Electrical synapse, 46
Electroacupuncture, 85–86, 214
Electrogalvanic stimulation, 319
Elevator muscle pain, 314
Emotional state, 96–97
Emotional stress, 97
Endoneurium, 14
Endorphins, 51, 84–85
Enkephalins, 51, 84
Entrapment neuropathy, 489–490

Ephapse, 15
Epineurium, 13
Episodic neuropathic pain
  cranial neuralgias. *See* Cranial neuralgias.
  description of, 137–138, 179f
  paroxysmal neuralgia. *See* Paroxysmal neuralgia.
Episodic neuropathic toothache, 281
Ergotamine, 424–425
Esophagitis, 388
Examination. *See* Clinical examination; Muscle examination.
Excitatory neurons, 21
Exercise, 217, 221
Expectancy, 96
Experimental pain, 108
Exteroceptors, 16–17
Extracranial tumors, 119–120
Eye evaluation, 160

F

Facial expression muscles, 305, 307f
Facial nerve
  anatomy of, 36f, 38–39
  evaluation of, 158
  neuritis of, 473
Facial pain, atypical, 431, 433–435, 522–523
Facilitation, 78
Famciclovir, 210, 253
Fasciitis, 311
Fast pain, 57
Fibromyalgia
  description of, 290, 313
  management of, 323–324
Fibrous ankylosis, 361
Fight-or-flight reaction, 34, 97
5HT receptors, 209
Flare, 56, 110
Free nerve endings, 17–19
Frontal lobe, 25
Functional activities, 149
Functional disc displacement
  clinical features of, 340f
  description of, 336–338, 337f, 340, 340f
  with reduction, 340–341, 341f
  without reduction, 341–343, 342f
Fungal infections, 247, 250f

G

GABA, 50
Gabapentin, 464, 498
Gag reflex, 159

Ganglia
  basal, 26
  definition of, 14
Gate control theory, 76–77, 77f
Generalized anxiety disorders, 528
Geniculate herpes, 479
Geniculate neuralgia, 391, 459
Giant cell arteritis. *See* Cranial arteritis.
Gigantocellular nucleus, 81
Gingiva, 172
Gingivitis
  acute necrotizing ulcerative, 247, 250f
  pregnancy-related, 250, 251f
Ginglymoarthrodial joint, 331
Glandular pain, 396f, 397
Glossodynia, 254
Glossopharyngeal nerve
  anatomy of, 36f, 38–39
  evaluation of, 158
Glossopharyngeal neuralgia, 364–365, 457–459
Glossopharyngeal neuritis, 473, 475, 477f
Glutamate, 49–50
Glycerol, 211
Glycine, 50
Golgi tendon organs, 17–18
G-protein–linked channel, 48
Gyrus
  definition of, 25
  parahippocampal, 26–27

H

Headache
  biofeedback for, 223
  cluster. *See* Cluster headache.
  features of, 429t
  hypnic, 430
  International Headache Society classification
    of, 130t, 130–131, 404f
  migraine. *See* Migraine.
  mixed, 418
  new daily-persistent, 430
  pain caused by, 121–122
  primary, 130t
  primary cough, 430
  primary exertional, 430
  primary stabbing, 429–430
  primary thunderclap, 430
  secondary, 130t
  sinus, 394
  SUNCT syndrome, 427–428, 429t
  tension-type. *See* Tension-type headache.
Hearing evaluations, 158f

Hemicrania continua, 430
Herpes simplex infection, 251–253
Herpes zoster, 116–117, 256, 478–481, 496
Heterotopic pain
  central pain, 67
  definition of, 66, 109
  diagnosis of, 179–180
  differential diagnosis, 255
  in eye, 397
  nondental origin of, 273–274
  preauricular pain, 396
  projected pain, 67–68
  referred pain, 68–69, 71–73, 313
  toothaches caused by
    cardiac, 279–281
    description of, 277
    muscular, 277–278
    neurovascular, 277, 279
  types of, 66–68
Hippocampus, 26
Histamine, 50
History taking
  aggravating factors, 149–150
  alleviating factors, 149–150
  behavior of pain, 147–148
  characteristics of pain, 147–148
  chief complaint, 145–150
  concomitant symptoms, 148
  description of, 144, 145
  elements of, 145t
  forms of, 144
  intensity of pain, 148
  litigation, 150
  location of pain, 145, 146f
  manner of flow of pain, 148
  medical history, 150
  onset of pain, 145, 147
  oral, 144
  past consultations, 150
  past treatments, 150
  psychologic assessment, 150–151
  quality of pain, 147
  review of systems, 150
  summary of, 151–152
  written, 144
Horner syndrome, 159
Hydrotherapy, 214
Hyperalgesia
  definition of, 64
  localized, 246
  primary, 64, 246
  secondary, 73-74, 179, 273, 297, 306, 392

Hypernoceptors, 113
Hypersensitivity, 255
Hyperuricemia, 359
Hypnic headache, 430
Hypnotherapy, 222
Hypochondriasis, 151, 533, 535
Hypoglossal nerve
  anatomy of, 36f, 39
  evaluation of, 158
Hypothalamic-pituitary-adrenal axis, 24
Hypothalamus, 24–25
Hypothyroid neuropathy, 506
Hypoxia/reperfusion theory, 345

I

Iatrogenic pain, 122
Indomethacin
  for cluster headache, 425
  for paroxysmal hemicrania, 427
Infection
  herpes simplex, 251–253
  mucogingival pain caused by, 247, 250f
  periosteal pain caused by, 384
  upper respiratory, 393–395
Inferior alveolar nerve block, 204f
Inferior lateral pterygoid
  anatomy of, 165
  myofascial pain referral to, 300–301, 301f
  pain referral to, 314–315, 348
  trigger points in, 301, 301f
Inflammation
  neurogenic, 56, 113
  of periosteum, 384
  pain caused by, 110–111, 181–182
  periarticular, 357, 360
Inflammatory arthritis, 353, 354f
Inflammatory fibrous ankylosis, 361
Inframylohyoid cellulitis, 385
Infraorbital anesthesia, 149
Infraorbital nerve block, 188, 190f
Inhibition, 79
Inhibitory neurons, 20
Injectable anesthetic agents, 203–206
Injury
  pain and, 7
  pain-producing substances released secondary
    to, 52–53, 53f
Insula, 26–27
Intensity of pain, 108, 147–148, 287
Intermittent pain, 147
Interneurons, 15, 21
Interocclusal appliances, 223–224, 224f

Interoceptors, 17
Interview
  history taking. *See* History taking.
  preliminary, 142–144
Intra-articular injections, 191
Intracapsular injections, 190–191, 191f
Intracranial pain, 119–120
Inverse stretch reflex, 18, 217
Ion channels
  description of, 47
  G-protein–linked, 48
  ligand-gated, 49
  voltage-gated, 48
Iontophoresis, 368
Isometric jaw exercises, for centrally mediated
    myalgia, 322, 323f

L

Laminae, 20
Lamotrigine, 464–465
Lancinating, 148
Lateral pterygoid, 165
Learned behavior, 228
Lemniscal system, 21
Leukotrienes, 54
Ligand-gated channels, 49
Lipoxygenase pathway, 54
Local anesthetic injections, 319–320, 320f
Local infections, 247, 250f
Local muscle soreness
  characteristics of, 291, 293–294, 311
  management of, 316–317
Localization behavior of pain, 148
Localized hyperalgesia, 246
Location of pain
  anesthetic techniques, 155f
  clinical examination to determine, 152–153
  dental pain, 262
  history taking regarding, 145, 146f
  mucogingival pain, 246
  periodontal pain, 271
  provocation for, 154f, 274, 275f
Locus ceruleus, 81, 410
Low-threshold mechanosensitive neurons, 20,
    30–31
Lymphadenitis, 397

M

Macrotrauma, 343–344
Maladaptive health behavior, 535, 537
Malingering, 535
Malocclusion, acute, 295

Mammillary bodies, 26
Mandible
  movement evaluation for, 167–169
  opening of
    deflection in, 168, 169f
    deviation in, 168, 169f
    extracapsular restrictions, 168
    intracapsular restrictions, 168–169
    pain production during, 169
    restricted, 167
Mandibular block anesthesia, 149
Mandibular positioning appliance, 370–372
Manic-depressive illness, 528
Manner of flow of pain, 148
Massage, 216–217, 319
Masseter
  injection of, 187f
  myofascial pain referral to, 298f, 298–299
  palpation of, 164, 164f
  trigger points in, 298f
Masticatory arthralgia, 329, 330f
Masticatory evaluation
  criteria used in, 167
  mandibular movement, 167–169
  oral structures, 171–174
  temporomandibular joint, 169–171
Masticatory pain
  case studies of, 302–303
  cycling, 302, 434
  events, 291–292
  local muscle soreness, 291, 293–294, 316–317
  model of, 290f, 290–291
  neuralgic pain vs., 462–463
  neurovascular pain vs., 435
  protective co-contraction, 291–293, 315–316
  referred pain vs., 313
  sympathetically maintained pain vs., 501
  tension-type headache and, 418
  types of, 289–290, 314–315
Maxillary sinusitis, 474
McGill Pain Questionnaire, 143
Mechanical vibration, 213–214
Mechanistic model, 98–99, 100f
Mechanoreceptors, 259
Medial pterygoid muscle, 299–300, 300f
Medical consultation, 176
Medical history, 150
Medulla oblongata, 22
Meissner's corpuscles, 17
Mental disorders
  anxiety disorders
    classification of, 529f

generalized anxiety disorder, 528
    posttraumatic stress disorder, 530, 543
  bipolar disorder, 526, 528
  classification of, 527f
  depression, 526
  description of, 526
  mood disorders, 526, 528
Merkel's corpuscles, 17
Mesencephalon, 23
Metabolic polyneuropathies
  alcoholism and, 506, 508
  characteristics of, 116, 506, 508
  classification of, 507f
  diabetes mellitus and, 506
  diagnosis of, 508
  electrophysiologic testing of, 508
  management of, 508–509
  pathophysiology of, 508
  precipitating factors, 508
  tricyclic antidepressants for, 509
Microtrauma, 344–347
Microvascular decompression, 465–466
Midbrain, 23
Middle cranial fossa tumors, 119
Migraine
  with aura
    description of, 405–406
    diagnosis of, 413–414
  cerebral blood flow during, 410
  characteristics of, 403–406, 429t
  description of, 403
  diagnosis of, 411–414
  epidemiology of, 403–404
  management of
    calcium channel blockers, 415–416
    dihydroergotamine, 415
    nonpharmacologic methods, 414
    patient education, 414
    pharmacologic methods, 414–416
    preventive medications, 415–416
    serotonin antagonists, 416
    tricyclic antidepressants, 416
    triptans, 415
  neurophysiology of, 407f–408f
  onset of, 404
  pathophysiologic features of, 406–411
  phases of, 404–406
  precipitating factors, 411, 413t, 414
  prodromes of, 405
  tension-type headache vs., 417–418
  triggers of, 411, 413t, 414

without aura
  description of, 406
  diagnosis of, 411, 413
Migrainous neuralgias, 279
Mitochondria, 46
Mixed headache, 418
Monoamine oxidase inhibitors, 207
Mood disorders, 139, 526, 528
Mucogingival pain
  behavior of, 243
  causes of
    allergic responses, 247
    burning mouth disorders, 253–255
    herpes simplex infection, 251–253
    local infections, 247, 250f
    recurrent aphthous stomatitis, 250–251,
      252f
    stomatitis medicamentosa, 247, 249f
    stomatitis venenata, 247, 249f
    systemic conditions, 250–253
    trauma, 246–247
  characteristics of, 246
  differential diagnosis, 255–256
  localization of, 246
  of mouth, 245–255
  referred pain vs., 246
Multidimensional Pain Inventory, 151
Multiple sclerosis, 461
Muscle co-contraction, 74, 112
Muscle examination
  description of, 161–162
  masseter, 164, 164f
  palpation, 162–166
  posterior cervical muscles, 164–166, 165f–166f
  sternocleidomastoid, 164, 165f
  temporalis, 162–164, 163f
  trigger points, 166–167
Muscle injections, for pain diagnosis confirma-
    tion, 184–186, 185f
Muscle pain
  behavior of, 289
  central nervous system effects on, 294
  centrally mediated myalgia
    characteristics of, 112, 291, 311, 313
    management of, 321–322, 323f
  characteristics of, 287, 289
  chronic myalgia, 294
  classification of, 288f
  cyclic, 293–294, 363
  fibromyalgia
    description of, 290, 313
    management of, 323–324

intensity of, 287
masticatory
  case studies of, 302–303
  cycling, 302, 434
  events, 291–292
  local muscle soreness, 291, 293–294,
    316–317
  model of, 290f, 290–291
  neuralgic pain vs., 462–463
  neurovascular pain vs., 435
  protective co-contraction, 291–293, 315–316
  referred pain vs., 313
  sympathetically maintained pain vs., 501
  tension-type headache and, 418
  types of, 289–290, 314–315
  myofascial. See Myofascial pain.
  myospasm, 295
  origins of, 287
Muscle relaxants, 207, 321
Muscle soreness, local
  characteristics of, 291, 293–294, 311
  management of, 316–317
Muscle spindles, 17
Muscle splinting, protective, 291–293
Muscular toothache, 277–278, 313
Musculoskeletal pain
  characteristics of, 109, 112, 136
  description of, 381
  diagnosis of, 181
  osseous-related, 381–384
Myalgia
  centrally mediated
    characteristics of, 291, 311, 313
    management of, 321–322, 323f
  chronic, 294
  description of, 272–273
  tonic contraction, 295
Myelin sheath, 14
Myelination, 14
Myofascial pain
  cervical muscles referral of, 306, 308
  co-contraction associated with, 297
  definition of, 295
  description of, 74, 291, 295–296
  digastric muscles referral of, 304f, 305f
  etiology of, 296
  facial expression muscles referral of, 305, 307f
  inferior lateral pterygoid muscle referral of,
    300–301, 301f
  management of, 319–321
  masseter muscle referral of, 298f, 298–299

medial pterygoid muscle referral of, 299–300, 300f
occipitofrontalis muscle referral of, 305, 306f
origins of, 296
postural factors, 321
referral patterns of, 298–308
sternocleidomastoid muscle referral of, 304f, 305
temporalis muscle referral of, 299, 299f
tension-type headache and, 308, 311
trapezius muscle referral of, 305, 305f
trigger points associated with, 296–297
Myofascial pain dysfunction syndrome, 296
Myofascial trigger points
autonomic effects produced by, 297–298
central excitatory effects created by, 297–298
definition of, 295
dental pain caused by, 273–274
description of, 74–75
latency of, 297
management of, 319–321
pain associated with, 295–297
Myogenous pain, 289
Myositis, 311
Myospasm
characteristics of, 112, 291, 295–296
management of, 317–319
Myotactic reflex, 41
Myotoxicity, 183, 205

N

Naloxone, 85–86
Narcotic analgesics, 201–203
Nasal mucosa pain
central excitatory effects, 392–393
characteristics of, 391–392
inferior turbinate, 392, 392f
upper respiratory infections as cause of, 393–395
Nasal mucosal toothache, 283–284
Neck mobility, 160–161, 161f
Neoplasm pain, 120
Neospinothalamic tract, 21
Nerve action potential, 45–46
Nerve block injections, 186, 188–190, 189f–190f
Nerve cell body, 14
Nerve fibers
anatomy of, 13–15
myelination of, 14
Nervi nervorum, 18
Nervous system
autonomic. See Autonomic nervous system.

central. See Central nervous system.
definition of, 10
Nervus intermedius neuralgia, 459–460
Neural pathways, 11
Neuralgia
characteristics of, 462–463
cranial. See Cranial neuralgias.
geniculate, 391
glossopharyngeal, 364–365
migrainous, 279
paroxysmal. See Paroxysmal neuralgia.
paroxysmal trigeminal, 114–115, 115f, 255
postherpetic, 116–117, 495–496
trigeminal, 114–115, 115f, 281
Neuritic pain
characteristics of, 282, 470
classification of, 471f
peripheral neuritis, 472–478
symptoms of, 470
Neuritis
description of, 116–117, 256
glossopharyngeal, 473, 475, 477f
peripheral, 472–478
Neuroanatomy
neurons, 13–15
nociceptors, 17–18
overview of, 13, 15–16
sensory receptors, 16–17
Neurogenic inflammation, 56, 113
Neurokinin A, 466
Neurolemma, 14
Neurolytic agents, 211
Neuroma
definition of, 117, 484
traumatic. See Traumatic neuroma.
Neurons
afferent, 11, 15, 69, 71–74
anatomy of, 14–15
autonomic, 75–76
classification of, 19t
convergence of, 65
efferent, 74–75
first-order, 11, 15, 19–20
inhibitory, 20
low-threshold mechanosensitive, 20, 30–31
postganglionic, 32
preganglionic, 15
primary afferent, 11, 15, 19–20
second-order, 11, 20–21, 29, 57, 68
sensitization of, 55–56
structure of, 14f
wide dynamic range, 20, 29–30, 68, 118, 499

Neuropathic pains
  behavior of, 450
  characteristics of, 137, 177, 179
  classification of, 179f, 244f, 260f, 288f, 330f,
    382f, 402f,449–450
  continuous
    atypical odontalgia, 490, 492–493
    burning mouth disorders, 253–255, 493–495
    centrally mediated, 490–506
    complex regional pain syndrome, 138,
      496–498
    deafferentation pain. *See* Deafferentation
      pain.
    description of, 116–119, 138, 179, 179f, 466
    entrapment neuropathy, 489–490
    herpes zoster, 478–480
    mechanisms of, 466–470
    metabolic polyneuropathies. *See* Metabolic
      polyneuropathies.
    neuritic pain. *See* Neuritic pain.
    peripherally mediated, 470–490
    sympathetically maintained pain. *See*
      Sympathetically maintained pain.
  definition of, 109, 114, 137, 449
  diagnosis of, 177, 179
  episodic
    cranial neuralgias. *See* Cranial neuralgias.
    description of, 137–138, 179f
    paroxysmal neuralgia. *See* Paroxysmal
      neuralgia.
  etiology of, 449
  metabolic polyneuropathy, 116
  neuritis, 116–117
  paroxysmal, 114–115, 115f
  sympathetically maintained, 118–119, 138
  in temporomandibular joint, 364
  toothache caused by, 281–283
  treatment of, 199
Neuropeptides, 49
Neuroplasticity
  chronic pain and, 120–121
  definition of, 47, 69, 467
  importance of, 121
Neurotransmitters
  acetylcholine, 49
  aspartate, 50
  bradykinin, 51–53, 63
  definition of, 49
  dopamine, 50
  endorphins, 51, 84–85
  GABA, 50

  glutamate, 49–50
  glycine, 50
  histamine, 50
  in migraine pathophysiology, 406
  nitric oxide, 50
  norepinephrine, 49
  rapid-acting, 49–50
  serotonin, 50, 84–85, 409
  slow-acting, 51–52
  substance P, 51, 55, 57, 64, 406
  synaptic removal of, 52
Neurovascular pain
  behavior of, 401
  classification of, 402f
  cluster headache. *See* Cluster headache.
  description of, 113–114, 137–138
  migraine. *See* Migraine.
  paroxysmal hemicrania, 425–427, 429t
  SUNCT syndrome, 427–428, 429t
  tension-type headache. *See* Tension-type
    headache.
Neurovascular toothache, 277, 279, 431–433
Neurovascular variants
  characteristics of, 430
  definition of, 430
  diagnosis of, 433–436
  management of, 436–437
  pathophysiology of, 430–431
  types of, 431–433
New daily-persistent headache, 430
Nitric oxide, 50
NMDA receptors, 69, 120, 466
Nociception
  central processing of, 65–76
  definition of, 8, 520
  description of, 141, 520
  initiation of, 63-64
  neurochemistry of, 52–55
  trigeminal terminals, 71–72
Nociceptive reflex, 18, 261
Nociceptive-specific neurons, 20, 30, 57
Nociceptors, 17–18
Nodes of Ranvier, 14
Noninflammatory pain, 111–112
Nonnarcotic analgesics, 201
Nonsteroidal anti-inflammatory drugs,
  369–370
Norepinephrine, 49, 209
Nucleus, 14
Nucleus raphe, 81
Nucleus raphes magnus, 28, 82

O

Occipital lobe, 25
Occipital neuralgia, 460
Occipitofrontalis, 305, 306f
Occlusal appliance therapy, 370–373
Occlusal disengagement, 223–224
Ocular pain, 397
Oculomotor nerve
  anatomy of, 36f, 38
  evaluation of, 156, 157f
Olfactory nerve
  anatomy of, 36f
  evaluation of, 153
Oligemia, 410
Onset of pain, 145, 147
Open bite, anterior, 353, 354f
Optic nerve
  anatomy of, 36f
  evaluation of, 153, 156
Orbicularis oculi, 307f
Orthodromic, 63
Orthopedic instability of temporomandibular
    joint, 345
Osseous pains
  classification of, 382f
  description of, 381, 383
  dry-socket pain, 383–384
  factors associated with, 381, 383
  of inflammatory origin, 384
  osteitis, 383
  osteomyelitis, 383
Osteitis, 383
Osteoarthritis, 329, 353–354, 354f, 357f, 358
Osteoarthrosis, 356
Osteomyelitis, 383
Oxcarbazepine, 463–464

P

Pacinian corpuscles, 17
Pain
  acute. See Acute pain.
  anatomic considerations, 10–11
  central influences on, 110
  changing concepts of, 6–7
  characteristics of, 4, 147–148
  chronic. See Chronic pain.
  components of, 6–7
  cutaneous sensation of, 19–20
  deep somatic. See Deep somatic pain.
  definitions of, 6–8
  denial of, 219, 538–539

  dental practitioner's responsibility, 4–5
  description of, 3, 107
  descriptors for, 143
  diagnosis of. See Diagnosis.
  dimensions of, 6
  economic costs of, 3
  emergency nature of, 7–8
  emotional significance of, 102–103
  heterotopic. See Heterotopic pain.
  historical description of, 5–6
  injury and, 7
  intensity of, 108
  location of. See Location of pain.
  masticatory. See Masticatory pain.
  modulation of, 11
  mucogingival. See Mucogingival pain.
  myofascial. See Myofascial pain.
  nasal mucosa. See Nasal mucosa pain.
  neural pathways of, 11
  neuropathic. See Neuropathic pains.
  neurovascular. See Neurovascular pain.
  noninflammatory, 111–112
  noxious stimulation-induced, 121
  osseous. See Osseous pains.
  periodontal. See Periodontal pain.
  peripheral origins of, 40–41, 110
  phylogenic considerations for, 9–10
  prevalence of, 4
  primary. See Primary pain.
  processing of, 8-9
  protective nature of, 6
  psychologic elements of. See Psychologic
    factors.
  psychologic intensification of, 122, 138–139,
    522
  secondary. See Heterotopic pain.
  site of, 65–67
  somatic. See Somatic pain.
  source of, 65–67, 152–153
  suffering and, 7
  surgical, 3
  sympathetically maintained. See Sympatheti-
    cally maintained pain.
  temporomandibular joint. See Temporo-
    mandibular joint pains.
  transmission of, 11, 13
  treatment-induced, 122
  types of, 107–109
  vascular. See Vascular pain.
  visceral. See Visceral pain.
Pain behavior, 8-9, 141–142, 220, 520, 524

Pain categories
  diagnosis of, 177–182
  multiple, 193
Pain classification
  axis I. *See* Axis I.
  axis II. *See* Axis II.
  chart of, 178f, 244f, 260f, 288f, 330f, 382f, 402f
  description of, 129
  symptomatology-based, 132
Pain complaint, 142
Pain cycling, 205
Pain experience
  behavioral traits associated with, 97–98
  description of, 76
  emotional state and, 96–97
  factors that affect, 95–98
  prior experiences' effect on, 96
Pain modulation
  by endorphins, 85
  gate control theory, 76–77, 77f
  of descending inhibitory system, 82–85
  principles of, 76–79
  by psychologic factors, 86–87
  in reticular formation, 81–82
  transcutaneous electrical nerve stimulation and, 79–81
  in trigeminal spinal tract nucleus, 79
Palatal reflex, 159
Paleospinothalamic tract, 21
Palpation
  of muscles, 162–166
  of temporomandibular joint, 170, 171f
Parafunctional activities, 149
Parahippocampal gyrus, 26–27
Paranasal sinus pain, 395–397
Parasympathetic nerves, 40
Parasympathetic nervous system, 33f, 33–34
Parasympathetic tone, 34
Parietal lobe, 25
Paroxysmal hemicrania, 425–427, 429t
Paroxysmal neuralgia
  characteristics of, 451
  classification of, 452f
  cranial neuralgias. *See* Cranial neuralgias.
  diagnosis of, 461–463
  management of
    baclofen, 464
    carbamazepine, 463
    gabapentin, 464
    lamotrigine, 464–465
    neurosurgical, 465–466

oxcarbazepine, 463–464
    pharmacologic, 463–464
    topiramate, 464
  masticatory pain vs., 462–463
  of auriculotemporal nerve, 454f
  of trigeminal nerve, 455f–456f
  pathophysiology of, 460–461
  precipitating factors, 461
Paroxysmal pain
  characteristics of, 148
  neuralgic, 137
  neuropathic, 114–115, 115f
Paroxysmal trigeminal neuralgia, 114–115, 115f, 255
Passive distraction, 369
Past consultations, 150
Perception, 11
Percutaneous stimulation, 215
Periapical pain, 270
Periaqueductal gray area, 28, 82
Periarticular inflammation, 357, 360
Perineurium, 13–14
Periodontal abscess, 264, 265f
Periodontal ligament, 259
Periodontal pain
  causes of, 270f, 271
  description of, 269–270
  localization of, 270
  occlusal overloading associated with, 271–272
  radiographic findings, 271f
Periodontal receptors, 269–270
Periosteal pains, 384–385
Periosteitis, 384–385
Periosteum, 121
Peripheral neuritis, 472–478
Peripheral nociceptive pathways
  considerations for, 40–41
  description of, 34–35
  trigeminal nerve, 35, 35f–36f
Peripheral sensitization, 466
Perpetuating factors, 227–228
Personality traits, 535
Phantom pain, 117–118, 490, 492–493
Pharyngeal mucosa pain, 390–391
Pharyngitis, 388, 391
Phentolamine, 506
Phlebitis, 437
Phonophoresis, 216
Physical activity, 217–218
Physical dependence, 202
Physical self-regulation, 221, 224–226, 315, 539–541

Placebo therapy, 176–177, 192
Platysma, 307f
Polarization, 45
Polymyalgia rheumatica. *See* Cranial arteritis.
Polyneuropathies, metabolic
  alcoholism and, 506, 508
  characteristics of, 116, 506, 508
  classification of, 507f
  diabetes mellitus and, 506
  diagnosis of, 508
  electrophysiologic testing of, 508
  management of, 508–509
  pathophysiology of, 508
  precipitating factors, 508
  tricyclic antidepressants for, 509
Pons, 22–23
Posterior cervical muscles
  injection of, 187f
  palpation of, 164–166, 165f–166f
Postganglionic neurons, 32
Postherpetic neuralgia, 116–117, 495–496
Posttraumatic stress disorder, 530, 534
Potassium channels, 48
Preauricular pain, 396
Preganglionic neuron, 15
Preliminary interview, 142–144
Preoptic nucleus, 24
Pressure algometry, 162
Presynaptic terminals, 46
Pre-trigeminal neuralgia, 457
Primary afferent neuron, 11, 15, 19–20
Primary cough headache, 430
Primary exertional headache, 430
Primary hyperalgesia, 64, 246
Primary pain
  description of, 65, 108–109
  diagnosis of, 179–180
  injectable anesthetic agents for, 204–205
  referred pain vs., 152–153, 274, 277
Primary stabbing headache, 429–430
Primary thunderclap headache, 430
Progressive relaxation, 221–222
Projected pain, 67–68
Projection tracts, 25
Proopiomelanocortin, 82
Proprioceptive re-education, 226, 541
Proprioceptors, 17
Prostaglandin, 53–54, 111
Prostaglandin E_2, 201
Protective co-contraction
  characteristics of, 291–293
  management of, 315–316

Protective muscle splinting, 291–293
Provocation, 154f, 274, 275f
Psychogenic intensification, 101
Psychogenic pain, 76
Psychogenic toothache, 284
Psychologic assessment, 150–151, 176–177
Psychologic factors
  anxiety disorders
    classification of, 529f
    generalized anxiety disorder, 528
    posttraumatic stress disorder, 530, 543
  biopsychosocial model, 98–99, 100f, 520
  bipolar disorder, 526, 528
  classification of, 527f
  depression, 526
  description of, 86–87, 98, 520, 525, 526
  mechanistic model, 98–99, 100f
  medical conditions affected by, 535, 537
  mood disorders, 526, 528
  somatization, 103
  somatoform pain disorder, 103–104, 139, 151, 284, 533–534
Psychologic intensification, 122, 138–139, 522
Psychotherapy, 219–220
Pterygoids
  inferior lateral
    anatomy of, 165
    myofascial pain referral to, 300–301, 301f
    pain referral to, 314–315, 348
    trigger points in, 301, 301f
  lateral, 165
  medial, 299–300, 300f
  superior lateral, 301, 301f, 338
Pulpal necrosis, 264
Pulpal pain
  acute, 263–264, 265f
  chronic, 265–266, 266f
  diagnosis of, 268–269
  identification of, 268–269
  obscure causes of, 267–268
  radiographic findings, 269, 269f
  recurrent, 266–267, 267f

Q

Quality of pain
  dental pain, 262
  history taking regarding, 147

R

Ramsay Hunt syndrome, 391, 479
Receptive field, 17

Receptors
  nociceptors, 17–18
  sensory, 16–17
  specialized, 18–19
Reciprocal click, 338, 339f
Reciprocal inhibition, 217
Recurrent aphthous stomatitis, 250–251, 252f
Recurrent pulpal pain, 266–267, 267f
Red nucleus, 23
Referred pain
  characteristics of, 68–69, 71–73
  dental, 272
  differential diagnosis, 255
  from dry-socket pain, 383
  from trigger points, 166–167
  masticatory pain vs., 313
  mucogingival pain vs., 246
  primary pain vs., 152–153, 274, 277
  in temporomandibular joint, 364
Reflex arc, 16
Reflex sympathetic dystrophy, 119, 496,
    498–499. See also Complex regional pain
    syndrome.
Reflex testing, 159
Relaxation training, 221–224
Repolarization, 46
Reticular formation
  anatomy of, 81
  definition of, 22
  pain modulation in, 81–82
Reticular inhibitory area, 59
Retrodiscal pains, 347–350
Retrodiscitis, 348–349
Review of systems, 150
Rheumatoid arthritis, 353, 354f
Rhizotomy, 465
Ruffini's corpuscles, 17

S

Secondary gain, 103, 228
Secondary hyperalgesia, 73–74, 273, 297, 306,
    392
Secondary pain. See Heterotopic pain.
Second-order neuron, 11, 20–21, 29, 57, 68
Selective serotonin reuptake inhibitors, 208
Sensitization
  central, 68–76
  definition of, 120
  neuronal, 55–56
Sensory receptors
  description of, 16
  exteroceptors, 16–17

interoceptors, 17
proprioceptors, 17
Sensory stimulation
  cutaneous stimulation, 212–214, 213f
  description of, 212
  percutaneous stimulation, 215
  transcutaneous stimulation, 214–215
Septum pellucidum, 26
Serotonin, 50, 84–85, 409
Serotonin receptors, 409
Silent nociceptor, 20
Sinus headache, 394
Sinus toothache, 283–284
Sleep disturbances, 149, 228, 323–324, 528
Slow pain, 57
Sodium channels, 45, 48
Sodium hyaluronate, 190–191
Soft connective tissue pains, 385
Somatic pain
  characteristics of, 132, 134
  classification of, 180f, 244f, 260f, 288f, 330f,
    382f, 402f
  deep
    cervical causes of, 308
    characteristics of, 109, 112–114, 135–137,
      180–181
    diagnosis of, 180–181, 363
    differential diagnosis, 385–386
    primary, 387
    treatment of, 386
  definition of, 109
  diagnosis of, 177, 179
  neural structures involved in, 132
  superficial, 112, 134
  treatment of, 198, 256–257
Somatic structures, 10–11
Somatization, 103
Somatization disorder, 531
Somatoform disorders
  conversion disorders, 531, 533
  hypochondriasis, 533, 535
  somatoform pain disorder, 103–104, 139, 151,
    284, 533–534
  undifferentiated, 531
Spinal nerves, 38
Splenius capitis
  injection of, 187f
  palpation of, 165, 166f
Split tooth, 267–268
Spontaneous pain, 109, 121
Spray and stretch technique, 217, 319, 320f,
    368

State-dependent sensory processing, 87–89
Stellate ganglion block, 188, 190, 206, 388
Sternocleidomastoid
  injection of, 187f
  myofascial pain referral to, 304f, 305
  palpation of, 164, 165f
Stimulus-evoked pain, 109
Stomatitis medicamentosa, 247, 249f
Stomatitis venenata, 247, 249f
Streptococcal pharyngitis, 391
Stress
  continued levels of, 228
  description of, 97, 149
  physiologic response related to, 537
  reduction of, 220–221
  tension-type headache precipitated by, 420
Stretch reflex, 18
Submandibular salivary gland pain, 396f, 397
Subnucleus caudalis, 28
Substance P, 51, 55, 57, 64, 406, 466
Substantia gelatinosa, 79, 82
Substantia nigra, 23, 81
Suffering
  definition of, 8, 520
  pain and, 7
Sumatriptan
  for cluster headache, 424
  for neuromuscular variants, 436–437
SUNCT syndrome, 427–428, 429t
Superficial pain
  definition of, 109
  diagnosis of, 180–181
Superficial reflexes, 159
Superficial somatic pain, 134
Superior laryngeal neuralgia, 460
Superior lateral pterygoid, 301, 301f, 338
Supramylohyoid cellulitis, 385
Supraoptic nucleus, 24
Sympathetic blockade, 206
Sympathetic nerves, 39–40
Sympathetic nervous system, 31–33, 32f
Sympathetic tone, 34
Sympathetically maintained pain
  case studies of, 504f–505f
  characteristics of, 498–499
  description of, 118–119, 138
  diagnosis of, 501
  management of, 501, 503
  masticatory pain vs., 501
  pathophysiology of, 499, 501, 503f
  precipitating factors, 501
  toothache caused by, 501

Symptom Check List 90, 151
Synapse
  anatomy of, 15, 46, 47f
  neurotransmitter removal from, 52
Synovitis, 350
Systemic conditions
  mucogingival pain caused by, 250–253
  muscle function affected by, 292

T

Teeth
  description of, 259
  evaluation of, 172
  functions of, 259
  innervation of, 261
Temporal behavior of pain, 147–148
Temporal lobe, 25
Temporal summation, 65
Temporalis
  injection of, 187f
  myofascial pain referral to, 299, 299f
  palpation of, 162–164, 163f
Temporomandibular disorders
  description of, 218, 224–225, 289, 313
  management of, 540
Temporomandibular joint
  anatomy of, 331–335, 332f–333f
  arthralgia of
    as capsular pain, 351
    description of, 346
    hyperuricemia as cause of, 359
    inflammatory, 363
    inflammatory fibrous ankylosis, 361
    intermittent, 363
    malignant tumors, 362
  articular disc of, 331, 332f
  Class II malocclusions of, 347
  closed lock of, 342f, 342–343
  condyle-disc complex, 331, 333–334, 334f
  crepitation in, 170
  distraction of, 369
  evaluation of, 169–171
  function of, 331–335
  functional dislocation of, 340, 340f
  imaging of, 174, 175f
  ligamentous structures of, 335
  loading of, 345
  orthopedic instability of, 345
  osseous resorption of, 355, 355f
  pain in, 136, 169–170
  palpation of, 170, 171f
  passive distraction of, 369

physical therapy for improve function of, 368–369
radiographs of, 174, 175f
sounds of, 170–171, 371
stable position of, 172, 173f
Temporomandibular joint pains
  arthritic
    characteristics of, 353
    description of, 353
    osteoarthritis, 353–355, 354f, 357f, 358
    periarticular inflammation, 357, 360
    rheumatoid, 353
    traumatic, 356
  behavior of, 329, 331
  capsular
    capsulitis, 350
    causes of, 350
    fibrosis, 350, 352
    synovitis, 350
  cervical spine injury and, 344
  chronic mandibular hypomobilities, 360
  description of, 335
  differential diagnosis, 365
  disc derangement, 338–343
  disc-interference disorders, 365–373
  Eagle syndrome, 364
  functional disc displacement
    clinical features of, 340f
    description of, 336–338, 337f, 340, 340f
    with reduction, 340–341, 341f
    without reduction, 341–343, 342f
  growth-related, 360, 362
  ligamentous, 336–343
  macrotrauma, 343–344
  microtrauma, 344–347
  neuropathic, 364
  reciprocal click, 338, 339f
  referred, 364
  retrodiscal, 347–350
  treatment of
    analgesic medications, 369–370
    anterior mandibular positioning appliance, 370–372
    anti-inflammatory medications, 370
    coolant therapy, 368
    occlusal appliance therapy, 370–373
    overview of, 365–366
    patient education, 367
    pharmacologic, 369–370
    physical therapy modalities, 367–369
    rationale for, 365
Tender teeth, 273

Tendonitis, 311, 313
TENS. See Transcutaneous electrical nerve stimulation.
Tension-type headache
  analgesics for, 420
  botulinum toxin injections for, 420–421
  characteristics of, 308, 416–417, 429t
  chronic, 417, 419
  diagnosis of, 418–419
  electromyographic findings, 417
  epidemiology of, 416–417
  frequent episodic, 419
  infrequent episodic, 418–419
  management of, 419–421
  masticatory pain and, 311, 418
  migraine vs., 417–418
  myofascial pain and, 308, 311
  neurovascular pain and, 113–114
  pathophysiologic features of, 417–418
  precipitating factors, 418
  stress and, 420
Tetrodotoxin, 48
Thalamus, 24
Tic douloureux. See Trigeminal neuralgia.
Tolerance, 202
Tonic contraction myalgia, 295, 317–319.
  See also Myospasm.
Tonsillitis, 391
Tools-Hunt syndrome, 475
Toothache
  cardiac, 279–281
  deafferentation, 282, 483
  differential diagnosis, 275f–276f, 284
  heterotopic, 277
  mandibular, 476
  muscular, 277–278, 313
  nasal mucosal, 283–284
  neuritic, 472–473
  neuropathic, 281–283
  neurovascular, 277, 279, 431–433
  of dental origin. See Dental pain.
  of nondental origin, 273–284, 501
  provocation of, 274, 275f
  psychogenic, 284
  signs and symptoms of, 284
  sinus, 283–284
  treatment of, 285
Topical anesthetics, 203, 204f
Topiramate, 464
Transcutaneous electrical nerve stimulation
  acupuncture vs., 86
  electroacupuncture vs., 85–86, 214

principles of, 79–81, 214–215
therapeutic uses of, 214–215
Transduction, 11, 13
Transmission cell, 79
Trapezius
injection of, 187f
myofascial pain referral to, 305, 305f
palpation of, 165, 166f
Trauma
cluster headache caused by, 422–423
iatrogenic, 344
mucogingival pain caused by, 246–247
pain induced by, 145, 147
posttraumatic stress disorder secondary to, 530, 543
temporomandibular joint, 343–344
Traumatic arthritis, 353, 356
Traumatic neuralgia, 256
Traumatic neuroma
case studies of, 486–487
characteristics of, 481–482, 484
diagnosis of, 485, 488
management of, 488–489
mucogingival scars associated with, 485
pathophysiology of, 484–485
precipitating factors, 485
Treatment
considerations for, 537–539
dental practitioner's responsibility, 5
description of, 212
dietary changes, 211–212
history taking regarding, 150
interocclusal appliances, 223–224, 224f
manual techniques for
exercise, 217
massage, 216–217
physical activity, 217–218
spray and stretch, 217, 319, 320f, 368
neuropathic pain, 199
overview of, 197–198
pain caused by, 122
pharmacologic
adjuvant analgesics, 203
analgesic agents, 201–203
anesthetic agents, 203–206
antianxiety agents, 208
anticonvulsive agents, 210
antidepressants, 207–208
antihistamine agents, 210
anti-inflammatory agents, 206–207
antimicrobial agents, 209–210
antiviral agents, 210

considerations for, 200–201
mechanism of action, 199–201
muscle relaxants, 207
narcotic analgesics, 201–203
neurolytic agents, 211
nonnarcotic analgesics, 201
norepinephrine blockers, 209
overview of, 199–201
uricosuric agents, 211
vasoactive agents, 208–209
physical self-regulation, 221, 224–226, 315, 539–541
physical therapy modalities
deep heat therapy, 216
EGS, 216
transcutaneous electrical nerve stimulation, 214–215
ultrasound, 216, 216f
psychologic modalities
behavioral modification training, 220–226
counseling, 218–220
realistic expectations regarding, 219–220, 539
sensory stimulation, 212–215
somatic pain, 198
temporomandibular joint pains. See Temporomandibular joint pains, treatment of.
Trial placebo therapy, 176–177, 192
Tricyclic antidepressants
for metabolic polyneuropathies, 509
for migraine, 207–208
for traumatic neuralgia, 488
Trigeminal nerve
anatomy of, 28–31, 35, 35f–36f, 39, 56–57
evaluation of, 156, 157f
paroxysmal neuralgia of, 455f–456f
Trigeminal neuralgia
characteristics of, 114–115, 115f, 281, 451, 453
classification of, 461
posttraumatic, 482, 484
pre-, 457
triggers of, 453
Trigeminal system, 28–31
Trigeminovascular reflex, 411
Trigeminovascular system, 406, 407f, 412f
Trigger points
examination of, 166–167
features of, 297
in inferior lateral pterygoid, 301, 301f
injection of
myalgia treated with, 319, 320f
pain diagnosis confirmation by, 184–186, 185f

therapeutic uses for, 205, 205f
in masseter, 298f
myofascial
  autonomic effects produced by, 297–298
  central excitatory effects created by, 297–298
  definition of, 295
  dental pain caused by, 273–274
  description of, 74–75
  latency of, 297
  management of, 319–321
  pain associated with, 296–297
referred pain from, 166–167
in superior lateral pterygoid, 301, 301f
Triptans, 415
Trochlear nerve
  anatomy of, 36f, 38
  evaluation of, 156, 157f
Tryptophan, 212
Tympanic plexus neuralgia, 457

U

Ultrasound, 216, 216f, 319
Upper respiratory infections, 393–395
Uricosuric agents, 211

V

Vagus nerve
  anatomy of, 36f, 38–39
  evaluation of, 158
Vapocoolant therapy, 213
Vascular pain
  behavior of, 401
  carotidynia, 439–440
  classification of, 402f, 438f
  cranial arteritis, 437, 439
  description of, 437

Vasoactive agents, 208–209
Venlafaxine, 208
Ventricles of brain, 27–28
Vestibulocochlear nerve. *See* Acoustic nerve.
Visceral pain
  behavior of, 387–388
  central excitatory effects of, 388
  characteristics of, 109, 113–114, 136–137
  classification of, 389f
  description of, 387
  diagnosis of, 181
  mucosal causes of
    description of, 390
    nasal, 391–395
    paranasal, 395–397
    pharyngeal, 390–391
  types of, 388
Vital signs, 153
Voltage-gated ion channels, 48

W

Wernicke's area, 25
Wheal, 56, 110
Wide dynamic range neuron, 20, 29–30, 68, 118, 499

X

Xerostomia, 254, 256

Z

Zolmitriptan, 425
Zygomaticus major, 307f